PROF. G. A. GRESHAM
HISTOLOGY LABORATORY
ADDENBROOKES HOSPITAL
HILLS ROAD, CAMBRIDGE

Systemic Pathology

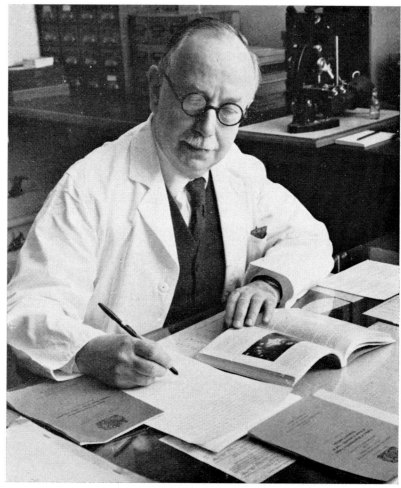

Photograph of George Payling Wright reproduced by permission of Mrs Payling Wright and of the holders of the copyright, the Shell International Petroleum Company Limited, London

GEORGE PAYLING WRIGHT

4th April 1898 : 4th April 1964

Authors

C. W. M. Adams

B. S. Cardell

J. B. Cavanagh

K. G. A. Clark

C. A. G. Cook

*T. Crawford

A. R. Currie

P. M. Daniel

W. M. Davidson

I. M. P. Dawson

I. Doniach

B. Fox

*I. Friedmann

H. Haber

D. G. F. Harriman

*B. E. Heard

Kristin Henry

*R. E. B. Hudson

P. E. Hughesdon

M. L. Lewis

R. B. Lucas

W. H. McMenemey

J. A. Milne

G. Morgan

B. C. Morson

*D. A. Osborn

*K. A. Porter

H. A. Sissons

J. C. Sloper

W. Thomas Smith

Sabina J. Strich

W. St C. Symmers

A. C. Thackray

K. Weinbren

*C. P. Wendell-Smith

E. D. Williams

*G. Payling Wright

A. H. Wyllie

* Contributors to Volume 1

Editor

W. St C. Symmers

Systemic Pathology

SECOND EDITION

by THIRTY-EIGHT AUTHORS

VOLUME 1

Cardiovascular System
Respiratory System

CHURCHILL LIVINGSTONE
Edinburgh London and New York 1976

CHURCHILL LIVINGSTONE
Medical Division of Longman Group Limited

Distributed in the United States of America by Churchill Livingstone Inc., 19 West 44th Street, New York, NY. 10036, and by associated companies, branches and representatives throughout the world.

First Edition (edited by G. Payling Wright and W. St. Clair Symmers) 1966

Second Edition 1976
Reprinted 1980

ISBN 0 443 01330 6

Library of Congress Cataloging in Publication Data

Main entry under title:

Systemic pathology.

    First ed. edited by G. P. Wright and W. St. C. Symmers.
    Includes bibliographical references.
    CONTENTS: v. 1. Cardiovascular system, respiratory system.
    1. Pathology. I. Wright, George Payling,
1898-1964, ed. Systemic pathology. [DNLM:
1. Pathology. QZ4 S995]
RB111.W76 1976 616.07   75–35746

Printed in Great Britain by
T. & A. Constable Ltd., Edinburgh

Preface to the Second Edition

The first edition of *Systemic Pathology* was published by Longmans on the 31st December 1966, and went out of print four years later. The publishers had expected that the second edition would appear about four years after the first: it is deplorable that a succession of delays has more than doubled this interval. Fortunately, the cooperation of contributors has made it possible to ensure that the book is more up to date on publication than is usual for texts that are the joint work of many authors. Most of the contributors have had the vexatious necessity of reviewing their chapters at least twice during the preparation of the new edition: the publishers' appreciation and thanks, and mine, are due to all those who recognized the inevitability of the delays and generously helped to offset their effects, at the cost to themselves of much extra work and inconvenience.

There have been several changes in the panel of authors since 1966. Their other commitments made it necessary for two contributors to refuse the invitation to revise their chapters—Professor Robert H. Heptinstall, who wrote on the kidneys, and Dr J. H. Shore, who wrote on the gall bladder and bile ducts: it is a pleasure to acknowledge their work for the first edition and to thank them for their participation. Doctor B. S. Cardell has written the new chapter on the gall bladder and bile ducts in addition to revising his chapter on the pancreas; the new chapter on the kidneys is by Professor K. A. Porter, who joins the panel of contributors. Doctor Kristin Henry, who has written the chapter on the thymus, and Professor E. D. Williams, who has written the chapter on the parathyroid glands, have also joined the panel, taking over from contributors to the first edition who wanted to reduce the number of chapters that they are responsible for. Other contributors to the first edition asked that the revision of their chapters might be shared, or undertaken, by colleagues: among the latter are nine further new members of the panel—Dr K. G. A. Clark (diseases of blood), Professor I. M. P. Dawson (small intestine), Dr B. Fox (adrenal glands), Dr D. G. F. Harriman (skeletal muscle), Dr M. L. Lewis (diseases of blood), Professor J. A. Milne (skin), D r Gwyn Morgan (eyes), Professor W. Thomas Smith (central nervous system) and Dr A. H. Wyllie (pituitary gland).

Sir Theo Crawford has revised the chapter on the heart that was written for the first edition by its editor, Professor George Payling Wright. This chapter stands in the new edition as a memorial to Professor Payling Wright's humanity and scholarship and to his unique stature as a pathologist. His death, in 1964,* deprived much of the book of the advantages that it should have gained from final revision under his editorship and in the light of his lifetime of experience of the practical application of the principles of pathology. Professor Payling Wright did not consider textbooks to be a medium appropriate for the publication of memorial eulogies: it is in deference to this view that no formal appreciation of his life and work is included here, and it is in accord with his belief that the use of eponyms in the title of textbooks is undesirable that this book appears with the simple name, *Systemic Pathology*, implicitly acknowledging that it is the contributors who have written it.

The text has been so extensively amended during the preparation of the new edition that the type has had to be completely reset. This has made it possible to produce the book in four volumes instead of two, with greater convenience for the reader. The contents of all four volumes are listed at the beginning of each volume.

The only major change in the presentation of the text is that the references are no longer printed as footnotes. Instead, they are numbered serially as they occur and are collected at the end of the chapter. As before, the names of periodicals are abbreviated in accordance with the practice of the World Medical Association in its publication, *World Medical Periodicals* (third edition, New York, 1961; supplement,

* Cameron, G. R., GEORGE PAYLING WRIGHT: 4 APRIL 1898–4 APRIL 1964, *Journal of Pathology and Bacteriology*, 1966, **92**, 613–630.

New York, 1968). The intention to give the title and inclusive pagination of all articles cited in the new edition had to be dropped because of the impossibility of meeting the cost of the professional bibliographical help that would have been necessary. This, like the change in the method of presenting the references, is one of several consequences of the increasing cost of production that have had to be taken into account in preparing this edition. If, as I believe, economies have not diminished the usefulness of *Systemic Pathology* on this occasion, this is in part thanks to substantial, outright and unconditional financial support from a pathologist who, anonymously, considers the book to deserve such help. The future for books of this type is uncertain, in view of the limited circulation that results from the high price at which they have to be marketed if the expenses involved are to be covered: it may be that the time is coming when they will be publishable only if they have independent, non-commercial, financial backing.

*   *   *   *   *

As a consequence of the reorganization of the publishers' medical interests, this edition appears over the imprint of Churchill Livingstone, the Medical Division of Longman Group Limited. It is an editor's privilege to acknowledge the help of the members of the staff of the publishing house who have worked most closely on a shared undertaking, although house policy may prevent him from thanking all of them by name. Miss E. M. Bramwell, the publishers' senior house editor assigned to *Systemic Pathology*, has been uncommonly helpful and constructive in preparing the edited chapters for the printers and in eliminating difficulties that could have arisen from the fact that our complementary work was carried out in cities four hundred miles apart.

Many people, in many centres, have been involved in the preparation of this book. I cannot write personally about most of those whose technical, photographic, secretarial and other professional skills assisted the contributors, but I am sure that the latter would acknowledge the book's dependence on this help. It is a special pleasure to thank the senior members of the technical staff of the Department of Histopathology of Charing Cross Hospital and Medical School, London, for their interest—Mr F. D. Humberstone (Pathology Museum), Mr K. R. James (Hospital), Miss P. Naidoo (Medical School) and Mr H. Oakley (Mortuary). Their work is represented in many chapters, along with that of their colleagues in pathology departments of other hospitals and schools. Mr R. S. Barnett, in charge of the photographic laboratories of the Department of Histopathology at Charing Cross, has prepared many of the new illustrations, taking upon himself the responsibility of maintaining standards set in the first edition, to which his former chief, Miss P. M. Turnbull, head of the School's Department of Medical Illustration, contributed so notably. My thanks are also due to Miss S. M. Bennett, secretary of the Department of Histopathology of Charing Cross Hospital and Medical School, who not only produced much of the final typescript of the edited text—a classic exercise in decipherment—but also gave much other practical help in the preparation of the book.

In sum, as editor I owe much to many who have furthered *Systemic Pathology* by making it easier for me to work on it. They may not all be named, but I am glad to acknowledge their support. In particular, I would thank the histopathologists at Charing Cross, who have generously accepted, without remarking on it, the increase in their own work that resulted from my commitment to the book.

May the book prove useful, at least to the extent that what it has cost shall not be counted too great.

Northwood, Middlesex   William St Clair Symmers
England
November 1975

Contents

Volume 1

CONTENTS

Volume 4

Volume 5

Volume 6

Authors of Volume 1

SIR THEO CRAWFORD, BSc (Glasgow), MD (Glasgow), FRCP (London and Glasgow), FRCPath
Emeritus Professor of Pathology in the University of London; Honorary Consulting Pathologist, St George's Hospital, London; formerly Director of Pathological Services, St George's Hospital and Medical School; Past President of the Royal College of Pathologists; Honorary Fellow of the Royal College of Pathologists of Australia.

I. FRIEDMANN, DSc (London), MD (Prague), DCP (London), FRCS (England), FRCPath
Emeritus Professor of Pathology in the University of London; Honorary Consulting Pathologist, Royal National Throat, Nose and Ear Hospital, London; Honorary Consultant Pathologist, Northwick Park Hospital and Clinical Research Centre, Harrow, Middlesex; Research Fellow, Imperial Cancer Research Fund, London; Consultant in Electron Microscopy, Ear Research Institute, Los Angeles, California; formerly Director of the Department of Pathology and Bacteriology, Institute of Laryngology and Otology, University of London.

B. E. HEARD, BSc (Wales), MD (Wales), FRCP (London), FRCPath
Professor of Histopathology in the University of London at the Cardiothoracic Institute; Honorary Consultant Pathologist, Brompton Hospital, London;

R. E. B. HUDSON, Honorary DSc (Emory), MD (London), BPharm (London), FRCPath, PhC, FPS
Emeritus Professor of Pathology in the University of London at the Cardiothoracic Institute; Honorary Consulting Pathologist, National Heart Hospital, London.

D. A. OSBORN, MD (London), FRCPath
Reader in Pathology in the University of London at the Institute of Laryngology and Otology and Deputy Director of the Department of Pathology and Bacteriology of the Institute; Honorary Consultant Pathologist, Royal National Throat, Nose and Ear Hospital, London.

K. A. PORTER, DSc (London), MD (London), FRCPath
Professor of Pathology in the University of London at St Mary's Hospital Medical School; Honorary Consultant in Pathology, St Mary's Hospital, London.

C. P. WENDELL-SMITH, PhD (London), MB, BS (London), DObstRCOG, FACE
Professor of Anatomy in the University of Tasmania; Honorary Anatomist to the Royal Hobart Hospital, Hobart, Tasmania, Australia.

The late G. PAYLING WRIGHT, BA (Oxford), DM (Oxford), FRCP (London)
Emeritus Professor of Pathology in the University of London; Consulting Pathologist, Guy's Hospital, London.

Editor

W. St C. SYMMERS, DSc (London), MD (Belfast), PhD (Birmingham), FRCP (London, Ireland and Edinburgh), FRCS (England), FRCPA, FRCPath

Professor of Histopathology in the University of London at Charing Cross Hospital Medical School; Honorary Consultant Pathologist, Charing Cross Hospital, London; Honorary Fellow of the Royal College of Pathologists of Australia.

1: *The Heart*

by the late G. PAYLING WRIGHT

Revised by T. CRAWFORD

CONTENTS

1: *The Heart**

by the late G. PAYLING WRIGHT

Revised by T. CRAWFORD

THE PERICARDIUM

The pericardial sac serves two functions in the physiology of the heart. First, its smooth meso-thelium-covered inner surface facilitates the movements of the heart. Ordinarily, the visceral and parietal surfaces of the sac are separated by some 20 to 30 ml of limpid straw-coloured fluid—virtually a protein-free filtrate of plasma—the low viscosity of which renders it an excellent lubricant for the moving heart. Second, through its mechanically strong connective tissue matrix, the sac tends to preserve the myocardium from the injurious effects of any sudden excessive dilatation by preventing overfilling during diastole. That this latter function is probably of lesser importance seems to be shown by the fact that no cardiac disabilities manifest themselves in people who have the rare congenital abnormality of total absence of the pericardial sac.[1]

Abnormal Fluids in the Pericardial Sac

In consequence of the great resistance of the sac to any sudden stretching force, any abrupt increase of its fluid contents, such as may be brought about by a rapidly forming exudate or intrapericardial haemorrhage, may so severely restrict the diastolic filling of the heart that acute circulatory failure may soon follow. This condition is known as *cardiac tamponade*, and is met with most frequently in clinical work as a manifestation of haemoperi-cardium—the result of rupture of a myocardial infarct or of an aneurysm of the aorta or the accompaniment of some serious injury to the heart or chest wall. The sudden entry of some 200 to 300 ml of blood under high pressure into an intact pericardial sac will cause death almost at once. Should the haemorrhage follow some injury to the

thorax—especially if ribs are fractured—the accompanying laceration of the wall of the sac may allow the escape of some of this blood into the pleural cavity or the mediastinal tissues. The relief afforded by this leakage may prolong the period before the heart becomes irremediably embarrassed and thus may allow time for effective surgical measures. Should the patient survive, the residual blood in the sac coagulates and in time undergoes organization, with partial or complete obliteration of the pericardial cavity.

Although the pericardial sac yields little to a sudden stretching force, it distends gradually when the tension is applied continuously over periods of weeks or months. In slowly developing cardiac and renal failure—in which venous pressure may be raised or plasma protein concentration lowered—fluid often accumulates gradually in all the main serous cavities; in such cases, as much as 500 ml or more may collect slowly in the pericardial sac without serious hindrance to the diastolic filling of the atria. An excessive pericardial transudate of this kind, whatever its volume, is known as a *hydropericardium*. Eventually, however, the limit may be reached beyond which the sac can expand no further; after this stage has been attained, the pressure within it begins to build up and when it reaches about 10 mmHg the incoming veins suffer compression, the return of blood to the heart is impaired and cardiac output falls in consequence. The effects of progressive cardiac tamponade in raising venous pressure and lowering systemic arterial pressure were shown very clearly by Cohnheim when he introduced gradually increasing amounts of oil into the pericardial sacs of dogs.[2] Clinically, in man, an improvement in the circulation follows almost at once when hydropericardium is relieved by paracentesis.[3] As with transudates in general, the fluid that collects in hydropericardium

Congenital diseases of the heart are the subject of Chapter 2 (page 73).

is clear and pale yellow and contains very little protein. Its presence does not injure the mesothelial lining of the sac and its removal is not followed by pericardial adhesions such as commonly follow the absorption or paracentesis of an inflammatory exudate.

Blood-Stained Effusions

Blood-stained pericardial effusions (as distinct from frank pericardial haemorrhage) are strongly suggestive of invasion of the pericardium by a malignant tumour. A useful diagnostic guide may be obtained by examination for the presence of tumour cells in fluid removed by paracentesis but it is necessary to warn that skilled interpretation is needed to avoid confusion between tumour cells and desquamated mesothelium.

Further causes of blood-stained effusion include leukaemia and other blood diseases associated with a haemorrhagic tendency. A small blood-stained effusion may be found in association with myocardial infarction.

Pericardial 'Milk Spots'

Opaque fibrous thickenings of the visceral pericardium, 1 to 3 cm in diameter, are frequently found on the anterior surface of the ventricles, oftener on the right than on the left side. They are commonly referred to as 'milk spots' and were formerly termed the 'soldier's patch' in the belief that they resulted from mechanical trauma by knapsack-straps. The notion that trauma is the causative factor is almost certainly erroneous, but nothing better has replaced it. The patches are of no clinical significance but it is to be noted that they are more numerous on hypertrophied hearts and on those with valvular disease than on hearts of normal size.[4]

Acute Pericarditis

Aetiology

Acute inflammation of the pericardial sac, which may be fibrinous, serofibrinous or purulent in character, may result from a wide variety of causes, some infective, others toxic or allergic.

Bacterial infections of the pericardium, notably those due to pneumococci, streptococci and staphylococci, have become less common since the introduction of antibiotics.[5] Such pyogenic organisms, however, may enter and infect the sac through perforating wounds of the chest wall. Occasionally, too, they may extend into it from some infection of the pleura or peritoneum, or from some infected neoplasm in the thorax, such as a carcinoma of the oesophagus or bronchus. In cases of pyaemia, the sac may be infected either by the escape of pus from a superficial abscess in the myocardium or directly from the blood stream. Although suppurative pericarditis is thus an occasional complication of acute bacterial endocarditis,[6] it usually follows some purulent lesion in other parts of the body: notable among these are carbuncles and acute osteomyelitis, and thrombosis of the cavernous or lateral sinus in cases of facial sepsis or otitis media.

In recent years, various forms of pericarditis have been described of which the pathogenesis is still in question. Sometimes, pericarditis develops acutely, with precordial pain and a local friction rub. This form may run a prolonged course, often with periods of exacerbation and remission.[7] In many cases, the serum titre against some strain of Coxsackie B virus has been found to rise during the course of the disease, and there thus seems a likelihood that this may be the responsible organism.[8] During an outbreak of Coxsackie virus meningitis in Melbourne an increased incidence of 'idiopathic' pericarditis was noted: Coxsackie virus type B5 was isolated from 2 of 14 cases studied, and other cases showed serological evidence of a similar infection.[9] In other cases, acute pericarditis of a relapsing kind has been associated with cardiac infarction, and the suggestion has been made that the inflammation may be part of a local reaction to cardiac muscle proteins that have escaped from the necrotic fibres.[10]

Acute pericarditis has also long been recognized as a frequent accompaniment of acute rheumatic carditis. Two variants of this form may be distinguished—one with and one without an effusion of fluid into the sac; the former has much the worse prognosis.[11] A sterile, apparently toxic, form of pericarditis also develops commonly as a terminal complication in acute and chronic renal failure with uraemia.[12]

The term 'malignant pericarditis' is sometimes used to describe the condition when the pericardial sac is involved by tumour: it is better avoided, however, as the lesion is essentially non-inflammatory and is characterized by a blood-stained effusion (see above).

Morphological Changes

In acute serofibrinous pericarditis, especially that associated with acute rheumatism or the early stages of bacterial infection, the lining of the sac, especially over the posterior surface of the atria, presents the features typical of inflammation of a serous membrane.[13] The smaller blood vessels in the subserosa of both the visceral and parietal surfaces are much dilated, and this hyperaemia gives them a dusky redness. The early erythema is often obscured by a rough, tawny, overlying film of fibrinous exudate—the 'bread and butter' appearance described by Laënnec, or 'cor villosum' of other writers (Fig. 1.1). In the early stages of

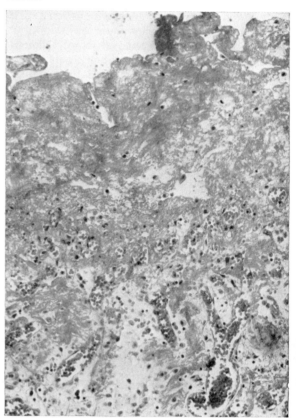

Fig. 1.2. Acute fibrinous pericarditis. The section is of the superficial zone of the visceral layer of the pericardium. The mesothelium has disappeared, and the pericardial surface is covered by a thick layer of fibrin in which there are only very scanty leucocytes. Vascular granulation tissue has begun to appear deep to the fibrin; dilated capillaries are conspicuous. *Haematoxylin–eosin.* × 140.

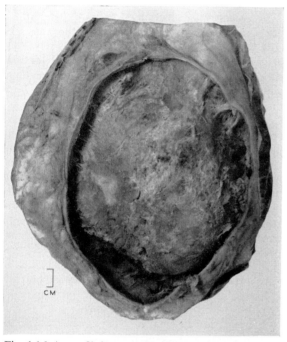

Fig. 1.1.§ Acute fibrinous pericarditis. The pericardial sac has been opened by cutting a window in its parietal aspect, exposing the thick, rough layer of fibrinous exudate on the visceral surface, and the stringy, fibrinous connexions between the apposed surfaces.

the inflammation this fibrin layer can usually be peeled away to expose the still glistening but injected red serosa beneath. If the inflammatory reaction has been present for several days, however, organization will have begun, so that the fibrinous exudate adheres much more firmly to the subserosa on which it lies. If it is detached forcibly, the surface of the heart can be seen to have lost its smooth, shiny appearance, and this change is reflected histologically in the loss of its mesothelium (Fig. 1.2).

When acute pericarditis is of recent origin, little

§ See *Acknowledgements*, page 71.

or no excess of fluid is found on opening the sac: this is the 'dry' form, in which friction rubs are usually audible clinically over the precordium. In cases of longer duration, much yellowish fluid, rendered turbid by many suspended shreds of fibrin, may be present. The protein content of such fluids, like that of all inflammatory exudates, is much raised—often to 4 or 5 per cent—and the many leucocytes add further to the turbidity. Should the inflammation subside, the gradual absorption of the excess of fluid which separated the visceral and parietal walls of the sac allows the two rough, fibrin-covered surfaces to come again into contact. Over the apposed areas, particularly when they lie near the base of the heart where the excursion of the chamber walls is small, the two surfaces may then become adherent to one another. Organization, which proceeds simultaneously from both surfaces (Fig. 1.3), finally completely replaces the exudate, adhesions forming that lead in time to partial or complete obliteration

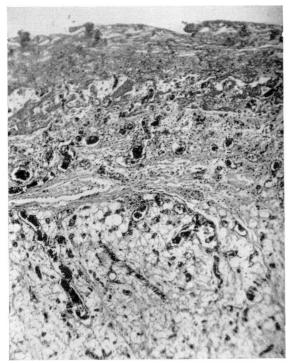

Fig. 1.3. Acute fibrinous pericarditis. The condition is at a stage later than that shown in Fig. 1.2. There is a well-formed zone of vascular fibrous tissue between the inflamed epicardial adipose tissue and the fibrinous exudate on the surface. Vascular dilatation is a prominent feature (the red blood cells appear black in the photograph). *Haematoxylin–eosin.* × 50.

of the cavity of the pericardium. Adhesions in this sac, however, never acquire the sclerotic character of those that form as a result of inflammation in the other serous cavities, for the constant movement of the heart tends to stretch them and so preserve their flexibility.

Suppurative Pericarditis

When the pericarditis is caused by such pyogenic bacteria as the staphylococcus, the streptococcus or the pneumococcus, the initial serofibrinous exudate soon assumes a frankly purulent character. Leucocytes, particularly neutrophils, emigrate in large numbers from the hyperaemic vessels in the inflamed serosa and the fluid gradually becomes more viscous and correspondingly more difficult to remove by paracentesis. Purulent pericarditis, with its clinical features of general intoxication,

swinging fever and high leucocytosis, has a serious prognosis, for the inflammatory reaction beginning in the serosa may extend into the underlying muscle and give rise to a superficial myocarditis. Moreover, even in patients who are recovering, resolution of the inflammation may be delayed through the survival of bacteria in pockets of exudate. If the infection is overcome and the exudate eventually undergoes organization, constrictive pericarditis is likely to result (see below).

Chronic Pericarditis

The nomenclature of chronic pericardial diseases has long been confused, partly through uncertainty as to their aetiology and partly through the use by different authors of the same term for conditions that differ significantly in character and pathogenesis.[14] The following main varieties can be distinguished:

(a) adherent pericardium
(b) mediastinopericarditis
(c) tuberculous pericarditis
(d) constrictive pericarditis (Pick's disease).

Adherent Pericardium

In this not uncommon condition, which succeeds an earlier episode of serofibrinous inflammation, the cavity of the sac may be partially or wholly obliterated through the organization of the original exudate. The resulting adhesions vary widely in character: sometimes they merely connect the two layers of the pericardium with one or more tenuous fibrous bands ('synechiae cordis'); oftener, they fill much or all of the space between the visceral and parietal layers with a fine and rather lax connective tissue. In cases of this kind, the sac wall is neither thickened nor firmly attached to nearby rigid structures, and so the adhesions, even when they enclose the heart, hardly impede its contractions and its musculature shows no hypertrophy. The condition gives rise to no symptoms and is often first recognized at necropsy.

Mediastinopericarditis

When the original inflammation has involved the connective tissues of the mediastinum as well at the serosal lining of the pericardial sac, the succeeding fibrosis often unites all these structures firmly together. Consequently, each contraction of the ventricles pulls on the now adherent chest wall, and this is seen clinically as a systolic retraction of the sternum and lower ribs. This additional and wasteful mechanical effort adds materially to the work of the heart, and in time results in myocardial hypertrophy and, eventually, cardiac failure. Since this uncommon form of pericarditis is generally of rheumatic origin, other chronic cardiac lesions, particularly in the valves, may also contribute to enlargement of the heart.[15]

Tuberculous Pericarditis

Tuberculosis of the pericardium is the most frequent form of tuberculosis of the heart.[16] In most cases, the sac is invaded by bacilli that have traversed lymphatic channels between infected mediastinal lymph nodes and the base of the heart: the pericardial infection is almost invariably the sequel to some preceding tuberculous disease of the lungs or pleura.[17]

When seen in its early, active phase, tuberculous pericarditis shows the changes typical of serofibrinous inflammation, though should fluid be present the exudate is usually more copious and likelier to be bloodstained in tuberculosis than in other infections. If the visceral and parietal layers of the pericardium are separated, the remains of the serosal surface of each are seen to be covered with thick fibrin, often mingled with caseous material; when this is removed, small grey or yellow tubercles are disclosed. On microscopical examination, this lining granulation tissue is distinctive in that it contains many tubercles;[18] their presence, together with areas of caseation, is strongly suggestive of tuberculosis, though occasionally a similar histological reaction can be found in other conditions, for example, in blastomycosis. Acid-fast bacilli can sometimes be detected in sections, but proof of the tuberculous nature of the infection depends upon the results of the inoculation of the exudate into guinea-pigs or of its culture upon suitable culture media.

It is now believed that in some patients a tuberculous pericarditis, after following a chronic course, can heal through the absorption of much of the exudate and the organization of the residual, partly caseous lesions. If this takes place, the fibrous tissue formed in the much thickened and adherent sac wall can gradually contract and give rise to the condition known as 'constrictive pericarditis' (see below).

Constrictive Pericarditis (Pick's Disease)

It has been known for more than a century that in certain forms of chronic pericarditis in young and middle-aged adults, the sac wall may be much thickened and may press not only on the heart, limiting diastolic expansion, but also on the main veins, which, as they approach the atria, become compressed and distorted. In consequence of the obstruction to the venous return to the heart, many of the clinical features of congestive cardiac failure appear.[19] This condition, now known as 'constrictive pericarditis', is often amenable to surgical treatment. The resection of much or all of the thickened sac leads to a marked fall in venous pressure, and to a return of the cardiac output toward a more normal value as a result of the greater stroke volume of the ventricles, now freed from the enveloping fibrous sheath; as a result, most or all of the clinical features that arose from the circulatory congestion disappear.[20]

When seen at operation or necropsy, the pericardium in this condition is seen to be grossly thickened—sometimes to 10 mm or more—and its cavity to be completely obliterated by dense adhesions.[21] It is as though the heart had been enclosed in a strait-jacket that restricted every movement. Sometimes, large areas of calcification or collections of cholesterol crystals are embedded in the dense, hyaline, avascular fibrous tissue. There are seldom any discernible signs of a preceding infective process. Though the wall of the sac is so greatly altered, adhesions between the pericardium and the adjacent mediastinal structures are rarely present. In this important respect, and in the associated absence of myocardial hypertrophy, constrictive pericarditis differs from mediastinopericarditis.

Occasionally, as a result of compression of the inferior vena cava by the coarse fibrous tissue, a syndrome known as 'polyserositis' (Concato's disease) develops in which fluid gradually collects in the pleural and peritoneal cavities. The liver and spleen become enlarged, and their surfaces, and often the serosal covering of the underside of the diaphragm, may be patchily or uniformly thickened by an opaque, white mass of hyaline fibrous tissue. This material, which may form a layer several millimetres in thickness, is covered by mesothelium; it is debatable whether it represents a reactive subserosal fibrosis, with hyaline changes in the collagenous tissue and its matrix, or whether it is the end-result of the deposition of fibrin from the peritoneal effusion and its eventual organization on the serosal surface.

Although the aetiology of constrictive pericarditis is still in some respects obscure, there are cogent reasons for believing that in many cases the condition is tuberculous in origin.[22] This view rests on three pieces of evidence: (i) known cases of tuberculous pericarditis when followed clinically can in time progress into the constrictive form; (ii) the occasional finding of histological appearances suggestive of tuberculosis in portions of the sac wall; and (iii) the occasional recovery of tubercle bacilli by animal inoculation. In a minority of cases, the dense fibrous tissue may be the remains of an old suppurative pericarditis that has healed. Rarely, the condition is the outcome of pericardial involvement in the course of systemic lupus erythematosus (see below).

Pericarditis in the 'Collagen Diseases'

The occurrence of pericarditis in association with *rheumatoid arthritis* was described by Charcot,[23] and, in the juvenile form of the disease, by Still.[24] Wilkinson[25] observed this complication in four among 197 patients. Usually the layers of the pericardium are markedly thickened and adhesions are present. Microscopy shows degenerate collagen and non-specific chronic inflammatory changes. Occasionally vasculitis and fibrinoid necrosis are seen. Progression to constrictive pericarditis has been observed[26] and beneficial results from pericardiectomy have been reported.[27]

The pericardium is usually abnormal in *disseminated lupus erythematosus*. A study[28] of 27 cases coming to necropsy showed pericardial involvement in 20. In most the sac was obliterated by adhesions but some showed effusion or fresh deposits of fibrin. Microscopy showed fibrinoid areas and numerous haematoxyphile bodies amongst the degenerate collagen and chronic inflammatory tissue. Progression to constrictive pericarditis has been observed.[29]

Scleroderma of the progressive systemic type (systemic sclerosis) is not infrequently accompanied by pericardial effusion, the fluid being rich in protein but having a low cell content. [30, 31]

Other Forms of Chronic Pericarditis

Among the rarer forms of chronic pericarditis, with thickening of the wall of the sac by granulation tissue, are actinomycosis[32] and amoebiasis.[33] The actinomyces usually invades the pericardium from the lungs or pleural cavity; it gives rise at first to a copious effusion and later, if the patient survives, to extensive obliteration of the sac—in both forms the

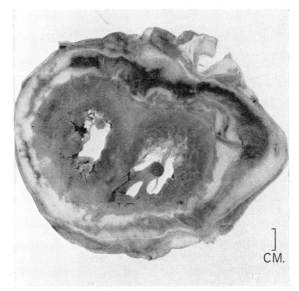

Fig. 1.4.§ Carcinomatous invasion of the pericardium. The two layers of the pericardium are covered by a thick, irregular growth of cancerous tissue. The layers of tumour on the visceral and parietal surfaces are in part separated by haemorrhagic exudate. The primary tumour was a bronchial carcinoma.

action of the heart is seriously embarrassed. Amoebiasis of the pericardium almost invariably follows from the extension of an abscess of the liver through the diaphragm; the condition is generally fatal unless chemotherapy is accompanied by surgical drainage.

Neoplasms of the Pericardium[34]

Primary neoplasms of the pericardium[35] are rare and when they occur may present considerable difficulty in diagnosis to both the clinician and the pathologist. Among benign tumours, lipomas, myomas and fibromas are most frequently recorded. The least rare malignant tumours are fibrosarcoma and mesothelioma: in recent years the latter diagnosis has been made with increasing frequency and the probability is that many tumours formerly regarded as fibrosarcomas would today be categorized as mesotheliomas.

Primary *mesothelioma* may involve the pericardium diffusely or as one or more localized nodules.[36] In the diffuse type the heart may be sheathed in greyish-white rather slimy tumour tissue, a centimetre or more in thickness, and there may be a loculated blood-stained effusion. Microscopically, the tumours may be predominantly of

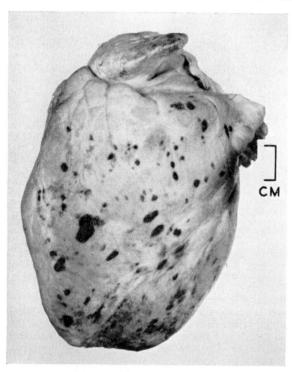

CM

spindle-cell type, or mainly 'epithelial' in appearance. A review of 25 cases showed 14 spindle-cell tumours, 6 of 'epithelial' type and 5 of mixed type.[37] About half the tumours metastasize to the lymph nodes, pleura or lungs: when this occurs it is difficult to be certain of the primary site.[38] There is as yet no evidence that primary pericardial mesotheliomas, as distinct from pleural and peritoneal tumours, are particularly associated with exposure to asbestos (see page 407).

Invasion of the pericardium is a relatively common feature of the late stages of *carcinoma* of the bronchus (Fig. 1.4), oesophagus, breast and stomach. It occurs also with *thymoma*.

In *leukaemia*, the pericardium, like the other serous sacs, may show numerous petechial haemorrhages (Fig. 1.5).

Fig. 1.5.§ Petechial haemorrhages and ecchymoses in the visceral layer of the pericardium of a boy, aged 12 years, who died of monocytic leukaemia.

THE HEART

ISCHAEMIC HEART DISEASE

The term 'ischaemic heart disease' is now applied to those conditions in which the nutrition of the heart is impaired as a result of some abnormality of its coronary arteries. Rarely, the abnormality is congenital, as when these arteries arise from the pulmonary artery instead of from the aorta, but in the vast majority of cases it is acquired and takes the form of atherosclerosis in their main trunks. The effect of such arterial obstruction on the myocardium can readily be appreciated: the milder forms result in some reduction in the capacity of the heart to meet the circulatory stresses of exercise; severer obstruction leads to local necrosis of myocardial fibres (myocardiolysis) and their replacement by scar tissue (replacement fibrosis) and often eventually, especially when complicated by thrombosis, to gross infarction.[39]

In the past, obstructive lesions in the main coronary arteries had long been recognized as occasional post-mortem findings, sometimes associated with sudden death after angina pectoris—as in the case of the great surgeon-pathologist John Hunter. It was only after the first world war, however, that the clinical syndrome of coronary arterial occlusion became sufficiently defined for the disease to be diagnosed with confidence. Formerly, many cases of ischaemic heart disease were unrecognized either clinically or at necropsy, and as a consequence it is only in recent years that mortality statistics have disclosed its prevalence.[40] In the Registrar General's *Statistical Review of England and Wales for the Year 1973* rather more than a quarter of all deaths were attributed to 'ischaemic heart disease'. Most of those who died from this cause were men of 45 years or over, but in recent times the incidence of this type of heart disease among women and younger men has shown a significant and disturbing rise. Coronary disease is particularly prevalent among professional men: it was named in more than a third of 500 obituaries of American physicians who died in 1969 in which the cause of death was stated. On the whole, as Morris and his colleagues have pointed out, it tends to be less common among the physically more active men of the labouring classes.[41, 42]

The Anatomy of the Main Coronary Arteries

Our knowledge of the distribution of the two main coronary arteries and of their wide variations from person to person has become better appreciated through the use of coronary angiography in both the living individual and the necropsy specimen.[43-46] The technique of first injecting a lead-agar preparation into the arteries and then opening the organ before it is radiographed has made it possible to identify all the coronary branches with a calibre of a millimetre or more (Fig. 1.6). Such studies have shown that about one-third of all hearts

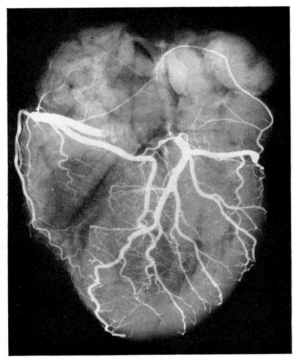

Fig. 1.6.§ Post-mortem coronary angiograph in the case of a man, aged 25 years, who had been killed in a road accident. The arteries are free from significant atheroma.

possess left and right main arteries of about the same size—the right coronary artery then supplies almost the whole right ventricle and the posterior part of the left ventricle and of the interventricular septum, while the left coronary artery is distributed to most of the left ventricle and the anterior part of the septum. In the other two-thirds, however, one of the main arteries, usually the right one, is larger—often considerably so—and supplies proportionately more of the cardiac muscle. It should be noted that the effects of atherosclerosis tend to be more serious in hearts with a preponderating left coronary artery.

During early life the anastomoses between the terminal branches of the two coronary arteries, although numerous, are very small, so that in the event of an obstruction to one of the main trunks neither can take over the function of the other. They are 'end arteries' in Cohnheim's sense of that term. The size and number of these anastomoses have been estimated in various ways, most of which depend on the examination either of histological material or of radiographs of injected hearts. The method that has probably provided the best estimate of their calibre, however, is that employing the perfusion of the coronary arteries with suspensions of glass or wax spherules and the subsequent determination of the size of the largest spherules capable of passing from one main artery to the other.[47] Even this method probably underestimates the effective size of these small precapillary anastomotic channels during life. Though differing in detail, all the methods that have been employed for determining the size and number of these anastomotic vessels agree in indicating that both increase with advancing years (Fig. 1.7). In young people they are few and small, but in the older they may become large enough to contribute materially to maintaining the blood supply to a portion of myocardium rendered ischaemic by an obstruction of the major artery by which it is ordinarily supplied.[48]

Injection studies have further shown that small arteries round the ostia of the aorta and pulmonary arteries and of the systemic and pulmonary veins form tortuous anastomoses with the two coronary arteries.[49] Although their contribution to the myocardial circulation is normally insignificant, even these small pre-existent vessels can, if the need arises, gradually undergo very considerable enlargement and provide a functionally important collateral circulation for the heart.

The major coronary arteries in their course in the epicardium are often partially or wholly embedded in its adipose tissue. At frequent intervals they give off branches which pass more or less perpendicularly into the underlying myocardium; their calibre becomes smaller and their walls thinner as they approach the lining of the ventricles.[50-52] It is these finer ramifications of the arterial tree that are compressed or even obliterated by the contraction of surrounding cardiac muscle fibres during systole.

The Physiology of the Coronary Circulation

The investigation of the coronary circulation provides problems of peculiar technical difficulty, yet

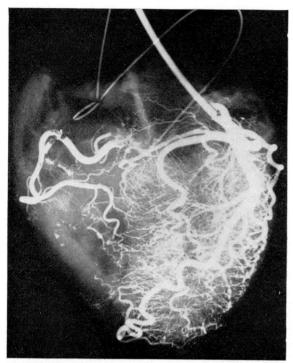

Fig. 1.7.§ Post-mortem coronary angiograph in the case of a woman, aged 60 years, who died of gastric cancer. There was only trivial vascular disease in any part of the body. The angiograph shows the remarkable extent of the meshwork of fine branches of the coronary arteries that may be found in older people. In order not to make the picture too complex, only the main branches of the right coronary artery have been injected. Some gas bubbles introduced with the radio-opaque medium are still present in these vessels.

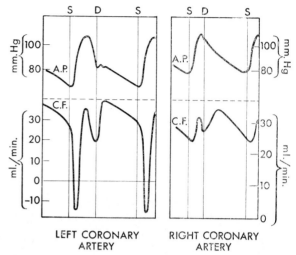

Fig. 1.8.§ Curves showing the blood flow recorded from the anterior descending branch of the left coronary artery of a small dog (left) and from the right coronary artery of a large dog (right). A.P., aortic pressure; C.F., coronary flow. The beginning of cardiac systole (S) and diastole (D) is marked by vertical lines. There is a sharp fall in the velocity of the blood flow through the left coronary artery as the pressure within the aorta rises during systole; transient reversal of the direction of flow is shown (see text). In the right coronary artery, in contrast, there is only little slowing of the flow during systole. In both arteries the blood flow is greatest during diastole. [*Redrawn from:* Gregg, D. E., *Coronary Circulation in Health and Disease*, Fig. 39; London, 1950.]

sufficient is now known of its physiology to make it clear that the circulation of blood through the small vessels of the myocardium, especially those in the wall of the left ventricle, differs radically from that of any other organ. In the vessels of other organs, the rate of flow of blood is greatest during cardiac systole, when arterial pressure is at its highest. In the heart, on the other hand, the closure of many of the smaller arteries and arterioles by nearby contracting heart muscle fibres during each systole is accompanied by a correspondingly intermittent fall in the circulation through the myocardium. The only comparable physiological event is the ischaemia of skeletal muscle that is in a state of vigorous sustained ('tetanic') contraction.

Much of our knowledge of the variations in the rate of the coronary blood flow during the different phases of the cardiac cycle has come from the experiments of Gregg and his colleagues, who inserted a flow-meter into an artificial anastomotic channel which they created by joining a small

branch of the aorta and one of the coronary arteries.[53] Their general conclusion, shown in Fig. 1.8, has been confirmed by more refined techniques of measuring blood-flow.[54] It can be seen that as the pressure within the aorta rises, during systole, there is no immediate forward flow of blood through the left coronary artery; indeed, blood is actually forced backwards in its larger branches by the compression of the distal vessels lying in the substance of the ventricular wall. Shortly after this initial reflux, some degree of forward movement is resumed, but the greater part of the myocardial circulation takes place during the diastolic phase of the cardiac cycle, at a time when the aortic pressure is still high and the ventricular muscle has become soft and relaxed. In the right side of the heart these phasic variations in blood flow are less marked: because of the much lower systolic pressures normally generated in the right ventricle there is no backward movement of blood in its coronary vessels during systole, and in fact only a small reduction in the forward flow. Should the systolic pressure in the right ventricle rise sub-stantially as a result of cardiac or pulmonary disease—for example in the severer grades of mitral stenosis—its myocardial fibres become hypertrophied and therefore lose this advantage over those of the left ventricle. The consequent deterioration in the supply of oxygen probably contributes to the development of the terminal right-sided cardiac failure so common in this disease.

The coronary circulation is impeded when there are lesions of the aortic valve. When this valve is stenotic, the pressure in the left ventricle rises during systole to a height that may be more than 100 mmHg above that in the arch of the aorta, so that the small vessels in the myocardium of this chamber are correspondingly more severely compressed. With aortic regurgitation, the low diastolic aortic pressure lessens the coronary flow during the time when the flaccidity of the myocardium permits the passage of blood through its capillaries. Yet despite these mechanical handicaps, the dilatation of the coronary arteries usually more than compensates for these disadvantages and permits an adequate flow of blood to be maintained.[55]

These studies on the haemodynamics of the coronary circulation are important for an understanding of certain features in the pathogenesis of ischaemic heart disease, for they disclose three very material points. First, it seems that if there is no compensatory vasodilatation the blood supply to the myocardium is likely to suffer as the heart rate increases, because the duration of diastole becomes reduced proportionately more than that of systole. Second, the myocardium of the left ventricle is much more vulnerable to ischaemia than that of the right. Third, the damage following progressive arterial occlusion, which may result from the growth of plaques of atherosclerosis, is likely to be more pronounced in that portion of the myocardium closest to the cavity of the ventricle, for it is in this layer of its wall that the smaller vessels are most compressed.

In a healthy man, about 200 ml of blood pass through the coronary arteries every minute while he is at rest.[56, 57] From observations on dogs it seems likely that in moderately severe exercise the flow rate may be raised materially, largely as a result of arterial dilatation.[58] But even this circulation rate, high in proportion to the weight of tissue when compared with other organs, is barely sufficient to provide the oxygen needed by the myocardium.[59] In no other organ except the liver —which, with its portal circulation, provides a special case—is the blood so deoxygenated by the time that it reaches the venous system. Of the oxygen that is present in coronary arterial blood,

over 70 per cent is abstracted by the heart. There is thus little possibility that the heart's increased need for oxygen during exercise can be met by the more complete removal of oxygen from the blood as it passes through the capillaries of the myocardium. The 'factor of safety' even in the healthy heart is already low—a feature of cardiac physiology which emphasizes the gravity of any arterial lesion, such as atherosclerosis, which diminishes the supply of blood to the myocardium.

Little is yet known of the momentary pressure fluctuations that may occur at particular sites in the coronary arterial system, though more is likely to be learned of such transient changes by the employment of capacitance manometers, with their virtual absence of instrumental inertia and time-lag in recording. From what is known of 'superimposed waves' in other parts of the circulation,[60] however, it seems likely that, for very brief periods of the cardiac cycle, reflected waves passing backwards from the arterial branches that have become temporarily closed in the contracting myocardium may raise the local pressure at certain sites in the major coronary trunks to levels substantially higher than those which have been recorded in the aorta and other large arteries by means of conventional manometers. The notable frequency with which atherosclerotic plaques form in the first 3 to 4 cm of the course of the main coronary arteries may be the result of stresses in the wall that arise from the local impact of such superimposed waves.

The Aetiology of Ischaemic Heart Disease

Although ischaemic heart disease may be produced on rare occasions by congenital defects of the coronary arteries, syphilitic aortitis, polyarteritis nodosa, dissecting aneurysm or coronary artery embolism, the outstandingly dominant determinant of ischaemic disease is severe atherosclerosis in these vessels. It is evident, therefore, that the factors known or believed to influence the development of atherosclerosis will be similarly involved in the aetiology and pathogenesis of ischaemic heart disease. These factors are discussed at some length in Chapter 3 (page 130). There are, however, additional factors which seem particularly related to the development of coronary artery and ischaemic heart disease and these require separate discussion.

Geographical and Racial Factors

Variations in the prevalence and severity of atherosclerosis between different countries and races of mankind have long been known. They have recently been the subject of intensive study on a world-wide basis—the International Atherosclerosis Project.[61] This study strove to express in an accurate quantitative way the variations in the amount of involvement of the arteries by atherosclerosis in different geographical areas. It is interesting to find that although the death rates from ischaemic heart disease vary widely in different parts of the world, individual cases present, on the average, much the same amount of advanced atherosclerosis regardless of age, sex and geographical location.

In general terms, death rates from ischaemic heart disease are highest in so-called prosperous countries and are strikingly lower in underdeveloped areas. Thus the highest rates are recorded in North America and North-West Europe (Finland and Scotland occupying an unenviable position at the top of the table) and the lowest in the Far East and Central Africa.

The relative roles of race and environment in determining these differences are not entirely clear though studies on migrant populations indicate that environmental factors may be dominant.

Age and Sex

Ischaemic heart disease is unusual before the age of 40. After this age its incidence rises steeply and the death rate from this cause increases with each succeeding decade up to the eighth.

A remarkable feature is the relatively low incidence in women during the child-bearing period. After the age of 50, however, this sex difference becomes much less apparent, and with advancing age the mortality rate from this cause in women approximates more and more closely to that in men. In spite of this rising death rate in later life the incidence of the disease among women never reaches that among men of the same age; it would seem that in their liability to this form of atherosclerosis women lag some 10 to 20 years behind their husbands and brothers.[62] A study of the insusceptibility of women to ischaemic heart disease before middle life, and of their liability to it later, might yield valuable clues to the pathogenesis of atherosclerosis in general. *Prima facie*, their relative freedom from the disease would seem to be more closely associated with the distinctive metabolism of steroid hormones, in particular the oestrogens, than with any other physiological difference between the sexes.[63] This inference is supported by the

finding that atherosclerosis appears much earlier in women whose ovaries have been removed.[64, 65]

Economic Factors

That the incidence of ischaemic heart disease is significantly correlated with economic prosperity is well attested by numerous statistical surveys and by national mortality returns. In England and Wales in 1951, after the numbers of deaths from this disease in various social groups had been corrected for variations in age distribution, the standardized mortality among men of the better-off classes was about twice that among unskilled manual workers.[66] It is a subject of speculation for epidemiologists at the present time whether this social gradient depends upon differences in physical activity or in supposed dietetic habits—especially as regards the consumption of fats—or upon one or more of the many other differences that are believed to distinguish the modes of life of these groups of men. One conclusion that has emerged is that among men in the same social group, those in occupations that require constant physical exertion are less prone to ischaemic heart disease than those who lead a sedentary life.

Recent epidemiological studies have disclosed a curious inverse relationship between death rates from cardiovascular disease (of which ischaemic heart disease is the major component) and hardness of water—the 'harder' the water supply the lower the death rates. This observation has been confirmed in the United States,[67] Great Britain[68, 69] and Sweden[70] and there can now be no doubt as to the validity of the statistical relationship: its interpretation, however, remains uncertain. A comparative study of hearts in a hard-water area (London) and a soft-water area (Glasgow) suggested that in the soft-water area myocardial damage occurred with a lower degree of arterial disease than was required to lead to myocardial damage in the hard-water area.[71] Clearly, more investigations are needed to elucidate the nature and mode of action of the 'water factor'.

Lastly, there is good evidence that people, particularly women, who suffer from hypertension or diabetes mellitus are liable to develop coronary atherosclerosis prematurely and to die at a relatively early age from ischaemic heart disease. The nature of the association with diabetes mellitus is still conjectural: the link may well be provided by the disturbances in lipid metabolism that complicate its course.

The Structural Features of Coronary Atherosclerosis

With age, the coronary arteries undergo a definite sequence of changes, and a progressive development of lesions in these vessels which may later culminate in atherosclerosis has been well described.[72-74] During childhood, the intima becomes steadily thickened by hyperplasia of its connective tissue, until by early adult life it has become thicker than that of any muscular artery elsewhere in the body. It is in the deeper parts of this layer, at the junction of intima and media, that deposits of lipid first make their appearance; they are often recognized in childhood or adolescence as small, yellow, pin-head spots. The relation of these deposits to later atherosclerotic plaques is, however, still obscure, for there is some evidence that at these stages the lipids can be reabsorbed and the lesions regress. These spots appear first in the descending branch of the left coronary artery, then in its main trunk and still later in the right coronary artery and the circumflex branch of the left one. By middle life, clearly defined, smooth atherosclerotic plaques are usually present in the main coronary arteries; later, the plaques tend to become confluent over considerable areas of the intima and their central areas commonly calcify. From then onwards the greater rigidity of the wall of the artery and the reduction in lumen that generally occurs at the same time combine to render the vessels less and less capable of supplying the metabolic needs of the heart during exercise.

It is unnecessary to describe in detail here the successive changes in the arterial wall as atherosclerosis develops—the subject is considered elsewhere (page 123). The alterations, however, are summarized in Table 1.1.

Post-mortem angiographic studies in which the coronary vasculature has been filled with radio-opaque material have much extended our knowledge of the distribution and extent of the atherosclerotic lesions in ischaemic heart disease.[75, 76] They have shown that, while there is no single 'artery of coronary occlusion', the anterior descending branch of the left coronary artery close to its origin is the vessel usually most severely affected (Fig. 1.9). The extent of the plaques varies much from case to case, but frequently many centimetres of the artery are affected; it is uncommon for less than 5 cm of the vessel to be diseased. When a heart is examined in the post-mortem room, few sites of obstruction will be overlooked if cross-cuts, about 5 mm apart, are made in the

Table 1.1. *The Progressive Development of Atherosclerosis*

Portion of arterial wall	Stage of atherosclerosis		
	Early	Moderate	Advanced
Intima:			
(a) endothelium	Intact	Intact	Often lost
(b) connective tissue	Progressive hyperplasia with increase of mature collagen and smooth muscle		
(c) lipids	Progressive increase of cholesterol		
(d) vascularity	None	Marginal and basal	
(e) calcification	None	Present	Often extensive
Media:			
(a) internal elastic lamina	Some splitting	Frayed	Largely lost
(b) other elastic laminae	——Progressive calcification——		
(c) muscle	Little change	Some thinning	Much atrophied

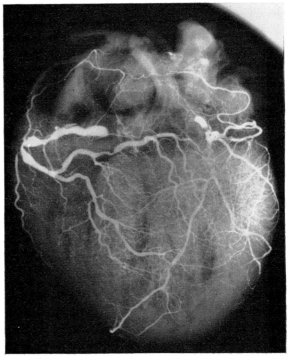

Fig. 1.9.§ Post-mortem coronary angiograph in the case of a man, aged 62 years, who died six months after a left ventricular infarction. The vessels show the irregularity of calibre characteristic of advanced atheroma; the anterior descending branch of the left coronary artery is occluded close to its origin.

major arteries throughout the first 6 or 7 cm of their course.

As atherosclerotic plaques increase in size, the wall of the artery becomes progressively thickened and its lining endothelium is often partially shed, so that the likelihood of the local deposition of thrombus increases. Indeed, in cases of sudden death from cardiac ischaemia, it is usual to find freshly formed thrombus on such areas. There is evidence that thrombosis may in many instances be initiated as a result of rupture of the inner surface of an atheromatous plaque.[77] When this occurs blood may be forced into the plaque (see below) and atheromatous debris prolapse into the lumen of the artery.[74]

Among the morphological changes in coronary atherosclerosis which have attracted attention in recent years one of the more notable has been the progressive vascularization of the plaques with age, and the possible contribution that this may make to the production of the terminal occlusion by thrombosis. In the wall of normal arteries of this size only the adventitia and outer two-thirds of the media are furnished with nutrient vessels, but as atherosclerosis progresses the capillaries advance until they penetrate the substance of the thickened intima. From the frequency with which small haemorrhages have been seen in close proximity to sites of recent thrombosis it has been supposed that thrombosis is liable to supervene in an artery the lumen of which, already narrowed by atherosclerosis, is suddenly further obstructed by the lifting of the plaque through the formation of a haematoma by leakage from capillary loops beneath it. Attractive though this supposition may appear at first sight, however, there are reasons for questioning its validity. Serial sections made at sites of coronary thrombosis usually disclose some small rupture in the intima of the artery itself, and the collection of blood in the plaque probably results from an influx from the lumen of the artery rather than from an extravasation from capillaries within its substance.[78] Further, it seems unlikely that any blood that might escape from minute vessels of the intima, with their relatively low internal pressure, could exert a force sufficient to displace an overlying plaque against a higher pressure inside the main artery itself.

It is hardly possible yet to decide the order of events in the origin of such small mural haematomas—whether a local haemorrhage precedes and perhaps contributes to the thrombosis, or whether the advent of the thrombus and its ischaemic sequelae in the myocardium lead to some reactive

dilatation of the artery, with tearing of its endothelial lining or of the delicate capillary network in its wall. In the second case the haemorrhage might well be a terminal feature of the lesion rather than a primary causative one.

The Effects of Ischaemia on the Myocardium

Chronic Ischaemic Myocardial Fibrosis

The effect of uncomplicated coronary atheroma on the heart is to lessen progressively its range of adaptation to the demands of exercise by limiting the maximum rate of the flow of blood through the myocardium. At first such limitations manifest themselves in lowered exercise tolerance and in the readier occurrence of dyspnoea on exertion. Often, too, circumstances of minor stress are accompanied

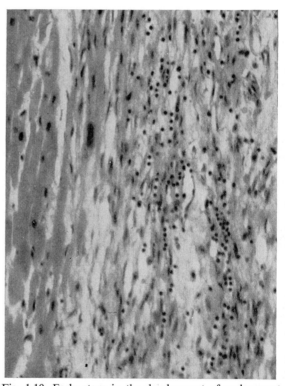

Fig. 1.10. Early stage in the development of replacement fibrosis of myocardium of the left ventricle, consequent on persistent ischaemia due to coronary atheroma. The surviving myocardial cells to the left of the microscopical field show some variation in nuclear size, and there is atrophy of many of the cells. The muscle has disappeared from the rest of the field, its place being taken by a loose-textured, collagenous tissue. Fibroblasts are numerous in this part and there is also a rather sparse accumulation of lymphocytes, with an occasional neutrophil among them. (See also Figs 1.12 to 1.15.) *Haematoxylin–eosin.* × 165.

by a sense of constriction in the chest or even by retrosternal pain. Later, when the vascular obstruction has become more pronounced, the onset of any unusual physical activity may be quickly followed by the pain of angina pectoris—typically about the upper part of the sternum, but often radiating to the left shoulder and arm. There seems little doubt now that the syndrome of angina

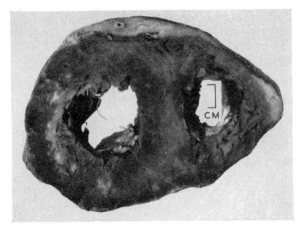

Fig. 1.11.§ This heart, in addition to hypertrophy and dilatation of both ventricles, shows many patches of fibrosis, particularly within the wall of the left ventricle. The fibrotic foci are seen as pale areas. Note the marked atheromatous thickening of the wall of the coronary arteries in the sub-epicardial adipose tissue.

pectoris is brought about by a temporary inadequacy of the myocardial circulation to meet the raised metabolic demands of the heart, though through what mechanism—local hypoxia itself or the products of glycolytic metabolism under hypoxic conditions—is not known. It is prone to occur in conjunction with anaemia,[79] and its mechanism seems to bear some relationship to that of the severe pain that develops in a limb during exercise if its circulation is temporarily interrupted by a compression cuff.[80]

In its milder forms, the ischaemia of coronary atheroma probably leads to few changes in the myocardium, and these are for the most part likely to be reversible when the temporary ischaemia ends. As the deprivation of blood becomes more persistent and severer, focal structural changes appear; while the hardier connective tissue cells can survive prolonged periods of ischaemia, the metabolically more active muscle fibres die and eventually disappear through autolysis ('myocardiolysis'). This differential mortality of stromal and parenchymatous cells has been expressed in the phrase 'elective parenchymatous necrosis'.[81, 82] In

time, the loss of muscle cells and the multiplication of fibroblasts lead to the condition known at 'replacement fibrosis' (Figs 1.10, 1.11 and 1.12). As might be anticipated from the anatomical arrangement of the arteries in the myocardium, the muscle cells that lie closely beneath the endocardium of the left ventricle near its apex are those most endangered by hypoxia; it is this inner layer of the ventricular wall that most commonly presents the silvery scars of replacement fibrosis. The sequence of events is illustrated in Figs 1.13 to 1.15,[83] which, though from a case of the rare disorder known as thrombotic thrombocytopenic purpura (see Chapter 8), exemplify the effects of focal myocardial ischaemia due to occlusion of the smallest arterioles.

As the occlusive changes of coronary atherosclerosis progress, the slow piecemeal replacement

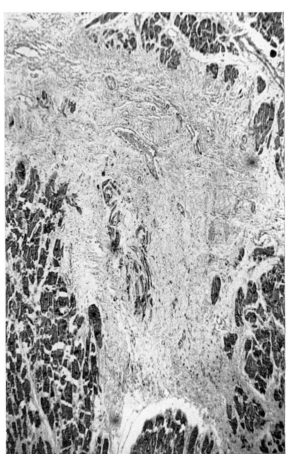

Fig. 1.12. A large focus of interstitial fibrosis in the wall of the left ventricle, the result of ischaemia due to coronary atheroma. This is the sort of picture that is seen microscopically in fibrotic areas such as are seen in Fig. 1.11. *Haematoxylin–eosin.* ×40.

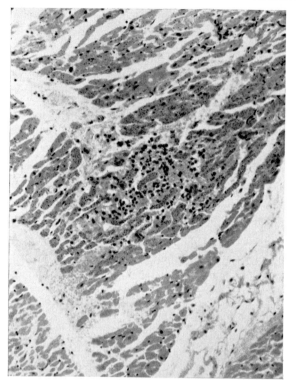

Fig. 1.13.§ Microscopical focus of fresh necrosis of ventricular myocardium, with accumulation of neutrophils among the dead cells. The lesion is identical with that caused by ischaemia due to coronary atheroma: in the case illustrated it is due to occlusion of a terminal arteriole by platelet thrombus in the course of thrombotic thrombocytopenic purpura. See also Figs 1.14 and 1.15. *Haematoxylin–eosin.* × 145.

fibrosis of the myocardium may be followed suddenly by infarction of a large mass of the ventricular wall. In the great majority of examples of myocardial infarction the precipitating cause is closure of the already narrowed vessel supplying the area by a deposit of thrombus. In the presence of a fairly recent myocardial infarct a careful examination of the coronary arteries will disclose such a thrombus in 80 per cent or more of the cases.[84] Such interference with the oxygen supply of cells that are metabolically as active as heart muscle fibres is promptly followed by their death and the creation of a gross lesion in the myocardium. Thrombosis, however, is not the only circumstance by which the coronary blood flow to large portions of the myocardium may suddenly become insufficient for the survival of the muscle cells: two others may be mentioned here in both of which a fall in the coronary blood flow follows a sharp fall in the aortic blood pressure. In the

first, in patients who are persistently hypertensive, the blood pressure may drop suddenly to normal or subnormal values as a result of the administration of a ganglion-blocking drug or from collapse associated with surgery or trauma. In the second, the blood pressure of elderly people, previously normal, may decline sharply under similar conditions.[85] In both cases, it may be surmised that large portions of the myocardium that had long been rendered vulnerable through pre-existing chronic disease of the cardiac vasculature succumb to the added stress of an acutely imposed local hypoxia.

Gross Changes in Myocardial Infarcts

It is important to realize that, in many instances in which ischaemia is quickly followed by the patient's death, no gross lesion may be recognizable in the myocardium at necropsy. It is only after some 8 to 10 hours that changes become apparent. On examining the heart when death has occurred after

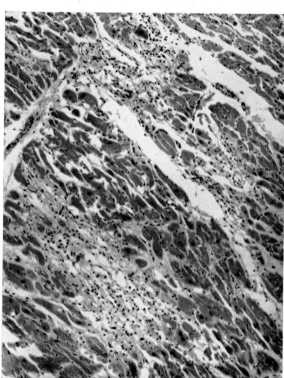

Fig. 1.14.§ Three microscopical foci of 'myocardiolysis' in the ventricular myocardium in the case illustrated in Figs 1.13 and 1.15. These lesions are at a stage slightly more advanced than that shown in Fig. 1.13: the dead muscle cells have disappeared, leaving the defects shown. *Haematoxylin–eosin.* × 90.

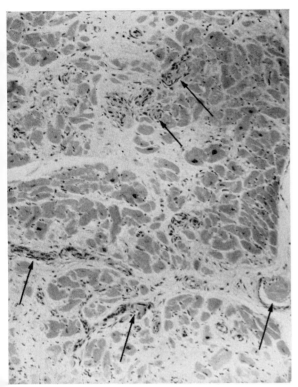

Fig. 1.15.§ Multiple foci of fibrosis in the ventricular myo-cardium in the case illustrated in Figs 1.13 and 1.14. These fibrotic foci are the outcome of focal necrosis and subsequent myocardiolysis such as are shown in the two preceding figures. The arrows indicate lesions of the thrombotic microangiopathy that is characteristic of thrombotic throm-bocytopenic purpura. As mentioned in the caption of Fig. 1.13, the changes in the myocardial parenchyma in this case are identical with those of ischaemia due to atheroma. *Haematoxylin–eosin.* × 90.

this interval the rather swollen and lustreless appearance of the ischaemic muscle contrasts with neighbouring unaffected areas. As the age of the infarct increases the morphological alterations become more easily recognizable. Within a few days the infarcted muscle becomes pale, soft and easily torn—the condition termed 'myomalacia cordis' by Ziegler—and it is often demarcated from the rest of the heart by a zone of confluent haemorrhages (Fig. 1.16). In mechanically inactive organs, such as the kidneys, the blood that escapes from injured vessels at the margin of an infarcted area remains close to the site of leakage but in the heart the beating muscle continually massages the flaccid, dying tissues so that any extravasated blood becomes dispersed more widely.

When the patient survives for several weeks the necrotic myocardium is progressively replaced,

first by granulation tissue and later by a fibrous scar (Fig. 1.16). Occasionally, such a scar, which often forms a silvery, band-like zone beneath the endocardium of the left ventricle, may bulge externally to form a 'cardiac aneurysm'. Although the fibrous walls of such aneurysms may stretch considerably with time, especially when subjected to the high systolic pressures of the left ventricle, they rarely rupture. If rupture occurs, it is usually through the myocardium immediately adjoining the fibrotic wall of the aneurysm and not through the latter itself.

In many hearts which have been injured by ischaemia, both old and recent lesions may be found at necropsy, and it is not always easy to correlate the morbid anatomical findings with the clinical history. When confronted with the problem of dating such lesions the pathologist must fall back on the general principles of morbid anatomy and histology—the fact that necrobiotic and auto-lytic changes take place relatively rapidly in

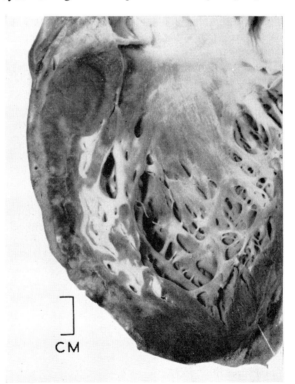

Fig. 1.16.§ Left ventricle opened to show anterior wall adjacent to septum. There is dense white scar tissue im-mediately under the endocardium at the site of an infarct that occurred nine months before death. The blotchy appearance of the myocardium superficial to the scar is due partly to fibrosis and partly to fresh infarction that led to rapidly fatal congestive heart failure. From a woman, aged 71 years.

metabolically active cells; the brief survival of extravasated red blood cells and neutrophile leucocytes; the comparative vascularity of recently formed granulation tissue and of young fibrous tissue; and the silvery, avascular nature of the strong scars, which may be from a few months to many years old. Some of these guides to the chronological assessment of such lesions will be considered in the next section.

Histochemical enzyme studies have shown that succinic dehydrogenase is lost from infarcted muscle some 6 to 8 hours after the onset of ischaemia.[86] This enzyme loss can be well displayed in both gross and microscopical specimens, and may prove helpful in timing the onset of the infarction.

Histological Features of the Development and Healing of Myocardial Infarcts

The need to tide patients suffering from cardiac infarction over the early critical period in which sudden death from rupture of the ventricle may occur has encouraged a close study of the rate of development of the hoped-for reparative fibrosis. Only from knowledge of the likely mechanical strength of the cicatricial tissues at various stages in their formation is it possible to estimate the delay desirable before subjecting the patient's heart to the added stresses inseparable from his again becoming ambulatory.

Our knowledge of the sequence of histological changes that follow infarction in the heart has been obtained from two sources: first, experiments on dogs and other large animals killed at various intervals after ligation of a major branch of a coronary artery;[87] and second, human patients in whose cases the time of occurrence of the infarction and the time of death were both accurately known. Fortunately, the conclusions that can be drawn from these sources corroborate one another, though some differences—mainly in the rate at which repair progresses—are naturally to be expected in findings derived for the most part from previously healthy experimental animals on the one hand and from chronically diseased and elderly men and women on the other.

In man, the progressive changes in cardiac infarcts have been studied in detail, and the following account summarizes the sequence of events that takes place in the structures affected and the practical conclusions that may be drawn for clinical guidance.[88] Within a few hours of the onset of complete local ischaemia the muscle fibres

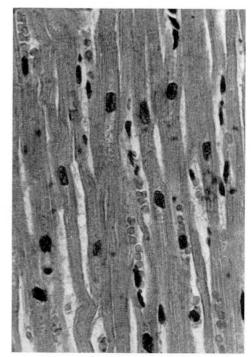

Fig. 1.17A. Normal myocardium of anterior wall of left ventricle of a healthy middle-aged man. For comparison with Fig. 1.17B. *Haematoxylin–eosin.* × 350.

die—their death is recognizable histologically by swelling, blurring and coarsening of cross-striations and the assumption of a deep eosinophilia (Figs 1.17A and 1.17B). Very soon afterwards the infarcted tissue becomes progressively, but temporarily, infiltrated from its margins by neutrophile leucocytes (Fig. 1.17B). The second week sees the beginning of the fixed cell reaction in the form of a zone of proliferating granulation tissue which surrounds the necrotic area. In small infarcts—those up to a few millimetres across—most of the necrotic muscle cells will have disappeared by the end of this period, partly as a result of autolysis and partly through ingestion by immigrant macrophages. In the third week the earliest signs of the formation of collagen fibres can be seen, first near the edges of the infarct but deeper within the area as the days pass. From this time onwards the usual reparative reaction known as 'organization' proceeds without interruption, unless a further ischaemic episode occurs; the remnants of any residual muscle fibres gradually disappear, while the replacement of the infarcted area by granulation tissue advances steadily. By the end of the second month, in all but the largest infarcts,

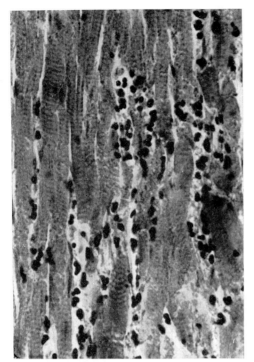

Fig. 1.17B. Infarcted myocardium of anterior wall of left ventricle of a middle-aged man who died 23 hours after thrombosis of the anterior descending branch of the left coronary artery. The muscle fibres are swollen and their cross-striations are blurred and coarsened; the nuclei have disappeared (karyolysis), but there is darkening of the cytoplasm at their site, presumably due to the persistence of some soluble product of the haematoxyphile nucleoproteins. There is also an irregular increase in the affinity of the muscle cytoplasm for eosin. Neutrophils are conspicuous in the interstitial tissue. Compare with the normal appearances shown in Fig. 1.17A. *Haematoxylin–eosin.* × 350.

the many stout collagen fibres by that time laid down provide a cicatrix of sufficient mechanical strength to obviate any likelihood of cardiac rupture. As bed-rest is succeeded at suitable intervals by ambulation and mild bodily exercise, the growing strength of the myocardial scar enables the patient to resume with safety a more normal mode of life. The current tendency is to encourage earlier physical activity in patients with myocardial infarction than was formerly advised.[89] It seems that this practice brings certain benefits in terms of an earlier return of cardiovascular postural reflexes to normal and of a diminished risk of embolic events: but physicians planning such a regimen should bear in mind that a large infarct is not fully replaced by firm, mature collagen for a period of 6 to 12 weeks from the onset.

Complications of Cardiac Infarction

Intracardiac Thrombosis

One of the common, and potentially grave, complications is the deposition of thrombus on the endocardium overlying the infarcted muscle.[90] Such mural thrombotic masses, which often present a laminated structure when cut through, may come to occupy a large part of the cavity of the ventricle and to present a rough surface to the interior of the chamber on which fresh thrombus becomes deposited (Fig. 1.18). If the process comes to an end, often through the use of anticoagulant drugs, the mass may become slowly organized from the underlying ventricular wall, and may remain for months and years afterwards as a white fibrous plaque. But sometimes, more especially in the early days of its deposition, small pieces of thrombus may become detached and are then carried as emboli which may lodge in important organs such as the brain and kidneys. This mural thrombosis and its attendant risk of embolism add to the hazards of cardiac infarction and must be borne in mind in prognosis.

Pericarditis

Frequently, the visceral pericardium over an infarcted area becomes mildly inflamed, perhaps as a result of irritation excited by some autolytic product diffusing from the necrotic muscle beneath. This sterile pericarditis, which appears about the second day, is sometimes recognizable clinically by a transient, localized friction sound (the 'friction rub'). It is seldom more than a mild serofibrinous reaction, which at necropsy can be recognized naked-eye by the dulling of the usually smooth and glistening epicardium covering the affected muscle and the deposition of an easily detachable film of fibrin. In itself, though an occasional aid in diagnosis, this manifestation is of little moment, for the volume of fluid that collects in the pericardial sac as a result of the inflammation is too small to embarrass the movements of the heart. Occasionally, when the infarct becomes cicatrized, fibrous adhesions may form between the visceral and parietal surfaces of the pericardial sac; they, too, are without functional significance.

Conduction Defects

When death quickly follows the onset of the ischaemia, there are reasons for believing that ectopic centres of excitation are set up in the

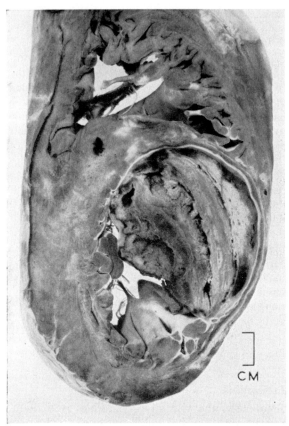

Fig. 1.18.§ The greater part of the anterior wall of the left ventricle is very thin, as a result of fibrous replacement of a large infarct; the anterior half of the interventricular septum is also affected. A large, laminated thrombus has formed over the fibrotic endocardium.

especially of the left ventricle, may so weaken the wall of the heart that it may rupture—often through a ragged tear several centimetres long—and bring about death suddenly from haemopericardium and cardiac tamponade (Fig. 1.19). This fatal complication is not uncommon, especially in patients who are hypertensive, and almost always occurs within the first few days of the infarction. Its incidence is highest in elderly women: it has been calculated that some 5000 cases occur annually in Great Britain.[93]

In one large series, about two-thirds of the ruptures took place within the first seven days and hardly any after the end of the second week.[94] Rupture of a papillary muscle[95] and rupture of the interventricular septum[96] are rare complications of myocardial infarction which, when not rapidly fatal, produce puzzling clinical manifestations.

Cardiac Aneurysm

In patients who have survived for many months after the infarction of a large part of the myocardium, the fibrous tissue which replaces the lost muscle often becomes stretched and thinned, so that the area forms a saccular bulge from the original contour of the heart. Such dilatations are termed 'cardiac aneurysms'; they are generally situated in the apical region of the left ventricle. They rarely rupture (see page 2). Although laminated thrombus usually forms on their endocardial surface, embolic phenomena are not

myocardium close to the affected area. In consequence, the orderly spread of the normal excitation wave from its source in the sinuatrial node is suspended, and fibrillation develops in the muscle fibres of the damaged ventricle. The cessation of their simultaneous contraction prevents the chamber from emptying normally and brings the circulation suddenly to an end.

Partial and complete heart block are not infrequent complications, arising acutely during the first few days following infarction. Unless rapidly fatal the heart block soon passes off—chronic heart block is rarely a sequel to infarction. The acute block appears to result from anoxia or some other reversible factor.[91, 92]

Rupture

All major infarcts that involve the whole or the greater part of the thickness of the myocardium,

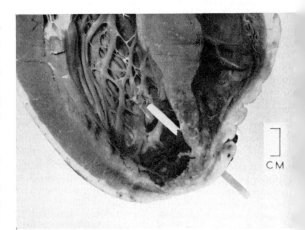

Fig. 1.19.§ Infarction of the apical part of the heart, involving both ventricles, has been followed by perforation of the softened tissue. The patient died of cardiac tamponade due to the massive haemopericardium that resulted. There is also fresh thrombus formation over the endocardial aspect of the infarcted part of the left ventricle wall.

common. The aneurysms cause important and sometimes puzzling haemodynamic and clinical effects.[97]

General Manifestations of Cardiac Infarction

The rapid autolysis of the muscle cells in an infarcted portion of the heart leads to the prompt escape into the circulation of a variety of breakdown products of the dying fibres. It seems likely that two of the common clinical manifestations of acute cardiac ischaemia, namely, pyrexia and leucocytosis—and possibly also the shock-like lowering of arterial blood pressure—may be attributable to the effect of pharmacologically-active substances released from the damaged tissues. Recently, various enzymes, among them transaminases and lactic dehydrogenase (see below) have attracted interest, because a rise in their concentration in the serum may be of value in the early diagnosis of cardiac infarction.

Pyrexia

Most patients who suffer from a major infarction of the heart develop pyrexia during the first few days of the acute attack. The fever is transitory and moderate in degree; in the absence of any complicating infection the temperature usually returns to normal within a week. Because this rise in temperature is generally associated with leucocytosis, and with pain that may be referred to the abdomen, it may be misinterpreted: the occurrence of acute cardiac ischaemia can consequently be mistaken for some other acute illness, with potentially disastrous results if the patient is subjected unnecessarily to the additional strain of a laparotomy.

Leucocytosis

Cardiac infarction is almost always followed by a rise in the leucocyte count in the blood to some 15 000 to 20 000 cells/μl.[98] The leucocytes, which are nearly all neutrophils, begin to enter the circulation during the first day, and the count usually reaches and passes its peak on the third or fourth day. As might be expected from its pathogenesis, the height to which the count rises is related to the size of the infarct; consequently, it is of some prognostic value.

Serum Enzymes[99]

Severe cardiac ischaemia is followed by the release of intracellular enzymes from degenerating and necrotic fibres. Two of these enzymes, transaminase and lactic dehydrogenase, can be readily estimated in the serum, and the degree and duration of their elevation provide some indication of the extent of the necrosis.

Serum transaminase catalyses a biochemical reaction which involves the exchange of an amino group of an amino acid for a keto group of another acid.[100] In most clinical laboratories, glutamic acid is used as the amino-group donor and oxalacetic acid as the amino-group recipient. The enzyme estimated in this way is serum aspartate-aminotransferase, also known as glutamic-oxalacetic transaminase (GOT). Its level in the serum rises earlier and more steeply than that of the associated enzyme, glutamic-pyruvic transaminase (GPT).[101] The value of the serum transaminase determination for the diagnosis of cardiac infarction depends on the fact that the concentration of this enzyme in the myocardium is higher than it is in any other organ. The disintegration of the heart muscle cells that follows infarction frees large amounts of transaminase and brings about a marked increase —often 10 to 15 times the normal value—in its concentration in the serum. As might be expected from the rapidity with which autolytic processes develop in the necrotic myocardium, this rise in the serum enzyme level, like the rises in temperature and leucocyte count, takes place within a few hours of the infarction, and similarly is quite transitory.

Serum lactic dehydrogenase catalyses the conversion of pyruvic acid to lactic acid. Its estimation is not difficult and has an advantage over that for serum transaminase since the enzyme does not disappear so quickly from the blood and its persistence accordingly facilitates diagnosis.[102] This test may be still further refined by substituting α-oxobutyric acid for pyruvic acid.[103]

RHEUMATIC HEART DISEASE

Rheumatic carditis is by far the most serious manifestation of acute rheumatic fever, of which, with varying degrees of gravity, it is probably an invariable accompaniment. Its hazards are all the greater because the disease is very liable to recurrences in each of which the heart may be damaged still further. For long, the mortality from acute rheumatic fever in England and Wales has been falling: only 22 deaths from this cause were recorded in 1969, representing a death rate of less than one-hundredth of that of 50 years before; the figure had risen somewhat by 1973, when there were 46 deaths.

B

But although deaths from rheumatic fever in the acute stage are much less common now than formerly, those from the more chronic forms of rheumatic carditis—and more particularly from mitral stenosis—have not fallen to a comparable extent. It seems that the disease is now much less likely than a few decades ago to prove fatal during its acute stages, and correspondingly likelier to progress into chronic heart disease. Even so, the decreasing incidence of acute rheumatism in children today must in time be reflected in a fall in the incidence of chronic rheumatic carditis when their generation reaches middle life.

But although chronic rheumatic carditis is becoming less frequent, especially in younger age groups, it still accounts for a very large proportion of all cases of heart disease. Not only is its mortality high —it was the recorded cause of death of 7075 people in England and Wales in 1973—but its long and often disabling course greatly handicaps such patients for many years before they die. Probably some hundred thousand people—more women than men—in Britain at the present time are seriously incapacitated physically by this disease.

Aetiology

The Infective Element

Evidence from a variety of sources indicates strongly that rheumatic fever is a post-infective state which is closely associated with streptococcal infections, especially those of the throat and upper respiratory tract.[104-107] Many outbreaks have been described, often from schools and military training camps, in which some of the children or young men who contracted such infections developed acute rheumatic fever two or three weeks later. A further significant observation is that in some young people who have suffered a previous attack of rheumatic fever, a subsequent pharyngitis or tonsillitis has been followed promptly by a sharp recrudescence of rheumatic manifestations.

The likelihood that some causal connexion exists between streptococcal infections of the nasopharynx and acute rheumatic fever is further supported by circumstantial evidence from three sources. First, scarlatina and rheumatic fever both have a very similar seasonal incidence—a fact first pointed out by Newsholme in England many years ago,[108] and well borne out by a comparison of the monthly incidence of the two diseases in United States naval personnel.[109] Second, there was a close correlation between the incidence of scarlatina and that of rheumatic fever in several

military training camps in the United States during the second world war, as is shown in Table 1.2. Third, the incidence of rheumatic fever at a large United States naval station was substantially lower in a group of men who were given sulphonamide drugs as prophylaxis against epidemic infections of the upper respiratory tract than in a similarly exposed control group.[109]

Since scarlatina, as well as most other forms of acute tonsillitis and pharyngitis, results from infection of the throat with beta-haemolytic streptococci of Lancefield's Group A, the possible relationship of one or more types of this organism to rheumatic fever has naturally attracted much attention. It must be pointed out at once, however,

Table 1.2. *Comparisons of Scarlatina and Rheumatic Fever Morbidity Rates at Selected U.S. Naval and Marine Corps Stations in 1945*

Station	Average strength	Comparable rates*	
		Scarlatina	Rheumatic fever
Parris Island, S.C.	16 784	1·4	0·6
San Diego, Calif.	92 063	27·7	4·1
Bainbridge, Md.	31 424	80·1	18·8
Sampson, N.Y.	31 027	111·2	16·7
Great Lakes, Ill.	66 466	148·6	19·2

* Computed on an annual basis per 1000 of the average strength of the personnel of the stations.
Figures from: Coburn, A. F., Young, D. C., *The Epidemiology of Hemolytic Streptococcus during World War II in the U.S. Navy;* Baltimore, 1949.

that if there is any such connexion—and, as has already been stated, there are persuasive reasons for believing that one does exist—it is of an indirect nature. The many attempts to recover this organism from acute rheumatic lesions of the heart and from the inflamed joints have been almost uniformly unsuccessful. Also, the species of bacteria isolated in the occasional instances of bacteriaemia in rheumatic fever do not differ in any important respects from those recovered from other patients suffering from acute upper respiratory tract infections.[110] Furthermore, the histological character of the acute lesions in rheumatic fever (see below) bears no resemblance to any of those known to be provoked by the presence of this pyogenic streptococcus in the tissues.

Many years ago, Schick described a characteristic relationship in time between scarlatina and acute tonsillitis on the one hand and the onset of subsequent acute nephritis and acute rheumatic fever on the other.[111] This temporal association has since been frequently confirmed.[112] Three phases in the sequence can be distinguished: first, an acute nasopharyngeal infection due to beta-haemolytic streptococci; second, an interval of about two weeks during which the signs of infection usually subside; and third, the appearance of nephritis or rheumatic fever. Whenever a time lapse of this duration is recognized in the clinical course of an infectious disease, the hypothesis may reasonably be advanced that the secondary complicating lesions are not caused directly by the localization of the pathogenic organism but arise indirectly as an undesirable immunological response to some product of its metabolism that is released at its initial site of lodgement. Such an explanation of pathogenesis is in keeping both with the sterile nature of these secondary lesions in the heart or kidneys and with the time interval needed for the production of specific antibodies to products of the haemolytic streptococcus. This concept of acute rheumatic fever as an allergic manifestation that may complicate infections by this organism will be considered further below.

The Element of Personal Susceptibility

Many instances have been described of local epidemics of streptococcal tonsillitis and pharyngitis during which some of the patients developed acute rheumatic fever. Invariably, however, the proportion in which this complication developed was small, as can be seen from a few typical examples set out in Table 1.3.

Table 1.3. *The Frequency of Rheumatic Fever as a Complication in Institutional Epidemics of Acute Tonsillitis and Pharyngitis*

Type of Institution	Number of patients		
	Tonsillitis and pharyngitis	Rheumatic fever	%
Boys' school[113]	2000	39	2
Boys' school[114]	775	7	1
Boys' cadet camp [115]	1466	162	11
Army training camp[116]	410	15	4

From such records it would seem likely that there is some element of personal susceptibility in those who develop rheumatic fever rather than some distinctive property of the responsible strain of the streptococcus, which is presumably common to all who contract the initial throat infection in the course of a given outbreak. What personal factor may be responsible for this vulnerability has hitherto escaped recognition. In the past, as with many other infectious diseases, emphasis has been laid on the aetiological importance of heredity in rheumatic fever. In recent times, however, there has been a clearer appreciation of the fact that families are intimately associated in their environment as well as in their genetics, so that a more cautious interpretation has been placed on the inferences to be drawn from family outbreaks.[117] Likewise, there is not sufficient evidence to support the hypothesis that specific dietary deficiencies, for instance of ascorbic acid, play any part in the pathogenesis of the disease—a hypothesis essentially founded on the fact that the disease formerly had a high incidence among children in the poorer classes.

The Social Distribution

Among widespread endemic diseases there are some, such as tuberculosis, in which prevention depends chiefly on the protection of susceptible people from the primary infective agent. In others —and among these is rheumatic fever—a strong suspicion may attach to some particular microorganism, though its direct responsibility has not been convincingly demonstrated. For these latter diseases, as long as the primary factor remains uncertain, preventive measures must continue to be directed toward mitigating such secondary aetiological factors—for example, adverse social conditions—as are suspected from comparative epidemiological studies.

Rheumatic fever is not a notifiable disease in Britain, and mortality figures have in consequence been the only guide to differences in its incidence in various communities. These figures have served to show that for many years the disease has had an indisputable social gradient.[118] Adverse conditions in housing, in nutrition and in other necessaries and amenities of life have long been regarded as contributory factors in the causation of rheumatic fever.[119] At the present time, the social gradient in Britain is appreciably less steep than formerly, and the participation of those general factors customarily included in the concept 'social conditions' is not nearly so evident as it was even half a century ago. Indeed, it seems likely that the great reduction in the mortality of children from rheumatic fever in England and Wales during the past 25 years (from

43 to less than one death per million) is mainly to be attributed to the amelioration of living conditions in those strata of society in which the disease was formerly rife. Similar declining rates have been recorded in the West of Scotland where formerly they were particularly high.[120] But in many parts of the world, where the primary needs of life are less uniformly distributed, these social factors may still have an important aetiological role.

Pathogenesis of Rheumatic Disease—The Allergic Concept[121]

Failure to recover micro-organisms from active rheumatic foci in the heart or the affected joints has led to alternative suggestions as to the way in which these very widely dispersed lesions are brought into being. The hypothesis which regards them as allergic in character, and perhaps similar in their mode of origin to the lesions in acute post-scarlatinal nephritis, has received much support.

In its essentials, this allergic hypothesis supposes that the potentially antigenic products of the streptococci multiplying in the throat are absorbed through the blood vessels and lymphatics of the inflamed tissues and distributed by the blood stream to the whole body. These antigens disappear from the circulation, partly through removal by the reticuloendothelial system and partly, after escape into the tissue fluids in many parts of the body, through attachment to various extravascular tissue elements, among which the fibrous tissues of the heart and joint capsules are particularly noteworthy. After a lapse of some 10 to 14 days, specific antibodies formed during this period are released from the cells which produce them and enter the blood stream. Escaping thence into the tissue fluids—which they do more readily at sites of mechanical stress or minor injury—they combine with the streptococcal antigen already attached to local structures and a local inflammatory reaction results. Studies on the distribution in the tissues of fluorescein-labelled antigens which have been injected into the circulation lends support to this allergic hypothesis, which in many features parallels the now well-established theories on the pathogenesis of 'serum sickness'.

The allergic hypothesis of the pathogenesis of rheumatic fever requires that antibodies to streptococcal metabolites shall be present in the blood of patients suffering from the disease. Such antibodies have been found: probably the most important is antistreptolysin O, though others—antihyaluroni-

dase, antistreptokinase and antistreptococcal-nuclease—may also be present.[122-124] (In parenthesis, it may be pointed out that streptolysin O is a haemolysin produced by beta-haemolytic streptococci and reversibly inactivated by oxygen—hence the designation O.) Many serologists have followed the changes in the titre of antistreptolysin O during attacks and remissions of acute rheumatic fever. Their general conclusions can be summarized fairly by stating that the titre of this antibody rises materially during an attack—notably during a relapse—and subsides during remissions to values little above those found in the serum of normal people. Cross-reactions have been demonstrated between sarcolemmal antigen in human myocardium and strains of Group A haemolytic streptococci, both of which reacted with antibodies in the blood of patients with rheumatic fever.[125, 126]

The possibility of an aetiological connexion between beta-haemolytic streptococcal infections and acute rheumatic fever, and more particularly the possible pathogenesis of the lesions as allergic reactions to streptococcal products, have led to many attempts to produce a comparable disease in animals. The closest replica of the human disease has resulted from repeated small inoculations of beta-haemolytic streptococci into the skin of rabbits.[127] In many of these animals, lesions developed in the heart and joints that bore a close resemblance to the small granulomas found in these sites in acute rheumatic fever in man (see below). Moreover, the allergic pathogenesis of these experimental lesions is supported by the appearance of specific antistreptolysin O in the blood.

In many diseases in the pathogenesis of which allergy is believed to play an important part, the severity of the process may be lessened by the use of corticotrophin or of a corticosteroid, preferably one with preponderant glucocorticoidal activity, so that sodium retention is not increased unduly. In rheumatic fever, their administration, although not always devoid of troublesome side-effects, has been found to be valuable: the duration of the disease and the severity of the damage to the heart both appear to be reduced by their use.[128]

The Pathological Changes in Rheumatic Carditis

The Focal Reaction—The 'Aschoff Nodule'

It was in 1906 that Aschoff described small fusiform granulomatous structures in histological sections of the myocardium of patients who had died in the acute stage of rheumatic fever. These 'Aschoff nodules', which have since been widely accepted as the characteristic lesions of the disease,[129] can be found, sometimes easily, sometimes only after careful search, in the hearts not only of patients who die early in the disease, but also, as has been shown in specimens of atrial appendages removed in the course of operations on the mitral valve, in those in whom the disease has reached the chronic stage.[130]

The sequence of changes passed through by an Aschoff nodule (Figs 1.20 to 1.22) as it develops and regresses has been described very fully by Klinge.[131] The earliest sign of injury in the heart, sometimes apparent as soon as two weeks after the

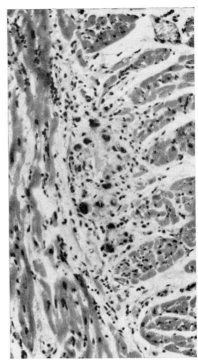

Fig. 1.21. Another small Aschoff nodule, showing the characteristic shape of the lesion, the peculiar cytology and the eosinophile swelling of the collagen fibres. There is some atrophy of the myocardial cells immediately adjoining this lesion. See also Figs 1.20 and 1.22 *Haematoxylin–eosin.* × 160.

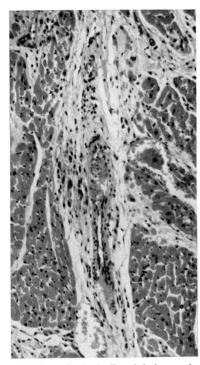

Fig. 1.20. A fairly early Aschoff nodule is seen in the interstitial connective tissue adjoining a small artery in the ventricular wall. Its spindle shape and the presence of large cells with large, hyperchromatic nuclei are seen. Swelling of the intercellular connective tissue fibres accounts for the grey background of the nodule. See also Figs 1.21 and 1.22. *Haematoxylin–eosin.* × 145.

onset of the disease, is in the collagen fibres of the affected area, usually close to small arteries. These fibres swell, lose their typical staining reactions, and come to stain in ways that were formerly believed to be characteristic of fibrin: for this reason, the change is often known as fibrinoid

degeneration. Histochemical studies on the reactions of fibrin and fibrinoid have disclosed differences, however, and have made it seem likely that this change in the staining reaction is due to an infiltration of the collagen fibre by some glycoprotein.[132] It is only after this degenerative change has taken place in the fibres that cells begin to accumulate in the nodule. These cells are of various kinds, but although neutrophils and lymphocytes may be conspicuous at first, macrophages are ultimately the most numerous and persistent. In time, small multinucleate cells, most of which may be formed by the fusion of macrophages, often enclose and apparently digest the remnants of the damaged collagen fibres; similar cells may be the remains of degenerating muscle fibres.[133] In its final stages, which it reaches some months after its first appearance, the nodule is colonized by fibroblasts from the surrounding connective tissues, and as a result of their activities new collagen fibres are laid down to form the eventual microscopical scar.

In rheumatic fever, small granulomas closely

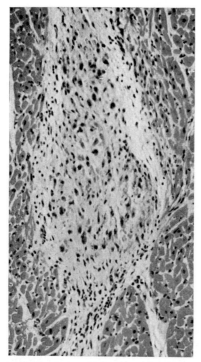

Fig. 1.22. An older Aschoff nodule, larger than those shown in Figs 1.20 and 1.21. *Haematoxylin–eosin.* × 145.

resembling Aschoff nodules develop in many other parts of the body. Those in the capsules of large joints, such as the knees and ankles, which are commonly affected, are associated with the inflammatory swelling and pain that are so characteristic a feature of the disease.[134] Others, often forming small clusters, are frequently palpable in the subcutaneous tissues in parts of the body, such as the elbows and knees, that are especially liable to minor trauma.[135] Careful search of the tissues of patients who have died from rheumatic fever has shown that these typical granulomatous nodules are dispersed very widely—few organs escape some sign of specific injury.[136]

The Heart in Acute Rheumatic Fever

Typical granulomatous nodules are commonly present in the pericardium, myocardium and endocardium in rheumatic fever; to emphasize the widespread extent of the lesions, the term pancarditis is often employed. The little granulomas may also be found in the wall of the aorta.[137] It must be remembered, however, that not all examples of acute rheumatic carditis exhibit characteristic Aschoff nodules: in some instances, particularly

in material from patients dying early in the disease, the nodules are scanty or absent. In these cases the changes found may be quite insignificant and consist mainly of diffuse interstitial oedema with a light exudate of lymphocytes, plasma cells and macrophages.

Pericardium

Inflammation of the pericardium is a common but not invariable accompaniment of rheumatic carditis. At necropsy, the lining of the sac can be seen to have lost its normal shiny surface and to have become covered with fine shreds of fibrin, which in the earlier stages are easily detachable, leaving a reddened serosal layer beneath. Sometimes, an amount of slightly turbid fluid has accumulated—serofibrinous pericarditis—but in the absence of complications it never becomes purulent or collects in sufficient amount to embarrass the movements of the heart. Occasionally, when much fibrin has been deposited on its surface, the heart may possess a shaggy appearance, to which the terms 'bread and butter heart' and 'cor villosum' have been given.

When examined histologically the epicardium may show areas of fibrinoid degeneration in the subserosal connective tissue in addition to the usual inflammatory changes typical of serofibrinous pericarditis. Aschoff nodules may form, and later undergo organization and fibrosis. If organization is extensive, and has been accompanied by the loss of many of the mesothelial cells which provide the shiny surface of the normal pericardium, the resulting fibrous tissue may form permanent adhesions between the visceral and parietal surfaces of the pericardial sac, and these may even obliterate the cavity completely. The adhesions that form, unlike the firm, dense ones that develop following pleural and peritoneal serositis, are usually lax in character. Unless the pericardial sac has become attached to the chest wall—which may happen if the inflammation has extended into the mediastinum—such intrapericardial adhesions add little or nothing to the mechanical load on the myocardium (see page 5).

Myocardium

Aschoff nodules tend to form in the connective tissue round small arteries in any part of the heart, though they are usually most numerous just beneath the endocardium—a feature which may account for the frequency with which defects develop in the conducting system in this disease. They often predominate on the left side of the heart, and in the posterior wall of the left atrium they may become so widespread and confluent as to form a sheet of granulation tissue in the deeper layers of the endocardium—the so-called 'MacCallum's patch'.[138] In the thin wall of the atrium such a high proportion of the muscle fibres may be damaged that the eventual reparative changes may lead to relatively more replacement of the myocardium by fibrous tissue than occurs in other chambers of the heart.

Endocardium

The naked-eye appearance of the valves in acute rheumatic carditis is characteristic. Along their line of closure an almost continuous series of small, brownish-grey, wart-like vegetations, each a millimetre or so in diameter, stretches from one commissure to the other (Fig. 1.23). Often they lie so

histological sections, they can be seen throughout the substance of the cusps, up to, and including, the fibrous rings. While most of these minute granulomas are situated within the substance of the valves and chordae tendineae, some develop close to their surface. When these superficial nodules are situated along the line of closure of the cusps, where the frictional forces are greatest, the endothelial cells are shed: the small and often flattened vegetations characteristic of rheumatic endocarditis result from the deposition of platelets from the blood passing over the minute raw areas so produced (Fig. 1.24). It is because of their small size and firm attachment to the connective tissues exposed at the site of erosion that the vegetations in acute rheumatic carditis do not become detached to form emboli—a common sequel with the larger, more friable vegetations of infective endocarditis. In time, the caps of thrombus formed over the

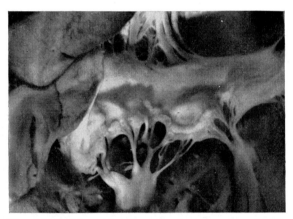

Fig. 1.23.§ Tricuspid valve, showing the characteristic appearance and distribution of the endocardial vegetations of acute rheumatic fever. The patient was a boy, aged 7 years, with severe rheumatic pancarditis.

close to one another that neighbouring vegetations fuse to form a rough and irregular ridge along the free margin of the cusps. Sometimes, too, they may be seen on the chordae tendineae. In the majority of cases the mitral and aortic valves, but particularly the former, are mainly affected, possibly because of the greater mechanical stresses to which the structures on the left side of the heart are subjected. The tricuspid and pulmonary valves seldom show these visible manifestations of involvement.

When the affected valves are examined in the fresh state at necropsy, Aschoff nodules can just be seen with the help of a good hand-lens as minute white spots in the endocardial tissues. In

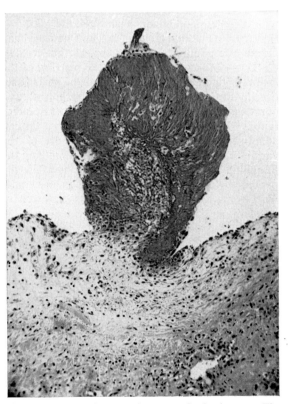

Fig. 1.24. Rheumatic vegetation on a mitral valve cusp. The vegetation consists mainly of fibrin that has formed over the collection of blood platelets that were deposited where the cusp was denuded of endothelium at its surface of contact with the opposed cusp. The distribution of the sparse inflammatory cells in the substance of the cusp has the characteristics of an Aschoff granuloma. *Haematoxylin–eosin*. × 85.

minute rheumatic granulomas exposed on the contact margins of the valve cusps become organized by fibroblasts that enter them from the underlying tissue, so that as the weeks and months pass the normally delicate free edges become coarsened and fibrotic.[139]

Although the changes in the endocardium of the mitral and aortic valves are the most conspicuous feature of acute rheumatic carditis, similar, but less obvious, alterations also take place in the lining of the chambers. This reaction tends to be most marked in MacCallum's patch (see above), with the result that the posterior wall of the left atrium may ultimately become coarsely roughened through the scarring in both endocardium and myocardium.

The Heart in Chronic Rheumatic Carditis

As with other diseases in which allergic reactions are believed to play an important part, rheumatic carditis often pursues for years a chequered course with alternating remissions and relapses. During the latter, successive crops of Aschoff nodules may follow one another, and the fibrosis that follows each crop adds progressively to the scarring of the heart. With growing incapacitation of such functionally important structures as the mitral and aortic valves, the effectiveness of the heart in maintaining the circulation inevitably lessens, though adaptive changes in the muscular walls of the various chambers have the effect of minimizing the disability. As long as these adaptations allow the patient to follow an ordinary, if physically somewhat restricted, life, the condition is referred to clinically as 'compensated', but in many cases—now less numerous than formerly[140, 141]—recurrent attacks of the disease ultimately lead to a state of 'decompensation' in which even mild exercise can no longer be tolerated and the patient becomes bedridden.

In reviewing the structural changes that take place in the heart over periods of months and years as a result of chronic rheumatic carditis, it is convenient to consider first the progressive induration of the valves and later the resulting changes—mainly compensatory—in the myocardium of the various chambers.

Valves

The possibility of greatly lessening the disability of mitral stenosis by surgical treatment has created new interest in the functional behaviour of the valve in health and the manner in which its aperture

becomes so greatly reduced in chronic rheumatic heart disease.[142] From direct digital palpation of the valve at operation, it is now known that in the great majority of patients, irrespective of the severity of their clinical condition, the orifice is reduced to a residual oval, usually from 12 to 20 mm in the longer dimension and about 5 mm in the shorter. The mildness or gravity of the circulatory symptoms is determined much less by the area of the aperture that remains than by the effectiveness of the myocardial adaptation to the added mechanical stresses.

From the study by Brock, the very uniform size of the orifice in mitral stenosis appears to be due to the anatomical arrangement and specialized functional behaviour of the chordae tendineae.[142] Although many of the chordae pass more or less obliquely from the tips of the papillary muscles to the undersurface of the valves, the shorter and stouter ones that lie in the direct line of pull of these muscles and are inserted into the cusps at distances of about 20 mm from the two commissures, and from each other, appear to have a distinctive role in cardiac physiology (see Fig. 1.25). They hold the two cusp margins particularly firmly together at these two sites of 'critical insertion', and, in the normal valve, are thus particularly effective in preventing regurgitation of blood into the atrium during ventricular contraction.

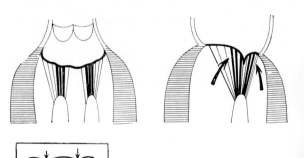

Fig. 1.25.§ Diagrams to show the mode of closure of the cusps of the mitral valve, and Brock's concept of critical areas of insertion of the chordae tendineae. The chordae tendineae that are in the direct line of the pull of the papillary muscles are thicker and stronger than the other chordae, as well as shorter. The left-hand diagrams show how these short and unyielding chordae pull two particular parts of each mitral leaflet strongly toward the corresponding parts of the opposed leaflet (only one leaflet is shown in the upper diagram). The right-hand diagram shows how the same chordae play a particularly important part in maintaining effective closure of the mitral valve during ventricular systole, when the blood is forced by the muscular contraction against the undersurface of the leaflets. [*Redrawn from:* Brock, R. C., *Brit. Heart J.*, 1952, **14**, 489 (Fig. 4).]

Because these short strong chordae tendineae cause the two cusps to be pressed together with particular firmness at the sites of critical insertion, it follows that, should rheumatic carditis develop and small vegetations form along the contact margins of the mitral valve, the ensuing organization of the vegetations is prone to cause adhesions to form between the two cusps at these points, so that the functional lumen of the valve becomes in effect reduced to a flattened oval, often only some 15 mm long, that remains as a pathway for the blood between these two areas of primary fusion (Fig. 1.26). Gradually, and as a secondary process, the now virtually immobilized edges of the two opposing cusps, between the areas of 'critical insertion' and the commissures, become attached to one another by the fibrosis that follows organization of their opposed vegetations. A feature of mitral stenosis that has an important bearing both on

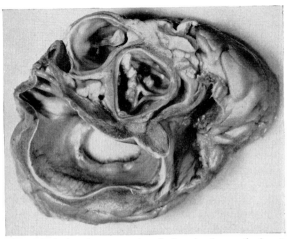

Fig. 1.27.§ Another example of chronic rheumatic heart disease. The mitral valve is both stenotic and incompetent, the rounded orifice being rigidly fixed in the shape seen. There is also marked stenosis of the aortic valve.

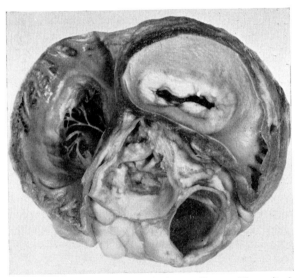

Fig. 1.26.§ Chronic rheumatic heart disease. The mitral valve (upper right of picture) is stenotic, and shows the characteristic 'button-hole' appearance—the slit in this case was 32 mm long, about 4 mm wide, and quite rigid in outline. Note the thickening of the lining of the dilated left atrium, which consequently is opaque, in contrast to the normally transparent lining of the right atrium. The aortic valve is also affected, being both stenotic and incompetent.

the pathogenesis and the surgical treatment of the condition is that the fibrous attachments between the cusps over this portion of their contact margins are rarely so strong as those at the sites of critical insertion. As a result of these successive phases of the fibrotic reaction, the mitral orifice becomes reduced to a small opening, often with a rigid

ring-like margin, the area of which when patent may be only one-tenth to one-twentieth of the aperture of a normal valve.

In more advanced grades of mitral stenosis, the entire cusp may become grossly thickened, so that the valve comes to form a stiff fibrous diaphragm with a small and, generally, central opening (the 'button-hole' deformity). Less often, the chordae tendineae become much involved, and their consequent shortening and mutual adhesion draw the margin of the orifice downwards (the 'funnel' deformity). It is in cases in which the cusps have been extensively sclerosed and the chordae tendineae much shortened that the functional disability that arises from the stenosis is likely to be augmented by the even more serious circulatory disturbances that follow from mitral regurgitation. In all types of mitral stenosis it is common for the functional activities of the damaged cusps to be still further impaired by deposits of calcium salts within their substance. Usually, these masses form in the parts of the cusp that are near to the ring, but sometimes they produce craggy projections at the margins of the stenosed orifice or on the surfaces of the sclerotic cusps.

Chronic rheumatic disease of the aortic valve (Fig. 1.27)—which may occur alone but more usually is associated with involvement of the mitral valve—leads in time, through the organization of the verrucose vegetations on its contact edges, to comparable coarsening and reduced mobility of its cusps. As a result, both obstruction and insufficiency may supervene, and if, as is common, the damaged cusps become extensively calcified, the already severe mechanical stress thrown on the left ventricle is still further augmented by the rigidity of the stenosed valve.

Myocardium

The alterations in the muscle walls of the heart that result from defects of the valves are essentially dilatation, hypertrophy and atrophy, the distribution of these changes being determined by the particular valves that are involved, and by the redistribution of work between the various chambers that results from the effects of the valve lesions on the blood flow.

When the mitral valve becomes stenosed, the effect of the obstruction falls at first mainly on the left atrium. This chamber consequently fails to empty completely during its systole, becomes in consequence dilated, and may in time develop some hypertrophy, though with so thin-walled a structure the degree of the latter change is difficult to assess. Occasionally, when the atrial muscle has been severely injured and the wall scarred as a result of earlier and extensive rheumatic inflammation, the dilatation of the now largely fibrous tissue sac may become so great—sometimes up to a litre in capacity—that the remaining three chambers are dwarfed by comparison.[143] When it is so greatly enlarged, the left atrium may displace the neighbouring organs and vessels and seriously embarrass their functions. In many patients with chronic rheumatic carditis the blood pressure in the pulmonary arteries rises to values three or four times the normal, and necrosis of the walls of the small vessels may follow[144] (see page 282). The additional mechanical work thus imposed on the right ventricle often causes it also to enlarge and the pulmonary conus to dilate; sometimes the chamber hypertrophies to such an extent that in weight and thickness of wall there is little difference between the two ventricles (see Table 1.4).[145]

Chronic disease of the mitral valve not only causes the flow of blood from the left atrium to the left ventricle to be impeded, but—especially in the 'funnel' deformity—may also permit considerable regurgitation owing to the incompetence of the valve in ventricular systole. With this added load, the left ventricular muscle, too, may undergo some degree of hypertrophy, though its extent is generally small in comparison with that developing when the aortic valve becomes seriously affected.

When the aortic valve is grossly deformed by chronic fibrosis—often associated with much irregular calcification—the demands made on the left ventricle are greatly increased. Not only is the outflow into the aorta during systole impeded by the stenosis, but during ventricular diastole blood that has just been expelled regurgitates, often in considerable volume. Consequently, if the circulation rate is to be maintained, the stroke volume must increase, and this can only take place if the diastolic capacity of the ventricle is enlarged by adaptive dilatation and the obstruction at the valve orifice compensated for by hypertrophy of the ventricular muscle.

Table 1.4. *Weights of the Two Ventricles in Uncomplicated Mitral Stenosis and in Uncomplicated Aortic Regurgitation**

Condition	Weight of muscle (g)			
	Both ventricles and septum	Right ventricle (R)	Left ventricle (L)	Ratio L to R
Normal heart	168	53	87	1·64
Mitral stenosis	202	88	82	0·93
Aortic regurgitation	462	121	267	2·20

* Lewis, T., *Heart*, 1914, **5**, 367.

The nature, extent and combinations of the valvular lesions that develop in chronic rheumatic heart disease vary widely from patient to patient, and the resulting functional defects are accompanied by a corresponding range of alterations in the various chambers of the heart as regards both dilatation and hypertrophy. The connexion between these valvular defects and the myocardial adaptations that arise from them is clearly shown by the comparative weights of the two ventricles in a series of hearts with uncomplicated mitral stenosis and uncomplicated aortic regurgitation respectively (see Table 1.4). These variations in their absolute and relative weights show how the various portions of the myocardium respond by hypertrophy to the additional stresses imposed by the mechanical inefficiencies of the respective valves. They also demonstrate that when heavy mechanical demands are made continuously on the left ventricle, as in aortic regurgitation, the myocardium of the right side of the heart also shares in the hypertrophy. This possibly unexpected feature may be accounted for by the anatomical structure of the myocardium, for many of its muscular bands are arranged in a spiral form and so contribute to the contractions of both the ventricles.

The Common Sequelae of Rheumatic Carditis

At any stage, rheumatic carditis may be associated with disturbances of cardiac rhythm. Some degree of heart block due to the proximity of the inflammatory process to the conducting system is not unusual during acute rheumatic fever, but it is in the chronic stages that the most characteristic arrhythmia, atrial fibrillation, is usually found. It would seem that damage to the atrial muscle, often associated with the presence of active Aschoff nodules, leads to the development of ectopic foci of excitation from which waves of contraction pass in an uncoordinated fashion through the atrial myocardium. As a result, the normal, almost synchronous contraction of the atria is replaced by an irregular twitching of their muscle fibres. Not only do these chambers then fail to empty into their respective ventricles at the proper phase in the cardiac cycle, but the consequent irregular stimulation of the atrioventricular node leads to an accelerated and irregular rhythm of the ventricles. It is probable that this arrhythmic tachycardia—in which many ventricular beats being premature are both wasteful of the metabolic resources of the myocardium and mechanically ineffective in promoting the circulation—contributes materially to the progressive failure of the heart in many cases of chronic rheumatic carditis.

The combination of chronic injury to the lining of the left atrium and the stasis that accompanies atrial fibrillation often leads to the formation of large mural thrombi within the chamber and thus to one of the gravest of the complications of chronic rheumatic carditis.[146] Usually, thrombosis begins in the atrial appendage, but it often extends over much of MacCallum's patch on the posterior wall of the chamber.[147] The detachment of fragments from such friable masses is inevitably followed by their ejection as emboli into the main arterial system; sometimes the mass is so large that the aorta becomes blocked at its bifurcation.[148] While many of these emboli finally lodge in 'silent' areas with little harm resulting from their presence, others settle in organs in which any sudden interruption of blood supply promptly leads to infarction. Since the brain receives a very large fraction—nearly one-quarter—of the blood expelled by the heart in a resting person, and is of all organs the one most vulnerable to anoxia, it is readily understandable that such sequelae of cerebral infarction as hemiplegia occur with distressing frequency as complications of atrial fibrillation. This grave complication is, moreover, particularly likely to follow the administration of quinidine or other similarly acting drugs which, by restoring the normal synergistic contraction of the musculature of the atria, are likely to bring about the dislodgement of any thrombus that may be insecurely attached.

A further and much feared sequel to chronic rheumatic carditis is the infection of a part of the damaged endocardium, particularly the valve cusps, by any organism that may be present in the blood stream during a temporary bacteriaemia. This grave condition of infective endocarditis is discussed in the next section of this chapter.

Common Manifestations of Acute Rheumatism in Other Organs

Only brief mention need be made here of the lesions in the three other situations that are particularly liable to be affected in the course of acute rheumatic fever—the brain, the joints and the subcutaneous tissue. Involvement of these tissues, together with the all-important carditis, comprises the well-known syndrome of acute rheumatism.

It has been known for many years that Sydenham's chorea is a manifestation of rheumatic disease in children: this form of chorea, in parallel with acute rheumatic fever itself, has now become quite rare. Sometimes the nervous symptoms are found apparently alone, but if the clinical course of those affected is followed during the ensuing months, a considerable proportion is found to show signs of cardiac involvement. Thus, while the great majority of such children escape any serious neurological aftermath, the occurrence of chorea should always be regarded with apprehension, for it is a warning of possible injury to the heart.

The acute and painful inflammation of the synovial membranes of some of the joints, especially the larger joints of the limbs, is a frequent but by no means invariable accompaniment of rheumatic fever. Indeed, grave damage can occur in the hearts of children who have never suffered arthralgia, or even 'growing pains', at any stage of their illness.

The subcutaneous tissues have long been known to be subject to involvement in rheumatic fever. Firm, painless nodules, some millimetres in diameter, often appear in the skin, subcutaneous tissue and aponeuroses, particularly on the exposed extensor surfaces of the limbs. These run their course for several weeks, and then subside.

In evaluating the relative importance of the various clinical manifestations of rheumatic fever, Carey Coombs's remark should be borne in mind: 'The joint lesions attract immediate attention by the pain they cause; the movements of chorea are not likely to escape notice; but it is the cardiac lesion which shortens life'.[149]

INFECTIVE ENDOCARDITIS

Infective endocarditis, formerly known as bacterial endocarditis,* is a grave disease in which the endocardium has become infected by organisms which can be isolated during life from the circulating blood and after death from the vegetations that have formed on the heart valves. Cases of the disease present themselves in two main forms, acute and subacute, which are separable both clinically by their rate of progress and pathologically by the organisms responsible. In the former, known as 'acute', 'malignant' or 'ulcerative' endocarditis, the disease, when not treated with effective antibiotics, runs a rapid course, and death as a rule takes place within a few weeks or months. At necropsy, the lesions in the heart, and more particularly those in its valves, are severe; often little of the substance of the affected cusps remains. In the 'subacute' form, the deterioration of the untreated patient's health is more gradual, and a year or more may elapse before the almost invariably fatal outcome. The cardiac lesions, too, are less extensive, and the destructive processes in the affected valve cusps can be seen microscopically to be to some extent countered by efforts at repair.

Although the clinical and pathological features of the various forms of infective endocarditis are now well delineated, the more slowly progressive subacute variety was long confused with rheumatic endocarditis.[150, 151] Many circumstances contributed to rendering the differentiation between these two forms of heart disease one of the most perplexing problems in cardiology. In the first place, most cases of subacute infective endocarditis were known to occur as a delayed complication of rheumatic endocarditis. Secondly, both were soon regarded (correctly, it is now thought) as in some way associated with streptococcal infections, but confusion arose because the techniques for the differentiation of the many species in this group of organisms were insufficiently developed at the time. Lastly, some of the early investigators of infective endocarditis recorded their inability to recover any infecting organism from their patients. This frequent lack of success in isolating the responsible organism arose mainly for two reasons: first, the unreliability of the methods of blood culture then in use; and second, the lack of appreciation by pathologists at that time of the intermittent character of the bacteriaemia in many slowly advancing cases and of the need for repeated efforts at culture. The position was still further obscured by the reported discovery of a bacterium—to which the name '*Micrococcus rheumaticus*' was given—that could be recovered from the blood and heart valves in rheumatic carditis. From morphological and other considerations, there seems now little doubt that this organism was a streptococcus—possibly *Streptococcus viridans*—and that the hearts from which it was obtained were affected by subacute infective endocarditis and not by uncomplicated rheumatic fever.

Today, although the problems of the pathogenesis of rheumatic fever and its cardiac manifestations are still not completely resolved, those surrounding the origins of the various forms of infective endocarditis have with few exceptions been successfully clarified.

Incidence

Although infective endocarditis is still an important disease in Britain—it was the certified cause of 259 deaths in England and Wales during 1973—its mortality is steadily declining. To some extent, this may be attributed to the falling incidence of rheumatic heart disease and to the much improved standards of dental hygiene (see below), but the introduction of antibiotic drugs has been an important contributory factor. The antibiotics have proved successful in terminating infection in many established cases of the disease, though residual scarring of the valve is to be anticipated as an outcome of the infection. Further, the prophylactic administration of antibiotics to patients known to be suffering from any form of chronic valvular disease or congenital abnormality of the heart shortly before they undergo dental extractions, tonsillectomy or such minor genitourinary operations as cystoscopy, has greatly reduced the danger that is inherent in the temporary bacteriaemia that often follows such traumatic procedures involving potentially infected tissues.

While no age group is immune, most cases of infective endocarditis in Britain occur among the middle-aged and elderly. Males are affected oftener than females, and no social or economic factors apart from those influencing the incidence of

---

* The term *bacterial endocarditis* ceased to be appropriate once it became recognized that some infections were caused not by bacteria but by fungi or by the rickettsial organism, *Coxiella burnetii* (see below).

rheumatic heart disease and the standard of oral hygiene seem to have any bearing on its aetiology.

Pathogenesis

Many kinds of micro-organisms have been isolated from patients with infective endocarditis, but the great majority of cases is accounted for by only a small number of bacterial species.[152] In acute infective endocarditis, the responsible organism is usually a beta-haemolytic streptococcus, a pneumococcus, a gonococcus or a coagulase-positive staphylococcus. Unfortunately, in recent years, many of the strains of staphylococcus recovered from these cases have proved resistant to antibiotic treatment, so that this organism is now responsible for an increasing proportion of the fatal cases.[153] Occasional cases of acute infective endocarditis are due to a meningococcus or a coliform organism. In the commoner subacute form of the disease, Streptococcus viridans is outstandingly the most important single pathogen;[154] in all recorded series of this disease in which the causative organism has been identified, this bacterium has been found in well over three-quarters of the cases. The remaining organisms that may cause subacute infective endocarditis form a miscellaneous collection in which, inter alia, the following figure—the enterococcus (Streptococcus faecalis), brucellae,[155] the haemophilus group of organisms, and Coxiella burnetii,[156] the cause of Q fever.

In recent years, increasing numbers of fungal infections of the heart valves have been recorded, among them those due to Histoplasma capsulatum[157] and Candida albicans.[158] Endocardial candidosis occurs particularly in three types of patients—as a complication of intravenous self-administration of drugs of addiction, due to failure to take aseptic care; as a complication of open-heart surgery; and as an 'opportunistic infection' when chronic debilitating diseases are treated with corticosteroids or cytotoxic drugs, which lower resistance to infection, or with broad-spectrum antibacterial antibiotics, which encourage overgrowth of the candida in the intestinal contents and elsewhere, and thus increase the chances of its invading the tissues through mucosal ulcers or by contamination of fluids given intravenously.

In every patient with bacterial endocarditis, the infection of the heart has been preceded by a bacteriaemia, though this may have been only transient or intermittent. In acute cases of the disease, the cardiac complication is often secondary to some readily recognized acute infective lesion elsewhere, such as furunculosis, pneumonia or puerperal sepsis. Occasionally, it occurs in narcotic addiction, when the drug is injected directly from a contaminated syringe into a vein.[159, 160] The frequency with which Streptococcus viridans can be isolated from the blood and vegetations in cases of subacute infective endocarditis suggested that some trauma to the mucosa of the mouth provides the portal of entry, since this organism is almost always present as a commensal in the saliva. This expectation was confirmed when it was found that Streptococcus viridans could be recovered from the blood in a large proportion of cases during the few minutes following dental extractions[161, 162] or tonsillectomy.[163] Further, the more heavily infected the gingival margins at the time, and the larger the number of teeth extracted on a single occasion, the greater is the likelihood of a bacteriaemia. Other infected tissues may also provide portals of entry. Transitory bacteriaemia occurs in nearly half of all cases of perurethral prostatectomy, and bacterial endocarditis due to Streptococcus faecalis has followed this operation.[164]

It must be realized that in cases of bacterial endocarditis the numbers of circulating bacteria are small—seldom more than a few hundred organisms in each millilitre of blood;[165] it is necessary, therefore, to take a sample of not less than 5 to 10 ml of the patient's blood, and, in view of the unknown nature of the supposed pathogen, to cultivate it under both aerobic and anaerobic conditions. The blood drawn should be inoculated into about 20 times its own volume of nutrient broth; this large volume of medium, to which the anticoagulant, sodium citrate, should be added, is needed partly to lessen the likelihood that the blood will form a clot in the culture bottle and so imprison any bacteria it may contain, and partly to dilute the patient's serum and thus to minimize the antibacterial effects of specific immune bodies, which may be present there in considerable concentrations. Because of the small number of bacteria in many such samples, several—sometimes many—days may elapse before any growth can be recognized in the culture medium. No culture should be discarded before the end of the third week of incubation.

It is usual for the heart affected by acute infective endocarditis to have been normal before the onset of the infection. In contrast, subacute infective endocarditis is almost always a complication of a congenital or acquired lesion. In most instances, scarring which has resulted from rheumatic fever is the predisposing condition,[166] so that the valves on the left side of the heart and the posterior wall of the left atrium (MacCallum's patch) are particularly vulnerable. Much less frequent, but also important, is infection of a bicuspid aortic valve—a structural deformity that may be either a congenital anomaly[167] or acquired as a sequel to some longstanding local inflammation.[168] Rarer still, and in general seen only in older patients, is infective endocarditis developing on aortic valves damaged by syphilis[169] or atheroma. Today, when many cases of infective endocarditis are cured with antibiotics, the resulting scarring in the valve cusps renders them liable to re-infection; second attacks of the disease—often caused by a different organism—are consequently being reported with increasing frequency.

Since some earlier damage to a valve seems to be an antecedent in the great majority of cases of subacute infective endocarditis, there has been considerable speculation as to the reason for the greater vulnerability of the injured cusps. It has long been known from injection studies that chronically inflamed valve cusps have an unusually extensive vasculature within their fibrous stroma. Minute vessels may even extend to their free margins,[170] and it was formerly suggested that the infection of the cusp follows the lodgement of the responsible organism at some site in this leash of capillaries. It now seems more probable, however, that during their passage through the chambers of the heart, the circulating organisms become deposited on the endothelium covering the affected cusp, and that, if circumstances favour their survival and multiplication, they establish themselves at the site of implantation.[171, 172] It is known that microscopical aggregations of platelets may form from time to time on the exposed surface of the valve cusps, especially the lines of their contact during closure. While platelet aggregations may form occasionally on an apparently normal valve, they do so much more readily on one that is sclerotic. Should the formation of these miniature thrombi coincide in time with a transient bacteriaemia, the organisms may first become attached to circulating platelets—a well-known phenomenon which has been called 'platelet-loading'[173]—and later become incorporated in deposits of these elements as they adhere to the surface of the valve cusp. Further, the presence of the organisms in these incipient thrombi may have a detrimental action on the endothelium nearby and so promote the adherence of more platelets.

The likelihood of the implantation hypothesis is supported by the superficial character of the early lesions, especially those found in the subacute form

of the disease, and by the absence of any serious disturbance in the deeper structures of the cusps near their attachment to the valve ring, where the vasculature is more profuse. Occasionally, elongated pendulous vegetations on the free edge of a valve cusp, swung in various directions by the alternations in the direction of the blood flowing past them, give rise to further vegetations at those relatively distant sites where their free end strikes against the previously unaffected endothelium of the endocardium or aortic intima.[174] Even this slight trauma to the lining of the heart or aorta at such points of impact permits organisms to lodge and give rise to satellite vegetations.

The Cardiac Lesions in Infective Endocarditis

Gross Appearances

Since in virtually all cases of subacute infective endocarditis, and in some cases of acute infective endocarditis, the infection is superimposed on an earlier cardiac lesion, and especially on chronic rheumatic carditis, the affected heart generally presents evidence of the primary disease. Since these predisposing lesions occur almost exclusively on the left side of the heart, the vegetations of infective endocarditis are typically met with on the cusps of the mitral and aortic valves—on the former rather oftener than on the latter, though both are not uncommonly involved at about the same time. Occasionally, a persistently patent ductus arteriosus or a traumatic arteriovenous aneurysm may become infected and vegetations indistinguishable from those that form on the heart valves may arise on the intimal lining at such sites.

On naked-eye examination, the vegetations of infective endocarditis are typically large, tawny to greenish, irregular and crumbly (Fig. 1.28). As a rule, they can easily be distinguished from those of acute rheumatic endocarditis by their much greater size, fungating appearance, surface friability and local destructiveness. It is the prominence of this last feature in the acute forms of the disease that gave rise to the term 'ulcerative endocarditis'. Although the vegetations usually seem first to form on the valve cusp near its line of closure, at the time of death they may have spread so widely that their site of origin can no longer be determined. Much of the atrial aspect of the mitral valve may eventually be obscured by irregular, rough, greenish-grey nodules, and in advanced cases the vegetations may have extended to cover much of MacCallum's patch on the posterior wall of the atrium. Some-

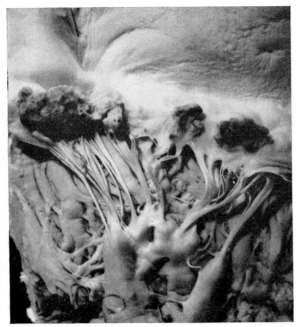

Fig. 1.28.§ Acute infective endocarditis of the mitral valve, due to *Staphylococcus aureus*. The patient was a woman, aged 59, with chronic staphylococcal osteomyelitis and terminal septicaemia. Examination showed no evidence of antecedent disease of the infected valve. The lack of destructive changes in the valve may be due to the short duration of the endocarditis before the patient's death.

times, vegetations which have begun on the mitral valve may spread downward on to the chordae tendineae and cause their erosion and even rupture (Fig. 1.29); similarly, those formed on the aortic valve may extend downward on to the endocardium of the left ventricle or upward into the sinuses of Valsalva. Weakening of the fibrous stroma of any infected valve may lead to aneurysmal pouching; when this occurs on the aortic cusps, which are particularly subject to sudden and severe stresses, perforation or rupture may follow (see Fig. 1.30).

Large vegetations close to the openings of the mitral and aortic valves interfere with their function and add appreciably to any mechanical inefficiency that may have resulted from the predisposing disease. Although as the vegetation grows it progressively narrows the orifice of the valve and impedes the passage of blood, its injurious effects on cardiac function are usually due more to the regurgitation that results from the associated incomplete closure of the orifice. This incompetence may be further augmented, suddenly and gravely, by the ulcerative perforation of one of the cusps.

Since the introduction of antibiotic and chemotherapeutic agents, patients suffering from infective endocarditis have often recovered from the infection—a result rarely known before the discovery of these drugs. But although the infection is overcome, the structural damage to the affected valves may be substantial, and the final scarring of the cusps, sometimes accompanied by much calcification, can lead both to serious functional inefficiency and to a risk of recurrence of the endocarditis, perhaps through infection with a different type of organism.

When treatment is delayed and the vegetations have become large, stenosis of the mitral valve, and stenosis and incompetence of the aortic valve are often the ultimate local effects. Although the prognosis for patients with infective endocarditis is now much better than in the pre-antibiotic era, their expectation of life is below normal.[175]

Microscopical Changes

Histological examination of a typical vegetation of infective endocarditis shows that it is composed of several structurally distinct zones (Figs 1.31A to 1.31C). The rough, finely granular, eosinophilic material which forms its outer layer or cap—and which provides most of the smaller emboli that are so commonly given off in this disease—is made up of conglutinated platelets held together partly by mutual adhesiveness and partly by interlacing strands of fibrin. Immediately beneath this layer

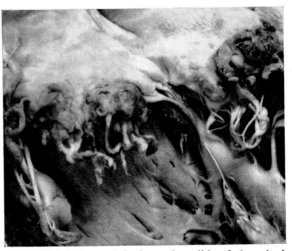

Fig. 1.29.§ Subacute infective endocarditis of the mitral valve, due to *Streptococcus viridans*. There was antecedent rheumatic disease of the valve. The extent of destruction of the chordae tendineae, many of which have broken and retracted or knotted, is unusual in a case of subacute infective endocarditis.

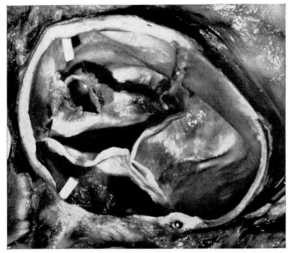

Fig. 1.30.§ Subacute infective endocarditis of the aortic valve, due to *Streptococcus viridans*. The infection was thought to have occurred as a complication of a spontaneous tear in the cusp, perhaps at the site of a congenital fenestration. There was no other abnormality of the heart.

is the zone occupied by the masses of causative organisms; this zone is usually deeply haematoxyphile unless the bacteria have died and lost this characteristic staining property. The bacterial component of the vegetation may be lacking altogether, particularly in treated cases. Deep to the bacterial zone is the inflamed tissue of the cusp itself, and in the subacute form of the disease this commonly shows evidence of repair.

In subacute infective endocarditis, the reparative changes in the valve cusps are generally conspicuous, and much of the deeper portion of the vegetation is composed of young granulation tissue in which fibroblasts and macrophages are present in large numbers. Sometimes, too, large multinucleate giant cells are created by the fusion of several macrophages, and not infrequently granular haematoxyphile deposits of calcium salts form in the deeper parts of the cusps. In acute infective endocarditis, on the other hand, there is usually widespread destruction of the substance of the cusp and little evidence of any repair. Further the virulent species of bacteria responsible for this rapidly progressive form of the disease excite a more obvious inflammatory response in the valve, and neutrophile leucocytes tend to accumulate in large numbers in the close vicinity of the bacteria.

Although the conspicuous valvular changes in infective endocarditis naturally attract most attention, the lesions that accompany them in the myocardium are also important and may assume

various forms. First, local destruction of the muscle may be brought about by the extension of the infection from the endocardium into the underlying myocardium. Second, embolism of some of the smaller coronary arteries may result from the fragmentation of friable vegetations (Fig. 1.32). This is particularly apt to happen with lesions of the aortic valve, for the abrupt reflux of blood into the sinuses of Valsalva at the end of systole may detach small particles and carry them into the coronary openings.[176, 177] Last, and perhaps most important, are the many small localized areas of myocarditis which probably result from the lodgement of dead or living organisms in the smaller vessels of the heart (Fig. 1.33). These inflammatory foci often take the form of minute abscesses or granulomas and are variants of the heterogeneous group of myocardial lesions formerly known as 'Bracht–Wächter bodies'. These are quite different from Aschoff nodules, some of which may also be seen if the predisposing rheumatic disease is still active.[178] In the vicinity of Bracht–Wächter bodies the myocardial fibres show signs of degeneration or even of necrosis, and neutrophile leucocytes and macrophages often collect near them in large

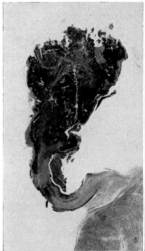 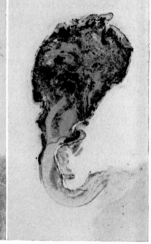

Fig. 1.31A. Vegetation of subacute infective endocarditis. The bulbous mass at the margin of the valve leaflet consists mainly of bacteria and fibrin. Its dark appearance in this preparation is due to the haematoxyphilia of the bacteria. See also Figs 1.31B and 1.31C. The organism was *Streptococcus viridans*. *Haematoxylin–eosin*. × 5.

Fig. 1.31B. A section adjoining that shown in Fig. 1.31A, stained by Gram's method. There is a narrow but distinct covering of Gram-negative material (mainly blood platelets and fibrin) over the mass of bacteria and fibrin forming the bulk of the vegetation. See also Fig. 1.31C. *Gram preparation*. × 5.

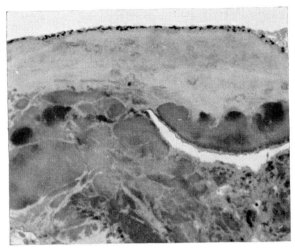

Fig. 1.31C. Higher magnification of part of the surface of the vegetation illustrated in Fig. 1.31B. There is a line of neutrophils at the surface of the vegetation (above). The superficial zone, which appears pale and homogeneous, consists of conglutinated blood platelets, with some fibrin (the slightly darker material). Deep to this there are the masses of streptococci: the staining of the bacteria varies in intensity, for many of the organisms are dead and have lost their capacity to give a positive Gram reaction. Note the fissure in the bacterial mass, indicative of the friability of the vegetation, crumbling of which gives rise to embolism. *Gram preparation.* × 140.

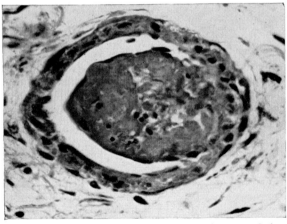

Fig. 1.32. This small coronary artery contains an embolus that was detached from a vegetation on the aortic valve in a case of subacute infective endocarditis due to *Haemophilus parainfluenzae.* The embolus is adherent to the wall of the artery over part of its extent; elsewhere, it has shrunk away from the wall, and its surface has acquired a covering of endothelium. *Haematoxylin–eosin.* × 350.

numbers. There is little doubt that these myocardial lesions, though small individually, are important cumulatively in weakening the heart, for functional deterioration is often indicated by abnormalities in the electrocardiogram.[179] Indeed in untreated or unsuccessfully treated cases of infective endocarditis, these widespread myocardial injuries are probably largely responsible for the cardiac failure that often supervenes terminally.

Complications

Although in the early clinical stages of infective endocarditis the lesions are for the most part confined to the heart, in its subsequent progress other organs become increasingly involved. Indeed, few diseases exhibit a closer correlation between their clinical and pathological features, or at necropsy present a picture that can be predicted with greater confidence from the previous history of the case. According to their pathogenesis, these complications can be classified as either embolic or toxic in origin.

Embolic Complications

The friability of the typical vegetation, its constant exposure to the rapid to and fro movements of the streaming blood, and the recurring mechanical shocks which arise from the impacts of the valve cusps on closure are collectively responsible for the frequency with which small fragments are thrown off from its surface into the general circulation. In acute infective endocarditis such particles may contain pyogenic organisms capable of creating metastatic abscesses wherever they come to rest.

In almost all cases of the subacute form of the disease, and in some cases of the acute form, the embolic particle is dislodged from the most superficial layer of the vegetation, where organisms are lacking. Consequently, as it is not infective, its impaction at some peripheral site merely leads to a bland infarct. While such emboli may be carried into any terminal branch of the systemic circulation, the very high proportion of the resting cardiac output that passes through the brain and kidneys, together with the end-artery distribution of the main vasculature of these organs, largely accounts for the frequency with which they suffer infarction.

Occasionally, in subacute bacterial endocarditis, an embolus contains viable streptococci, and although the bacteria are not sufficiently virulent to produce a metastatic abscess, they may nonetheless survive in the thrombus particle when it lodges at some site of arterial narrowing or bifurcation. At such sites, the bacteria may proliferate slowly, and, by a process similar to that by which they progressively injure the heart valve, they may

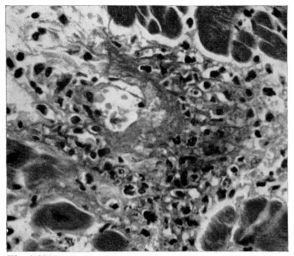

Fig. 1.33. Bracht–Wächter body in the myocardium in a case of subacute infective endocarditis due to *Streptococcus viridans*. A minute necrotic focus has formed in the vicinity of a terminal arteriole: the wall of the vessel is necrotic, there is fibrinous exudate in the tissue round it, and neutrophils and macrophages have accumulated. *Haematoxylin–eosin.* × 350.

gradually erode the wall of the artery and give rise to what is termed a 'mycotic aneurysm'.[180, 181] These aneurysms, though seldom more than a few millimetres in diameter, have a serious prognosis, for should they rupture—as is not uncommon— death from haemorrhage may quickly follow.[182]

Toxic Complications

The prolonged bacteriaemia which is so typical a feature of subacute infective endocarditis is associated with many manifestations of a toxic character that are brought about by bacterial products liberated from the many sites in the reticuloendothelial system where ingested organisms are undergoing destruction. Quite early in the disease the patient may suffer from intermittent attacks of pyrexia, and as the condition progresses these are likely to become severer and more frequent. Anaemia, sometimes marked, is frequently present and is one of the factors responsible for the distinctive '*café au lait*' colour of the skin in this disease. Moderate leucocytosis is often present and may increase when infarcts occur. The spleen is often enlarged to three or four times its normal size, and so becomes palpable below the costal margin. The splenomegaly is often related to the presence of infarcts in the organ, though it is partly due to the hyperplasia of the reticuloendothelial cells in the

splenic pulp—a result, perhaps, of the long continued ingestion of bacteria from the blood.

Of all the changes encountered, those that follow from the increased fragility of blood capillaries are among the most significant for clinical diagnosis.[183] This raised fragility is usually first apparent from the appearance of small petechial haemorrhages in the mucous membranes and the skin, particularly the skin of the flexor surface of the forearm. That these extravasations are to be attributed to abnormal weakness of the walls of the small vessels is demonstrable from the readiness with which a crop of fresh petechiae can be evoked in these patients by raising the venous pressure in the arm by partially inflating a manometer cuff placed well above the elbow.

Renal Lesions. Among the most noteworthy of the small haemorrhages in various parts of the body are those in the glomeruli of the kidneys. In subacute infective endocarditis, the kidney is often spoken of as 'flea-bitten', because of the many small red spots, a millimetre or so in diameter, that are visible when its subcapsular surface and exposed cortex are examined. These minute haemorrhages were at first thought to be the result of impaction of microemboli in the glomerular vessels; it was this interpretation that led Löhlein many years ago to term the condition 'focal non-suppurative embolic nephritis'—it is still occasionally referred to by this name. There is no reason, however, to believe that these small glomerular lesions, which usually appear in only a minority of the nephrons, are actually microscopical infarcts.[184] Typically, only a portion of the tuft is affected (see Chapter 24), while the circulation continues through the other vascular loops. Rather, it would seem that these tuft capillaries, which are relatively unsupported by surrounding tissues and which are ordinarily subjected to higher internal blood pressures than those in vessels of comparable character elsewhere, occasionally rupture like those in the skin. This allows blood to escape first into the glomerulus itself and thence through its epithelial covering into Bowman's capsule and the emergent tubule. It is these small haemorrhages that are visible to the naked eye as 'flea-bites'. Such individually small but collectively numerous haemorrhages in the nephrons are responsible for the mild grade of more or less continuous haematuria that is a common feature of this disease and renders the microscopical examination of urinary deposits so valuable a diagnostic procedure.

Many patients with infective endocarditis develop

a more serious renal lesion in the form of a generalized glomerulonephritis.[185] This was the cause of death in 14 per cent of one series of fatal cases.[186] The glomerular lesions are similar to those of immune-complex-mediated glomerulo-nephritis complicating other forms of strepto-coccal infection and presumably they have a similar pathogenesis (see Chapter 24).[187]

Causes of Death in Treated Infective Endocarditis

The success that has followed the use of antibiotics in infective endocarditis has led to the appearance of sequelae that were rarely, if ever, seen before the introduction of these drugs. Heart failure and infarction of important organs still remain the commonest complications in the earlier phases of treatment and account for a large proportion of the deaths. Even after the infection has been overcome and reparative changes have taken place, however, the valvular defects produced or aggravated by the disease continue to place stresses on the already damaged myocardium and lead in time to congestive cardiac failure. Functional disabilities are particularly likely to follow diffuse calcification of the affected cusp—a change which is liable to occur in the centre of an incompletely organized vegetation. The lesions in the kidneys may be so widespread that renal insufficiency and uraemia eventually develop. All the many records of successful therapy in infective endocarditis go to show, however, that the sooner and more energetically such patients are treated effectively with antibiotics, the less the likelihood of serious complications and the better the ultimate prognosis.

SYPHILIS OF THE HEART[188]

The clinical manifestations of cardiovascular involvement appear in the later stages of syphilis—often 20 years or more after the infection was contracted. Prompter and more effective treatment—particularly, in recent times, with penicillin—has resulted in a steady decline in tertiary syphilis in the United Kingdom, though the rise in the incidence of the acute disease during the second world war may well have an aftermath in the number of chronic lesions seen a decade or so hence. It should be noted, too, that as regards the late manifestations of syphilis, the improvement in incidence has been much more apparent in its neurological than in its cardiovascular forms. In England and Wales in 1961, the mortality from the neurosyphilitic diseases (general paresis and tabes dorsalis) was only a quarter of that 10 years earlier, while that of cardiovascular syphilis, typified by syphilitic aneurysms of the aorta, had hardly changed during the same period.[189] By 1969, deaths from both these forms of late syphilis had declined in the two countries to half the 1961 levels; in 1969 there were 148 deaths from cardiovascular syphilis and 73 from neurosyphilis: in 1973 the respective figures were 85 and 38.[190]

Morphologically, the cardiac lesions in acquired syphilis fall into two distinct categories: (1) those of a chronic granulomatous nature in the myocardium; and (ii) those which begin in the aortic ring and valve and lead in time to grave insufficiency of the valve. Although gummas—the localized syphilitic granulomas—sometimes occur in the heart, it must be stressed that they are comparatively rare and are greatly surpassed both in number and in importance by the lesions that develop in the vicinity of the aortic ring. The numerical disparity between the two forms is borne out by necropsy studies: in a series of 126 syphilitic hearts, only three had gummas.[191]

Granulomatous Syphilitic Myocarditis

While gummas have no clearly distinctive site of election in the myocardium, they tend to occur in the interatrial septum or the upper portion of the interventricular septum. Because of their proximity to the atrioventricular node, they may disturb the conducting system of the heart and provide one of the less common causes of the Stokes-Adams syndrome (complete heart block).[192] Myocardial gummas are usually single and range in size from the microscopical to masses several centimetres in diameter. In these larger and usually older lesions, the central, pale, rubbery, necrotic area is surrounded by fibrous granulation tissue that often has a capsule-like character. In the earlier and more active stages of its development, macrophages, plasma cells and fibroblasts form the bulk of the cells in the marginal zones, while eosinophils and giant cells of the Langhans type may occasionally be present.[193]

Syphilitic Lesions in the Aortic Ring and Valve

In syphilis of the aorta, the severest lesions are usually in the aortic ring and the ascending part of the arch, possibly because the vasa vasorum with their circumvascular lymphatics are most numerous in these portions of the vessel.[194] Since the main features of the aortic lesions in this disease are discussed on page 136, it will suffice here to point out that the chronic stages of syphilis are associated with a patchy loss of muscle fibres and elastic tissue from the media, with replacement first by granulation tissue and later by collagenous fibrosis. Occasionally, the centres of such lesions may be necrotic, microscopical gummas being seen in the wall of the aorta.[195] Focal destruction of those elements in the media that are specially adapted to resist mechanical stresses and their substitution by ordinary fibrous connective tissue lead to dilatation of the root of the aorta, especially at the commissures between the attachments of the aortic valve cusps. It is at these points in the aortic ring that the stretching forces, magnified by the shortening of the free edges of the cusps (see below), act most powerfully during cardiac diastole.

Dilatation of the ring, however, is not the only cause for the incompetence of the aortic valve in this disease, for the cusps, too, suffer damaging changes of a distinctive kind. Whereas in the normal cusp the fibrous stroma gradually thins as it extends from its aortic attachments to its free edge, in syphilis the normally delicate margin is thickened to create the typical, rounded, cord-like 'rolled edge', which often passes uninterruptedly from one commissure to the other (Fig. 1.34).[195] When such a cusp is cut from its free edge to its aortic attachment, its cross-section is seen to have a club-shaped outline; the rounded 'head' at the free margin is formed of dense and often hyaline fibrous tissue.

This highly characteristic 'rolled edge' deformity of the aortic valve cusps is produced by the ingrowth of fibroblasts from the intima of the aorta along the normally thin margin. That the coarsening has this origin is shown by the fact that in its earlier stages of development the rolling is most marked in the vicinity of the commissures. The replacement of the delicate pliable cusp edge by a coarse fibrous band naturally limits the freedom of movement so that during systole the cusps fail to open fully and in diastole they are unable to close completely to prevent the backward flow of blood into the left ventricle.

The aortic valvular incompetence so typical of cardiovascular syphilis is thus brought about in two ways: firstly, by dilatation of the aortic ring, mainly through the stretching of its commissures; and secondly, by the deformity of the cusps due to the fibrosis and shortening of their free edges (Fig. 1.35).

Changes due to syphilis in the root of the aorta may also affect the heart adversely in still another

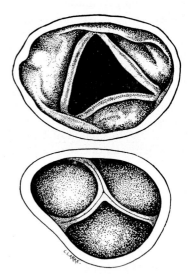

Fig. 1.35.§ Diagrammatic drawings of models of the aortic orifice in a case of severe syphilis of the valve (above) and in a normal heart (below). Both diagrams represent the condition of the cusps during ventricular diastole. The incompetence of the syphilitic valve is due to dilatation of the aortic ring and thickening and retraction of the valve cusps, which fail to approximate, leaving a triangular opening (compare with the perfect coaptation of the leaflets in the healthy valve). The models were made by pouring molten paraffin wax into the aorta, and then preparing plaster of Paris casts from the wax plugs after solidification. [*Redrawn from:* Scott, R. W., *Arch. intern. Med.*, 1924, **34**, 645 (Figs 5 and 6).]

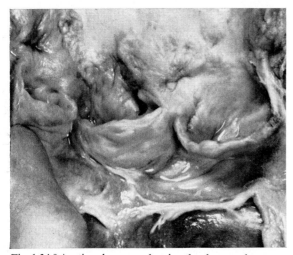

Fig. 1.34.§ Aortic valve cusps showing the changes characteristic of syphilis—thickening and rolling of the free edge, retraction of the cusp as a whole, and widening of the commissure between adjacent cusps. There are also well-marked changes of syphilitic aortitis.

way, for the granulomatous lesions often involve the openings of the coronary arteries. This complicating arteritis tends to occur in patients in whom, as a developmental anomaly, these vessels arise above the level of the sinuses of Valsalva and consequently nearer to the region of greatest damage to the aorta.[196] The effect of the chronic inflammatory reaction round these arteries is to reduce their size during their course through the wall of the aorta and for a few millimetres beyond;[197] this narrowing may be so severe that their lumen over this short distance may fall to pin-hole size. Such coronary stenosis, coupled with the low diastolic pressure accompanying the valvular insufficiency, gravely lessens the supply of blood to the myocardium. The resulting ischaemia may be so severe that on mild exertion the patient develops the pain of angina pectoris;[198] sudden death is by no means uncommon, and cardiac infarcts are sometimes found at necropsy. Furthermore, any estimate of the impairment in the coronary vasculature in this disease must take into account the increased demands on the coronary circulation resulting from the myocardial hypertrophy which develops as a consequence of the incompetence of the aortic valve (see below).

The aortic insufficiency that results from syphilis leads to dilatation and hypertrophy of the heart. In many cases, the weight of the whole heart is more than doubled, and dissection of its chambers shows that this increase is due mainly to hypertrophy of the left ventricle. The work required from this chamber is materially and continuously raised; studies on the volume of the systolic output and of the diastolic regurgitation indicate that in pure aortic insufficiency the leakage of blood backward through the valve may be two to three times the volume that is propelled usefully into the systemic circulation—the work performed by the left ventricle is increased proportionately.[199]

MISCELLANEOUS MYOCARDIAL ABNORMALITIES

The Metabolism of Heart Muscle

The technique of introducing a catheter into the coronary sinus and thus collecting samples of venous blood from the human heart has enabled much light to be thrown on the metabolism of the myocardium. By comparing the concentrations of different nutrient substrates in the systemic arterial blood and in the emerging venous blood, the extraction of these substances by the cardiac muscle can be determined. While this procedure

probably gives a reasonably accurate estimate of the consumption of such substances by the muscle during the work it is undertaking at the time, there inevitably remains an element of uncertainty, for such arteriovenous differences can take no account of the deposition or utilization of such stored metabolites as neutral fat and glycogen. However, the errors which result from such shortcomings of the method are probably of slight importance.

Coronary catheterization studies have disclosed the metabolic versatility of cardiac muscle—fatty acids, lactic acid, pyruvic acid, ketones and carbohydrates can be used for the production of mechanical energy in the myocardium.[200, 201] After fasting, when the blood sugar is low and the respiratory quotient for the whole body is only slightly above 0·7, the heart obtains most of its energy from the aerobic oxidation of fatty acids—mainly saturated fatty acids—which it obtains directly from the blood. When the blood sugar is high, however, the concentration of the free fatty acids in the plasma falls, and cardiac metabolism becomes mainly one of carbohydrates. It is noteworthy that cardiac metabolism is almost wholly aerobic; even in exercise, when the work of the heart is increased, the concentrations of lactic and pyruvic acids in the coronary venous blood hardly rise.

Many of the metabolic problems of the failing heart still await investigation. In most cases of heart failure due to hypertension or valvular defects the chemical energy released seems to be little changed.[202] It appears that in these cases the disturbance lies in the utilization of this energy for mechanical work, and that this reduction in efficiency may be due to changes in those muscle proteins, notably actomyosin, shortening of which is responsible for the contraction of the muscle fibre.[203]

It is only occasionally that cardiac failure results from some depression of the chemical metabolic processes in the muscle fibres: thiamin deficiency (beri-beri) and hyperthyroidism are probably instances of such basic biochemical disturbances.[204]

Hypertrophy and Atrophy of the Myocardium

The weight of the normal heart depends mainly on the sex, age and physique of the individual. Table 1.5 sets out the mean values for adults of different heights and weights, and by appropriate interpolation it is possible to estimate whether or not the weight of the heart in any particular instance is abnormal.[205, 206]

In infants and children the weight of the normal heart depends mainly upon age. Some guiding figures are given in Table 1.6.[207]

Apart from age and sex, it is the average amount of mechanical work that the muscular elements of the heart are called upon to perform daily over long periods that mainly determines the weight of the heart. For this reason, the continuous stress imposed by essential hypertension or aortic stenosis produces severer grades of hypertrophy than the intermittent one of temporary bouts of physical exertion.

Table 1.5. *Heart Weight in Normal Men and Women of Various Heights and Weights*

Height (cm)	Body weight (kg)		Heart weight (g)	
	Men	Women	Men	Women
152	67	63	288	250
160	70	66	302	263
167	73	69	316	276
175	77	73	330	290
183	80	77	346	304
190	84	80	360	317

* These estimates were obtained by weighing more than a thousand hearts obtained from patients aged over 21 years who showed no apparent abnormality of the cardiovascular system either clinically or at necropsy (Smith, H. L., *Amer. Heart J.*, 1928, **4**, 79; Zeek, P. M. *Arch. Path.* (*Chic.*), 1942, **34**, 820).

Table 1.6. *Normal Heart Weight of Infants and of Children of Various Ages*

Age	Heart weight (g)	Age	Heart weight (g)
1 month	20	4 years	73
3 months	24	6 years	94
6 months	31	8 years	110
1 year	44	10 years	116
2 years	56	12 years	124

* Coppoletta, J. M., Wolbach, S. B., *Amer. J. Path.*, 1933, **9**, 55.

The adaptability of heart size to alterations in the demands of the circulation can be clearly demonstrated in animal experiments. If through some procedure the circulatory demand is raised, the heart weight increases, and if the demand is later reduced, the weight reverts to its former normal value. If, for example a rat has one kidney excised and the main artery to the other partially obstructed by a clip, it develops persistent hyper-

tension of a kind that is reversible only when the normal renal circulation is re-established. In one such experiment it was found that the mean systolic arterial pressure in a large group of rats was 116 mmHg, that it rose in the course of a few weeks to 171 mmHg when the artery was partially occluded, and that it soon fell back to 119 mmHg when the clip was removed.[208] In samples of these animals killed at various stages of the experiment, the average weight of the heart rose by about one-half at the height of the hypertension and had reverted to its initial value when the blood pressure had been normal for some weeks.

In an experiment of a different kind on rabbits, the cardiac output, and hence the work of the heart, was much increased by the creation of an arteriovenous fistula (between the carotid artery and the jugular vein).[209] In the course of three months, the heart weight rose steadily, and by the end of that period in some cases it had more than doubled. When the anastomosis was subsequently resected, so that the work of the heart was restored to normal, the heart weight reverted to its original figure in the course of the ensuing few weeks.[210]

In man, the work required of the myocardium may be increased in several ways. The commonest causes are persistent systemic hypertension, defects of the valves, congenital cardiovascular anomalies and severe anaemia. Much less frequent causes are the high cardiac output that is a feature of Paget's disease of bone and of thiamine deficiency ('wet beri-beri'), or the raised blood viscosity that accompanies severe degrees of polycythaemia. In all these conditions the stress falls unequally on the different chambers, which in consequence undergo differing degrees of hypertrophy. In mitral stenosis, for example, which in its later stages is often associated with a much elevated pulmonary arterial blood pressure, the load falls almost wholly on the right ventricle. In aortic valvular disease, either stenosis or incompetence, the left ventricle is mainly affected, though the right ventricle may share in the hypertrophy to a lesser extent.

When the heart undergoes *hypertrophy*, there is usually no increase in the number of its cells, the change being due solely to enlargement of the individual fibres (but see page 174). Rarely, mitosis is seen in cardiac muscle cells, but only in young people and after some local injury to the myocardium. With *atrophy*, on the other hand, there is a shrinkage in size and possibly sometimes a loss in number of the muscle fibres, although in neither respect is the reduction likely to be very pronounced: whereas in hypertrophy the heart weight may double or even treble, in atrophy it seldom declines by more than a quarter or a third.

In the absence of cardiovascular disease the weight of the heart tends to fall with increasing age and lessened bodily activity. This fall may become more pronounced if the effects of wasting diseases such as cancer are added to the normal changes of ageing. In such atrophic hearts, the individual fibres shrink and the lipofuscin pigment granules, which always increase in amount with age, become so concentrated in the muscle cells that they give the organ a distinctive brown colour. In this condition, known as *brown atrophy of the heart*, the golden-brown pigment can be seen microscopically, lying mainly as small granular caps at the two poles of the nucleus of each muscle cell. The pigment is best seen when the sections are stained with haematoxylin alone.

Primary Amyloidosis

Little is yet known of the circumstances under which primary amyloidosis develops: this contrasts with the well-known association of the secondary form with chronic suppurative lesions in the lungs or bones.[211] The two forms differ not only in their pathogenesis but also in the distribution of the abnormal material in the various organs. In the less common primary amyloidosis the deposits tend to occur more in muscular structures, and notably often in the myocardium. In its milder grades, some degree of amyloidosis is not uncommon in the hearts of elderly people, perhaps especially those dying from neoplastic disease.[212] But occasionally the degree of infiltration may be severer and brings about progressive deterioration in the contractile power of the heart, which may terminate in congestive cardiac failure.[213] Although sometimes suspected from electrocardiograms, the involvement of the heart is usually first recognized at necropsy, by which time the infiltration has generally led to a substantial increase in the weight of the organ through the uniform thickening of the walls of all its chambers.[214] As in advanced cases of secondary amyloidosis, the deposits confer a distinctive waxy translucency and firmness on the organ. The latter feature is particularly notable in the atria, which may be so rigid that they fail to collapse when emptied of blood. On histological examination, the infiltration, which often appears to originate near reticulin fibres, is mostly found lying patchily between groups of muscle cells (Fig. 1.36); sometimes it forms a ring enclosing such fibres and leads to their atrophy, and sometimes

it lies mainly in and around the walls of small vessels. In the more advanced cases the amyloid deposit may also be found in the endocardial and epicardial connective tissues; occasionally, it extends into the valve rings, but it seldom involves the substance of the cusps.

Amyloidosis of the Heart in Old Age.—Deposits of amyloid are a familiar histological finding in the heart in elderly people. They form in the myocardial fibres themselves, in the interstitial tissue of the myocardium or in the wall of myocardial arterioles, or in any combination of these tissues. The cardiac involvement, while usually predominant, is commonly accompanied by deposition of

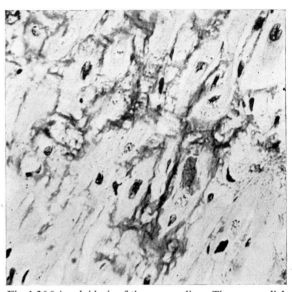

Fig. 1.36.§ Amyloidosis of the myocardium. The myocardial fibres are outlined by irregular deposits of amyloid, and amyloid is also seen forming transverse bars across some of the fibres. From a case of primary amyloidosis. *Congo red and Mayer's haemalum.* × 375.

amyloid in the wall of blood vessels, often including veins, in other parts of the body. The condition, which appears to be a particular form of primary amyloidosis associated with ageing, is usually of only microscopically recognizable extent; in exceptional cases it is so severe that the heart is considerably enlarged, and progressive heart failure is then likely to be the cause of death.

The frequency of this manifestation of amyloidosis has been variously reported as 2·5 to 90 per cent. In the tenth decade about 65 per cent of men and about 47 per cent of women have been found to have cardiac amyloidosis.[215]

Glycogen Storage Diseases[216]

It is mainly as a result of the work of Gerty T. Cori[217] that at least six distinct defects of glycogen metabolism are now known to have been erroneously regarded as a single entity under the name of 'glycogen storage disease' (von Gierke's disease). Each of these defects appears to result from deficiency of a different enzyme. The topic is pertinent to this chapter because hitherto it has usually been stated that 'von Gierke's disease' occurs in two forms, characterized by the accumulation of large amounts of glycogen respectively in the liver and kidneys and in the heart. In fact, the heart is never affected in the disease described by von Gierke,[218] which is now known to be an inborn error of metabolism characterized by failure of the liver and kidneys to synthetize glucose-6-phosphatase. This—the original von Gierke's disease, and the only condition that may properly be referred to by this eponym—is now also known as glucose-6-phosphatase deficiency hepatorenal glycogenosis and as *glycogen storage disease Cori type I*. It is inherited as a completely recessive trait involving a single autosomal gene.

Glycogen Storage Disease Cori Type II (Pompe's Disease)[219]

It is only in three of the less frequent glycogen storage diseases that the heart is affected. The least rare of these is glycogen storage disease Cori type II (Pompe's disease,[220] idiopathic generalized glycogenosis), in which glycogen accumulates in excess in all tissues that normally contain this carbohydrate —particularly myocardium (Fig. 1.37), tongue and other muscles, liver, kidneys and the central nervous system (see Chapter 34). In some cases cardiac involvement predominates clinically, and in others the involvement of the nervous system is more conspicuous. Death usually occurs within a year or two of birth. The disease is hereditary and appears to be transmitted through a single recessive autosomal gene. The nature of the defect underlying the metabolic disturbance has not yet been recognized.

Histology.—Microscopical examination shows the cytoplasm of the affected cells to be greatly distended with glycogen (Fig. 1.37). This carbohydrate can be demonstrated readily by staining sections of appropriately fixed tissue with Best's carmine. The periodic-acid/Schiff method may also be used, and the Schiff-positive material can be shown to be glycogen by its disappearance from sections that have been incubated with diastase.

Other Glycogen Storage Diseases with Cardiac Involvement

Myocardial involvement also occurs in two other glycogen storage diseases. These are Cori type III (Forbes's disease),[221] an inborn error of metabolism characterized by deficiency of amylo-1,6-glucosidase activity in the liver and in heart and skeletal muscle, and the even rarer Cori type IV (Andersen's disease[222, 223]), in which the defect is more generalized, with correspondingly more widespread accumulation of glycogen within the cells.

Involvement of the heart has not been recorded in glycogen storage disease Cori type V (McArdle's disease[224]), which affects skeletal muscle, and Cori type VI (Hers's disease[225]), which affects the liver and the leucocytes.

Beri-Beri (Thiamin Deficiency)

In many oriental countries in which highly milled rice deprived of germ and pericarp has provided the staple diet, beri-beri has long been a scourge of the poor. The disease may appear in various forms: in one—the 'dry' form—the syndrome is mainly neurological, while in others it is of a predominantly cardiovascular character, such cases being either acute or chronic in their course. The acute form of cardiovascular beri-beri is often rapidly fatal and is comparatively rare. The slowly progressive chronic cardiovascular form—'wet' beri-beri—is characterized by oedema, which develops chiefly as a result of cardiac failure

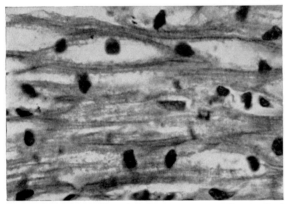

Fig. 1.37.§ Myocardium in glycogen storage disease Cori type II (Pompe's disease). The muscle fibres of the heart are distended by the accumulation of an excess of glycogen in their cytoplasm. In the fresh specimen the clear spaces were filled with the carbohydrate. *Haematoxylin–eosin.* × 400.

though the low concentrations of plasma proteins often found in such patients may further promote its formation. Although the very restricted diets on which these patients subsist is deficient in many essential ingredients, especially animal proteins, it is lack of thiamin (vitamin B$_1$; aneurin) that is responsible for the main features of all types of beri-beri. In occidental countries, deficiency of this vitamin is rare, and is usually met with among chronic alcoholics, in whom both neurological and cardiovascular disorders may coexist.[226]

There now seems no doubt that the cardiac failure of 'wet' beri-beri results from the effect of the deficiency both on the heart and on the peripheral vasculature. In fatal cases, the heart is often enlarged through both dilatation and hypertrophy, though on histological examination there is very little or no evidence of structural change.[227] From dietetic studies on animals, it is known that the carbohydrate metabolism of the myocardium is adversely affected in thiamin deficiency, a biochemical lesion developing in which the effectiveness of the enzyme system concerned in the oxidation of lactic and pyruvic acids is impaired.[228] The lack of the vitamin also leads to dilatation of arterioles, and the resulting diminution in peripheral resistance in the circulation causes the resting cardiac output to become much raised.[229] This increase in its work throws a heavy and continuous strain on the heart, and beri-beri provides one of the best examples of high-output cardiac failure. A dramatic consequence of thiamin therapy in this disease is the rapid reduction in the circulation rate to within normal limits.[230]

Diphtheria

When diphtheria was common in Britain, a large proportion of the deaths from the disease resulted from acute cardiovascular failure. The hearts from patients who had survived for more than a few days generally showed morphological evidence of widespread intoxication of the myocardium.[231, 232]

The powerful exotoxin produced by all three types of *Corynebacterium diphtheriae* appears to act primarily on the cardiac muscle fibres, many of which show parenchymatous or fatty degeneration. These areas of parenchymatous injury are patchy and usually microscopical in size; they soon become surrounded and infiltrated by leucocytes, among which macrophages are numerous and eosinophils not uncommon. Should the patients survive for more than a week, signs of fibroblastic repair appear in these foci, and in those who recover the

place of the lost muscle cells is eventually taken by a microscopical scar. However, from long-term follow-up studies of survivors—whose hearts had presumably been less damaged by the toxin—there is little evidence that these myocardial lesions are succeeded by any serious cardiac disability.[233]

Viral Diseases

In recent years, instances have been recorded in which injuries to the heart muscle have developed in the course of some of the commoner viral infections. These cardiac complication are often indicated by electrocardiographic abnormalities. If the patient dies while the infection is active, many minute inflammatory foci may be found in the myocardium. Of the viral diseases that are prevalent in Britain, poliomyelitis is probably the most important in this respect, though there is evidence that comparable lesions may sometimes develop in measles and mumps.

It is now known that a viraemia occurs in the preparalytic stage of *poliomyelitis*, and it seems likely that the infection of the myocardium takes place during this comparatively brief period. The pathogenesis of the typical lesion can be inferred from comparative studies of hearts from early and late cases. It appears probable that the lesion begins with localized degeneration and necrosis of a few muscle fibres.[234] An inflammatory reaction develops in their immediate neighbourhood, and neutrophile leucocytes, followed quickly by a much larger number of lymphocytes and macrophages, collect round the autolysing cells.[235] Should the patient recover, these lesions presumably disappear after the dead cells have undergone digestion, or they may be replaced by minute scars as a consequence of local fibroblastic hyperplasia. Neither sequel seems to be of functional importance, for there is no evidence that any permanent cardiac disability remains.[236]

Several *epidemics of myocarditis* in very young infants—some with a high case fatality rate and often associated with meningoencephalitis—have been recorded in recent years; one in Munich, during the second world war, caused over 50 deaths.[237] Similar outbreaks—though on a smaller scale—have been described in Holland and in South Africa, and in some of the fatal cases Coxsackie B virus—a recognized cause of epidemic myalgia and pericarditis in older children and adults—has been recovered (Fig. 1.38.)[238, 239] Since myocarditis can be induced experimentally in mice, rabbits and monkeys by the inoculation of certain viruses, it is possible that the application of modern techniques for the isolation of such pathogens might throw light on some of the still obscure forms of myocarditis in man.

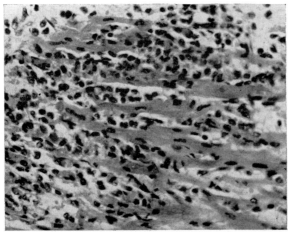

Fig. 1.38.§ Acute myocarditis due to Coxsackie B3 virus (case of: Butler, N., Skelton, M. O., Hodges, G. M., MacCallum, F. O., *Brit. med. J.*, 1962, **1**, 1251). The patient was a baby, nine days old, who collapsed suddenly and died eight hours later. Both parents had very recently had a transient, feverish illness that might have been caused by the same virus. There is infiltration of the myocardium by lymphocytes and macrophages, with occasional neutrophils. *Haematoxylin–eosin.* × 300.

Toxoplasmosis[240]

Both in infants and in adults, infection with *Toxoplasma gondii*, an organism with a world-wide distribution in domestic and wild animals, can cause distinctive areas of myocarditis with local infiltration by lymphocytes, macrophages, plasma cells and eosinophils. The parasites, often in large numbers, may be seen inside the cardiac muscle fibres, but their presence seems hardly to incommode the affected cell (Fig. 1.39). Although intracellular parasitization may be conspicuous in histological sections, it seldom leads to clinical signs or symptoms, though cases with death following cardiac failure are occasionally recorded.[241, 242]

Trypanosomiasis (Chagas's Disease)

Trypanosomiasis is endemic in large areas of Africa and of Central and South America. African trypanosomiasis affects the central nervous system predominantly (see Chapter 34). In the Americas, where the species of trypanosome is *Trypanosoma*

cruzi, the infection is known as Chagas's disease and is generally transmitted to man by blood-sucking bugs of the genus *Triatoma*, in the intestine of which it multiplies; the reservoir of infection is among wild animals, mainly armadillos, opossums and bats. Man tends to become infected when the wild animals of an area are reduced in number, as by forest clearing, and the bugs are obliged to go in search of a new host. Infection takes place when the insect bites: the puncture in the skin is contaminated by its faeces, which it excretes as it starts to suck the victim's blood. The bugs are often especially numerous in the crevices of the walls of the mud huts in which the rural population lives.

In infants, Chagas's disease usually runs a fatal course, the symptoms being those of acute meningo-encephalitis. In those children who survive, and in people infected later in life, who may have acquired some immunity, the disease becomes chronic, and its effects then fall notably on the central nervous system and the heart. In the heart the trypanosomes invade the muscle fibres, multiplying freely in their cytoplasm, where they may be demonstrable, although it is often difficult to find them (Fig. 1.40). Disruption of infected fibres releases the organisms, which can then colonize adjacent fibres. The resulting areas of necrosis of the myocardium evoke

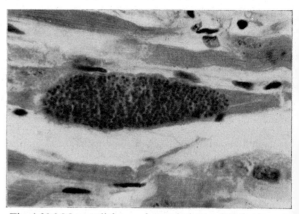

Fig. 1.39.§ Myocardial toxoplasmosis (case of: Scheidegger, S., *Schweiz. Z. allg. Path.*, 1957, **20**, 697). The patient was a man, aged 72 years. The granular-looking structure in the distended muscle fibre is a 'pseudocyst' of *Toxoplasma gondii*: the pseudocyst, which has no distinct wall, is a large collection of toxoplasmas—when it bursts, the individual parasites are liberated into the surrounding tissue. The absence of apparent reaction to the infection in this field is striking, but elsewhere there was a conspicuous accumulation of lymphocytes and neutrophils, particularly in parts of the myocardium in which pseudocysts had recently ruptured. *Haematoxylin–eosin.* × 650.

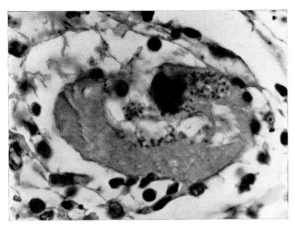

Fig. 1.40.§ Myocarditis of South American trypanosomiasis (Chagas's disease). Cross-section of a heart muscle fibre parasitized by *Trypanosoma cruzi*. The patient was a Brazilian visitor to London who died of acute congestive heart failure. [Unpublished case (W. St C. Symmers, 1963).] *Haematoxylin–eosin.* × 750.

a local accumulation of macrophages and lymphocytes, and later fibrosis occurs. There is often particularly heavy involvement of the myocardium of the apical region of the left ventricle (Fig. 1.41), which becomes thin and may undergo aneurysmal dilatation.[243] Eventually, heart failure develops, and in certain cases its onset and progress are rapid. A notable feature of chronic myocardial trypanosomiasis is destruction of the nerve cells in the cardiac ganglia.[244] The infection may cause a nodular subepicardial lymphangitis (Fig. 1.42).

Sarcoidosis[245, 246]

The heart is affected directly or indirectly in about one-fifth of all cases of generalized sarcoidosis. In most of these cor pulmonale develops, as a consequence of extensive involvement of the lungs. In a minority, however, the heart muscle itself contains sarcoid granulomas. While sarcoidotic changes may develop in any part of the myocardium, the conducting system seems to be particularly vulnerable: abnormalities of cardiac rhythm are frequent features of these cases.

Acute Idiopathic Myocarditis

It has been recommended that the term idiopathic or primary myocarditis designate examples of acute inflammation involving the myocardium as an isolated phenomenon in the absence of an identifiable cause.[247] It is better to avoid the use of

eponyms such as *Fiedler's myocarditis* as there is probably a group of conditions to be considered rather than a single nosological entity. As knowledge advances, an increasing proportion of these cases is likely to be ascribed to specific causative agents.

These forms of myocarditis, which usually are not accompanied by either pericarditis or endocarditis, may develop acutely in patients of any age, though they are most frequent in early adult life. The clinical condition of the patients deteriorates rapidly, the heart becomes increasingly dilated, and death occurs, often suddenly, from cardiac failure.

On microscopical examination, the myocardium may present one of two typical appearances. In the first, and commoner, form, there is a diffuse inflammatory reaction in the interstitial tissues accompanied by a pleomorphic infiltrate of leucocytes among which eosinophils may figure prominently (Fig. 1.43). In the other, or granulomatous, form, larger and more discrete foci develop, each containing many lymphocytes and macrophages, and sometimes multinucleate giant cells (Figs 1.44 and 1.45). In both forms, the muscle fibres may show evidence of injury, and their degeneration and

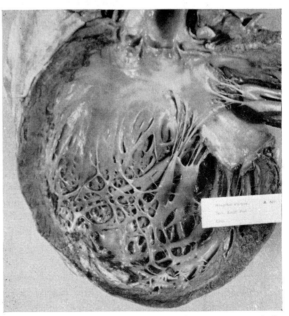

Fig. 1.41.§ Myocarditis of South American trypanosomiasis (Chagas's disease). There is a very striking dilatation of the left ventricle, with marked thinning of the myocardium, particularly toward the apex—these findings are characteristic of this form of myocarditis. See also Figs 1.40 and 1.42.

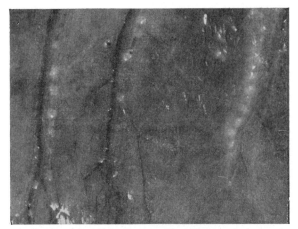

Fig. 1.42.§ Granulomatous subepicardial lymphangitis in South American trypanosomiasis (Chagas's disease). The smooth, glistening, quite sharply demarcated nodules are characteristic. See also Figs 1.40 and 1.41.

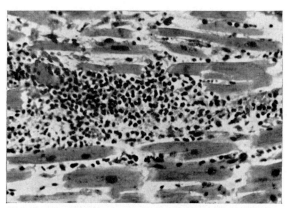

Fig. 1.43.§ Acute interstitial myocarditis. The interstitial tissue of the myocardium is infiltrated by lymphocytes, neutrophils and eosinophils. The patient was a middle-aged man who was found dead in his seat at the end of a cinema show. There was no macroscopical abnormality to account for his death. Epidemics of poliomyelitis and influenza were current, but no evidence of either disease was found on post-mortem examination (virological studies were not made). [Unpublished case (W. St C. Symmers, 1962).] *Haematoxylin–eosin.* × 250.

necrosis are probably responsible for the rapidly progressive cardiac failure.

In spite of careful search, no infective agent has yet been identified in the heart in these cases. Various suggestions have been made as to the pathogenesis but none has received acceptance. In recent years, more has become known of the development of myocarditis in viral diseases, and it is not unthinkable that some of the conditions now included in the category of acute idiopathic

myocarditis may in time acquire a place among the effects of viruses (see page 45).

Myocardial Disorders in Friedreich's Ataxia and in Progressive Muscular Dystrophy

In Friedreich's ataxia (hereditary spinal and cerebellar ataxia), a heredodegenerative disease of young adults, the heart is often hypertrophied, and its ventricles show a progressive, interstitial myocarditis that may culminate in cardiac failure.[248] Muscle fibres throughout the heart undergo degeneration and necrosis, with gradual replacement by collagenous fibrous tissue. Many lymphocytes can be seen between the disintegrating muscle fibres. Nothing is known of the pathogenesis of the cardiac lesions, though the participation of some toxic agent has been suggested.[249]

In a large proportion of cases of progressive muscular dystrophy the myocardium becomes involved. Resulting heart failure may be the cause of death. At necropsy, the heart muscle is frequently seen to be streaked with grey flecks. Histologically, fibrosis of the ventricular walls ranges from a mild, diffuse sclerosis to marked scarring; much of this reaction seems to follow the piecemeal degeneration and death of the muscle fibres.[250] The pericardium and endocardium are unaffected, and there is no coronary arterial disease that might cause myocardial ischaemia.

Disorders of the Conducting System

The Sinuatrial Node of Keith and Flack

This node, which normally discharges about seventy times a minute, lies in the sulcus terminalis on the anterolateral aspect of the vena cava close to its entry into the right atrium. It is a crescentic, neuromyocardial structure—a plexus of distinctive, fusiform muscle cells—embedded in an envelope of fibroelastic tissue through which pass the numerous fibres of the right vagus nerve and the sympathetic nerves which control its rhythm. Although this nodal tissue is not very close to those parts of the myocardium that are most frequently injured organically, it occasionally becomes involved in chronic rheumatic heart disease, in myocardial ischaemia (especially when the right coronary artery is markedly atherosclerotic) or in cardiac metastases of malignant tumours.[251] Under these circumstances, the normal rhythm of the heart is disturbed, and other foci of excitable tissue may take over the initiation of cardiac systole.

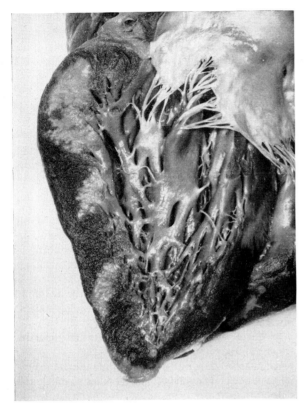

Fig. 1.44.§ Giant cell (tuberculoid) myocarditis. The pale tissue in the wall of the left ventricle showed the microscopical features of a non-caseating, fibrosing, tuberculoid granuloma. The patient was a middle-aged man who died suddenly, without premonitory symptoms of illness. Apart from sparse and minute tuberculoid foci in the lungs and spleen there were no other abnormal findings. [Unpublished case (G. A. C. Summers, Bristol and York, 1956).]

The Atrioventricular Node of Tawara

This structure lies in the lower part of the atrial septum, close to the orifice of the coronary sinus and the fibrous ring of the tricuspid valve. From its lower aspect the bundle of His passes downwards into the interventricular septum to divide and radiate over the inner aspect of both ventricles. Like the sinuatrial node, the muscle fibres of the atrioventricular node are paler than the surrounding myocardial fibres and also possess fewer myofibrils in their cytoplasm. Fibres from the left vagus nerve and sympathetic nerves enter the nodal area and modify its rhythm. Normally, this node has a slower rate of spontaneous discharge than the sinuatrial node, and consequently it follows the faster rhythm of the latter; after a brief interval— the P-R interval—it relays the wave of systole to both ventricles through the bundle of His.

The atrioventricular node is the more vulnerable of the two nodes, and, with its emergent bundle, is not infrequently injured in various organic disorders of the myocardium, notably in rheumatic disease of the heart,[252] by chronic lesions involving the bases of the aortic and mitral valves,[253] by ischaemia of the nearby myocardium[254] and by sarcoidosis of the heart.[255] The result is a form of arrhythmia known as heart-block (Stokes-Adams syndrome), in which a period of ventricular asystole results in a brief state of unconsciousness due to transient cerebral ischaemia.

The pathology of heart-block has received increasing attention since the introduction of electronic methods for artificial 'pacing' of the heart. These have enabled patients with heart-block to survive for indefinite periods. A recent study has clarified the pathological basis of the lesions in most of these patients.[256] Transient heart-block is nearly always associated with myocardial infarction and, if the patient survives, normal rhythm will soon be restored in the majority of cases. Chronic (or permanent) heart-block, on the other hand, has a wide variety of causes. Of 100 such cases coming to necropsy, 46 were found to be associated with unexplained (non-ischaemic) fibrosis of the bundle of His, 15 resulted from ischaemic destruction of the bundle or of the atrioventricular node, and 13 were associated with cardiomyopathy. The remaining 26 cases included a variety of associations, among them calcific valve disease (8), myocarditis (4), connective tissue diseases (3), amyloidosis (3), gumma (3), congenital lesions (3) and siderosis (2).

The Cardiomyopathies

The term cardiomyopathy was introduced in 1957 to cover unusual or unexplained diseases involving

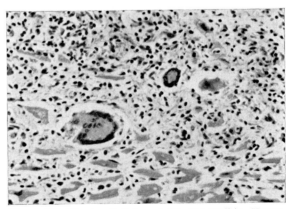

Fig. 1.45.§ Giant cell (tuberculoid) myocarditis. *Haematoxylin–eosin.* × 125.

the myocardium.[257] Unfortunately the word has come to be used in different ways by different authorities and a good deal of confusion has arisen: for instance, nothing is gained from such expressions as 'amyloid cardiomyopathy' or 'ischaemic cardiomyopathy'. It is proposed to restrict the use of the word here to a number of conditions in which disturbed heart muscle function is associated with pathological changes that are poorly understood or of uncertain nature.

Classification

Many attempts have been made at a logical classification of the cardiomyopathies, and some of the results are very intricate and comprehensive (for example, that of Hudson[258]). There are obvious advantages in a classification that takes into account the classic features as they present to the cardiologist: for that reason a modification of Goodwin's[259] system is used here. In this classification the main subdivision is into:

(a) *Congestive cardiomyopathy*, presenting with left ventricular failure and chronic venous congestion of unknown cause. The cases in this group may be further subdivided into idiopathic, familial and tropical forms and they include examples associated with skeletal myopathies, Friedreich's ataxia and acromegaly as well as those related to a high intake of alcohol and those developing in the puerperium.

(b) *Hypertrophic obstructive cardiomyopathy*, characterized by obstruction to the outflow tract of the left ventricle and presenting with features suggestive of aortic stenosis.

(c) *Obliterative cardiomyopathy*, presenting usually with reduction in volume of the ventricles and ventriculoatrial regurgitation. The classic type under this heading is the mainly tropical condition, endomyocardial fibrosis.

Congestive Cardiomyopathy

Patients with this form of cardiomyopathy usually show left ventricular failure that progresses fairly rapidly to right ventricular failure and chronic venous congestion. The average duration from onset to death is around three and a half years. Causative factors are usually not in evidence but in Goodwin's 74 cases alcohol may have been a factor in 17, seven presented in the puerperium and 13 were preceded by respiratory infections.[259] Idiopathic cases are reported most frequently from tropical and subtropical lands, notably Nigeria, South Africa, India, Brazil and Jamaica, but in recent years cases have been recognized in increasing numbers in temperate areas, including Britain, North America and Japan. There is a familial incidence in about one quarter of the cases:[260] the mode of inheritance is variable and may be that of an associated skeletal myopathy or Friedreich's ataxia.

Functional studies show that the greatly enlarged left ventricle changes size only slightly between systole and diastole. This implies a high residual volume and low ejection fraction.

Necropsy Findings.—Typically, the heart is enlarged and increased in weight, though in cases that follow a rapid course the weight may be little raised. The shape of the heart is characteristically globular and all four chambers are enlarged. Muscle hypertrophy, as judged by ventricular wall thickness, is masked by dilatation, and indeed the dilated chambers may appear abnormally thin-walled: however, assessment of muscle mass will usually disclose at least a moderate increase. In the later stages of the disease dilatation of the mitral and tricuspid valve rings leads to incompetence of these valves. The endocardium is thickened and pale and in many cases mural thrombi are found in the ventricles and atria. The coronary arteries are usually free from any significant degree of atherosclerosis: indeed, Davies[261] stated that he had never been able to establish the coexistence of coronary artery disease and idiopathic cardiomyopathy.

In addition to the changes in the heart the systemic features of congestive cardiac failure are present. There may also be evidence of pulmonary and systemic embolism.

Histology.—The microscopical features of the heart vary considerably from case to case but comprise a mixture of muscle fibre degeneration, irregular hypertrophy of surviving fibres and interstitial fibrosis (Fig. 1.46). Degenerate fibres appear swollen and vacuolated and their nuclei are enlarged, irregular and hyperchromatic. Ultimately, empty sarcolemmal sheaths are found surrounded by cell debris, macrophages, lymphocytes and often a few Anitschkow myocytes. Surviving fibres undergo irregular hypertrophy so that a stage is reached when slender degenerating fibres and plump hypertrophied fibres are randomly intermingled. Irregular overgrowth of interstitial fibrous tissue completes the picture of a severely disturbed myocardium. The endocardium is usually thickened

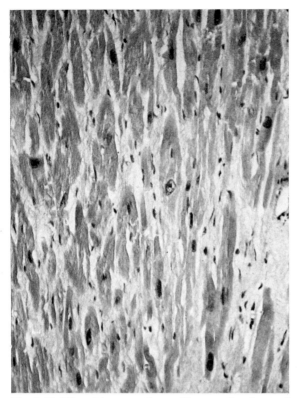

Fig. 1.46. Idiopathic congestive cardiomyopathy. Some of the muscle fibres are atrophic and others are irregularly enlarged. Aberrant hyperchromatic nuclei are conspicuous and there is diffuse interstitial fibrosis. *Haematoxylin–eosin.* × 140.

Men and women are about equally often affected and in about 30 per cent of cases there is a familial history. In the familial cases death tends to occur at an earlier age than in non-familial cases. The first cases to be recognized[262] presented as sudden deaths: today, the disease is usually diagnosed clinically, by recognition of what are now known to be the characteristic features of the disease. Angiography shows narrowing of the left ventricular cavity, thickening of the ventricular wall and a normal end-diastolic volume. Outflow obstruction is usually, but not always, present.

Necropsy Findings.—The heart is enlarged and increased in weight. These changes, except when death has been preceded by a period of cardiac failure, are accounted for almost entirely by the increased bulk of the left ventricular muscle. The cavity of the left ventricle is normal or reduced in size, and certainly it appears minute in relation to the strikingly increased thickness of the wall (Fig. 1.47). This hypertrophy is characteristically asymmetrical and usually affects the septum more than the external walls of the ventricle. The thickened septum may swell markedly into the cavity of the ventricle, accounting for the earlier designation of rhabdomyoma: it is also easy to see how the outflow obstruction ('subaortic stenosis') is produced. Over the swollen septum the endocardium is often white and thickened where it comes in contact with the anterior cusp of the mitral valve in systole. Less frequently the hypertrophy is most developed in

by a layer of subendothelial fibrous tissue varying in thickness from place to place, while here and there mural thrombus may be found in varying stages of organization. Haemosiderin deposits are sometimes conspicuous.

Hypertrophic Obstructive Cardiomyopathy

This condition masquerades in medical literature under a remarkable profusion of synonyms. Many old specimens in museums are labelled as rhabdomyomas of the heart. Names that have been used since the condition was more clearly recognized include asymmetrical hypertrophy of the heart[262] and hypertrophic subaortic stenosis[263] and occasionally the eponym, Teare's disease. The term hypertrophic obstructive cardiomyopathy was introduced in 1964[264] and is now generally preferred in the United Kingdom (see also page 80).[265]

The disease may present at any age but most frequently between the ages of 25 and 50 years.

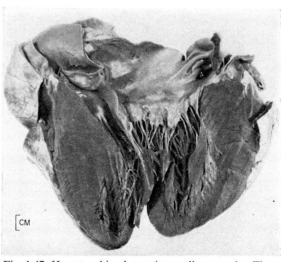

Fig. 1.47. Hypertrophic obstructive cardiomyopathy. There is marked asymmetrical hypertrophy of the upper part of the interventricular septum.

the anterior or posterior wall of the ventricle; sometimes it is symmetrical—these are the cases likeliest to be overlooked unless careful histological studies are undertaken. No distinctive changes are found in the valves or in the coronary arteries.

Histology.—The histological features (Figs 1.48 and 1.49) include: irregular hypertrophy of muscle fibres, some of which are very broad but apparently short; interruption of muscle bundles by bands of fibrous tissue; overgrowth of interstitial fibrous tissue; degenerative changes in individual fibres; bizarre, large and hyperchromatic nuclei; and a disorderly arrangement of the muscle fibres with irregular whorl formation. These abnormalities are not confined to the area of greatest thickening of the myocardium; moreover, the affected parts may be separated by more normal areas.

None of these changes can be regarded as specific or diagnostic of the disease, though the whorling of the muscle fibres perhaps comes close

to being so. The fibre degeneration takes the form of juxtanuclear vacuolation that progresses to cytoplasmic disruption, with the result that empty sarcolemmal sheaths may be seen, usually in areas where fibrosis is developing. Histochemical[266] and ultrastructural[267] studies likewise show non-specific changes that do not serve to distinguish the condition from other causes of muscle fibre hypertrophy and degeneration. It will be appreciated that experience of typical material is needed before a pathologist may be sure of himself in making this diagnosis in doubtful cases.

Obliterative Cardiomyopathy

This subdivision of the cardiomyopathies comprises the single fairly well defined entity of *endomyocardial fibrosis*. This condition was first observed by Bedford and Konstam[268] among African troops serving in the Middle East during the second world war, but detailed studies of its pathology were not published until 1954[269] and subsequently when

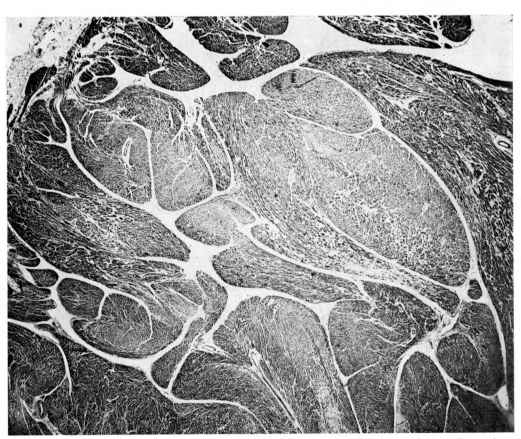

Fig. 1.48.§ Hypertrophic obstructive cardiomyopathy. The muscle bundles show irregular whorling and are separated by fibrous septa. See also Fig. 1.49. *Haematoxylin–eosin.* × 7.

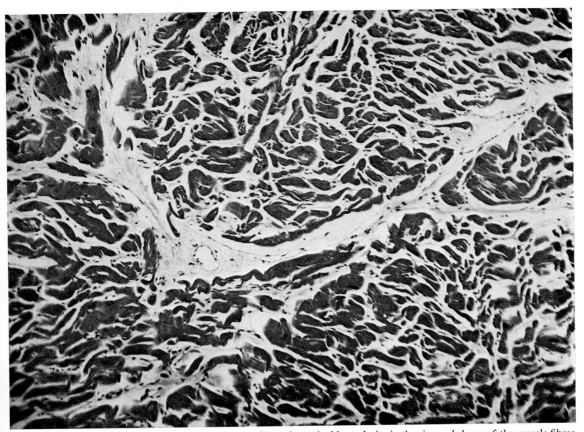

Fig. 1.49.§ Hypertrophic obstructive cardiomyopathy. There is marked irregularity in the size and shape of the muscle fibres. There is also some excess of interstitial fibrous tissue. *Haematoxylin–eosin.* × 80.

Davies and his colleagues, working in Uganda, described the findings in a large series of cases.[270, 271]

The geographical distribution of endomyocardial fibrosis is striking. The main areas with a high endemic rate are Uganda and western Nigeria, but cases occur in most other parts of Africa and in Sri Lanka, southern India, Malaysia and parts of tropical South America. Europeans long resident in endemic areas may develop the disease: a review in 1967 recorded its occurrence in 23 Europeans whose symptoms appeared while they were living in Britain after residence in Africa.[272]

Endomyocardial fibrosis is unlikely to be diagnosed until a late stage of the disease, though, in endemic areas, it is frequently found at necropsy in cases of death from other causes. Sometimes the clinical manifestations[273] are ushered in by a febrile illness, but usually the history is of gradually developing symptoms and signs of cardiac failure, and often ascites is prominent by the time the patient is first seen. Confirmation of the diagnosis requires selective angiocardiography which demonstrates the characteristic deformity of one or both ventricles.

Necropsy Findings.—The findings vary markedly from case to case: most characteristically the ventricles are reduced in size while the atria are hypertrophied and dilated. The heart weight is often around the normal figure but may be as much as 600 grams. The overall size of the heart may be further increased by the presence of a pericardial effusion.

The ventricles may be involved singly or together, the right being affected alone in some 10 per cent of cases, the left alone in 40 per cent and the two together in half the cases.[274] The essential lesion is an overgrowth of dense white fibrous tissue that thickens the endocardium and spreads for a varying distance into the adjacent myocardium (Fig. 1.50). The inflow tract of either or both ventricles is

C

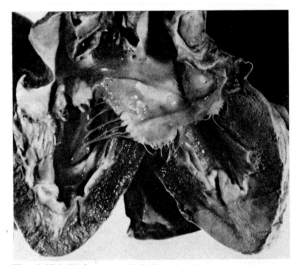

Fig. 1.50.§ Endomyocardial fibrosis. The left ventricle is lined by thickened, glistening, white endocardium. The papillary muscles are partly embedded in this fibrous tissue, which also involves some of the chordae tendineae, with consequent distortion of the mitral valve cusps. As is usual, however, the greater part of the cusps appears normal.

Histology.—Microscopical examination of the affected parts of the heart confirms that the endocardium is thickened by dense, relatively avascular collagenous fibrous tissue which also spreads out among the muscle fibres of the inner third of the myocardium. Here and there flattened mural thrombi will be seen in varying states of organization. A few elastic fibres may be seen amongst the collagen strands but they are not conspicuous. The subjacent muscle fibres show degenerative changes of non-specific character; there may be foci in which empty and disintegrating sarcolemmal sheaths are seen (myocytolysis—Fig. 1.51).

Aetiology.—The cause of endomyocardial fibrosis remains obscure though numerous factors have been regarded as contributing to its development. The geographical distribution has already been mentioned. The disease is seen predominantly in the lower socio-economic groups of the population, and malnutrition has been postulated as a factor. However, the disease is certainly not limited to the

mainly involved. Often the fibrosis is grossest at the apex of the ventricle and extends upward on the posterior wall behind the posterior cusp of the mitral or tricuspid valve. The papillary muscles and chordae tendineae are involved and become retracted and thickened so that gradually the valves become severely incompetent, though the cusps themselves escape. In the left ventricle the fibrous thickening of the endocardium usually extends only a short way up the interventricular septum, ending in a thickened, sharply defined edge.

In spite of the incompetence of the atrioventricular valves, the ventricles are prevented from dilating by the rigidity conferred upon them by the overgrowth of fibrous tissue—indeed, considerable reduction of the size of the ventricular cavities is usual. The atria, on the other hand, are under no such restriction and their expected hypertrophy and dilatation often attain an impressive degree and may predispose to the development of mural thrombi or even large ball thrombi occupying much of the cavity. Mural thrombi are often found too on the affected parts of the ventricular endocardium, and embolic incidents are a feature of the late stages of the disease in about 15 per cent of cases. Bacterial endocarditis is an unusual complication but is said to be present at necropsy in about 2 per cent of cases.[274]

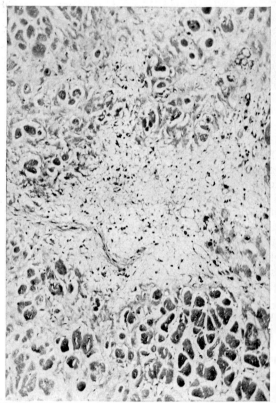

Fig. 1.51.§ Endomyocardial fibrosis, illustrating myocytolysis —the central area shows well the characteristic 'falling out' necrosis, only the sarcolemmal sheaths remaining recognizable. *Haematoxylin–eosin.* × 180.

undernourished, and no specific deficiency can be substantiated. Excessive consumption of bananas, which may contain serotonin and give rise to urinary excretion of large amounts of 5-hydroxy-indoleacetic acid,[275] has been suggested as a possible causative factor, for there is some superficial resemblance between the lesions of endomyocardial fibrosis and the cardiac manifestations of the argentaffinoma (carcinoid) syndrome (see Chapter 16): however, consumption of bananas has not proved to be a constant feature of the history of patients with the disease. The possibility that endomyocardial fibrosis is a sequel of viral or parasitic disease lacks supporting evidence. An immunological basis for the disease has also been postulated: the scanty evidence is unconvincing.[276]

As regards the pathogenesis of the lesions there is some indication that the fibrosis results at least in part from recurrent deposition of fibrin in the affected areas, with subsequent organization and collagen formation. This observation leaves us still in need of an explanation for such selective fibrin deposition.

MISCELLANEOUS ENDOCARDIAL ABNORMALITIES

Fibroelastosis of the Endocardium

Occasionally, death from cardiac failure in infancy or early childhood is associated with the formation of a diffuse layer of fibrosis, often several millimetres thick, in the mural endocardium, particularly of the left atrium and left ventricle.[277, 278] This thickening imparts a rigidity to the walls of these chambers which usually leads to gross myocardial hypertrophy, the heart developing a typical globular shape. The sclerosis is usually fairly evenly distributed as a smooth, sometimes porcelain white, layer over the interior of the affected chamber (Fig. 1.52). In extreme cases this layer may obscure the normal trabecular structure of the underlying myocardium. Thrombus may sometimes form over portions of these sclerosed areas. In about half the cases of fibroelastosis of the endocardium, the aortic and mitral valves are similarly coarsened by fibrosis, so that to the functional embarrassment created by the thickened endocardium is added the handicap of sclerotic valve cusps.

Histologically, the endocardial plaques are composed of dense deposits of interlacing connective tissue fibres, mostly of the elastic type but with some accompanying collagen, all lying in bundles more or less parallel to the wall of the chamber.[279] The cells from which these fibres have formed

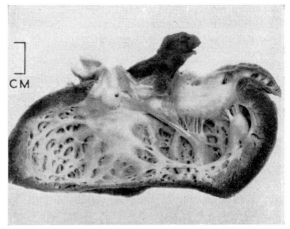

Fig. 1.52.§ Fibroelastosis of the endocardium. The opaque, white appearance of the endocardium of this child's heart is due to the diffuse fibrosis of the subendothelial tissue. The valves were not affected in this case.

appear to be few in number, and lie inconspicuously in their interstices. The entire layer is devoid of blood vessels and presents no sign of past or present inflammation. The myocardial fibres for the most part show little change except for hypertrophy, but some of the muscle fibres lying just under the thickened endocardium may present signs of degeneration such as are commonly seen when there is local ischaemia. This alteration may result from the obliteration of the Thebesian vessels (venae cordis minimae), which some authorities believe may contribute to the supply of oxygen to this layer of the myocardium.

Little is known of the aetiology and pathogenesis of fibroelastosis of the endocardium; there is nothing in the appearance of the affected structures to support the former view that it has an infective origin. It is a congenital condition, and the great majority of affected infants die within their first year. Death may sometimes be accelerated by accompanying congenital abnormalities, the most notable among them being aberrant origins of the coronary arteries and coarctation of the aorta (see also page 110).

Although congenital fibroelastosis in some respects resembles endomyocardial fibrosis, several points of difference clearly distinguish these two conditions.[280, 281] The former is almost confined to young children—in whom it is often associated with other congenital abnormalities—and results in the formation of endocardial plaques that are mainly composed of elastic fibres. The latter, in contrast, develops in adults, and is associated with the loss of much of the normal endocardial elastic tissue and with the formation of masses of collagen typical of fibroblastic organization.

Non-Bacterial Thrombotic Endocardiopathy

In elderly people, especially those dying from chronic tuberculosis or cancer, small vegetations occasionally develop on the lines of closure of the mitral and aortic valves. When seen at necropsy most of these vegetations have an appearance not unlike that of the warty nodules of acute rheumatic endocarditis; occasionally they are larger and less regular, and resemble the vegetations found in Libman–Sacks endocardiopathy (see below) (Fig. 1.53). Histologically, too, these vegetations have certain features in common with rheumatic endocarditis, though in the latter disease the contribution made by the platelet thrombus is greater and that of degenerating collagen and local cellular reaction less.[282] These vegetations seldom evince any clinical sign of their presence; rarely they may be dislodged as emboli. In most instances, they can be regarded as a terminal development.[283]

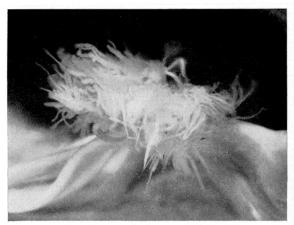

Fig. 1.54.§ Papillary 'tumour' of the endocardium of an aortic valve cusp. These lesions, which are 'giant' forms of Lambl's excrescences, are not neoplastic but organized fibrinous deposits. *Photographed under water; magnified* × 5.

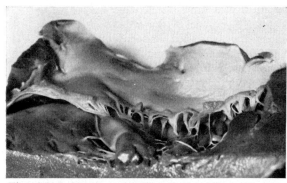

Fig. 1.53.§ Non-bacterial thrombotic endocardiopathy. Characteristic verrucose lesions on the closure line of the mitral valve leaflets.

Lambl's Excrescences

Careful examination of the mitral and aortic valve cusps in hearts from people of all ages has shown that small endocardial deposits of fibrin along the lines of closure are so common, even in early adult life, that they must be regarded as a normal age change.[284] Most of these minute tags become organized from below and covered with endothelium from the sides, so that they contribute to the slow progressive thickening of the cusps as age advances. Occasionally, however, the tag becomes pedunculated, and after organization

it forms one of the small, often tassel-shaped, filamentous appendages on the margin of the valve cusps which are known as 'Lambl's excrescences'. Sometimes these lesions become quite large—up to a centimetre across—and they have been referred to as 'papillary tumours' (Fig. 1.54). As indicated above, they are not neoplasms.

Libman–Sacks Endocardiopathy

Many years ago, Libman and Sacks drew attention to a form of sterile endocardial vegetation to which they gave the name 'atypical verrucous endocarditis', and which they carefully distinguished from rheumatic and bacterial endocarditis.[285] The structures they described usually form near the line of closure of the cusps of the mitral and tricuspid valves and are arranged in a more or less continuous chain of wart-like vegetations, larger than those found in acute rheumatic endocarditis but not otherwise unlike them. The condition differs significantly from rheumatic carditis, however, for no Aschoff nodules are found in the endocardium or myocardium. Less often, the vegetations appear as large, grey, rather smooth and flattened masses which, though typically occupying large areas on the atrial surfaces of the mitral and tricuspid valve cusps, may also occur on the endocardium of the chambers.

It is now realized that the characteristic Libman–Sacks lesions of the heart are one of the manifestations of systemic lupus erythematosus, systemic sclerosis, thrombotic thrombocytopenic purpura and other members of the group of so-called 'collagen diseases'. When studied histologically, the thrombus mass which forms the bulk of the vegetation can be seen to be superimposed on an area of degenerating collagen in the underlying endocardium.

The patients seldom show any clinical disabilities attributable to these cardiac changes. However, subacute infective endocarditis has been observed as a complication.[286]

CHRONIC CARDIAC FAILURE

The various and often progressive handicaps placed on the heart by acquired valvular defects, congenital abnormalities, ischaemic myocardial fibrosis, hypertension, or the metabolic disturbances that accompany certain intoxications and nutritional deficiencies, gradually lessen its ability to respond normally to any added demand on the circulatory system that may be made by increased physical exertion. The slow deterioration in the myocardial reserve, expressed as exercise tolerance, may long remain unnoticed, or may be accepted as an inevitable accompaniment of increasing age. In the case of many cardiac patients, however, the heart deteriorates so much that eventually the myocardium can no longer respond even to the ordinary demands of a sedentary life, and the clinical condition known as heart failure sets in. Often, with appropriate rest and treatment, failure can be arrested for a time, but such relief is usually limited and temporary.

This progressive deterioration, which passes through stages of diminished exercise tolerance to eventual cardiac failure, may take many years, especially if the patient adopts a form of life in which excessive physical activity can be avoided. But, in spite of care, a large proportion of cardiac patients must finally succumb to the effects of the abnormal stresses on the myocardium that for a time have been met successfully by its compensatory hypertrophy.

Myocardial Metabolism in Cardiac Failure

At least three stages can be distinguished in the conversion of the chemical energy of nutrient materials into the mechanical work that the heart performs in propelling the blood.[287, 288] The first stage comprises the succession of intermediate metabolic steps that culminate in the oxidation of carbohydrates, fatty acids and amino acids and the release of their chemical energy. In most cases of cardiac failure, to judge from the consumption of oxygen by the heart, these metabolic steps are little, if at all, affected. It is only in some deficiency diseases, notably thiamin deficiency, or in intoxications, notably thyrotoxicosis, that there is any serious disturbance in this normal oxidative metabolism. The second stage is the development of tension in the muscle fibres—an isometric event which probably depends on the reaction of adenosine triphosphate with the proteins actin and myosin present in these cells. The third stage is the conversion of this tension into the mechanical work of the chambers in expelling blood. In this sequence of stages, about 25 per cent of the chemical energy provided by the oxidation of the nutrient substances is converted into mechanical work by the normal heart.

It seems that in the forms of heart failure that follow from the mechanical stresses imposed by hypertension or severe valvular disease, the muscle fibres are less efficient than in a normal heart in transforming chemical energy into mechanical tension and thus in effecting the contraction of the chambers. The defect may lie in some alteration of the contractile proteins which decreases their ability to convert the energy liberated in metabolism into useful work.[289]

Left-Sided and Right-Sided Cardiac Failure

Since the damage in acquired diseases of the heart is usually at first mainly localized to one portion of the cardiovascular system, its effects generally fall more heavily on one side of the heart than on the other. This unilateral feature of cardiac failure is particularly evident during its incipient stages. For example, in the cardiac sequelae of rheumatic fever, in which the mitral and aortic valves are often seriously diseased, the left side of the heart is mostly affected, so that many of the symptoms and signs in this form of valvular disease arise mainly from congestion in the pulmonary circulation. The left side of the heart is also affected in those forms of failure that follow other types of stenosis or incompetence of the aortic valve, or the continuous stress imposed by prolonged systemic hypertension. Failure of the right side of the heart is less frequent, and occurs mainly as a result of pulmonary hypertension: this may be of the uncommon primary form, about the aetiology of which little is known (see page 283), or of the much commoner secondary form associated either with advanced disease of the lungs or stenosis of the mitral valve.

For some years, the terms 'forward failure' and 'backward failure' have been freely used in cardiological literature. The former emphasizes the adverse effects of a reduction in the output of the heart upon all those organs which are mainly supplied by the systemic arterial system. These effects are, in brief, the tissue changes which can be attributed to long continued partial ischaemia, and which become more apparent under the added stress of physical exercise. The term 'backward failure', on the other hand, lays emphasis on the congestive features that result from the relatively ineffective propulsive action of the heart, and covers in its scope the disturbances in the respiratory system that follow left-sided cardiac failure and the venous engorgement and peripheral oedema that come from failure of the right chambers of the heart. Whether the use of these terms has contributed to a better understanding of the fundamental functional pathology of cardiac failure is a point on which views may differ.

In the remainder of this section, some of the more conspicuous functional disturbances that accompany incipient or established heart failure will be considered in the light of modern knowledge of cardiopulmonary physiology. The technique of cardiac catheterization, and advances in cardiac surgery, by making it possible to obtain samples of blood for gas analysis from the various chambers of the heart and to record by direct measurement the blood pressure changes within them, have in recent years revolutionized our knowledge of this important field of functional pathology. By greatly increasing the range and accuracy of quantitative observations on the circulation, these procedures have enabled much light to be thrown on the pathogenesis of the symptoms and signs of advanced heart disease.

The Cardiac Output in Heart Failure

Since the function of the heart is to maintain a rate of circulation of the blood commensurate with the requirements of the body, it is to be expected that any serious disease of this organ will place increasing limitations on the extent to which this rate can be raised to meet the added metabolic demands of physical exercise. Much of our knowledge of circulation rates and their variations in health and disease has been acquired through the application of the principle originally suggested in 1870 by the Würzburg physicist and physiologist, Adolph Fick, whose methods have been supplemented in recent years by the less direct procedures of dye-dilution techniques and ballistocardiography. What is now termed 'Fick's direct method' depends on determining first, by ordinary spirometry, the amount of oxygen absorbed or of carbon dioxide excreted in any short but measured period of time, and second, the amounts of one or other of these gases in (a) the arterial blood, usually obtained from the radial artery, and (b) the mixed venous blood in the right side of the heart, collected with the aid of a suitable catheter inserted through one of the veins in the arm. Should oxygen be selected as the gas to be used, the cardiac output can be calculated from the simple formula:

$$\text{cardiac output} = \frac{O_2 \text{ consumption}}{\text{arteriovenous } O_2 \text{ difference}}.$$

Since individuals vary widely in size and in physique, it is customary to express cardiac output in terms of litres per minute per square metre of body surface —this last is a value that can be readily obtained for either sex from appropriate height-weight tables such as those employed in the study of basal metabolism. Rates so adjusted are known as the 'cardiac index'; in healthy adults this has values that range closely between 3 and 4 litres per minute per square metre of body surface at rest and rise to some five to six times as much during short bouts of vigorous exercise.

Although observations have now been made on the cardiac index in several types of cardiovascular disease, none has been studied so often or with such care as uncomplicated mitral stenosis. The investigations of Wade and his associates may be taken as a model for such studies.[290] Because several of their observations will be further discussed below in relation to other aspects of cardiac failure, some of their findings are set out in Table 1.7. These show very clearly the correlation between the progressive incapacitation of the cardiopulmonary apparatus and the exercise tolerance of the patients in three groups separated for their degrees of disability.

From Table 1.7 it is apparent that in mitral stenosis the 'stroke volume'—the quantity of blood expelled at each heart-beat—falls steadily with the growing physical disability of the patient, and almost certainly in consequence of the obstacle presented by the narrowed mitral orifice to the filling of the left ventricle during diastole. The cardiac index, however, declines less rapidly; its continuance at a value higher than might be inferred from the reduction in the stroke volume is brought about by a rise in the heart rate, so that the incompleteness of diastolic filling is partially offset by

Table 1.7. *Functional Cardiorespiratory Studies on Patients with Varying Grades of Disability Due to Mitral Stenosis**

Degree of limitation of activity	Number of patients	Cardiac index	Stroke volume (ml)	Mean pulmonary arterial pressure (mmHg)	Capillary blood pressure (mmHg)	Arteriovenous O_2 difference (ml/dl)
Little or none	8	4·1	84	17	13	3·5
Considerable	9	2·7	56	31	20	5·3
Discomfort even at rest	4	2·2	38	52	27	6·9

* Wade, G., Werkö, L., Eliasch, H., Gidlund, A., Lagerlöf, H., *Quart. J. Med.*, 1952, N.S. **21**, 361.

more frequent emptying. This adaptation, however, is not without its drawbacks, for the cardiac acceleration is necessarily accompanied by a shortening of the duration of diastole, the phase of the cardiac cycle in which the flow of blood through the coronary circulation is greatest (see page 10). The heart muscle is thus under a two-fold handicap—increased demands on its contractile powers to compensate for the valvular defect and reduction in the supply of oxygen for its own metabolic requirements.

In mitral stenosis, the inadequacy of the heart to meet the demands of everyday life is naturally most clearly apparent when the patient is set to undertake some suitably graded exercise. A very full study has been made by Hoiling and Venner of the extent to which patients with varying grades of disability are able to cope with increased physical effort.[291]

In mitral stenosis, two further complications may arise which still further burden the already over-stressed heart: first, the advent of atrial fibrillation, and second, the development of increasing incompetence of the valve with progressively greater regurgitation of blood into the left atrium during ventricular systole. With the heart in atrial fibrillation, ventricular systole frequently occurs before the full stroke volume of blood has entered the ventricles: such beats are therefore correspondingly less effectual and the already impaired powers of the myocardium are wasted in unproductive contractions. The degree to which this added cardiac burden has lessened the exercise tolerance of such patients often becomes apparent clinically when, through therapy, normal sinus rhythm is restored.

Regurgitation of blood into the left atrium during ventricular systole places a heavy additional burden of useless work upon the already injured heart. This valvular incompetence is likely to reduce cardiac efficiency most when the orifice, surrounded by rigid and partially fused mitral cusps, is still large in comparison with that leading into the aorta, for then a large proportion—sometimes more than half—of the blood in the ventricular cavity at the beginning of systole is expelled backward into the atrium instead of forward through the aortic valve.[292]

In recent years, the application of certain haemodynamic principles has made it possible to gauge fairly closely in the living patient the area of the orifice of the mitral valve during ventricular filling. Accurate estimates of this area are naturally of much value to cardiac surgeons when they are balancing the advantages and drawbacks of mitral valvotomy. It has been found that in patients with advanced stenosis the orifice may be one-tenth or less of the 6 cm^2 of the fully open aperture of the normal adult valve. It is hardly surprising that the reduction of the cardiac index in such patients (Table 1.8) is correlated with the degree of stenosis, and that if the latter is relieved at operation, the former, and with it the patient's clinical condition, is in most cases materially improved.[293]

Table 1.8. *Comparison of the Size of the Valve Orifice and the Cardiac Index in Mitral Stenosis**

Number of records	Size of orifice (cm^2)	Mean of cardiac indexes
9	0·4–0·7	2·0
5	0·8–1·2	2·8
6	1·3–1·7	3·2

* Donald, K. W., Bishop, J. M., Wade, O. L., Wormald, P. N., *Clin. Sci.* 1957, **16**, 325.

Although studies on the functional disturbances found in mitral stenosis much outnumber those carried out in other forms of heart disease, enough have now been made in other conditions to show that in them also cardiac failure is usually accompanied by some reduction in the cardiac index. In aortic stenosis and in aortic insufficiency, and when these defects are combined, the cardiac index is generally lowered, but the decline is not as a rule serious as long as the patient is at rest. Indeed, the area of the aperture of the stenosed valve may fall from its normal of 3 cm² to 0·5 cm² without any substantial reduction in the stroke volume. The reason why the cardiac index is maintained so well in such severe grades of stenosis of the aortic valve, whereas it falls so greatly in mitral stenosis, is to be found in the great difference between the muscular power of the left ventricle and that of the left atrium. But the maintenance of the circulation in aortic stenosis is brought about only through the development of very high left intraventricular pressures during systole—probably some 250 to 300 mmHg—with a fall of pressure at the aortic valve orifice of some 100 to 200 mmHg. The extra efforts of the left ventricular myocardium, however, make extra demands upon its metabolism: this induces its hypertrophy, which the coronary circulation may in time find it difficult or impossible to sustain. When aortic valvular insufficiency is added, as is often the case, the work required of the left ventricle to maintain an adequate circulation rate, even while the patient is at rest, may rise to three or more times that needed normally.[294]

In hypertension, the stress placed upon the myocardium differs in an important respect from that experienced in exercise in that it is maintained more or less without remission, day and night. In spite of the hypertrophy of the left ventricle—which may double or treble in weight—the cardiac index ultimately falls to values that are scarcely sufficient for the patient while at rest and become quite inadequate for even comparatively mild exercise.[295]

Before leaving the subject of abnormal circulation rates, mention may be made of the so-called 'hyperkinetic states' found in severe anaemia, arteriovenous shunts and advanced Paget's disease of bone, in all of which the cardiac index is abnormally high both at rest and during exercise.[296] That the heart can maintain such raised outputs for years without apparent damage from overloading probably follows from the fact that the peripheral resistance encountered—because of the lowered viscosity of anaemic blood or because of an abnormally dilated systemic vascular bed—largely, if not wholly, offsets the greater volume of the cardiac output. If any sign of heart strain develops, as it may with arteriovenous shunts or in Paget's disease, it is likely to present itself as right-sided failure, because on this side of the circulation the high level of the cardiac output finds no corresponding compensation such as an increased patency of the pulmonary vascular bed.

The Circulation Time in Heart Failure

In cardiac failure, not only is the cardiac index reduced but the time required for blood to pass from one point in the circulatory system to another —now usually measured from the left antecubital vein to the right brachial artery—is considerably prolonged. In the past, such measurements have been made by injections of various substances, the instant of arrival of which at some selected site can be immediately determined either subjectively by the patient or objectively by the observer. The dye uranin (the arrival of which can be detected with ultraviolet light), decholin (which produces a sudden bitter taste), histamine (which creates a malar flush) and many other substances have been employed, but latterly such studies have been made preciser by the use of radioactive isotopes, their gamma radiation passing readily through the skin to a suitable counting tube sited over the selected blood vessel. When human serum albumin to which radioactive iodine has been coupled is employed, a sharp inflection on a suitably shielded recording Geiger-Müller counter marks the arrival of the marked material at the site. Coupled with appropriate timing devices capable of determining the interval between injection and excitation of the counter, these instruments can be employed for timing the passage of blood by the shortest route over various pathways in the circulation. Such records can also be employed for estimating cardiac output, and thus provide an alternative to the more usual direct Fick technique (see page 58): the agreement between the methods is remarkably good.[297]

Of the many observations that have been made on the circulation time from one point in the vascular circuit to another, two examples are given in Table 1.9. In both, the time taken for the

Table 1.9. *Circulation Time from Arm to Arm in Mitral Stenosis*

Indicator substance	Time in seconds		
		Disability	
	Normal	Moderate	Severe
Radon[298]	18	21	38*
Evans blue[299]	23	21	36

* Patients with atrial fibrillation.

indicator to pass from the antecubital vein in one arm to the brachial artery in the other was determined—in one study with the radioactive element radon and in the other with the dye Evans blue. From them it can be seen that as long as the cardiac rhythm remains normal and the disability slight, there is little change in the time, but if atrial fibrillation develops or the disability becomes severe, the circulation time may even be doubled.

Changes in the Structure and Functions of the Lungs in Heart Failure

Structural Changes in the Lungs

In mitral stenosis, the check to the circulation develops close to where the blood emerges from the pulmonary vessels, so that it is to be expected that the effects of an obstruction at this valve should fall heavily on the lungs. In advanced cases, the grosser alterations due to this passive venous congestion may be recognizable when the thorax is opened, either at operation or at necropsy.[300] The lungs have a characteristic deep purple colour and fail to retract as completely as do the normal organs when the negative intrapleural pressure is lost. Occasionally, too, the pleural surface may present one or more rather prominent, dark plum-coloured areas—often several centimetres across—where the underlying lung has recently become infarcted. The lining of the bronchi is often a deep, dusky red and covered with a thick film of mucus or mucopus. The major pulmonary arteries and veins are generally distended, and the former often contain many raised, yellowish plaques of atheroma, on some of which mural, or even occluding, thrombi may have formed. The hilar lymph nodes, especially those just below the carina, are typically swollen, moist and hyperaemic.

When cut, the lung substance seems unusually resistant to the knife, and the freshly exposed surface generally possesses a rusty brown colour which soon loses a distinctive cyanotic tinge on exposure to the air. These typical features have led to the term *brown induration*, which is applied to lungs in the more advanced stages of passive venous congestion. Sometimes, especially in elderly patients with a long history of heart failure, the lower lobes are heavy from accumulation of fluid in the alveoli. When the lung is squeezed small beads of pus are extruded from the lesser bronchi —a manifestation of terminal bronchopneumonia.

The histological changes in such passively congested lungs are quite distinctive,[301] and usually increase in severity from the apical regions. The alveolar walls are much thickened, partly through the formation of many new collagen fibres and partly through the collection of oedema fluid between the small blood vessels and the alveolar lining. The blood capillaries appear unusually prominent, partly because of their dilatation and partly because their greater tortuosity conveys an exaggerated impression of an increase in their number. It now seems likely, however, that these histological signs of congestion may be a post-mortem artefact, for studies on patients with mitral stenosis have shown that even in chronic heart failure the quantity of blood in the pulmonary circuit is raised only slightly above the normal.[302]

The alveoli, especially those in the basal regions, are often filled with fluid, which, having the low protein content typical of transudates, stains only faintly with eosin. Many macrophages—the so-called 'heart failure cells'—are present, some heavily blackened with carbon dust and others coloured a golden brown by haemosiderin granules. Sometimes these siderotic macrophages (sidero-phages) fill particular groups of alveoli, forming pigmented nodules that are large enough to be conspicuous on the cut surface of the lungs and in radiographs of the chest.[303] The haemosiderin is probably derived from capillary haemorrhages in the mucosa of small bronchi and bronchioles: the escaping red cells are carried down into the dependent alveoli, where, after ingestion by macrophages, their haemoglobin is converted into the relatively soluble yellow haematoidin (bilirubin) and the insoluble golden-brown haemosiderin. Both at the exposed cut surface of the lungs at necropsy and in histological sections, the haemosiderin can readily be displayed by Perls's Prussian blue reaction.

A structural alteration which attracted little attention before the introduction of mitral valvotomy is to be found in the small arterioles and precapillary vessels in the lungs.[304-306] Normally, the walls of these vessels are thin and have an insignificant medial coat, but in advanced cases of mitral stenosis, when the size of the valve orifice has fallen to 1 cm² or less, their media is found to be much more conspicuous and their calibre reduced. This structural change has the effect of raising the resistance to the passage of blood through the lungs, and is followed by two further noteworthy changes—one advantageous to the patient, the other detrimental. The *benefit* that follows from the partial occlusion of these vessels lies in the protection that it affords to the lung

C*

capillaries against exposure to blood pressure so raised that it might lead to excessive transudation through their walls and to the consequent flooding of the lungs with oedema fluid. It is in the most advanced cases of mitral stenosis that this protective occlusion is most in evidence—the great rise in the mean pulmonary arterial pressure that is typical of patients with the greatest disability is not accompanied by any corresponding elevation in the pressure of the blood in the alveolar capillaries. The *handicap* that follows the arteriolar occlusion is that the systolic pressure in the right ventricle rises to three or four times that found normally, so that a great and continuous strain is placed upon its myocardium. It seems likely, too, that in their more advanced stages the changes in the arterioles and precapillaries are irreversible, and that the failure of mitral valvotomy to benefit certain patients is due to the fact that, although the surgeon can relieve the stenosis, the secondary pulmonary hypertension persists and consequently no relief is afforded to the overworked and hypertrophied right ventricle.

Functional Changes in the Lungs

The main clinical interest in the morphological changes found in brown induration of the lungs lies in the physiological changes that accompany them and the contribution that such functional disturbances make to the signs and symptoms of chronic heart failure.[307] An observation that has thrown light on the dyspnoea and cyanosis that are often conspicuous clinical features in such patients is the decline in the vital capacity that takes place concurrently with the increasing disability.[308] Several factors may contribute to this deterioration. Formerly, it was believed to be mainly attributable to the encroachment made by the supposedly distended capillaries on the air space in the alveoli, but modern studies have shown that during life the quantity of blood within the pulmonary circuit rises little in mitral stenosis.[309, 310] While in advanced cases of congestive heart failure the accumulation of cells and oedema fluid in the alveoli—especially those of the lower lobes—probably contributes materially to the reduction in vital capacity, the most important single factor in exciting dyspnoea would seem to be some limitation of the free movement of the lung parenchyma, due to a diminution in its normal power of elastic recoil during expiration. In recent times, the term 'compliance' has been introduced to denote this concept of pulmonary inertia. Its

significance in relation to the dyspnoea of mitral stenosis can be appreciated from the observation that whereas in normal people a change in pressure of 1 cm of water in the pleural cavity leads to a movement of about a quarter of a litre of air into or out of the lungs, in patients with this form of heart disease the same change in intrapleural pressure only effects the displacement of about half this volume of air.[311] The lungs thus appear to have become more rigid than before—perhaps because of an erectile effect caused by the rise in their capillary and venous blood pressure. The subjective sensation of dyspnoea that distresses many cardiac patients may result from the increased work constantly required of the thoracic muscles in maintaining pulmonary ventilation. When such patients undertake even minor forms of physical activity, the added respiratory exertion causes them disproportionate discomfort.

In spite of the morphological and functional evidence of pulmonary changes in advanced mitral valve disease, the gas content of the arterial blood is comparatively little altered and is unlikely to contribute significantly to the clinical manifestations. The arterial blood saturation in normal people is about 96 per cent; in a series of 10 patients with mitral stenosis, sometimes accompanied by atrial fibrillation, the corresponding saturation was on average 93 per cent, though the variation was considerable.[312] Such a small reduction in the quantity of oxygen in the arterial blood —and even this is often mitigated by some degree of polycythaemia—could contribute only very slightly to hypoxia in the peripheral tissues. There is seldom much change in the content of carbon dioxide in the blood leaving the heart:[313] only in the advanced stages of congestive failure, when the release into the blood of such non-volatile organic acids as lactic acid has reduced its bicarbonate reserve appreciably, does its carbon dioxide content tend to fall. Even in advanced heart failure, therefore, the lungs usually possess sufficient reserve to enable them to continue to cope adequately with the exchange of these gases so long as the patient remains quietly at rest.

Although in most patients with acquired heart disease the content of oxygen and carbon dioxide in the arterial blood differs little from that found in healthy people, the mixed venous blood that returns to the lungs after its slower passage through the peripheral tissue capillaries contains much less oxygen and more carbon dioxide than normally. Moreover, the already exaggerated arteriovenous difference typical of congestive failure becomes even more apparent when the patient is mildly exercised. It would seem that both at rest and on exercise the greater removal of oxygen from the blood in the tissue capillaries partially compensates for the inability of the heart to adjust the circulation rate to current metabolic needs. This increased abstraction of oxygen as the blood passes through the capillaries necessarily affects metabolism in many of the tissue cells, especially those in the vicinity of the venules. The adverse effects of chronic hypoxia are readily recognizable in the liver—the incoming portal blood, even in normal persons, is low in oxygen—and death of many of the parenchymatous cells round the hepatic venules in the central part of the lobule forms a conspicuous feature of the 'nutmeg' liver of prolonged passive venous congestion. But although many tissue cells are chronically short of oxygen, it is usually only under the stress of exercise that the concentration of the anaerobically-formed catabolite lactic acid undergoes any significant rise in the mixed venous blood.[314] In most patients, even when congestive failure is severe, it seems that as long as they remain at rest the tissue cells generally, although handicapped, are able to maintain their activities adequately through the ordinary processes of oxidative metabolism.

Oedema in Heart Failure

The gradual accumulation of oedema fluid, especially in the lowermost parts of the body—the legs in ambulatory patients, and the sacral region in the bedridden, is a characteristic and often conspicuous feature of the later stages of cardiac failure. Much oedema fluid can collect in the tissues, however, before its presence becomes detectable by the clinical 'pitting test', and it is only through periodic weighing of the patient that any minor degree of oedema can be recognized and its progress followed.

While there is little doubt that several physiological disturbances are ordinarily concerned in the pathogenesis of cardiac oedema, elevation of venous blood pressure, often associated with a rise in blood volume, is among the more important of the contributory factors. It has frequently been confirmed that the venous pressure rises as the severity of heart failure increases; in the graver cases, the rise is often apparent on clinical examination from the distension of the veins in the neck when the patient is sitting or standing. Typical pressures for such cases are set out in Table 1.10; they were obtained by inserting a manometer needle into the antecubital vein while the subject was in the recumbent position so that the vein and the right atrium were at the same level.[315]

The effects on the movement of fluid across the vessel wall of a rise in blood pressure within the veins, and of the greater concomitant rise within the capillaries drained by them, can be demonstrated by applying a sphygmomanometer cuff to

Table 1.10. *Pressure of the Blood in the Antecubital Vein in Normal People and in Patients in Various Grades of Congestive Cardiac Failure**

Condition	Venous pressure (mmHg)	
	At rest	On exercise
Normal control	3	5
Mild failure	7	13
Severe failure	13	22

* Albert, R. E., Eichna, L. W., *Amer. Heart J.*, 1952, **43**, 395.

a limb and partially inflating it so as temporarily to occlude the venous return. If such a compressed limb is placed in a plethysmograph to record changes in its volume, its rate of swelling at various venous pressures can be determined.[316, 317] When the venous pressure rises above about 12 mmHg, the first signs of excessive transudation become perceptible on the oncometer, and above that pressure the rate of swelling closely parallels the pressure applied through the cuff to the underlying vessels. After a time, if the obstruction is continued, the rate of accumulation of transudate declines in consequence of the rise in the pressure of the extravascular fluid opposing its further formation. When an elevated venous pressure is maintained for weeks and months as a result of cardiac failure, especially in elderly patients whose connective tissues have lost some of their former elasticity, the subcutaneous tissue spaces become stretched and large quantities of oedema fluid can collect.

In spite of the hypoxia of many of the peripheral tissues, there is no evidence that their capillaries become any more permeable than before to the plasma colloids. Estimations of the protein content of the oedema fluid of cardiac failure have shown that its concentration is little if at all in excess of what is believed to be characteristic of normal tissue fluid. In a series of 26 patients with cardiac oedema this concentration averaged 0·21 per cent,[318] and in another group, of 10 patients, 0·24 per cent.[319] Such concentrations of protein signify that mechanical forces alone are primarily concerned in the pathogenesis of the oedema of heart failure.

The concept of the mechanism of development of oedema in cardiac failure that was based upon Starling's theory of the factors controlling the movement of electrolytes through capillary walls has now been supplemented by the suggestion that some impairment in the excretion of sodium by the kidneys may lead to its retention and accumulation. That renal excretion is affected in cardiac failure has long been known, but its analysis in current physiological concepts has been achieved only comparatively recently.[320, 321] As cardiac failure develops, the output of the heart falls and the renal blood flow becomes reduced much more than proportionately. As a consequence, the rate of glomerular filtration declines substantially, and sodium ions, together with water, are retained in the body, first in the blood, which increases in volume, and later in the tissue fluid, into which they escape as a result of the raised hydrostatic pressure in the capillaries. It seems likely, too, that the lessened excretion of sodium may in part result from the increased liberation of the hormone aldosterone from the adrenal cortex, but further work remains to be done before the role of this endocrine mechanism is fully understood (see Chapter 30).

Cardiac Insufficiency in Hypertension and Aortic Valve Disease

Much of the foregoing discussion on congestive cardiac failure has centred on observations made on patients with advanced mitral valve disease, mainly because more studies have been made on this common condition than on any other form of heart disease. Failure may supervene, however, as a result of other acquired cardiac disabilities, among which prolonged systemic hypertension, chronic cardiac ischaemia from coronary arterial disease, and aortic valve lesions are the most frequent.

In systemic hypertension, congestive cardiac failure is the commonest terminal feature of the disease. By the time this stage has been reached, the output of the heart has become materially diminished, exercise tolerance is low and the other features of failure—a raised arteriovenous oxygen difference and an elevated pulmonary arterial pressure—have developed (see Table 1.11).[322] Clinically, such patients present the effects of left-sided failure on the respiratory system—dyspnoea (often paroxysmal and nocturnal in character), reduced vital capacity and pulmonary oedema: when the more advanced states are reached the signs of

peripheral congestive failure—venous distension and oedema—become increasingly manifest.

Studies on the stenotic aortic valve have shown that functional disturbances attributable to the defect become recognizable when the area of the orifice falls from its normal value of 3 cm^2 to about 0·5 cm^2, if the stenosis is pure, or to about 1·5 cm^2 if it is associated with regurgitation.[323] These changes inevitably involve abnormally high intraventricular systolic blood pressure, and consequently demand greater mechanical work of the left ventricle if the cardiac output is to be maintained at a level approximating to the normal—the work of the ventricles is about doubled with the grade of stenosis mentioned, and trebled if regurgitation is also present. It is this constant demand that brings about the very substantial and often closely correlated degree of hypertrophy of the wall of the chamber. In considering the

Table 1.11. *Functional Disturbances Associated with Moderate and Advanced Systemic Hypertension*[*]

		Hypertension	
	Controls	Moderate	Severe
Mean systemic arterial pressure (mmHg)	88	151	188
Cardiac index (output of blood in l/m^2/min)	4·42	3·72	3·05
Mean pulmonary arterial pressure (mmHg)	18	20	33
Mean resting arteriovenous oxygen difference (ml/dl)	3·21	3·92	5·51

[*] Taylor, S. H., Donald, K. W., Bishop, J. M., *Clin. Sci.*, 1957, **16**, 351.

effectiveness of this compensatory hypertrophy, however, it must be realized that in aortic regurgitation the aortic pressure is usually low in diastole, so that the coronary blood flow, which takes place chiefly in this phase of the cardiac cycle, may be insufficient to meet the greater requirements of the hypertrophied myocardium. Ischaemic changes in the heart—which are often associated with angina pectoris—may seriously handicap the already hypertrophied muscle and prevent it from maintaining ventricular output—a development that brings nearer the inevitable terminal stage of left-sided failure.

In many cases hypertrophy protects the patient for a long time from the development of heart failure; but later, when the efficiency of the heart muscle itself is deteriorating, a substantial volume of blood may remain in the left ventricular cavity at the end of systole. This may lead to a rise in the pressure needed in the left atrium to force blood through the mitral valve into the already partially filled ventricle. It is this rise in the pressure in the left atrium, transmitted backward into the pulmonary circulation, that eventually brings about the respiratory disturbances characteristic of left-sided cardiac failure.

TUMOURS OF THE HEART

Primary tumours of the heart are uncommon and in the past were usually first recognized at necropsy. Developments in angiography and in cardiac surgery, however, have led to greater interest in them for some can now be diagnosed during life and may be treated successfully by excision.

Much the most frequent primary tumour of the heart is the benign 'myxoma', which generally originates in the septal wall of the left atrium close to the rim of the fossa ovalis (Figs 1.55 and 1.56).[324, 325] It usually forms a pedunculate,

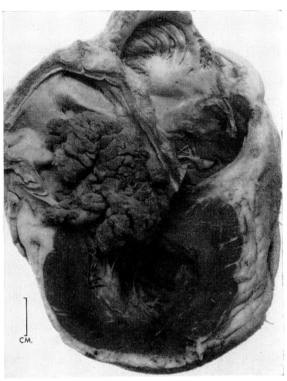

Fig. 1.56.§ The same specimen as in Fig. 1.55, after fixation in formol saline and preservation by Kaiserling's method. The tumour has shrunk and acquired a dry, opaque look.

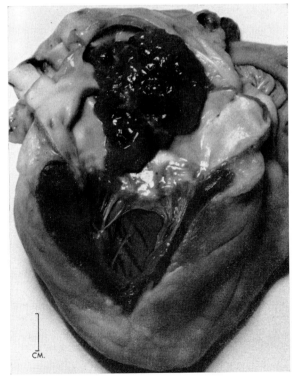

Fig. 1.55.§ 'Myxoma' of the left atrium, arising in the characteristic site on the septum. The photograph was made while the specimen was fresh (compare with Fig. 1.56).

globular or cauliflower-like mass, several centimetres in diameter, which protrudes into the chamber of the atrium. It causes little or no alteration in the adjacent myocardium. When large, it can obstruct the flow of blood through the mitral valve, and sometimes it causes sudden death through 'ball-valve' impaction in the orifice. Clinically, in addition to simulating mitral stenosis, an important feature of the atrial 'myxoma' is the frequency with which it is accompanied by embolic episodes in the systemic circulation. This complication is attributable to the exposed position and constant mechanical agitation of the tumour, both of which favour the detachment of small fragments of its substance or of overlying thrombus. In no sense is this dissemination of particles of tumour to be regarded as a manifestation of malignancy.[326] The emboli of 'myxoma' tissue do not grow at their site of impaction but undergo organization.

Microscopically (Fig. 1.57), cardiac myxomas are made up of loose connective tissue in which stellate cells lie widely separated in a matrix in which mucopolysaccharides can sometimes be identified.

The surface of the tumour is covered by endothelium on which small thrombotic masses often form. Because of their vulnerable situation, the delicate capillaries of the stroma may rupture and give rise to small haemorrhages which in time result in the local deposition of haemosiderin. The presence of these deposits of haemosiderin formerly encouraged the belief that the tumours were in reality thrombi

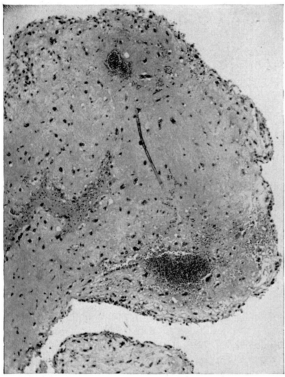

Fig. 1.57.§ Histological appearance of the tumour shown in Figs 1.55 and 1.56. The stroma appears homogeneous and opaque, due to precipitation of its mucoprotein content during histological processing. Apart from the small foci of haemorrhage, cells are scanty: most of them are large fibroblasts, some of which are of the stellate type associated with myxomatoid degeneration. The surface of the lesion has a definite endothelial covering. The appearances are consistent with oedema in an organized thrombus, and they have been so interpreted by some authorities; others regard these lesions as true myxomas. *Haematoxylin–eosin.* × 60.

which had undergone organization. In some examples of the tumour, endothelial cells are arranged in an acinar fashion round minute spaces; it is this appearance that suggested the term 'angiomyxomas' for such tumours.

Other benign tumours of the heart, among them fibromas and lipomas, are even rarer than the myxomas. The so-called 'congenital rhabdomyoma', in which single or multiple nodular collections of large, glycogen-filled, cross-striated cells distort the myocardium, was formerly considered to be a benign neoplasm of cardiac muscle. Its almost exclusive occurrence in infants and its usual lack of capsulation, however, have led to the abandonment of this view: the condition is now regarded as a hamartoma (a tumour-like mass of cells attributable to some error of development) rather than as a true neoplasm.[327] This belief is supported by the association of these myocardial nodules with comparable malformations in other organs, and more particularly with tuberose sclerosis of the brain (see also page 81, where the possible relation of the nodules to the abnormal storage of glycogen is noted).

The myocardial lesion of hypertrophic obstructive cardiomyopathy has sometimes been mistaken for a rhabdomyoma (see page 51).

Primary malignant tumours of the heart are even less frequent than benign ones. Most of them are so undifferentiated that they can only be described as 'round cell' or 'spindle cell' sarcomas: in at least some cases there is doubt as to the primary nature of such tumours—some of those in the older literature may well have been bronchial carcinomas that had spread to the heart. In rare instances cross-striation of the neoplastic cells provides a convincing demonstration of their kinship with cardiac muscle fibres (rhabdomyosarcoma). Sarcomas of the heart, like those that arise elsewhere, tend to occur in relatively young people, sometimes even infants, and to disseminate rapidly and widely to other parts of the body. Fibrosarcoma is an exception, usually occurring in middle age or later and seldom, if ever, metastasizing: it may arise in any part of the heart, but perhaps more frequently in the ventricular wall than elsewhere.[328]

Secondary tumours in the heart are by no means uncommon, and may reach a large size.[329, 330] With the rapidly rising incidence of bronchial cancer they are likely to be encountered more frequently in future. In many instances, the heart is involved by extension of the tumour first to the epicardium and later to the myocardium near the base. Invasion may result either directly from infiltration by the primary tumour in a nearby organ, or indirectly from extension through lymphatics from a secondary deposit in a mediastinal lymph node. It is no matter for surprise, therefore, that carcinomas of the bronchus and breast are among the commonest sources of secondary neoplasms in the heart. The presence of small secondary tumours in the myocardium appear to be well tolerated by the heart, for there is often little functional disturbance to its action. But if the deposits involve the endocardium, their exposed surface may become covered with thrombus. Should the nodules occur in the pericardium, they may lead to inflammatory changes in the serosa and to the accumulation of fluid, often blood stained, in the pericardial sac. Occasionally, haemorrhage from these deposits may be so severe that the patient dies from cardiac tamponade.

Pericardial tumours, including mesothelioma, are referred to on page 7.

REFERENCES

THE PERICARDIUM

1. Grant, R. T., *Heart*, 1926, **13**, 371.
2. Cohnheim, J., *Lectures on General Pathology*, vol. 1, p. 21. London, 1889.
3. Stewart, H. J., Crane, N. F., Deitrick, J. E., *Amer. Heart J.*, 1938, **16**, 189.
4. Nelson, A. A., *Arch. Path. (Chic.)*, 1940, **29**, 256.
5. Boyle, J. P., Pearce, M. L., Guze, L. B., *Medicine (Baltimore)*, 1961, **40**, 119.
6. Pyrah, L. N., Pain, A. B., *J. Path. Bact.*, 1933, **37**, 233.
7. Swan, W. G. A., *Brit. Heart J.*, 1960, **22**, 651.
8. Woodward, T. E., McCrumb, F. R., Carey, T. N., Togo, Y., *Ann. intern. Med.*, 1960, **53**, 1130.
9. Bennett, N. McK., Forbes, J. A., *Amer. Heart J.*, 1967, **74**, 435.
10. Dressler, W., *A.M.A. Arch. intern. Med.*, 1959, **103**, 28.
11. Thomas, G. T., Besterman, E. M. M., Hollman, A., *Brit. Heart J.*, 1953, **15**, 29.
12. Wacker, W., Merrill, J. P., *J. Amer. med. Ass.*, 1954, **156**, 764.
13. Friedberg, C. K., Gross, L⋅, *Amer. J. Path.*, 1936, **12**, 183.
14. Andrews, C. W. S., Pickering, G. W., Sellors, T. Holmes, *Quart. J. Med.*, 1948, N.S. **17**, 291.
15. Wood, P., *Diseases of the Heart and Circulation*, 2nd edn, page 673. London, 1959.
16. Diefenbach, W. C. L., *Amer. Rev. Tuberc.*, 1950, **62**, 390.
17. Harvey, A. M., Whitehill, M. R., *Medicine (Baltimore)*, 1937, **16**, 45.
18. Barr, J. F., *A.M.A. Arch. intern. Med.*, 1955, **96**, 693.
19. Paul, O., Castleman, B., White, P. D., *Amer. J. med. Sci.*, 1948, **216**, 361.
20. Sawyer, C. G., Burwell, C. S., Dexter, L., Eppinger, E. C., Goodale, W. T., Gorlin, R., Harken, D. E., Haynes, F. W., *Amer. Heart J.*, 1952, **44**, 207.
21. Armstrong, T. G., *Lancet*, 1940, **2**, 475.
22. Gimlette, T. M. D., *Brit. Heart J.*, 1959, **21**, 9.
23. Charcot, J. M., *Clinical Lectures on Senile and Chronic Diseases*, translated by W. S. Tuke, page 172 (New Sydenham Society, vol. 95). London, 1881.
24. Still, G. F., *Med.-chir. Trans.*, 1897, **80**, 47.
25. Wilkinson, M., *Brit. med. J.*, 1962, **2**, 1723.
26. Keith, T. A., *Circulation*, 1962, **25**, 477.
27. Kennedy, W. P. U., Partridge, R. E. H., Matthews, M. B., *Brit. Heart J.*, 1966, **28**, 602.
28. Brigden, W., Bywaters, E. G. L., Lessof, M. H., Ross, I. P., *Brit. Heart J.*, 1960, **22**, 1.
29. Yurchak, P. M., Levine, S. A., Gorlin, R., *Circulation*, 1965, **31**, 113.
30. Steinberg, I., Rothbard, S., *Amer. J. Cardiol.*, 1962, **9**, 953.
31. Meltzer, J. I., *Amer. J. Med.*, 1956, **20**, 638.
32. Cornell, A., Shookhoff, H. B., *Arch. intern. Med.*, 1944, **74**, 11.
33. Kern, F., *Arch. intern. Med.*, 1945, **76**, 88.
34. Mahaim, I., *Les Tumeurs et les polypes du cœur*. Paris, 1945.
35. Goldberg, H. P., Steinberg, I., *Circulation*, 1955, **11**, 963.
36. Thomas, J., Phythyon, J. M., *Circulation*, 1957, **15**, 385.
37. Dave, C. J., Wood, D. A., Mitchell, S., *Cancer (Philad.)*, 1953, **6**, 794.
38. Pietra, G. G., Silber, E., Levin, B., Pick, A., *Amer. Heart J.*, 1968, **75**, 545.

ISCHAEMIC HEART DISEASE

39. Crawford, T., in *Second Symposium on Advanced Medicine*, edited by J. R. Trounce, page 42. London, 1966.
40. Wilson, J. M. G., Heasman, M. A., *Mth. Bull. Min. Hlth Lab. Serv.*, 1959, **18**, 94.
41. Morris, J. N., Heady, J. A., Raffle, P. A. B., Roberts, C. G., Parks, J. W., *Lancet*, 1953, **2**, 1053, 1111.
42. Morris, J. N., Crawford, M. D., *Brit. med. J.*, 1958, **2**, 1485.
43. Schlesinger, M. J., *Arch. Path. (Chic.)*, 1940, **30**, 403.
44. Fulton, W. F. M., *The Coronary Arteries*. Springfield, Ill., 1965.
45. Mitchell, J. R. A., Schwartz, C. J., *Arterial Disease*. Oxford, 1965.
46. Baroldi, G., Scomazzoni, G., *Coronary Circulation in the Normal and the Pathological Heart*. Washington, D.C., 1967.
47. Prinzmetal, M., Simkin, B., Bergman, H. C., Kruger, H. E., *Amer. Heart J.*, 1947, **33**, 420.
48. Pitt, B., *Circulation*, 1959, **20**, 816.
49. Hudson, C. L., Moritz, A. R., Wearn, J. T., *J. exp. Med.*, 1932, **56**, 919.
50. Tandler, J., in *Handbuch der Anatomie des Menschen*, edited by K. von Bardeleben: *Anatomie des Herzens*, chap. 7, *Die Gefässe des Herzens*. Jena, 1913.
51. Whitten, M. B., *Arch. intern. Med.*, 1930, **45**, 383.
52. Lowe, T. E., *Amer. Heart J.*, 1941, **21**, 326.
53. Gregg, D. E., *Coronary Circulation in Health and Disease*. London, 1950.
54. Gregg, D. E., *Circulation*, 1963, **27**, 1128.
55. Gorlin, R., in *Modern Trends in Cardiology*, edited by A. Morgan Jones, page 191. London, 1960.
56. Bing, R. J., Hammond, M. M., Handelsman, J. C., Powers, S. R., Spencer, F. C., Eckenhoff, J. E., Goodale, W. T., Hafkenshiel, J. H., Kety, S. S., *Amer. Heart J.*, 1949, **38**, 1.
57. Essex, H. E., Herrick, J. F., Baldes, E. J., Mann, F. C., *Amer. J. Physiol.*, 1939, **125**, 614.

58. Maxwell, G. M., Castillo, C. A., White, D. H., Crumpton, C. W., Rowe, G. G., *J. clin. Invest.*, 1958, **37**, 1413.
59. Gorlin, R., in *Modern Trends in Cardiology*, edited by A. Morgan Jones, chap. 13. London, 1960.
60. Hamilton, W. F., *Amer. J. Physiol.*, 1944, **141**, 235.
61. *The Geographic Pathology of Atherosclerosis*, edited by H. C. McGill. Baltimore, 1968.
62. Lober, P. H., *A.M.A. Arch. Path.*, 1953, **55**, 357.
63. Barr, D. P., *J. chron. Dis.*, 1955, **1**, 63.
64. Oliver, M. F., Boyd, G. S., *Lancet*, 1959, **2**, 690.
65. Robinson, R. W., Higano, N., Cohen, W. D., *A.M.A. Arch. intern. Med.*, 1959, **104**, 908.
66. Ministry of Health, *Report for the Year 1957—Part II: On the State of the Public Health*, page 34. London, 1958.
67. Schroeder, H. A., *J. Amer. med. Ass.*, 1960, **172**, 1902.
68. Morris, J. N., Crawford, M. D., Heady, J. A., *Lancet*, 1961, **1**, 860.
69. Crawford, M. D., Gardner, M. J., Morris, J. N., *Lancet*, 1968, **1**, 827.
70. Biörck, G., Boström, H., Widström, A., *Acta med. scand.*, 1965, **178**, 239.
71. Crawford, T., Crawford, M. D., *Lancet*, 1967, **1**, 229.
72. Wolkoff, K., *Beitr. path. Anat.*, 1929, **82**, 555.
73. Ehrich, W., de la Chapelle, C., Cohn, A. E., *Amer. J. Anat.*, 1932, **49**, 241.
74. Crawford, T., in *Trends in Clinical Pathology*, page 63. London, 1969.
75. Schlesinger, M. J., Zoll, P. M., *Arch. Path. (Chic.)*, 1941, **32**, 178.
76. Crawford, T., Dexter, D., Teare, R. D., *Lancet*, 1961, **1**, 181.
77. Constantinides, P., *J. Atheroscler. Res.*, 1966, **6**, 1.
78. Drury, R. A. B., *J. Path. Bact.*, 1954, **67**, 207.
79. Pickering, G. W., Wayne, E. J., *Clin. Sci.*, 1934, **1**, 305.
80. Lewis, T., *Arch. intern. Med.*, 1932, **49**, 713.
81. Büchner, F., *Beitr. path. Anat.*, 1932, **89**, 644.
82. Büchner, F., *Dtsch. med. Wschr.*, 1957, **82**, 1037.
83. Symmers, W. St C., *Verh. dtsch. Ges. Path.*, 1953, **36**, 224.
84. Crawford, T., in *Second Symposium on Advanced Medicine*, edited by J. R. Trounce, p. 42. London, 1966.
85. Blumgart, H. L., Schlesinger, M. J., Zoll, P. M., *Arch. intern. Med.*, 1941, **68**, 181.
86. Nachlas, M. M., Shnitka, T. K., *Amer. J. Path.*, 1963, **42**, 379.
87. Karsner, H. T., Dwyer, J. E., *J. med. Res.*, 1916, **34**, 21.
88. Mallory, G. K., White, P. D., Salcedo-Salgar, J., *Amer. Heart J.*, 1939, **18**, 647.
89. Leading Article, *Lancet*, 1969, **1**, 821.
90. Wartman, W. B., Souders, J. C., *Arch. Path. (Chic.)*, 1950, **50**, 329.
91. Sutton, R., Davies, M. J., *Circulation*, 1968, **38**, 987.
92. Davies, M. J., Redwood, D., Harris, A., *Brit. med. J.*, 1967, **3**, 342.
93. Crawford, M. D., Morris, J. N., *Brit. med. J.*, 1960, **2**, 1624.
94. Mallory, G. K., White, P. D., Salcedo-Salgar, J., *Amer. Heart J.*, 1939, **18**, 647.
95. Sanders, R. J., Neuberger, K. T., Ravin, A., *Dis. Chest*, 1957, **31**, 316.
96. Barnard, P. M., Kennedy, J. H., *Circulation*, 1965, **32**, 76.

97. Mourdjinis, A., Olsen, E., Raphael, M. G., Mounsey, J. P. D., *Brit. Heart J.*, 1968, **30**, 497.
98. Selzer, A., *Arch. intern. Med.*, 1948, **82**, 196.
99. Wroblewski, F., *Advanc. clin. Chem.*, 1958, **1**, 313.
100. Hamolsky, M. W., Kaplan, N. O., *Circulation*, 1961, **23**, 102.
101. Cohen, L., *Mod. Conc. cardiov. Dis.*, 1967, **36**, 43.
102. Stewart, T. W., Warburton, F. G., *Brit. Heart J.*, 1961, **23**, 236.
103. Elliott, B. A., Jepson, E. M., Wilkinson, J. H., *Clin. Sci.*, 1963, **23**, 305.

RHEUMATIC HEART DISEASE

104. Waksman, B. H., *Medicine (Baltimore)*, 1949, **28**, 143.
105. Thomas, L., *Rheumatic Fever*. Minneapolis, 1952.
106. Bloomfield, A. L., *A.M.A. Arch. intern. Med.*, 1956, **98**, 288.
107. Coburn, A. F., *A.M.A. Arch. intern. Med.*, 1959, **104**, 1021.
108. Newsholme, A., *Lancet*, 1895, **1**, 589, 657.
109. Coburn, A. F., Young, D. C., *The Epidemiology of Hemolytic Streptococcus during World War II in the U.S. Navy*. Baltimore, 1949.
110. Leslie, C. J., Spence, M. J., *Amer. J. Dis. Child.*, 1938, **55**, 472.
111. Schick, B., *Jb. Kinderheilk.*, 1907, **65** (*Ergänzungsband*), 132.
112. Coburn, A. F., *Lancet*, 1936, **2**, 1025.
113. Glover, J. A., *Lancet*, 1930, **1**, 499.
114. Lovell, R., Straker, E. A., Wilson, J., *Lancet*, 1934, **1**, 205.
115. Green, C. A., *J. Hyg. (Lond.)*, 1942, **42**, 365.
116. Rantz, L. A., Boisvert, P. L., Spink, W. W., *Arch. intern. Med.*, 1945, **76**, 131.
117. Stevenson, A. C., Cheeseman, E. A., *Ann. Eugen. (Lond.)*, 1953, **17**, 177.
118. Morris, J. N., Titmus, R. M., *Lancet*, 1942, **2**, 59.
119. Coburn, A. F., *Amer. J. med. Sci.*, 1960, **240**, 687.
120. Scottish Health Services Council, *Rheumatic Fever in Scotland*. Edinburgh, 1967.
121. Vorlaender, K. O., in *Immunopathologie in Klinik und Forschung*, edited by P. Miescher and K. O. Vorlaender, 2nd edn, page 455. Stuttgart, 1961.
122. Bernhard, G. C., Stollerman, G. H., *J. clin. Invest.*, 1959, **38**, 1942.
123. McCarty, M., in *Rheumatic Fever*, edited by R. Cruickshank and A. A. Glynn, page 65. London, 1959.
124. Wannamaker, L. W., Ayoub, E. M., *Circulation*, 1960, **21**, 598.
125. Kaplan, M. H., Meyerstein, M., *Lancet*, 1962, **1**, 706.
126. Kaplan, M. H., Bolande, R., Rakita, L., Blair, J., *New Engl. J. Med.*, 1964, **271**, 637.
127. Murphy, G. E., Swift, H. F., *J. exp. Med.*, 1949, **89**, 687; 1950, **91**, 485.
128. Harris, T. N., Friedman, S., Needleman, H. L., Saltzman, H. A., *Pediatrics*, 1956, **17**, 11.
129. Aschoff, L., *Brit. med. J.*, 1906, **2**, 1103.
130. Enticknap, J. B., *Brit. Heart J.*, 1953, **15**, 433.
131. Klinge, F., *Ergebn. allg. Path. path. Anat.*, 1933, **27**, 1.
132. Glynn, L. E., Loewi, G., *J. Path. Bact.*, 1952, **64**, 329.
133. Murphy, G. E., *Medicine (Baltimore)*, 1960, **39**, 289.
134. Clawson, B. J., *Arch. Path. (Chic.)*, 1929, **8**, 664.
135. Bennett, G. A., Zeller, J. W., Bauer, W., *Arch. Path. (Chic.)*, 1940, **30**, 70.

136. Murphy, G. E., in *Rheumatic Fever—A Symposium*, edited by L. Thomas, page 28. Minneapolis, 1952.
137. Pappenheimer, A. M., VonGlahn, W. C., *J. med. Res.*, 1924, **44**, 489.
138. MacCallum, W. G., *J. Amer. med. Ass.*, 1925, **84**, 1545.
139. Tweedy, P. S., *Brit. Heart J.*, 1956, **18**, 173.
140. Bland, E. F., Jones, T. D., *Circulation*, 1951, **4**, 836.
141. Begg, T. B., Kerr, J. W., Knowles, B. R., *Brit. med. J.*, 1962, **2**, 223.
142. Brock, R. C., *Brit. Heart J.*, 1952, **14**, 489.
143. Bramwell, J. Crighton, Duguid, J. B., *Quart. J. Med.*, 1928, **21**, 187.
144. Symmers, W. St C., *J. clin. Path.*, 1952, **5**, 36.
145. Lewis, T., *Heart*, 1914, **5**, 367.
146. Fraser, H. R. L., Turner, R. W. D., *Brit. med. J.*, 1955, **2**, 1414.
147. Daley, R., Mattingly, T. W., Holt, C. L., Bland, E. F., White, P. D., *Amer. Heart J.*, 1951, **42**, 566.
148. Read, A. E., Ball, K. P., Rob, C. G., *Quart. J. Med.*, 1960, N.S. **29**, 459.
149. Coombs, C., *Rheumatic Heart Disease*, page 5. Bristol, 1924.

INFECTIVE ENDOCARDITIS
150. Bloomfield, A. L., *A.M.A. Arch. intern. Med.*, 1956, **98**, 288.
151. Kerr, A., Jr, *Subacute Bacterial Endocarditis*, page 135. Springfield, Ill., 1955.
152. Kellow, W. F., Dowling, H. F., *A.M.A. Arch. intern. Med.*, 1957, **100**, 322.
153. Finland, M., *New Engl. J. Med.*, 1955, **253**, 909.
154. Cates, J. E., Christie, R. V., *Quart. J. Med.*, 1951, N.S. **44**, 93.
155. Peery, T. M., Belter, L. F., *Amer. J. Path.*, 1960, **36**, 673.
156. Marmion, B. P., Higgins, F. E., Bridges, J. B., Edwards, A. T., *Brit. med. J.*, 1960, **2**, 1264.
157. Derby, B. M., Coolidge, K., Rogers, D. E., *Arch. intern. Med.*, 1962, **110**, 63.
158. Winner, H. I., Hurley, R., *Candida Albicans*, chap. 15. London, 1964.
159. Luttgens, W. F., *Arch. intern. Med.*, 1949, **83**, 653.
160. Louria, D. B., Hensle, T., Rose, J., *Ann. intern. Med.*, 1967, **67**, 1.
161. Okell, C. C., Elliott, S. D., *Lancet*, 1935, **2**, 869.
162. Hobson, F. G., Juel-Jensen, B. E., *Brit. med. J.*, 1956, **2**, 1501.
163. Rhoads, P. S., Sibley, J. R., Billings, C. E., *J. Amer. med. Ass.*, 1955, **157**, 877.
164. Merritt, W. A., *J. Urol. (Baltimore)*, 1951, **65**, 100.
165. Wright, H. D., *J. Path. Bact.*, 1925, **28**, 541.
166. Gross, L., Fried, B. M., *Amer. J. Path.*, 1937, **13**, 769.
167. Lewis, T., Grant, R. T., *Heart*, 1923, **10**, 21.
168. Gross, L., *Arch. Path. (Chic.)*, 1937, **23**, 350.
169. Wright, J., Zeek, P. M., *Amer. Heart J.*, 1950, **19**, 587.
170. Harper, W. F., *J. Path. Bact.*, 1945, **57**, 229.
171. Grant, R. T., Wood, J. E., Jones, T. D., *Heart*, 1928, **14**, 247.
172. Allen, A. C., *Arch. Path. (Chic.)*, 1939, **27**, 399.
173. Perla, D., Marmorsten, J., *Natural Resistance and Clinical Medicine*, page 662. Boston, 1941.
174. Grant, R. T., *Guy's Hosp. Rep.*, 1936, **86**, 20.
175. Friedberg, C. K., Goldman, H. M., Field, L. E., *Arch. intern. Med.*, 1961, **107**, 6.

176. De Navasquez, S., *J. Path. Bact.*, 1939, **49**, 33.
177. Brunson, J. G., *Amer. J. Path.*, 1953, **29**, 689.
178. MacIlwaine, Y., *J. Path. Bact.*, 1947, **59**, 557.
179. Saphir, O., Katz, L. N., Gore, I., *Circulation*, 1950, **1**, 1155.
180. Stengel, A., Wolforth, C. C., *Arch. intern. Med.*, 1923, **31**, 527.
181. Parkhurst, G. F., Decker, J. P., *Amer. J. Path.*, 1955, **31**, 821.
182. Cates, J. E., Christie, R. V., *Quart. J. Med.*, 1951, N.S. **44**, 93.
183. Lewis, T., Harmer, I. M., *Heart*, 1926, **13**, 337.
184. Bell, E. T., *Amer. J. Path.*, 1932, **8**, 639.
185. Libman, E., Friedberg, C. K., *Subacute Bacterial Endocarditis*, 2nd edn. New York, 1948.
186. Villarreal, H., Sokoloff, L., *Amer. J. med. Sci.*, 1950, **220**, 655.
187. Cordeiro, A., Costa, H., Laginha, F., *Amer. J. Cardiol.*, 1965, **16**, 477.

SYPHILIS OF THE HEART
188. American Heart Association: Symposium on Cardiovascular Syphilis, *Amer. Heart J.*, 1930, **6**, 1–162.
189. Ministry of Health, London, *Report for the Year 1961—Part II: On the State of the Public Health*, page 235. London, 1962.
190. *The Registrar General's Statistical Review of England and Wales for the Year 1973*, Part 1(A). London, 1975.
191. Clawson, B. J., Bell, E. T., *Arch. Path. (Chic.)*, 1927, **4**, 922.
192. Weinstein, A., Kampmeier, R. H., Harwood, T. R., *A.M.A. Arch. intern. Med.*, 1957, **100**, 90.
193. Sohval, A. R., *Arch. Path. (Chic.)*, 1935, **20**, 429.
194. Saphir, O., Scott, R. W., *Amer. Heart J.*, 1930, **6**, 56.
195. Gordon, W. H., Parker, F., Jr, Weiss, S., *Arch. intern. Med.*, 1942, **70**, 396.
196. Burch, G. E., Winsor, T., *Amer. Heart J.*, 1942, **24**, 740.
197. Moritz, A. R., *Arch. Path. (Chic.)*, 1931, **11**, 44.
198. Jones, E., Bedford, D. E., *Brit. Heart J.*, 1943, **5**, 107.
199. Gorlin, R., McMillan, I. K. R., Medd, W. D., Matthews, M. B., Daley, R., *Amer. J. Med.*, 1955, **18**, 855.

MISCELLANEOUS MYOCARDIAL ABNORMALITIES
200. Gordon, R. S., Cherkes, A. J., *J. clin. Invest.*, 1956, **35**, 206.
201. Messer, J. V., Wagman, R. J., Levine, H. J., Neill, W. A., Krasnow, N., Gorlin, R., *J. clin. Invest.*, 1962, **41**, 725.
202. Danforth, W. H., Ballard, F. B., Kako, K., Choudhury, J. D., Bing, R. J., *Circulation*, 1960, **21**, 112.
203. Blain, J. M., Schafer, H., Siegel, M. S., Bing, R. J., *Amer. J. Med.*, 1956, **20**, 820.
204. Olson, R. E., *J. chron. Dis.*, 1959, **9**, 442.
205. Smith, H. L., *Amer. Heart J.*, 1928, **4**, 79.
206. Zeek, P. M., *Arch. Path. (Chic.)*, 1942, **34**, 820.
207. Coppoletta, J. M., Wolbach, S. B., *Amer. J. Path.*, 1933, **9**, 55.
208. Byrom, F. B., Dodson, L. F., *Clin. Sci.*, 1949, **8**, 1.
209. Drury, A. N., Wightman, K. J. R., *Quart. J. exp. Physiol.*, 1940, **30**, 45.
210. Drury, A. N., *Quart. J. exp. Physiol.*, 1945, **33**, 107.
211. Symmers, W. St C., *J. clin. Path.*, 1956, **9**, 187.

212. Josselson, A. J., Pruitt, R. D., Edwards, J. E., *A.M.A. Arch. Path.*, 1952, **54**, 359.

213. Eliat, R. S., McGee, H. J., Blount, S. G., *Circulation*, 1961, **23**, 613.

214. Jones, R. S., Frazier, D. B., *Arch. Path. (Chic.)*, 1950, **50**, 366.

215. Pomerance, A., *personal communication*, quoted by Linzbach, A. J., Akuamoa-Boateng, E., *Klin. Wschr.*, 1973, **51**, 164.

216. Schmid, R., Manners, D. J., Illingworth, B., Brown, D. H., Hers, H. G., Larner, J., in *Ciba Foundation Symposium: Control of Glycogen Metabolism*, edited by W. J. Whelan and M. P. Cameron, pages 305–374. London, 1964.

217. Cori, G. T., *Mod. Probl. Pädiat.*, 1957, **3**, 344.

218. Gierke, E. von, *Beitr. path. Anat.*, 1929, **82**, 497.

219. Muller, O. F., Bellet, S., Ertrugrul, A., *Circulation*, 1961, **23**, 261.

220. Pompe, J. C., *Ann. Anat. path.*, 1933, **10**, 23.

221. Forbes, B. G. B., *J. Pediat.*, 1953, **42**, 645.

222. Andersen, D. H., *Lab. Invest.*, 1956, **5**, 11.

223. Sidbury, J. B., Jr, Mason, J., Burns, W. B., Jr, Ruebner, B. H., *Bull. Johns Hopk. Hosp.*, 1962, **111**, 157.

224. McArdle, B., *Clin. Sci.*, 1951, **10**, 13.

225. Hers, H. G., *Rev. int. Hépat.*, 1959, **9**, 35.

226. Weiss, S., *J. Amer. med. Ass.*, 1940, **115**, 832.

227. Rowlands, D. T., Viltek, C. F., *Circulation*, 1960, **21**, 4.

228. Passmore, R., Meiklejohn, A. P., in *Biochemical Disorders in Human Disease*, edited by E. J. King and R. M. S. Thompson, page 567. London, 1957.

229. Burwell, C. S., Dexter, L., *Trans. Ass. Amer. Phycns*, 1947, **60**, 59.

230. Weiss, S., Wilkins, R. W., *Ann. intern. Med.*, 1937, **11**, 108.

231. McLeod, J. W., Orr, J. W., Woodcock, H. E. de C., *J. Path. Bact.*, 1939, **48**, 99.

232. Gore, I., *Amer. J. med. Sci.*, 1948, **215**, 257.

233. Hoel, J., Berg, A. M., *Acta med. scand.*, 1953, **145**, 393.

234. Ludden, T. E., Edwards, J. E., *Amer. J. Path.*, 1949, **25**, 357.

235. Saphir, O., in *Pathology of the Heart*, edited by S. E. Gould, 2nd edn, page 809. Springfield, Ill., 1960.

236. Spain, D. M., Bradess, V. A., Parsonnet, V., *Amer. Heart J.*, 1950, **40**, 336.

237. Stoeber, E., *Z. Kinderheilk.*, 1947, **65**, 114.

238. Javett, S. N., Heymann, S., Mundel, B., Pepler, W. J., Lurie, H. I., Gear, J., Measroch, V., Kirsch, Z., *J. Pediat.*, 1956, **48**, 1.

239. Fechner, R. E., Smith, M. G., Middelkamp, J. N., *Amer. J. Path.*, 1963, **42**, 493.

240. Callahan, W. P., Russell, W. O., Smith, M. G., *Medicine (Baltimore)*, 1946, **25**, 343.

241. Potts, R. E., Williams, A. A., *Lancet*, 1956, **1**, 483.

242. Hooper, A. D., *A.M.A. Arch. Path.*, 1957, **64**, 1.

243. Bruni Celli, B., *Arch. Hosp. Vargas*, 1960, **2**, 558.

244. Köberle, F., *Virchows Arch. path. Anat.*, 1957, **330**, 267.

245. Porter, G. H., *New Engl. J. Med.*, 1960, **263**, 1350.

246. Pascoe, H. R., *Arch. Path. (Chic.)*, 1964, **77**, 299.

247. Hudson, R. E. B., *Cardiovascular Pathology*, vol. 3, page S.483. London, 1970.

248. Ivemark, B., Thorén, C., *Acta med. scand.*, 1964, **175**, 227.

249. Russell, D. S., *J. Path. Bact.*, 1946, **58**, 739.

250. Zatuchni, J., Aergerter, E. E., Molthan, L., Shuman, C. R., *Circulation*, 1951, **3**, 846.

251. Hudson, R. E. B., *Brit. Heart J.*, 1960, **22**, 153.

252. Gross, L., Fried, B. M., *Amer. J. Path.*, 1936, **12**, 31.

253. Crawford, J. H., Di Gregorio, N. J., *Amer. Heart J.*, 1947, **34**, 540.

254. Lev, M., Unger, P. N., *A.M.A. Arch. Path.*, 1955, **60**, 502.

255. Porter, G. H., *New Engl. J. Med.*, 1960, **263**, 1350.

256. Davies, M. J., *Pathology of Conducting Tissue of the Heart*. London, 1971.

257. Brigden, W., *Lancet*, 1957, **2**, 1179.

258. Hudson, R. E. B., *Cardiovascular Pathology*, vol. 3, page S.546. London, 1970.

259. Goodwin, J. F., *Lancet*, 1970, **1**, 731.

260. Emanuel, R., Withers, R., O'Brien, K., *Lancet*, 1971, **2**, 1065.

261. Davies, M. J., *personal communication*.

262. Teare, R. D., *Brit. Heart J.*, 1958, **20**, 1.

263. Braunwald, E., Morrow, A. G., Cornell, W. P., Aygen, M. M., Hilbish, T. F., *Amer. J. Med.*, 1960, **29**, 924.

264. Cohen, J., Effat, H., Goodwin, J. F., Oakley, C. M., Steiner, R. E., *Brit. Heart J.*, 1964, **26**, 16.

265. *Hypertrophic Obstructive Cardiomyopathy*, edited by G. E. W. Wolstenholme and M. O'Connor. London, 1971.

266. Van Noorden, S., Pearse, A. G. E., in *Hypertrophic Obstructive Cardiomyopathy*, edited by G. E. W. Wolstenholme and M. O'Connor, page 192. London, 1971.

267. Meessen, H., Poche, R., *Anglo-Germ. med. Rev.*, 1967, **4**, 73.

268. Bedford, D. E., Konstam, G. L. S., *Brit. Heart J.*, 1946, **8**, 236.

269. Ball, J. D., Williams, A. W., Davies, J. N. P., *Lancet*, 1954, **1**, 1049.

270. Williams, A. W., Ball, J. D., Davies, J. N. P., *Trans. roy. Soc. trop. Med. Hyg.*, 1954, **48**, 290.

271. Davies, J. N. P., Ball, J. D., *Brit. Heart J.*, 1955, **17**, 337.

272. Brockington, I. F., Olsen, E. G. F., Goodwin, J. F., *Lancet*, 1967, **1**, 584.

273. Somers, K., Fowler, J. M., in *Introduction to the Cardiomyopathies*, edited by A. G. Shaper, page 25. Basel, 1968.

274. Hutt, M. S. R., Edington, G. M., in *Introduction to the Cardiomyopathies*, edited by A. G. Shaper, page 22. Basel, 1968.

275. Crawford, M. A., *Lancet*, 1962, **1**, 352.

276. Shaper, A. G., Kaplan, M. H., Foster, W. D., MacIntosh, D. M., Wilks, M. E., *Lancet*, 1967, **1**, 598.

MISCELLANEOUS ENDOCARDIAL ABNORMALITIES

277. Rosahn, P. D., *Bull. N.Y. Acad. Med.*, 1955, **31**, 453.

278. Thomas, W. A., Randall, R. V., Bland, E. F., Castleman, B., *New Engl. J. Med.*, 1954, **251**, 327.

279. Gowing, N. F. C., *J. Path. Bact.*, 1953, **65**, 13.

280. Thomas, W. A., Randall, R. V., Bland, E. F., Castleman, B., *New Engl. J. Med.*, 1954, **251**, 327.

281. Hudson, R. E. B., *Cardiovascular Pathology*, vol. 1, page 863. London, 1965.

282. Allen, A. C., Sirota, J. H., *Amer. J. Path.*, 1944, **20**, 1025.

283. MacDonald, R. A., Robbins, S. L., *Ann. intern. Med.*, 1957, **46**, 255.

284. Pomerance, A., *J. Path. Bact.*, 1961, **81**, 135.

285. Libman, E., Sacks, B., *Arch. intern. Med.*, 1924, **33**, 701.
286. Muehrcke, R. C., Kark, R. M., Pirani, C. L., Pollak, V. E., *Medicine (Baltimore)*, 1957, **36**, 1.

CHRONIC CARDIAC FAILURE
287. Hajdu, S., Leonard, E., *Pharmacol. Rev.*, 1959, **11**, 173.
288. Katz, L. N., Feinberg, H., Shaffer, A. B., *Circulation*, 1960, **21**, 95.
289. Kako, K., Bing, R. J., *J. clin. Invest.*, 1958, **37**, 465.
290. Wade, G., Werkö, L., Eliasch, H., Gidlund, A., Lagerlöf, H., *Quart. J. Med.*, 1952, N.S. **21**, 361.
291. Holling, H. E., Venner, A., *Brit. Heart J.*, 1956, **18**, 103.
292. Novack, P., Schlant, R. C., Haynes, F. W., Phinney, A. O., *J. clin. Invest.*, 1957, **36**, 917.
293. Donald, K. W., Bishop, J. M., Wade, O. L., Wormald, P. N., *Clin. Sci.*, 1957, **16**, 325.
294. Gorlin, R., McMillan, I. K. R., Medd, W. D., Matthews, M. B., Daley, R., *Amer. J. Med.*, 1955, **18**, 855.
295. Taylor, S. H., Donald, K. W., Bishop, J. M., *Clin. Sci.*, 1957, **16**, 351.
296. Bishop, J. M., Donald, K. W., Wade, O. L., *Clin. Sci.*, 1955, **14**, 329.
297. Shackman, R., *Clin. Sci.*, 1958, **17**, 317.
298. Blumgart, H. L., *Medicine (Baltimore)*, 1931, **10**, 1.
299. Ball, J. D., Kopelman, H., Witham, A. C., *Brit. Heart J.*, 1952, **14**, 363.
300. Soulié, P., Baillet, J., Carlotti, J., Chiche, P., Picard, R., Servelle, M., Voci, G., *Arch. Mal. Cœur*, 1953, **46**, 393.
301. Zu Jeddeloh, B., *Beitr. path. Anat.*, 1931, **86**, 387.
302. Kopelman, H., Lee, G. de J., *Clin. Sci.*, 1951, **10**, 383.
303. Lendrum, A. C., Scott, L. D. W., Park, S. D. S., *Quart. J. Med.*, 1950, N.S. **19**, 24.
304. Broustet, P., Bricaus, H., *Arch. Mal. Cœur*, 1956, **49**, 234.
305. Heath, D., Whitaker, W., *J. Path. Bact.*, 1955, **70**, 291.
306. Symmers, W. St C., *J. clin. Path.*, 1952, **5**, 36.
307. Ebert, R. V., *Arch. intern. Med.*, 1961, **107**, 450.
308. Castaing, R., Bricaud, H., Broustet, P., Marty, J., *Arch. Mal. Cœur*, 1952, **45**, 725.
309. Kopelman, H., Lee, G. de J., *Clin. Sci.*, 1951, **10**, 383.
310. Rapaport, E., Kuida, H., Haynes, F. W., Dexter, L., *J. clin. Invest.*, 1956, **35**, 1393.
311. White, H. C., Butler, J., Donald, K. W., *Clin. Sci.*, 1958, **17**, 667.
312. Donald, K. W., Bishop, J. M., Wade, O. L., *Clin. Sci.*, 1955, **14**, 531.
313. Fraser, F. R., Harris, C. F., Hilton, R., Linder, G. C., *Quart. J. Med.*, 1928, **22**, 1.
314. Huckabee, W. E., Judson, W. E., *J. clin. Invest.*, 1958, **37**, 1577.
315. Albert, R. E., Eichna, L. W., *Amer. Heart J.*, 1952, **43**, 395.
316. Krogh, A., Landis, E. M., Turner, A. H., *J. clin. Invest.*, 1932, **11**, 63.
317. Landis, E. M., Gibbon, J. H., *J. clin. Invest.*, 1933, **12**, 105.
318. Bramkamp, R. G., *J. clin. Invest.*, 1935, **14**, 34.
319. Stead, E. A., Warren, J. V., *J. clin. Invest.*, 1944, **23**, 283.
320. Merrill, A. J., *J. clin. Invest.*, 1946, **25**, 389.
321. Mokotoff, R., Ross, G., Leiter, L., *J. clin. Invest.*, 1948, **27**, 1.
322. Taylor, S. H., Donald, K. W., Bishop, J. M., *Clin. Sci.*, 1957, **16**, 351.
323. Gorlin, R., McMillan, I. K. R., Medd, W. D., Matthews, M. B., Daley, R., *Amer. J. Med.*, 1955, **18**, 855.

TUMOURS OF THE HEART
324. Mahaim, I., *Les Tumeurs et les polypes du cœur*, Paris, 1945.
325. Diffording, J. T., Gardner, R. E., Roe, B. B., *Circulation*, 1961, **23**, 929.
326. Kroopf, S. S., Peterson, C. A., *A.M.A. Arch. intern. Med.*, 1957, **100**, 819.
327. Willis, R. A., *The Borderland of Embryology and Pathology*, page 375. London, 1962.
328. Symmers, W. St C., *unpublished series*, 1964–71.
329. Willis, R. A., *The Spread of Tumours in the Human Body*, 2nd edn, chap. 17. London, 1952.
330. Hanfling, S. M., *Circulation*, 1960, **22**, 474.

ACKNOWLEDGEMENTS FOR ILLUSTRATIONS

Figs 1.1, 4, 5, 18, 27, 29, 34, 53. Gordon Museum, Guy's Hospital, London; reproduced by permission of the Curator, Mr J. D. Maynard; photograph by Miss P. M. Turnbull, Charing Cross Hospital Medical School, London.

Figs 1.6, 9. Radiographs from St George's Hospital, London.

Fig. 1.7. Radiograph lent by Dr J. G. Jackson, Charing Cross Hospital Medical School, London, and Dr B. Murphy, Torbay Group Laboratories, Torquay, Devon.

Fig. 1.8. Redrawn from Fig. 39 in: Gregg, D. E., *Coronary Circulation in Health and Disease*, page 98; London, 1950. Reproduced by permission of Dr Donald E. Gregg, Walter Reed Army Institute of Research, Washington, D.C., and of the publishers, Messrs Henry Kimpton.

Fig. 1.11. Museum of the Department of Pathology, Guy's Hospital Medical School, London; photograph by Miss

P. M. Turnbull, Charing Cross Hospital Medical School, London.

Figs 1.13, 14, 15. Reproduced by permission of the editors from: Symmers, W. St C., *Verh. dtsch. Ges. Path.*, 1953, **36**, 224.

Figs 1.16, 19, 23, 26, 28, 52. Pathology Museum, Charing Cross Hospital Medical School, London; reproduced by permission of the Curator, Dr B. Fox; photographs by Miss P. M. Turnbull, Charing Cross Hospital Medical School.

Fig. 1.25. Redrawn from Fig. 4 in: Brock, R. C., *Brit. Heart J.*, 1952, **14**, 489. Reproduced by permission of Lord Brock and of the editor.

Fig. 1.30. Photograph provided by Dr G. A. K. Missen, Guy's Hospital, London.

Fig. 1.35. Redrawn from Figs 5 and 6 in: Scott, R. W., *Arch. intern. Med.*, 1924, **34**, 645. Reproduced by permission of the editor of the *Archives of Internal Medicine*, and of the Executive Managing Editor of the specialty journals of the American Medical Association, Chicago, Illinois.

Fig. 1.36. Reproduced by permission of the editor from: Symmers, W. St C., *J. clin. Path.*, 1956, **9**, 187.

Fig. 1.37. From a case in which the histological diagnosis was made by Dr B. McArdle, Guy's Hospital Medical School, London.

Fig. 1.38. Preparation provided by Dr M. O. Skelton, Lewisham Hospital, London.

Fig. 1.39. Preparation provided by Dr S. Scheidegger, Pathological Institute of the University of Basle, Switzerland.

Fig. 1.40. Photomicrograph provided by W. St C. Symmers.

Figs 1.41, 42. Photographs provided by Dr Blas Bruni Celli, Vargas Hospital, Caracas, Venezuela.

Fig. 1.43. Preparation provided by W. St C. Symmers.

Fig. 1.44. Specimen presented to Charing Cross Hospital Medical School, London, by Dr G. A. C. Summers, County Hospital, York; photograph by Miss P. M. Turnbull, Charing Cross Hospital Medical School.

Fig. 1.45. Preparation provided by Dr W. M. R. Henderson, Pembury Hospital, Kent.

Figs 1.48, 49. Reproduced by permission of the author and editor from: Teare, R. D., *Brit. Heart J.*, 1958, **20**, 1.

Figs 1.50, 51. Reproduced by permission of the authors and publisher, Edward Arnold, from: Edington, G. M., Gilles, H. M., *Pathology in the Tropics*, Figs 82 and 83; London, 1969.

Fig. 1.54. Photograph provided by Dr Ariela Pomerance, Northwick Park Hospital, Harrow, Middlesex.

Figs 1.55, 57. Photographs provided by Dr K. J. Randall, Orpington Hospital, Kent, who carried out the necropsy while at Guy's Hospital, London, in 1946. Reproduced by permission of Dr T. B. Brewin, Royal Infirmary, Glasgow, and of the editors, from: Brewin, T. B., *Guy's Hosp. Rep.*, 1948, **97**, 64.

Fig. 1.56. Photograph provided by Dr K. J. Randall, Orpington Hospital, Kent.

2: *Congenital Anomalies of the Heart and Great Vessels*

by R. E. B. HUDSON *and* C. P. WENDELL-SMITH

CONTENTS

2: *Congenital Anomalies of the Heart and Great Vessels*

by R. E. B. HUDSON *and* C. P. WENDELL-SMITH

MODERN METHODS OF DIAGNOSIS

Cardiac catheterization—first performed, on himself, by Forssmann[1] in Germany, in 1929, and developed as a practical investigative procedure some years later by Cournand[2, 3] and Richards[3] in the United States of America—is widely used in the study of congenital anomalies of the heart and great blood vessels. By its means, shunts between the systemic and pulmonary circulations can be detected, and the pressures in various parts of the heart and in the great arteries can be measured. Radio-opaque fluids can be injected directly into the chambers of the heart and recorded by cineradiography or on serial films, so that the spread of the material through abnormal apertures can be studied, and malformations, such as a narrowing of the outflow tract from the right ventricle, be delineated. Innocuous dyes or radio-active tracers can be injected into the heart or vessels and their appearance detected and graphically recorded with the help of an appropriate detector. Again, in the so-called retrograde studies, the catheter is inserted into a peripheral artery and pushed thence to the aorta and ventricle to enable the aortic valve or the coronary arteries to be studied by injecting dyes or radio-opaque fluid against the aortic blood stream.

These advances in diagnostic techniques laid the foundations for equally remarkable advances in surgery. The development of safe methods of producing hypothermia gave the surgeon time to open the heart and repair a defect or relieve a simple valve stenosis while the circulation is virtually arrested for a period of several minutes. Efficient machines have been devised by which the circulation of the blood and its gaseous exchanges can be maintained independently of the heart and lungs, which, in effect, are taken out of the circulation so that all kinds of intricate surgical procedures can be undertaken unhurriedly inside the opened heart; during these operations the beat of the heart can

now be halted temporarily and in safety. These techniques make it possible to resect diseased portions of arteries, or bypass them, using a homograft or a tube of synthetic material; similarly, abnormal valves can be replaced and by the insertion of baffles the direction of blood flow can be changed.

Comparable advances have been made in the accurate recording of heart sounds and murmurs by phonocardiography, which enables their precise relation to the cardiac cycle to be determined. Further, echocardiography, by which the size and thickness of the chambers of the heart and of the great arteries can be measured and the mobility of the atrioventricular valves determined, is a further means of establishing the presence and nature of congenital anomalies.

The knowledge accruing from these various diagnostic techniques has led to much greater comprehension of the significance of clinical signs of congenital cardiovascular disease that previously had been imperfectly understood. As a result, many congenital conditions can now be readily and accurately recognized by clinical methods alone.

The advances in diagnosis and treatment of congenital anomalies of the heart and great vessels have greatly increased the importance of these diseases in the teaching of pathology. In the account that follows, an attempt is made to explain the various anomalies in terms of the faults in embryonic development that they represent. Attention is directed mainly to those conditions that are consistent with the affected individual's extrauterine survival, and particularly those that are remediable by surgical means.

AETIOLOGY

Congenital anomalies of the heart may result from an abnormality of the zygote or an abnormal environment.

Abnormality of the zygote may or may not be inherited. Clear-cut examples of Mendelian inheritance are uncommon in congenital heart disease. Mendelian dominance is seen in *Marfan's syndrome*, a systemic disorder of connective tissue that is characterized by arachnodactyly and that may have cardiovascular components (see page 82).[4] The commonest cardiovascular anomalies in Marfan's syndrome are aortic valve disease and medial degeneration of the aorta, the latter predisposing to the development of dissecting aneurysm (see page 149). Mendelian recessive inheritance operates in the aetiology of *situs inversus*, the condition in which the viscera are situated on the side of the body opposite to that on which they are normally found. There is evidence that recessive inheritance may also account for some other malformations.[5] In many cases, however, the genetical factor merely determines susceptibility to malformation, other factors being responsible for its actual development; under these circumstances the occurrence of malformations in the family is sporadic, and the individual manifestations are variable.

Anomalies of Chromosomal Number.—Cardiovascular malformations may occur as a manifestation of abnormality of the chromosome content of the zygote, as in the *trisomies*, in which there is an extra autosome (which may be translocated—that is, joined to another chromosome). The most frequent trisomies are Down's syndrome (mongolism; trisomy-21; karyotype 47,XX,21+) (see Chapter 34), in which atrioventricular defects are common, and Patau's trisomy-13 (47,XX,13+) and Edwards's trisomy-18 (47,XX,18+), both of which are often accompanied by ventricular septal defect, persistent ductus arteriosus or double exit right ventricle. In the *monosomies* there is a missing chromosome: in the classic example, Turner's syndrome (karyotype 45,X) (see Chapter 26), stenosis of the aortic valve and, more rarely, coarctation of the aorta may occur.[6–8]

Twins.—Congenital heart disease is about twice as common in twins, both monozygotic and dizygotic, as in the general population.[9] If both of a pair of monozygotic twins are affected, the abnormality is usually the same in both. If only one of monozygotic twins is affected it is possible that the malformation concerned is caused by environmental factors in the womb.

The cardiovascular anatomy of *conjoined twins* may be highly abnormal and requires meticulous investigation before surgical separation can be contemplated. When the twins are joined in the thoracic region there may be two hearts, or two separated ventricles with one atrium, or a single heart: the type may be determined electrocardiographically.[10]

Local Factors.—Many embryologists believe that the flow of blood within the heart at any particular time in fetal growth is a determining force in its further development and provides a mechanism through which genetical forces can operate. Local deformities of the heart tube can produce anomalies of flow that reproduce the characteristics of any of the gamut of cardiac anomalies.[11] The external shape of the heart is probably little affected by internal flow. Abnormalities of shape may be associated with growth within a confined space, for it has been demonstrated that the asymmetry of the heart may be reversed by external pressure.[12]

During the active growth of the heart its cells have a high metabolic rate and mitotic division is conspicuous. Alteration in their environment may affect their metabolism directly, or possibly indirectly by interfering with the operation of normal genes. Environmental changes capable of acting thus may be induced experimentally.[13]

Viral Infections.—Of particular interest in recent years has been the observation that if the mother contracts *rubella* during the first hundred days of pregnancy the development of the fetus may be gravely affected.[14] Indeed, under these circumstances as many as a third of the infants born present some form of congenital anomaly, including blindness, deafness, hepatitis, haemolytic disease, thrombocytopenic purpura and cardiovascular lesions. The last include myocarditis, persistent ductus arteriosus, stenosis of the pulmonary and renal arteries and supravalvar aortic stenosis. Now that the virus of rubella has been isolated, vaccines are on trial for protecting susceptible children and also women of child-bearing age. Other viruses that can cross the placenta and may harm the fetus include those of measles, Asian influenza and mumps, cytomegalovirus and Coxsackie virus B.[15–17]

Drugs.—Drugs may also harm the fetus. Although this was well known from experimental evidence, it was not until the thalidomide disaster of the early 1960s, in which many hundreds of women who had taken this tranquilliser during pregnancy gave birth to deformed babies, that the potential danger of giving drugs, especially new and untried ones, to women in early pregnancy became widely recognized.[18]

Conclusion.—In considering the mode of operation of these various factors the concept of arrest of development has often been overemphasized;[19] many examples represent aberrant rather than arrested growth. It is worthy of note, too, that aberrant or arrested resorption of unneeded tissues may also play a part in the genesis of malformation.

FUNCTIONAL DISTURBANCES AND OTHER COMPLICATIONS ASSOCIATED WITH CARDIOVASCULAR ANOMALIES

Various functional disturbances in the circulation may be associated with congenital anomalies of the heart and great vessels. Some of the more important will be mentioned here.

Cyanosis.—Cyanosis results when a malformation allows access of venous blood to the systemic arterial circulation in considerable amounts. It is accompanied in its severer forms by polycythaemia, and by clubbing of the ends of the digits. The development of cyanosis after birth commonly indicates reversal of a shunt that at birth was arteriovenous (that is, from the arterial side of the circulation to the venous): thus, the shunt through a persistent ductus arteriosus reverses if pulmonary hypertension develops and the pressure in the pulmonary artery rises above that in the aorta.

Many cyanotic patients, and especially those with Fallot's tetrad, find the squatting position the most comfortable for resting; others prefer to lie supine. Various explanations have been suggested for such effects of posture. The oxygen saturation of the blood in these patients is higher in their position of preference[20] and this, perhaps, is a result of functional change at the site of the venoarterial shunt that accompanies the postural limitation of the blood flow to the legs.[21]

Severe attacks of dyspnoea, sometimes referred to as 'blue spells' and 'anoxic attacks', and even fatal syncope may occur in infants with Fallot's tetrad, especially when crying, feeding or defaecating. Various explanations of these attacks have been suggested, including an increase in the venoarterial shunt accompanying a further constriction of the right ventricular outflow caused by increased catecholamine stimulation; overheating and tachycardia have also been blamed. Prophylactic use of beta-adrenergic blocking drugs has proved successful in preventing this complication.[22]

Pulmonary Hypertension.—Anomalies such as atrial and ventricular septal defects and persistent ductus arteriosus may be complicated by pulmonary hypertension. This development profoundly alters the clinical picture and prognosis. It occurs in only a relatively small proportion of cases and its cause is obscure. At first, the pulmonary arteries show no more than simple hypertrophy of the medial coat: at this stage the condition may be reversible. Later, intimal proliferation, medial damage, thrombosis and recanalization occur. In the presence of such permanent structural changes pulmonary hypertension may rise high enough to reverse the shunt, causing cyanosis (the so-called 'Eisenmenger syndrome of Wood'[23]); at this stage surgical correction of the abnormality is useless, and, indeed, may be dangerous.

Thrombosis.—Thrombosis is not uncommon in the main pulmonary arteries as a complication of congenital malformations, particularly atrial septal defects. It seems to be related to the greatly increased blood flow to the lungs, and to the development of pulmonary hypertension, which tends to lessen this flow; repeated small episodes of pulmonary embolism may also be concerned. It has been observed that there may be a transient haemorrhagic state in the hypoxic newborn infant, with possible damage to vital organs from intravascular fibrin deposition.[24]

Myocardial Changes.—In the congenitally abnormal heart, hypertrophy of the myocardium occurs in the wall of the chamber that bears the greatest load. In addition, fatty changes are common, and in cases of severe malformation microscopical infarcts and scars may result from the supply of 'venous' blood to the myocardium.[25, 26]

Paradoxical Embolism.—Paradoxical embolism is said to occur when a thrombotic embolus from the systemic veins passes through a right-to-left shunt and thus lodges not in the pulmonary vasculature but in a systemic vessel. Very rarely, an embolus is found actually impacted in a shunt orifice, for example a valvular foramen ovale.[27]

Infection.—The risk of infection of a shunt channel or of a congenital stenotic lesion is constantly present. Antibiotic prophylaxis is a necessary safeguard whenever any such ordinarily minor procedure as a tooth extraction or catheterization of the urinary bladder is undertaken. The organism concerned is commonly *Streptococcus viridans*, and the changes that result at the site of the infection are completely comparable with those found in other cases of infective endocarditis (see page 34). In conditions like Fallot's tetrad, in which much venous blood enters the systemic circuit without filtering through the lungs, infarction of the brain may occur as an embolic complication of infective lesions in the right side of the heart.

ANOMALIES OF THE HEART AS A WHOLE

Development.—In the early somite embryo bilateral endothelial tubes are fusing to form a single primitive heart tube in the mesoderm, ventral to the foregut (Fig. 2.1A). Caudal to the heart tube is the mesoderm of the septum transversum. In this

the veins collect, forming the sinus venosus, which leads into a primitive atrium on each side. The atria lead to the single primitive ventricle, and thence to the bulbus cordis and ventral aortae, from which arises the first pair of aortic arches (Fig. 2.1B).

Ventral to the endothelial heart tube is the primitive pericardial cavity. Intervening is the myo-epicardial mantle, which is myogenic, and the myoendocardial space, which is filled with cardiac jelly—the precursor of cushion tissue (Fig. 2.1A). The cavity extends dorsally and then medially, so that the heart tube becomes suspended within it by a thin dorsal mesocardium. A spurt of growth results in looping of the bulboventricular segments ventrally (Figs 2.1C and 2.1D) and breakdown of the mesocardium dorsally, thus forming the trans-

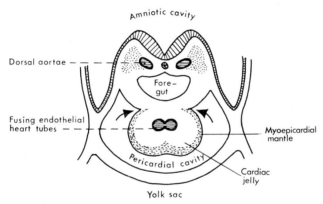

A. Cross-section of fusing heart tubes (third week of embryonic development).

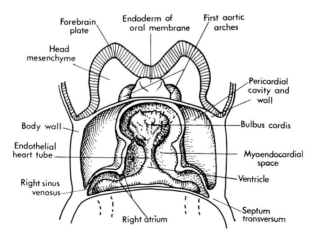

B. Ventral view of endothelial heart tubes early in the fourth week. The ventral body wall and myoepicardial mantle have been removed.

Fig. 2.1. Schematic diagrams of the heart at successive periods in embryonic development.

verse sinus of the pericardium. Meanwhile, the region between the bulbus and the aortic arches elongates outside the pericardium to form the truncus arteriosus (see page 103); the inflow from the sinus venosus is deviated to the right side, and a common pulmonary vein grows out to meet the pulmonary venous plexus (see page 83).

As growth proceeds, the atria fuse and rise out of the septum transversum: the bulboventricular loop is deflected caudally and twisted anticlockwise (when viewed from the ventral aspect), so that the ventricular limb comes to lie on the left of a bulboventricular notch and the bulbar limb on the right of this notch (Fig. 2.1C). The notch becomes shallower as the proximal bulbus merges into the ventricle, forming a common chamber. The atrium continues to rise and becomes subdivided. Parts of the sinus venosus and pulmonary venous tree are incorporated into the dorsomedial aspects of the right atrium and left atrium respectively, so that the primitive atria migrate ventrally and appear on each side of the bulbus cordis (Fig. 2.1D). The bulboventricular chamber soon shows external subdivision into right and left ventricles by interventricular sulci. These changes all take place between the third and the seventh week; by the end of this time the external form and the internal septal complexes (see pages 86 and 92) are established. At first the septal complexes lie roughly in the sagittal plane, but by mid-pregnancy the heart has rotated through some 45° to the adult position.

Pericardial Anomalies.—Pericardial defects are rare.[28] Failure of the pericardium to develop properly may leave its cavity in free communication with the left pleural cavity. A result of this is that infection of the left pleural cavity will necessarily be accompanied by pericarditis.

Another anomaly—such as persistent ductus arteriosus, tricuspid incompetence, atrial septal defect, bronchogenic cyst, pulmonary sequestration or diaphragmatic hernia—is present in 20 per cent of cases of pericardial defect.[29]

Diverticula of the pericardial sac are rare anomalies.

Ectopia Cordis.—Ectopia cordis is rare, the heart lying outside the thoracic cage as a result of faulty development of the sternum and pericardium. In some cases the condition can be corrected by surgery.[30]

Dextrocardia and Laevocardia

Dextrocardia.—Dextrocardia is the condition in which the apex of the heart is on the right side;*

* The term *dextroposition* is used to describe any secondary displacement of the heart to the right. Dextroposition is seldom a result of congenital faults. Its usual causes are a pleural effusion or diaphragmatic hernia on the left side or adhesions on the right, or collapse of the right lung.

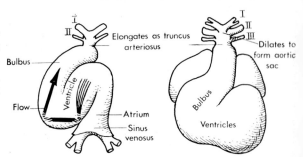

C. Ventral view of heart late in the fourth week.

D. Ventral view of heart in the fifth week.

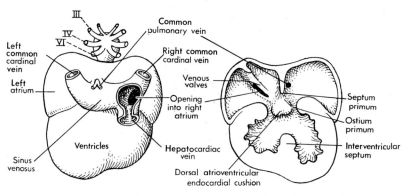

E. Dorsal view of heart at five weeks.

F. Coronal section of heart at five weeks, viewed from ventral aspect.

Fig. 2.1. Schematic diagrams of the heart at successive periods in embryonic development (see also pages 77 and 79).

there are four main types and an indeterminate group of variants.[31]

1. *Mirror-image dextrocardia* (*situs inversus totalis*). In this type of dextrocardia the form, position and connexions of the heart and abdominal viscera are the mirror image of the normal: otherwise the organs are usually structurally and functionally normal. The anomaly is genetically determined, and the asymmetry of the heart is reversed from the beginning of its development. As a result, the sinus venosus derivatives drain into the atrium on the left side and the pulmonary veins into the atrium on the right; the tricuspid valve is on the left side and the mitral valve on the right; the efflux from the left-sided ventricle passes to the pulmonary trunk and that from the right to the aorta. The transposition of the viscera—*situs inversus*—may be partial or complete; in partial

forms there are usually further abnormalities of the heart. Dextrocardia can be distinguished from dextroversion (see below) in the electrocardiogram.[32]

Some patients with dextrocardia have a predisposition to develop nasal sinusitis and bronchiectasis—this is *Kartagener's syndrome*.[33]

2. *Dextroversion* (pivotal dextrocardia). In dextroversion, the atria are normally placed but the ventricles are rotated so that the left ventricle is in front of and below the right ventricle: the rotation is usually associated with transposition of the great vessels.[32] An example that we studied showed, in addition, atrial and ventricular septal defects, pulmonary atresia and persistent ductus arteriosus, thus illustrating the multiplicity of malformations that may accompany the condition. Abdominal anomalies may also be present, including absence of the spleen and symmetrical heterotaxia—particularly, symmetrical disposition of the liver in relation to the median plane: such findings suggest that there has been suppression of left-sided structures, possibly as a result of external pressure. The position of the ventricles in dextroversion suggests that the anticlockwise twist of the bulboventricular loop has failed to take place.

3 and 4. '*Mixed dextrocardia*'. There are two forms of mixed dextrocardia: in one the atria are reversed and the ventricles are normal, in the other the ventricles are reversed and the atria are normal.

Laevocardia.—Laevocardia is a term that indicates that the apex of the heart is on the left side. There are four main types of laevocardia and an indeterminate group: these are the mirror-image counterparts of the corresponding forms of dextrocardia.[34] It will be appreciated that one type of laevocardia is the condition in the normal individual —the mirror image of *situs inversus totalis*. In all the other types the heart is always abnormal, often severely so. Sometimes the spleen is absent.

The counterpart of Kartagener's syndrome in cases of laevocardia with transposition of abdominal viscera is known as *Chandra's syndrome*.[35]

Asplenia and Polysplenia.—Cardiac anomalies, including atrial and ventricular septal defects, bilateral superior venae cavae and anomalous pulmonary veins, may be associated with asplenia (congenital absence of the spleen) or polysplenia (the presence of multiple spleens): these splenic anomalies may accompany complete *situs inversus abdominalis*, or the partial form in which the liver

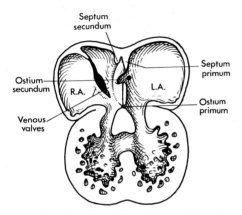

G. Coronal section of heart in seventh week.
L.A.—left atrium.
R.A.—right atrium.

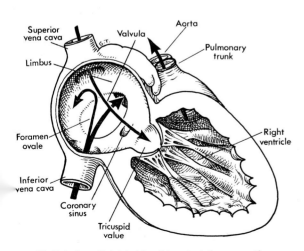

H. Interior of right side of heart at three months.

is medianly placed and there is malrotation of the bowel. Asplenia may be associated with trilobate lungs ('bilateral right-sidedness'), stenosis of the pulmonary valve, corrected transposition of the aorta and pulmonary artery, and absence of the duodenum. In contrast, polysplenia tends to be associated with bilobate lungs ('bilateral left-sidedness'), termination of the inferior vena cava in the azygos system, and absence of the gall bladder.[36]

Congenital Cardiomegaly

Enlargement of the heart in infants and children is usually secondary to a congenital structural defect. It may, however, result from infection or from abnormal vascular shunts,[37] or be a manifestation of certain hereditary nervous and muscular diseases (such as Friedreich's ataxia,[38] Refsum's syndrome,[39] muscular dystrophy[40] and dystrophia myotonica[41]). It may be due to primary myocardial disease,[42] such as storage diseases (see opposite), anomalies of the coronary arteries (see page 113), myocarditis and endomyocardial fibroelastosis. Sometimes it may be familial.[43]

Obstructive Cardiomyopathy.—This condition, which has attracted much attention since Teare's classic description of the necropsy findings in 1958,[44] has acquired various synonyms: these include asymmetrical hypertrophy,[44] hypertrophic obstructive cardiomyopathy,[45] idiopathic hypertrophic subaortic stenosis[46] and muscular subaortic stenosis.[47] It may become manifest at any age from birth. The characteristic finding (Fig. 2.2) is massive hypertrophy of the left ventricle, especially of the septum, causing resistance to ventricular filling and obstruction to the outflow from both ventricles, and interfering with the function of the mitral valve (some authorities consider mitral regurgitation to be the primary fault[45]). In studies of large series, 20 to 30 per cent of cases have been familial; the inheritance has been dominant in some families and recessive in others.[48] The sex incidence has been equal among familial cases; in contrast, males predominate by about two and a half to one among sporadic cases. In a rare autosomal dominant variety of the disease the condition is associated with the presence of multiple pigmented moles in the skin (lentiginosis).[49]

Biopsy of the ventricle has shown areas in which there are greatly enlarged muscle cells that have an 'empty' appearance, containing few myofibrils. The

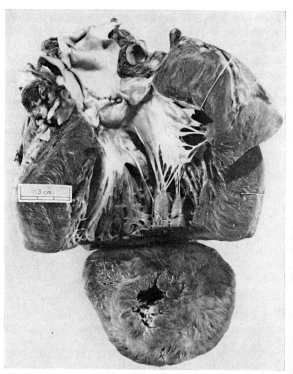

Fig. 2.2.§ Obstructive cardiomyopathy. The heart weighed 990 g. The patient was a boy of 16 years: he was short of stature and had dyspnoea and angina pectoris. Septal myotomy was performed. There is massive hypertrophy of the left ventricle; the septum projected into the right ventricle.

cells tend to be arranged in whorled fashion. Their nuclei are very large and of bizarre shapes. The interstitial fibrous tissue is increased in amount and there are areas where atrophy or necrosis of muscle—presumably ischaemic—has been followed by replacement fibrosis.[50]

Most patients with obstructive cardiomyopathy develop intractable heart failure eventually. Sudden death may occur at any time, particularly during strenuous exertion.

Miscellaneous Conditions

Infantile Endocardial Fibroelastosis.—Infantile endocardial fibroelastosis is a congenital condition in which the endocardium is markedly thickened. It may be primary, or secondary to stenotic or atretic lesions. The thickening results from an increase in the amount of collagenous and elastic fibrous tissue, particularly the latter. The left ventricle is affected oftener than the right. The sclerotic process occludes the vascular connexions between the cavity of the heart and the myocardial vessels; it may also involve the valves and chordae tendineae, which become thickened and adherent. Mural thrombosis may occur. When the thickening is marked it interferes with ventricular filling—this condition, which sometimes has been called constrictive endocarditis, leads to great enlargement of the heart. The electron microscope shows that the surface layers are composed of fibres indistinguishable from fibrin whereas in the deeper layers there are fewer of these fibres and a predominance of collagen.[51] These appearances suggest that the superficial layers are formed of fibrin, precipitated from the blood, and that the deeper layers represent organization of older similar deposits. Necrosis of muscle and replacement fibrosis at the myoendocardial junction may be due to vascular insufficiency.

The aetiology of the primary type of infantile endocardial fibroelastosis is unknown. Degenerative changes occur in the autonomic ganglia of the atria, and this, in association with subendocardial myocardiolysis, has been suggested as the primary cause.[52] Infection *in utero* by poliovirus, Coxsackie virus or mumps virus has also been postulated. Some workers have obtained a positive skin reaction to the intradermal inoculation of affected children with killed mumps antigen;[53] others have rejected the idea that there is any such association.[54] Familial factors may be concerned in some cases.[55]

Juxtaposition of the Atrial Appendages.—In this remarkable malformation the two atrial appendages lie either to the left (usually) or to the right of the great arteries instead of embracing them, one on each side. The condition results from anomalous folding of the primitive heart tube, and, not surprisingly, is accompanied by other cardiac anomalies and death in childhood, although survival to 25 years has been recorded. The commonest associated anomaly is transposition of the great vessels, with septal defects and various forms of valvar and subvalvar stenosis: 'corrected transposition' occurs, more frequently with right juxtaposition than left.[56]

'Parchment Heart'.—In this unexplained anomaly, first described by Osler,[57] the muscular tissue of the right ventricle is virtually absent so that the thin fibrous wall of the chamber resembles parchment.[58] The right atrium is greatly hypertrophied to assist the sluggish right ventricle.

Congenital 'Rhabdomyomas' (Nodular Glycogenic Infiltration).—According to Prichard,[59] no true diffuse rhabdomyoma of the heart has been

described, and most, if not all, reported examples are probably manifestations of glycogen storage disease (see page 44). The localized lesions that have been described as 'rhabdomyomas' are probably best regarded as hamartomas. They are usually multiple (Fig. 2.3), not encapsulate and not inva-

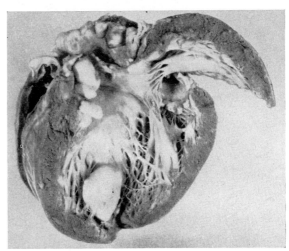

Fig. 2.3.§ 'Rhabdomyomas' in the heart of an infant, aged 13 days: left side of heart showing nodules protruding through the septum. The uppermost nodule is obstructing the aortic valve and impinges on a coronary ostium.

sive. Sometimes one of them is so situated that it interferes with the conducting system of the heart: surgical excision of such a nodule has been successfully accomplished.[60] Microscopically, the tissue is loose and sponge-like, due to conspicuous vacuolation. The vacuoles are mianly intercellular, and appear empty, through loss of the contained glycogen: some, however, are related to the so-called 'spider cells'—cells with many processes that suspend them within the vacuole (Fig. 2.4A), which then appears to be within the cytoplasm. The processes of the 'spider cells' and the walls of the vacuoles may show myostriation (Fig. 2.4B). It should be noted that the glycogen in this condition is not as resistant to aqueous solvents as the glycogen of von Gierke's disease[61]—in consequence, it may not be demonstrable histochemically in tissue that has been preserved in a watery fixative.

These tumours may occur in cases of tuberose sclerosis (epiloia) (see Chapter 34).

Storage Diseases.—The heart and vessels may be involved in storage diseases which, as inborn errors of metabolism, are germane to this chapter. Glycogen storage (see page 44) may produce cardiomegaly

§ See *Acknowledgements*, page 117.

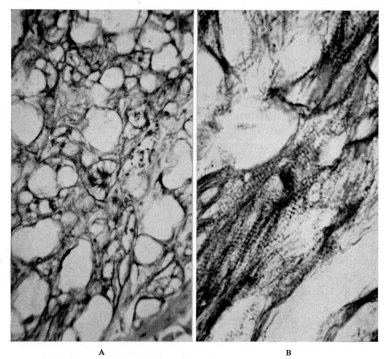

A   B

Fig. 2.4.§ Histology of 'rhabdomyoma' of the heart.
A. Sponge-like appearance of tumour, with a 'spider-cell' in the centre. × 385.
B. Area showing myocardial striations. × 760.
Both sections stained with phosphotungstic acid haematoxylin.

and a characteristic lacework appearance of the myocardium in histological sections (Pompe's disease).

Lipid storage diseases include Refsum's disease (in which the stored material is phytanic acid), Niemann–Pick disease (sphingomyelin), Hand–Schüller–Christian disease (cholesterol and neutral fat), Gaucher's disease (sphingosine, fatty acid, glucose), Fabry–Anderson disease (ceramide dihexose and trihexose) and lipoproteinosis. Most of them seldom involve the cardiovascular system seriously.

Mucopolysaccharide (glycosaminoglycan) storage diseases are familial and of many varieties, such as those that have been named after Hunter (sex-linked recessive polydystrophy), Hurler, Sanfilippo, Morquio and Ullrich, Scheie (autosomal recessive syndromes) and others. Dwarfism, mental deficiency and a gargoyle-like facies may be present, but many patients are free from such manifestations. The heart may be involved in all except Sanfilippo's type, being enlarged, with thickened deformed valves and narrowed coronary arteries. Excess of the stored material appears in the urine, providing a valuable means of screening those at risk.

Other Inborn Errors of Metabolism.—Haemochromatosis may give rise to pericarditis, disrhythmias and conduction disturbances. The myocardium is rusty brown because of the large amount of haemosiderin that has accumulated, particularly within the muscle cells. It is questionable whether the iron deposits in these cells seriously embarrass their function. The cardiac disturbances may be related to fibrosis developing round interstitial deposits of iron in proximity to the conducting system.

Primary oxalosis is characterized by the deposition of crystals of calcium oxalate in the kidneys, heart and other tissues. Myocardial fibrosis and sometimes heart block may result. The crystals can be seen in histological sections, particularly when examined in polarized light.

*Inherited Connective Tissue Diseases.—*Several of the inherited disorders of connective tissue involve the cardiovascular system. In *Marfan's syndrome,* an autosomal dominant condition, the patient is tall, thin and short-sighted and has long 'spider' fingers (arachnodactyly): the mitral and aortic valves may be enlarged and unusually lax and the aorta is often dilated and liable to develop medionecrosis with the attendant risk of dissecting aneurysm formation. Some patients with Marfan's syndrome also have homocystinuria, with mental deficiency, fatty change in the liver and liability to thrombosis; this is an autosomal recessive variant. *Ehlers–Danlos syndrome* (see Chapter 39), characterized by hyperelasticity of the skin, papyraceous scars and excessively mobile joints, is accompanied by a tendency to aneurysm formation and spontaneous rupture of arteries. Various congenital heart anomalies have been found in patients with the syndrome.

In *osteogenesis imperfecta* (see Chapter 37) the failure of collagen to mature adequately is manifested by multiple fractures, skeletal deformities, hyperextensible joints, blue sclerae and a tendency to develop hernias and to bleeding from defective vessels. The abnormality of collagen is seen in the heart in the form of occasional lesions of the aortic and mitral valves. *Pseudoxanthoma elasticum* (see Chapter 39) is a recessive, partly sex-linked, disease in which the skin of the neck, abdomen, groins, armpits and other flexures shows yellowish xanthoma-like plaques and papules, and becomes inelastic, redundant and sagging. The elastic tissue everywhere is coarse and fragmented. Involvement of blood vessels is manifested by claudication, angioid streaks in the optic fundi and other haemorrhages. The heart valves and atrial endocardium may be thickened, the appearances resembling those of chronic rheumatic disease.

Congenital Dysrhythmias.—These may be isolated disturbances. They sometimes prove fatal. *Ventricular tachycardia and fibrillation* may occur in children who have prolongation of the Q–T interval (Conor Ward's disease). When this disturbance is accompanied by congenital deafness it is sometimes referred to as the surdocardiac or cardioauditory syndrome of Jervell and Lange-Nielsen. The *Wolff–Parkinson–White syndrome* of bundle branch block, short P–R interval and a tendency to paroxysmal tachycardia in otherwise healthy young people may be due to a circus movement of the conduction impulse, which traverses the His–Tawara system and then re-enters retrogradely by an accessory pathway—for instance, a 'bundle of Kent'—connecting atria and ventricles. The circus movement may be in the opposite direction. If the disturbance endangers life its abolition may sometimes be effected by detection and surgical section of the anomalous pathway.

Congenital heart-block may affect otherwise normal hearts. It is usually due to fibrous interruption of the atrioventricular conducting system as it penetrates the central fibrous body of the heart in its passage from the atria to the ventricles.

Development.—The primitive sinus venosus of each side is a short venous trunk, lying horizontally in the septum transversum, receiving a vitelline and an umbilical vein and emptying into the corresponding atrium (Fig. 2.1B). Each sinus venosus later receives a duct of Cuvier, formed by the union of anterior and posterior cardinal veins draining the head end and hind end of the embryo respectively. After the rise of the atria from the septum transversum, the right and left horns of the sinus venosus—as they may now be called—also come to lie dorsal to the atria (Fig. 2.1E).

Initially, the sinuatrial junction is ill defined, but invaginations of the wall on each side appear as longitudinally disposed external grooves and internal folds. The left groove and fold are the more extensive, forming a sinuatrial septum that separates the left sinus horn from the atrium. This creates a transverse chamber, the body of the sinus venosus, linking the left and right sinus horns: it displaces the sinuatrial orifice to the right, between the right atrium and the right sinus horn. As the sinuatrial folds approach each other by increasing invagination, they form the right and left venous valves controlling the sinuatrial orifice; they meet cranially at the septum spurium and caudally at the dorsal atrioventricular cushion (Fig. 2.1F) (see also page 86).

Prior to this stage, an evagination from the sinus venosus has grown into the dorsal mesocardium and met the pulmonary venous plexus, forming the common pulmonary vein (Fig. 2.1E). To the right of its ostium is an elevation—the right pulmonary fold—that contributes to the interatrial septum: caudal to its ostium the sinuatrial septum grows across, defining a sinuatrial junction: as a result, the pulmonary venous drainage is directed to the left atrium. The common pulmonary vein and its right and left tributaries subsequently dilate and are incorporated into the left atrium as the smooth-walled vestibule: the primitive atrium with its ridged lining persists, becoming the atrial appendage.

Meanwhile, the left vitelline vein and the left and right umbilical veins lose their connexions with the sinus venosus. Thus, the right sinus horn receives cranially the right duct of Cuvier (superior vena cava), caudally the right vitelline vein (inferior vena cava) and from the left the body of the sinus venosus. The body of the sinus venosus receives the left sinus horn (coronary sinus), which receives the left duct of Cuvier (oblique vein of Marshall). The right horn dilates and is incorporated into the right atrium, forming the smooth-walled sinus venarum. The left venous valve fuses with the atrial septal complex; the right venous valve is reduced by resorption, until it is represented by the crista terminalis (separating the sinus venarum from the ridged primitive atrium), most of the valve of the inferior vena cava (Eustachian valve) and the valve of the coronary sinus (Thebesian valve): the Eustachian valve is completed by the spur of material (sinus septum) separating the orifices of the inferior vena cava and coronary sinus. The extent of resorption varies: the Eustachian and Thebesian valves may be absent, rudimentary, crescentic or fenestrated, or they may be surmounted or replaced by a *Chiari network*[62]—a meshwork of fibres extending from the margins of the valves to the taenia sagittalis (septum spurium) in the roof of the right atrium. These fibres may be the site of thrombus formation, and they may trap emboli from the systemic veins.

Rarely, the right venous valve of the sinus venosus evolves into a spinnaker-like flap: an instance of this was seen in a case of tricuspid atresia with atrial septal defect, the flap billowing into the defect or into the ostium of the coronary sinus, leading to syncopal attacks and eventually causing death.[63]

It may be noted here that the hepatic portion of the inferior vena cava may be obstructed by a congenital membrane:[64] this condition, which has been described as 'coarctation of the inferior vena cava', is amenable to surgery.[65]

Sinus Venosus (Superior Caval) Atrial Septal Defect.—In this condition a defect is found high in the interatrial septum, above the fossa ovalis, near or even within the orifice of the superior vena cava. Anomalous pulmonary venous drainage is a feature of the condition, which can be related to incomplete isolation of the vestibular part of the sinus venosus.[66, 67] If the developing interatrial septum fails to separate the vestibular part from the main sinus venosus, there will be a septal defect just below the entrance of the superior vena cava. When the pulmonary veins become incorporated into the vestibule the left veins are likely to be normal but the right veins will open near the defect. The

pattern shown in Fig. 2.5 is one commonly seen in this condition: a right upper vein enters the lower end of the superior vena cava, a middle vein enters the atrial wall opposite the defect and a lower vein enters the left atrium. The increased venous return to the right side of the heart causes compensatory dilatation and hypertrophy of the right atrium and ventricle. The flow of blood is always from left to right through the defect, unless pulmonary hypertension develops, in which case the shunt reverses and the patient becomes cyanosed. This condition can be corrected surgically and has therefore become of great importance.[68]

Occasionally, there is a defect in the fossa ovalis also (ostium secundum defect—see below), as in the example illustrated (Fig. 2.5).

Anomalous Pulmonary Venous Drainage.—Anomalous pulmonary venous drainage probably arises in different ways according to the site. Normal drainage depends on the appropriate evaginations from the sinus venosus reaching the pulmonary venous plexus, on the pulmonary venous plexus losing its primitive connexions with the vitelline and cardinal systems, and on the position of the interatrial septum. Connexion with too caudally placed an evagination would result in drainage into the sinus venarum or the coronary sinus. Failure to achieve connexion would result in persistent drainage into the cardinal system (left brachiocephalic vein, right or left superior vena cava), or into the vitelline system[69] (ductus venosus, portal vein, inferior vena cava). When drainage is into a left superior vena cava, only the distal part of the left duct of Cuvier persists: direct connexion with the heart being lost, blood passes up the left superior vena cava to the left brachiocephalic vein and thence by the right superior vena cava to the right atrium. If the elevation at the left of the ostium of the common pulmonary vein contributes to the interatrial septum, drainage will be into the right atrium.

Anomalous pulmonary venous drainage may be partial[70] or complete.[71] Partial forms involve only one lung or even one vein and are relatively harmless. An interesting variety is known as the 'scimitar syndrome':[72] the right inferior pulmonary vein in its course to join the inferior vena cava produces a scimitar-shaped radiographic shadow at the right border of the heart; there is dextrorotation of the heart and deviation of the mediastinum to the right.

When drainage is completely anomalous, a septal defect is essential, to enable some of the mixture of arterial and venous blood that enters the right

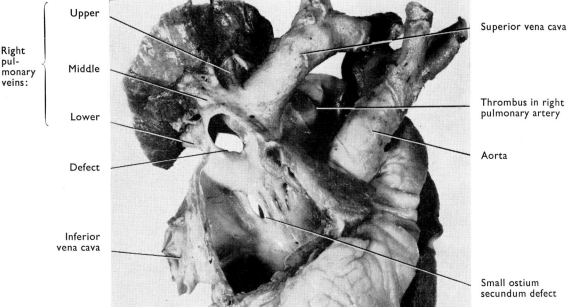

Right pulmonary veins:
- Upper
- Middle
- Lower

Defect

Inferior vena cava

Superior vena cava

Thrombus in right pulmonary artery

Aorta

Small ostium secundum defect

Fig. 2.5.§ Sinus venosus (superior caval) atrial septal defect with anomalous right pulmonary veins. View from right atrium. Note the small ostium secundum (fossa ovalis) defect and the massive thrombosis of the (right) pulmonary artery.

side of the heart to reach the left side of the heart. Many patterns have been described: they may be classified as intracardiac (drainage into the right atrium or coronary sinus), supracardiac (drainage into the left brachiocephalic vein or, on the right, into the superior vena cava), infracardiac (drainage into the portal vein or one of its tributaries) and combined (drainage in two or more anomalous situations).[73] The oxygen saturation of the blood is the same in samples from all chambers of the heart and from the great arteries: cyanosis is an inevitable consequence, although not always obvious.

If the blood flow is obstructed, as is common in the infradiaphragmatic types of anomalous drainage, the clinical picture resembles that of mitral stenosis, but without its murmur. The mortality of the obstructive forms in infancy may reach 75 per cent,[74] and early corrective surgery is advisable in all such cases: in the non-obstructive forms surgery may be delayed for a few years.[75]

Cor Triatriatum.—Cor triatriatum is a rare condition.[76] The term, which should mean a heart with three atria, is not strictly appropriate, the third chamber not being developmentally part of the atria. It may be either a greatly dilated coronary sinus receiving a persistent left superior vena cava (dexter or right-sided type of cor triatriatum—see

page 114) or the result of dilatation of the common pulmonary vein after its failure to be incorporated into the left atrium (sinister or left-sided type of cor triatriatum). In the left-sided type the extra compartment is dorsal to the rest of the heart and receives the pulmonary veins: one or more orifices in the membrane-like wall of this compartment provide for the blood flow into the left atrium. If the size of these openings impedes the circulation, as is usually the case, the clinical picture is identical with that of mitral stenosis, although the obstruction is above the mitral valve, which may be normal. The wall of the extra chamber is thickened, just as the wall of the left atrium is thickened in mitral stenosis. The condition can be remedied by surgical excision of the obstructing membrane.[77]

Left Superior Vena Cava.—An example of double superior vena cava is illustrated in Figs 2.6A and 2.6B, which show symmetrical right and left venae cavae. A double superior vena cava such as this is normal in some animals, such as the frog and the rabbit. The left superior vena cava passes anterior to the hilum of the left lung and enters the pericardium to join the coronary sinus, which is greatly dilated (cor triatriatum dexter—see page 114). The opening of the coronary sinus into the right atrium is often very large, owing to the much increased

D

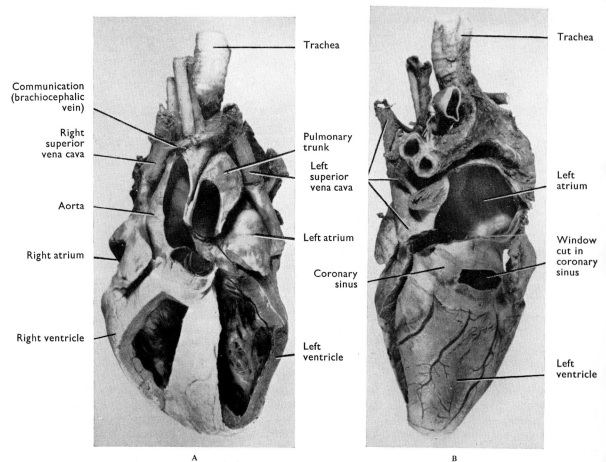

A

B

Fig. 2.6A.§ Double superior vena cava. Anterior aspect, showing the communication between the two vessels.

Fig. 2.6B.§ Double superior vena cava. Left lateral view of the specimen in Fig. 2.6A, showing the left vena cava joining the dilated coronary sinus.

volume of blood being carried. However, in one example that we studied the orifice was very small, and the direction of the blood flow in the coronary sinus was reversed, the stream having been directed up the left superior vena cava to reach the right superior vena cava through the left brachiocephalic vein.

A left superior vena cava by itself is of no importance: it may, however, be associated with other anomalies.[78] If the coronary sinus does not become separated from the left atrium by the atrioventricular fold, which normally effects this, the left superior vena cava will enter the left atrium directly and there will be no coronary sinus: these two anomalies and the presence of an atrial septal defect constitute a triad.[79]

THE INTERATRIAL SEPTUM

Development.—After rising from the septum transversum the atria lie dorsal to the bulbus cordis,

which lies in an interatrial sulcus on their ventral and cephalic aspect (Fig. 2.1D). A sickle-shaped fold of the myocardium grows in from the region of the interatrial sulcus and the dorsal and cephalic aspects of the atrial walls to form the septum primum, separating the atria (Fig. 2.1F). The right pulmonary fold is incorporated into the left side of the septum primum so that the common pulmonary vein lies on its left and the developing venous valves and septum spurium lie on its right (see page 83).

Meanwhile, the atrioventricular junction has narrowed to form a common canal, in which cushion tissue now accumulates to form the dorsal and ventral atrioventricular endocardial cushions: the dorsal and ventral horns of the sickle-shaped septum primum grow to reach the corresponding atrioventricular cushions. The cushions increase in size and meet, forming a broad partition that separates the narrow right and left atrioventricular canals (Fig. 2.12A). The advancing septum primum and the fused cushions bound a narrowing interatrial ostium primum, which eventually is closed by their union. A right-to-left shunt is maintained, however, because the cephalic part of the septum breaks down to form an ostium secundum.

A second sickle-shaped fold, the septum secundum, appears between the septum spurium and the septum primum. It carries the attachments of the latter and of the left venous valve on to its left and right sides respectively: the part of the septum primum that bounded the ostium secundum is now slung from the left side of the septum secundum, forming the flap-like valve of the foramen ovale, which is the residual orifice of the septum secundum. The dorsal and ventral horns of the septum secundum bound the foramen ovale as its limbus, thus completing the atrial septal complex, which permits a right-to-left shunt but prevents a left-to-right shunt (Fig. 2.1G).

A right-to-left shunt at atrial level is necessary throughout development for balanced growth of the chambers of the heart. The shunt is provided successively by the ostium primum, the ostium secundum and the foramen ovale. When the atrial septal complex is complete, oxygenated blood returning from the placenta forms the bulk of the inferior caval stream, which is directed forwards and to the left (Fig. 2.1H). The stream is then divided by the limbus of the foramen ovale (crista dividens): some three-quarters of the blood pass through the foramen ovale into the left atrium; the remainder joins the superior caval and coronary streams in the right atrium proper. At term, the inferior caval stream probably provides three-quarters of the intake of the left atrium, the remainder being pulmonary venous return. The mixture passes into the left ventricle and is ejected into the aorta, whence this comparatively highly oxygenated blood goes to the arteries of the heart, head, neck and arms: the residual stream flows through the isthmus of the aorta to join the stream from the ductus arteriosus (see page 105).

After birth, with the onset of respiration, the lungs are inflated, intrathoracic pressure and pulmonary vascular resistance fall, and the pulmonary blood flow increases perhaps tenfold in as many minutes. As the pulmonary venous return increases so does the left atrial pressure: in consequence the valvula foraminis ovalis is pressed against the septum, producing functional closure of the foramen ovale.

During the following months the connective tissue in the valvula increases and structural closure occurs. The part opposite the septum adheres to it and becomes integral with it; the part opposite the foramen ovale may now be termed the floor of the fossa ovalis. In 15 to 20 per cent of normal people the valve of the foramen ovale persists throughout life. In such cases there is normally no shunt, since the higher left atrial pressure keeps the valve closed. If, however, the pressure differential is reversed—as in cases of pulmonary stenosis, anomalous pulmonary venous drainage or ventricular septal defect—a right-to-left shunt may result. In the remaining 80 to 85 per cent, closure of the foramen ovale is completed during the first year of extrauterine life.

Closure of the foramen at an early stage in fetal development results in underdevelopment of the left ventricle, usually with atresia of the mitral or aortic valve or of both, so that blood entering the left atrium must escape by some other route, such as by a laevocardinal vein to a systemic vein, by bronchial veins, or by myocardial sinusoids to the coronary arteries and thence through a fistula to the coronary sinus (see page 114).[80] In contrast, when premature closure of the foramen ovale occurs late in fetal life the left side of the heart may develop normally.[81] In either case neonatal death is usual.

Common Atrium.—The form of trilocular heart that is characterized by a single, common atrium results when the interatrial septum is vestigial or absent (Fig. 2.7). In this rare anomaly, the anterior cusp of the mitral valve usually shows a deep, inverted-V notch, the apex of which may reach the atrioventricular ring and cause mitral regurgitation; this renders surgical correction difficult. Differential streaming of blood entering the common chamber prevents the complete arteriovenous mixing that might be expected.

Defects of the Endocardial Cushions.—In addition to fusing with the septum primum to close the ostium primum, the fused endocardial cushions form the septal leaflets of the mitral and tricuspid valves and the septum between them, and contribute to the interventricular septum (see page 92). Should the cushions fail to fuse, the ostium primum persists, the atrioventricular canal is undivided, a single atrioventricular valve has anterior and posterior cusps, and there is a defect of the interventricular septum continuous with the ostium primum defect. This condition is known as *atrioventricularis communis* (Figs 2.8A and 2.8B). It is one of the commoner anomalies of the heart in

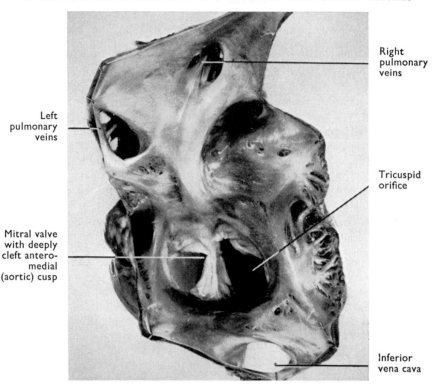

Left
pulmonary
veins

Mitral valve
with deeply
cleft antero-
medial
(aortic) cusp

Right
pulmonary
veins

Tricuspid
orifice

Inferior
vena cava

Fig. 2.7.§ Common atrium (cor triloculare biventriculare). View of single atrium from above, showing complete absence of the inter-atrial septum and the deeply-cleft anteromedial cusp of the mitral valve.

mentally defective children, and it has been associated particularly with Down's syndrome. In extreme examples the heart virtually has only two chambers (bilocular heart). An important consideration in the surgical treatment of atrioventricularis communis is the position of the conducting system. The atrioventricular node of Tawara lies just anterior to the orifice of the coronary sinus: from it the bundle of His runs along the margin of the ventricular septal defect for a variable distance before bifurcating; small filaments stream over the left side of the interventricular septum as the main bundle proceeds on its course and eventually, much reduced in size, constitutes the right branch. Some workers[82] have correlated relatively early electrocardiographic activation of the posterior part of the interventricular septum with early origin and posterior displacement of the left bundle branches, but this is debatable.

When fusion between the septum primum and the endocardial cushions fails to occur, the ostium primum fails to close (Fig. 2.9). An *ostium primum defect* lies immediately above the mitral and tricuspid valves. The anterior cusp of the mitral valve shows the deep notching that is found also when there is a common atrium. Since fusion of the endocardial cushions begins at the right and proceeds leftward, this defect is believed to indicate incomplete fusion.

Ostium primum defect has been called *endocardial cushion defect grade I* and atrioventricularis communis *endocardial cushion defect grade III*.[83] These terms stress the relationship of the two conditions. In an intermediate group—*endocardial cushion defect grade II*—although the cushions meet sufficiently to create separate mitral and tricuspid valves, the septal cusp of either or both valves may be deeply cleft at its midpoint; there is also an ostium primum defect and an insignificant ventricular septal defect. Clinically, this group cannot be distinguished from pure ostium primum defect.

Ostium Secundum Defect (Fossa Ovalis Defect).— If the valvula is inadequate to cover the foramen ovale, or if it is fenestrate, the floor of the fossa ovalis will be incomplete—hence the name 'fossa ovalis defect'. This is by far the commonest of all atrial septal defects; it may be only a few milli-

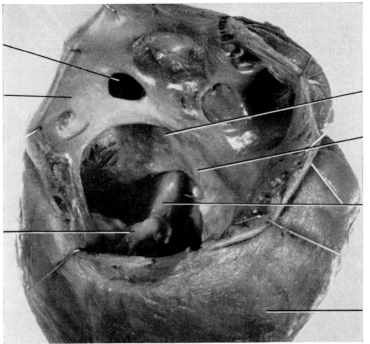

Small ostium
secundum defect

Interatrial
septum

Posterior cusp of
atrioventricular
valve

Large ostium
primum defect

Anterior cusp of
atrioventricular
valve

Upper border of
ventricular
septum

Right
ventricle

Fig. 2.8A.§ Atrioventricularis communis. View from right atrium to show the
large ostium primum and small ostium secundum atrial septal defects, and
the common atrioventricular valve cusps astride the upper rim of the interventricular septum.

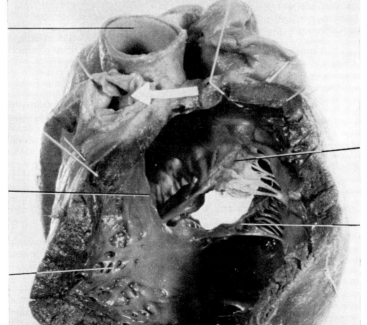

Aorta

Margin of
ventricular
septal defect

Left ventricle

Anterior cusp of
atrioventricular
valve

Posterior cusp of
atrioventricular
valve

Fig. 2.8B.§ Atrioventricularis communis. View from the left ventricle of
specimen illustrated in Fig. 2.8A, to show the rim of the interventricular
septum sweeping below the atrioventricular valve cusps. The white arrow
indicates the moderately stenotic pulmonary valve.

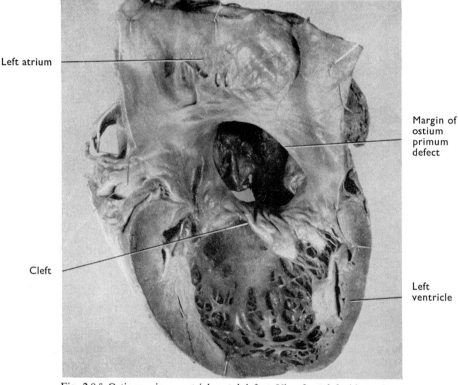

Left atrium

Margin of
ostium
primum
defect

Cleft

Left
ventricle

Fig. 2.9.§ Ostium primum atrial septal defect. View from left side to show
the deep cleft in the anteromedial cusp of the mitral valve.

metres across or it may occupy the whole extent of the fossa ovalis itself, which is then floorless (Fig. 2.10).

A well-developed Eustachian valve may be continuous with the anterior rim of an ostium secundum defect and create a surgical difficulty. The explanation is interesting. The Eustachian and Thebesian valves are both formed from the right venous valve, but the Eustachian valve is completed by the sinus septum (see page 84). The ventral horn of the septum secundum sweeps down across the fused endocardial cushions and bifurcates: one limb merges with the left venous valve; the other joins the sinus septum, giving continuity between the Eustachian valve and the limbus of the fossa ovalis (Fig. 2.11). In repairing a defect, a well-developed Eustachian valve must not be included in the closure, for this would result in diversion of the inferior caval stream into the left atrium.[84]

Inferior Caval Septal Defect.—This type of septal defect adjoins the entry of the inferior vena cava into the atrium. It has been interpreted as a failure in the formation of the posterior rim of the ostium secundum: however, the occasional presence of a fossa ovalis in the septal remnant is against this view. Another explanation is that the anomaly develops in relation to the formation of the ostium primum, with displacement posteriorly.[85]

General Observations on Defects of the Interatrial Septum

It is quite common for more than one type of atrial septal defect to be present or for two types to be combined: for instance, a fossa ovalis defect may lack a posterior rim, and, like a sinus venosus defect, it may be associated with anomalous right pulmonary veins.

In all atrial septal defects catheterization studies demonstrate that blood samples from the right atrium have an oxygen content higher than those from the superior vena cava.

The greatly increased blood flow through the right side of the heart that results from an atrial septal defect leads to dilatation and hypertrophy of the right atrium, right ventricle and pulmonary trunk, and there may be a functional diastolic murmur of pulmonary regurgitation (Graham Steell murmur). The intrapulmonary arteries are usually

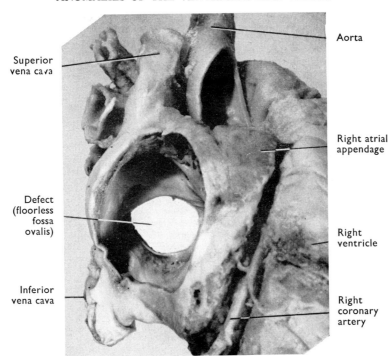

Superior
vena cava

Aorta

Right atrial
appendage

Defect
(floorless
fossa
ovalis)

Right
ventricle

Inferior
vena cava

Right
coronary
artery

Fig. 2.10. Ostium secundum (fossa ovalis) atrial septal defect seen through a window cut in the right atrium. The entire floor of the fossa ovalis is lacking.

hypertrophied, and in a proportion of cases permanent obstructive changes may occur and lead to pulmonary hypertension, which does not respond to surgical closure of the defect. Massive thrombosis in the main pulmonary arteries is not uncommon.

The mortality of atrial septal defect rises from 0·7 per cent in the second decade to 90 per cent in the sixth decade.[86] Ostium secundum defects usually have the best prognosis: however, there are occasional instances of long survival with other types of atrial septal deficiency, such as a patient who lived to 76 years with two large defects that had resulted from failure of both the ostium primum and ostium secundum to close.[87]

Occasionally, rheumatic mitral stenosis develops in a heart with an atrial septal defect (which may be of any type), producing the *syndrome of Lutembacher*.[88] The valvar stenosis results in augmentation of the left-to-right shunt and must be relieved before an attempt is made to close the septal defect surgically: failure to correct the stenosis before closing the septal defect may result in fatal pulmonary oedema.

Atrial Septal Defect in Association with Other Congenital Anomalies.—Atrial septal defect may be a component of various comparatively rare familial syndromes. These include the *Holt–Oram syndrome*, in which there are defects of the radial aspects of the forearms,[89] and the *syndrome of Ellis and van Creveld*,[90] in which polydactyly, chondrodystrophy and ectodermal dysplasia are commonly accompanied by an atrial septal fault.[91]

THE VENTRICLES AND VALVES

Development.—Within the bulboventricular loop (see page 77), the blood stream is directed first caudally, then to the right, and then cranially (Fig. 2.1C). Where the stream impinges on the wall, it is reflected and changes direction: loops and strands grow in from the myoepicardial mantle at these points, and interdigitate with the outpouchings from the endocardium that form the trabeculae of the primitive ventricles. The ventricles enlarge by deepening, leaving a region of stasis between: externally this appears as the interventricular sulcus and internally as the primitive ventricular septum.

The bulboventricular ridge is interposed—initially in the form of a spur—between the limbs of the bulboventricular loop; later it separates the

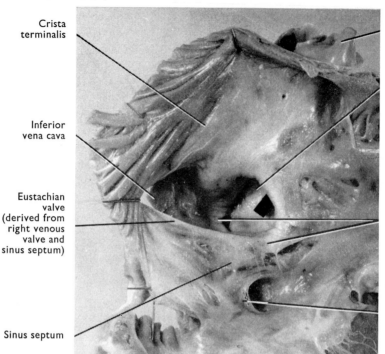

Crista terminalis

Inferior vena cava

Eustachian valve (derived from right venous valve and sinus septum)

Sinus septum

Superior vena cava

Normal fossa ovalis with well-formed limbus. The floor is derived from the septum primum. Black probe through valvular foramen ovale

Bifurcation of ventral horn of limbus (derived from septum secundum)

Coronary sinus and Thebesian valve

Fig. 2.11.§ Well-developed Eustachian and Thebesian valves in a normal heart. Note that the Eustachian valve extends between the inferior vena cava and the coronary sinus, there becoming continuous with an extension of the ventral horn of the limbus fossae ovalis; another extension of the ventral horn forms the lower rim bordering the fossa ovalis. A black probe is inserted into the valvular opening in the floor of the fossa ovalis.

atrioventricular canal from the bulbar orifice (Fig. 2.12A). With removal of the ridge, and merging of the bulbus into the ventricles, the right side of the atrioventricular canal comes to lie dorsal to the bulbar orifice (Fig. 2.12B). The crescentic ventricular septum has dorsal and ventral horns, which reach the corresponding atrioventricular cushions; it grows from below as the ventricles deepen on each side of it.

At this stage the ostium primum, atrioventricular canal and interventricular foramen form a continuous hiatus between the right and left sides of the heart (atrioventricularis communis, see page 87). After fusion of the atrioventricular cushions, the stream from the left atrioventricular canal enters the left ventricle and is ejected through the interventricular foramen into the dorsal part of the bulbar orifice. The right ventricular outflow passes into the ventral part of the bulbar orifice. The intersection of left dorsal and right ventral streams produces clockwise spiralling as the two streams traverse the bulbus and truncus to reach the

aortic sac (see page 105): the right ventral stream spirals to the dorsicaudal part of the aortic sac and the sixth aortic arches, whereas the left dorsal stream spirals to the ventricephalic part and the other aortic arches (Fig. 2.12B).

The bulbus and truncus are lined with deformable cushion tissue: this is moulded by the spiral streams, with the result that spiral ridges fill the relative deadspace between the streams. The ridges lie left and right in the aortic sac; when traced proximally through the truncus they rotate through 180°, so that the bulbotruncal junction—the site of formation of the semilunar valves—lies right and left (Figs 2.12B and C). Traced proximally, the right bulbar ridge crosses the right margins of the fused atrioventricular cushions to reach the dorsal horn of the ventricular septum; the left bulbar ridge reaches the ventral horn of the ventricular septum. Beginning distally, the spiral ridges meet, fuse and are reinforced by ingrowth of muscle tissue, forming a continuous spiral septum (Fig. 2.12D). The proximal part of the septum divides the bulbus into a major part, the infundibulum of the right ventricle, and a minor part, the aortic vestibule. A gap between this bulbar septum and the ventricular septum is closed by cushion tissue from the right side of the fused atrioventricular cushions. This grows along the crest of the ventricular septum, fusing with it and the bulbar septum, and eventually forms the pars membranacea, completing the separation of the ventricles.

At the bulbotruncal junction, the right and left ridges are elaborated to form localized cushions that fuse and then are bisected by the ingrowing muscle tissue (Fig. 2.12E). Thus, the dorsal halves present in the aortic channel and the ventral halves

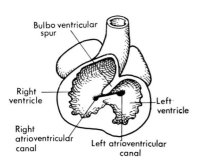

A. The interior of the ventricles in the fifth week of embryonic development (compare with Fig. 2.1D).

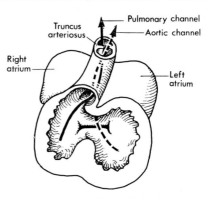

B.§ The interior of the ventricles early in the sixth week.

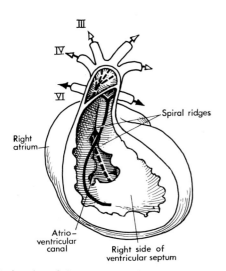

C. The interior of the right ventricle late in the sixth week.

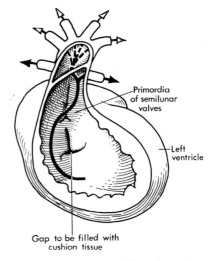

D. The interior of the right ventricle at the end of the sixth week.

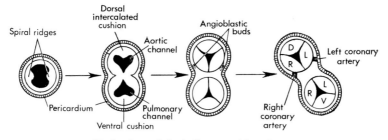

E. Sections of the bulbotruncal junctions.

Fig. 2.12. Schematic diagrams of the developing heart.

D*

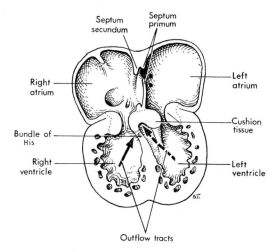

F. Coronal section of heart in eighth week.

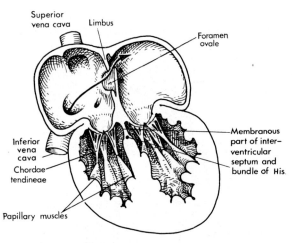

G. Coronal section of heart at three months.

Fig. 2.12. Schematic diagrams of the developing heart.

in the pulmonary channel as right and left valve cushions respectively. Each pair of right and left cushions is reinforced by further endocardial tissue and a third nonseptal cushion. The distal aspect of each cushion is then excavated, forming the cusps and sinuses of the semilunar valves (Fig. 2.12E).

After the atrioventricular cushions have fused, septal and lateral accumulations of cushion tissue present in the lumen of each atrioventricular canal (Fig. 2.12F). In the left canal, they form the leaflets of the mitral valve. In the right canal, the two lateral cushions are derived largely from the right bulbar ridge: they form the anterior and posterior leaflets of the tricuspid valve, whereas the third cushion and valve are septal in origin. Muscle trabeculae

extend into the bases of the cushions. As the cushions are excavated on their distal aspects, the trabeculae are stripped off the ventricular wall but retain their terminal attachments. Replacement of the muscle by collagen fibres completes the formation of the valve cusps and chordae tendineae, the mural ends of the trabeculae persisting as papillary muscles (Fig. 2.12G).

It should be remembered that all these complex events have taken place by the time the embryo is of little more than 2 cm in crown-rump length, and that consequently a minute aberration may have a very significant effect. Often several anomalies occur together: as many as eight have been found in one heart, although such gross malformation seldom permits survival for long. It is remarkable that faults are so infrequent.

Single Ventricle.—Like the common atrium form of trilocular heart (page 87), the common ventricle form is rare. The reduction in the number of chambers in the latter is due to the complete failure of the ventricular septum to develop, so that the mitral and tricuspid valves open into a single, large, thick-walled chamber. The aorta and pulmonary trunk arise from this common ventricle or from a rudimentary bulbar chamber,[92] and there may be cyanosis and digital clubbing. The malformation is seldom compatible with long survival, but in one remarkable instance the patient was 67 when he died. The probable explanation of this patient's exceptionally long survival was the association of stenosis of the pulmonary valve with the ventricular anomaly. The stenosis would protect the pulmonary circulation from the full effects of the systemic blood pressure, for which it is not adapted and which ordinarily causes irreversible pulmonary hypertension, with all its consequences. In this man's case, as in nearly all the cases in the literature,[93] the aorta and pulmonary trunk were transposed, the former arising in front of the latter. Because the ventricular septum is absent in such hearts, the lower free border of the bulbar septum, separating the orifices of the two great vessels, can be seen from the ventricular cavity.

Single ventricle in the conventional sense just described must be distinguished from absence or rudimentary development of one or other ventricle as a consequence of atresia of the corresponding atrioventricular valve. Further, some authorities distinguish single ventricle from common ventricle, using the latter term only in reference to the condition accompanying a large ventricular septal defect.[94]

The position of the heart is usually normal. Less commonly, there is dextrocardia or, rarely, mesocardia.[94] The great arteries may be transposed, either in the common fashion or in the mirror image of this; alternatively, they may be normal—this is known as 'Holmes's heart'—or their relations may be difficult to define precisely.

It is worth noting that in the frog, which has a single ventricle, the ventricular outlet (truncus) has a complicated system of semilunar valves arranged in two rows, one at the upper end of a spiral septum and one at its lower end: this valve functions in such a way that right atrial blood reaches the pulmocutaneous system and left atrial blood the systemic circulation at appropriate pressures and with minimal mixing.

Ventricular Septal Defect.—Formerly, the term *maladie de Roger*[95] was applied to any ventricular septal defect that was not associated with other anomalies. The eponym is now usually applied only to small harmless defects that cause no symptoms and are detected only by the characteristic systolic murmur of the local left-to-right shunt. The septal defect is commonly due to failure of the membranous part to develop: this probably results because the lower end of the bulbospiral septum does not approach near enough to the interventricular foramen for the gap to be filled from the atrioventricular cushions. Sometimes the defect is in the muscular part of the septum, in which case it probably results from faults in the embryonic meshwork that is the origin of the septal musculature. Defects in the muscular septum tend to be smaller during ventricular systole. They probably decrease in size as the heart grows: this may account for spontaneous closure of the defect, which has been reported by many observers. Campbell estimated that by their fortieth year 20 per cent of patients had closed their defect while 53 per cent had died.[96] Death before the age of 25 years is rare with uncomplicated single defects; multiple defects are not uncommon and may prevent successful surgery.

In infancy a large defect may allow torrential shunting, overloading the circulation in the lungs and causing heart failure: this necessitates urgent surgery, either to 'band' the pulmonary trunk with a ligature to control the flow[97] or, better, to close the defect, if possible. Rarely, such massive right ventricular hypertrophy develops in consequence of the shunt that the outflow to the lungs is constricted naturally, the clinical picture changing from that of ventricular septal defect to that of isolated infundibular pulmonary stenosis (acyanotic Fallot's tetrad).[98]

It is important to note that the bundle of His lies in the posterior rim of the defect and is thus at risk during operations to close the septum.

Incompetence of the aortic valve is a serious complication of ventricular septal defect. It is due to prolapse of one of the valve cusps (commonly the right cusp) into the defect. The herniated cusp may obstruct the outflow of the right ventricle. Successful closure of the defect and replacement of the valve by a homograft has been reported.[99]

Another serious complication is pulmonary hypertension. When this develops in association with ventricular septal defect the combination is known as *Eisenmenger's complex.*[100] The pulmonary hypertension results in hypertrophy of the right ventricle and dilatation of the pulmonary trunk. The cause of pulmonary hypertension in these cases is not clear. It may be a result of persistence of the fetal type of pulmonary arteries, with thick muscular walls. Normally, these vessels undergo an involutionary change during the first few weeks after birth and become transformed into the thin-walled postnatal type of vessel. The condition that Eisenmenger himself described was a ventricular septal defect with pulmonary hypertension. Other shunt anomalies, such as persistent ductus arteriosus, transposition of the great vessels, and sometimes atrial septal defect, may be associated with pulmonary hypertension: the term *Eisenmenger's syndrome*[101] has been introduced to include any reversed shunt due to pulmonary hypertension. The term Eisenmenger's complex may be reserved for the cases in which the shunt is a ventricular septal defect, as in Eisenmenger's own account of the condition.

Pulmonary Stenosis.—Pulmonary stenosis may affect the infundibulum (infundibular or subvalvar stenosis), the pulmonary valve (valvar stenosis) or the pulmonary trunk or branches (supravalvar stenosis).

Infundibular stenosis is characterized by a constriction in the musculature of the infundibulum (bulbus). This constriction is probably the result of some deviation at the lower end of the spiral septum, partially occluding the anterior division of the bulbus. Sometimes there is a chamber—the 'subvalvar chamber'—between the site of infundibular stenosis and the pulmonary valve. This represents the incompletely absorbed bulbar region.

In typical examples of *valvar stenosis*, the valve appears as a dome with a small central perforation surrounded by three small sinuses of Valsalva. The anomaly evidently results from fusion of the valve cushions and their failure to become properly hollowed out. Occasionally there is calcification of the malformed valve. Rarely, the cusps are thickened and myxomatoid ('pulmonary valvar dysplasia'), the cardiac anomaly then having a familial tendency and being associated with an abnormal facies.[102]

Supravalvar pulmonary stenosis affects the trunk of the pulmonary artery or its branches. It may be associated with supravalvar aortic stenosis, cardiac

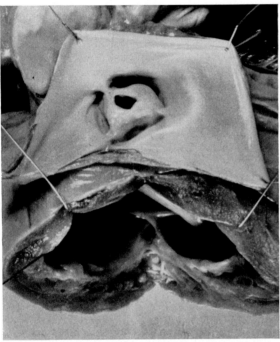

Fig. 2.13.§ Isolated congenital pulmonary valve stenosis. View from above showing the cusps fused into a dome with a central perforation. Note the hypertrophy of the right ventricle and the poststenotic dilatation of the pulmonary trunk.

anomalies and hypercalcaemia. Maternal rubella has been thought responsible in some cases. Familial cases have also been recorded.

Patients with uncomplicated pulmonary stenosis may survive into middle age and beyond, provided the stenosis is not severe. Dilatation and hypertrophy of the right atrium and ventricle result (Fig. 2.13), and poststenotic dilatation of the subvalvar chamber or of the pulmonary trunk is often present in cases of infundibular and valvar stenosis respectively. Central cyanosis may result if an atrial septal defect or valvular foramen ovale is present.

Fallot's Tetrad.—The complex malformation known as Fallot's tetrad is the commonest condition in which cyanosis and pulmonary stenosis are associated. The tetrad (see Figs 2.14A and 2.14B) consists of pulmonary stenosis (valvar or infundibular), ventricular septal defect, displacement of the aorta to the right so that it overrides the septal defect ('dextroposition') and right ventricular hypertrophy (which results from the pulmonary stenosis). Most of the anomalous features are explicable on the basis of abnormal deviation of the lower part of the bulbar septum.

Fallot described the condition in 1888.[103] However, it is now recognized[104] that the first description was more than 200 years earlier, by Niels Stensen,[105] the Danish anatomist. Many cardiologists give precedence to Peacock,[106] whose classic account appeared 22 years before Fallot's.

The patient with the classic Fallot tetrad is cyanotic and has clubbing of the fingers and toes and polycythaemia. The cyanosis is mainly due to the right-to-left shunt through the ventricular septal defect. If the pulmonary stenosis is very severe much of the blood flow to the lungs may be carried by dilated bronchial arteries.

Fallot's tetrad was the first cyanotic form of congenital heart disease to be operated upon surgically. It had been noted that the condition of affected neonates worsened when the volume of the shunt to the lungs fell in consequence of natural closure of the ductus arteriosus. It was then shown that improvement could be obtained by creating an artificial ductus between the subclavian and pulmonary arteries on one side (the Blalock–Taussig operation).[107] Most recently, it has proved possible in one operation to relieve the stenosis and close the defect, and—if necessary—even insert a homograft pulmonary valve.[108]

'Acyanotic Fallot's Tetrad'.—Cyanosis is not a feature of those cases of Fallot's tetrad in which the septal defect is large and the pulmonary stenosis mild, or of those in which the pulmonary stenosis is marked and the septal defect small. The picture in such cases is virtually that of simple ventricular septal defect or isolated pulmonary stenosis respectively.

Pulmonary hypertension does not occur in Fallot's tetrad. Indeed, the blood flow to the lungs is poor, and this has been blamed for the increased susceptibility of these patients to tuberculosis.

Since the pressure in the pulmonary trunk is low, it is difficult to understand why it and its main branches, particularly those on the left, are

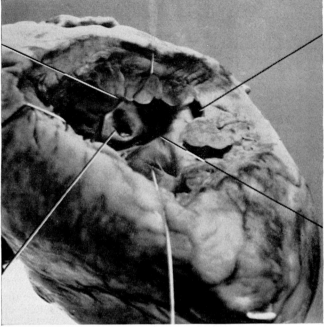

Upper margin of
defect (crista
supraventricularis)

Infundibular stenosis
in thick-walled right
ventricle

Lower margin
of defect

Coronary ostium
in aortic wall seen
through the ventri-
cular septal defect

Fig. 2.14A. Fallot's tetrad. View of infundibular type of stenosis and
the ventricular septal defect displayed by a window cut in the right
ventricle, which is greatly thickened. The aorta is visible through the
ventricular septal defect. (See Fig. 2.14B.)

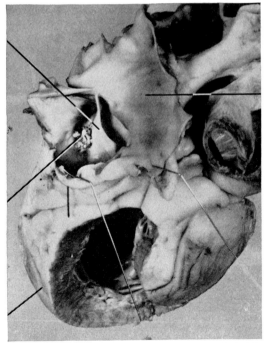

Pulmonary valve

Dilated, thin-walled
pulmonary trunk

Stenotic orifice
in floor of infundi-
bular chamber

Left ventricle

Fig. 2.14B.§ Fallot's tetrad. View of the stenosis in Fig.
2.14A, from above; it lies in the floor of a subvalvar
chamber. The valve is normal and the pulmonary trunk
dilated.

usually dilated. It is generally thought that the dilatation is due to abnormal forces produced within the vessel by turbulence set up by the jet of blood emerging from the stenotic orifice. The intrapulmonary arteries and veins are dilated also: there is atrophy of their medial coat and fibrosis of their intima, possibly from organization of mural thrombus.[109]

It is not common for patients with Fallot's tetrad to live to middle age. Marquis[104] recorded two cases with survival to the ages of 48 and 65 years respectively; he found records of only 10 other patients aged 40 years or over in the literature.

Fallot's 'Triad'.—Fallot's triad consists of pulmonary stenosis (valvar or infundibular), right ventricular hypertrophy, and an interatrial communication—either a septal defect or a valvular foramen ovale.[110] Although generally known by Fallot's name, this malformation was described by Palois in 1809,[111] long before Fallot's account.[103] Cyanosis is usually present early in life, but its appearance may be delayed a few years: it results from shunting of venous blood from the right atrium to the left, and it is accompanied by clubbing and polycythaemia. The expectancy of life is similar to that in cases of Fallot's tetrad. In an exceptional case the patient survived to the age of 75 years.[112]

Fallot's 'Pentad'.—This condition, which is often referred to simply as 'the pentad', may be regarded as a combination of Fallot's tetrad and triad—that is, the tetrad in association with atrial septal defect or valvular foramen ovale. The right-to-left shunt through the atrial septum may lead to left ventricular hypertrophy.[113]

Pulmonary Atresia.—Pulmonary atresia completely obstructs the blood flow between the right ventricle and the pulmonary arteries. The site of the obstruction is the pulmonary valve or the trunk of the pulmonary artery, or one or both of the main branches of the latter. There is an accompanying ventricular septal defect. Atresia of the main pulmonary branches is 'compensated'—sometimes overcompensated[114]—by the development of collateral 'bronchial' arteries arising directly or indirectly from the aorta; there is often persistence of the ductus arteriosus also.[115] These systemic arteries may in time virtually lose all connexion with the intrapulmonary arteries as a result of the development of obstructive changes accompanying pulmonary hypertension. The surgical treatment of pulmonary atresia is similar to that of Fallot's tetrad.

Double-Chambered Right Ventricle.—In this anomaly, often associated with ventricular septal defect and pulmonary stenosis, the right ventricle is partly or completely subdivided into a high-pressure proximal chamber and a low-pressure distal chamber by aberrant muscle bands joining the crista supraventricularis.[116] The condition may be indistinguishable from the infundibular stenosis with subvalvar chamber that is found in one of the varieties of Fallot's tetrad.

Aortic Stenosis.—Aortic stenosis, like pulmonary stenosis, may be subvalvar, valvar or supravalvar. Hypertrophy of the left ventricle is its inevitable accompaniment. The wall of the aorta beyond the stenosis may be abnormally thin.

(*a*) *Subvalvar aortic stenosis.* This occurs in two forms, membranous and muscular. The *membranous form* is probably due to deviation of the lower end of the bulbar septum to the left. A ridge or shelf of fibrous tissue runs more or less transversely on the wall of the ventricle below the aortic valve, sometimes extending on to the aortic cusp of the mitral valve. The aortic valve itself may be normal or, occasionally, stenotic. The stenotic area, or the valve beyond it, may become the site of infective endocarditis. The *muscular form* of subvalvar aortic stenosis is also probably congenital: it is discussed under 'obstructive cardiomyopathy' on page 80.

(*b*) *Congenital valvar aortic stenosis.*[117] Congenital stenosis of the aortic valve is only rarely of a type corresponding to the common type of stenosis of the pulmonary valve, in which there is a central dome with three small sinuses of Valsalva round it (page 95). The commonest obstructive condition of the aortic valve that has been considered to be of congenital origin is usually seen, paradoxically, in middle-aged or elderly people, and takes the form of a bicuspid valve with calcification. The bicuspid aortic valve, like the bicuspid pulmonary valve (with which it may coexist), is believed to originate in fusion of two of the valve cushions: these are commonly the two cushions adjoining the bulbotruncal septum, in which case both coronary arteries rise from the common sinus of Valsalva of the fused cusps. The double cusp is usually larger than the other: in its sinus of Valsalva a small raphe may mark the site of fusion of the cushions. In uncomplicated form this type of malformation is occasionally an incidental post-mortem finding in young adults: there is then no stenosis. Bicuspid aortic valve is not uncommon in cases of coarctation of the aorta, and its incompetence in these cases may result from stretching of the valve ring in consequence of the high blood pressure (see page 110).

When a bicuspid aortic valve becomes grossly distorted by calcification its differentiation from a calcified rheumatic valve may not be possible. Histological proof of this distinction is difficult and disputable. However, three observations are in favour of the congenital origin of a bicuspid aortic valve—the absence of a history of rheumatic fever, the absence of evidence of rheumatic involvement of any other valve, or of other sequels of rheumatic carditis, and the fact that the condition is usually seen at a much later age than rheumatic valvar disease. However, even if it is reasonably certain that rheumatic endocarditis can be ruled out as the cause of the lesion in any individual case, the possibility that the condition is the outcome of some other acquired disease cannot be excluded. For instance, it has been suggested that calcific aortic stenosis might be the end result of healed endocarditis due to infection by *Brucella abortus*.[118] Other authorities consider the condition to be merely an exaggerated manifestation of the phenomenon of ageing.

Replacement of a useless calcified valve by a prosthesis or graft is one of the most remarkable surgical advances of recent years.[119] The coronary arteries are often remarkably free of atheroma, so that the myocardium obtains full benefit from the improved coronary flow: as a result of the operation severe cardiac invalidism may give place to at least several years of active life.

(*c*) *Supravalvar aortic stenosis*. This usually takes the form of a fibrous shelf projecting just above the valve cusps. The shelf is sometimes partly fused to the cusps, shutting in a coronary ostium. The coronary arteries may be dilated and tortuous. The malformation is familial in some cases, and associated with mental deficiency and 'elfin' facies.[120] Other anomalies that may accompany it include peripheral pulmonary artery stenosis, hypercalcaemia,[121] and stenosis of other arteries, such as aortic arch branches and the coeliac, mesenteric and renal arteries. Maternal rubella has been responsible in some cases.

Supravalvar stenosis is distinct from aortic atresia in which there is uniform stenosis of the whole ascending aorta, as in the 'hypoplastic left heart syndrome' (see page 100).

Sinus of Valsalva Aneurysm.[122]—In a typical example of an aneurysm of an aortic sinus of Valsalva (Figs 2.15A and 2.15B) the appearance is as though a finger tip has been inserted into the sinus and then pushed outward against the aortic wall to make a diverticulum. One, two or all three of the aortic sinuses may be affected. The non-coronary (right posterior) sinus and the right coronary (anterior) sinus are involved most frequently, in that order: the aneurysm usually appears therefore as a swelling either in the right ventricle (at the site of the attachment of the septal cusp of the tricuspid valve) or in the outflow tract. An aneurysm of the left coronary sinus may protrude on the outside of the heart between the aorta and the left atrium. The wall of the aneurysm contains tissues of the site upon which it impinges, but little or no tissue of the aortic wall itself, presumably because the latter is poorly developed at the mouth of the aneurysm. Sinus of Valsalva aneurysm may accompany ventricular septal defect.[123]

A comparable aneurysm of the anterior sinus of the pulmonary valve has been described.[124]

Rupture, infection, and interference with the conducting system of the heart are the major complications. Although an aneurysm of a sinus of Valsalva may be symptomless until well into adult life, one or another of these complications develops in most cases: it is exceptionally rare to find an uncomplicated aneurysm at necropsy.

When rupture occurs, whether the outcome of simple distension or a result of infective endocarditis, a left-to-right shunt is suddenly established if the aneurysm concerned is situated in either of the cusps most frequently involved (see above). The patient may feel something give way and immediately notice a loud buzzing in the chest. If the shunt remains small, he may live for several years; usually, however, it puts a sudden strain on the right ventricle, which soon fails.

Infection is a common complication and leads to some of the most bizarre abnormalities to be found in the region of the aortic valve. The cusp of the involved sinus often becomes perforated. The aneurysm itself may burst into the right ventricle or its outflow tract, or into the right atrium, or it may form a sac between the left atrium and the left ventricle.

Complete heart block, with episodes of unconsciousness, may result if the aneurysm interferes with the bundle of His and its branches (Stokes–Adams attacks*).

* The familiar clinical syndrome that is commonly referred to by the term 'Stokes–Adams attacks' was mentioned first by Morgagni (in 1761) and described more fully by Spens (1793). In addition to Adams (1827), several others described the syndrome between 1827 and the time of Stokes's account (1846). The historically incorrect eponym that is generally used in English-speaking communities reflects Stokes's particularly outstanding contribution on this condition.

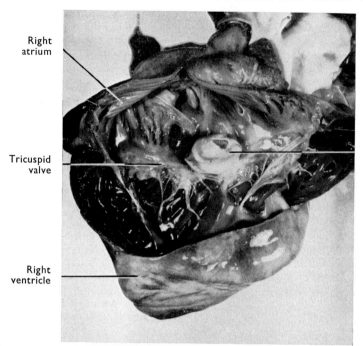

Right
atrium

Tricuspid
valve

Right
ventricle

Aneurysm
with
perforated
tip

Fig. 2.15A.§ Congenital aneurysm of a sinus of Valsalva, viewed
from the right side. The sac has a thin wall and protrudes at the
tricuspid valve ring; its apex is perforated. (See Fig. 2.15B.)

Closely related to aneurysm of the aortic sinuses
of Valsalva, and indeed possibly a complication
of the latter, is the condition awkwardly described
as 'aorto-left-ventricular tunnel'. This results when
a channel is burrowed, perhaps by extension of an
aneurysm, within the wall of the left ventricle and
opens into its chamber, producing signs of aortic
regurgitation.[125]

Fenestrate Semilunar Valves.—The commonest
anomaly of the pulmonary and aortic valves is
fenestration or reticulation of the cusps at one or
more commissures. While usually considered to be
congenital, the incidence of these lesions increases
with advancing age,[126] suggesting a degenerative or
traumatic origin. The anomaly is usually unimpor-
tant, for the condition never involves the central
part of the cusps, which therefore remain fully
competent. Rarely, rupture of one of the fine
fibrous cords that bound the defects allows the
cusp to prolapse sufficiently during diastole for
regurgitation to take place.

Other Anomalies of the Semilunar Valves.—The
pulmonary valve may be virtually absent,[127] being
reduced to flat mural ridges at the valve site. This
anomaly is usually accompanied by others, par-

ticularly Fallot's tetrad or ventricular septal defect.
The pulmonary trunk and main branches may be
greatly dilated but the pressure within them is
normal.[128]

The aortic valve is not uncommonly bicuspid,
usually as an isolated anomaly (page 98).[129] In
contrast, it is rare to see a bicuspid pulmonary
valve, and this anomaly is usually accompanied by
serious malformations, such as Fallot's tetrad.[130]
A quadricuspid pulmonary valve is much less rare
than a quadricuspid aortic valve: the four cusps
may be of equal size or one of them may be rudimentary. In cases of atresia of the aorta and atresia
of the pulmonary artery rudiments of valvar
elements may or may not be discernible.

Atresia of the Aorta.—Atresia of the aorta may
occur alone or be accompanied by atresia of the
mitral valve (see below): like the latter, it is usually
associated with hypoplasia of the left ventricle (the
'hypoplastic left ventricle syndrome'). The hypoplastic ascending aorta in the neonate may be only
1 to 2 mm in diameter: it has even been mistakenly
described as a single coronary artery arising from
the aortic arch. The arch and its branches are
normal. The ductus arteriosus is wide, appearing
as a continuation of the pulmonary trunk: it carries

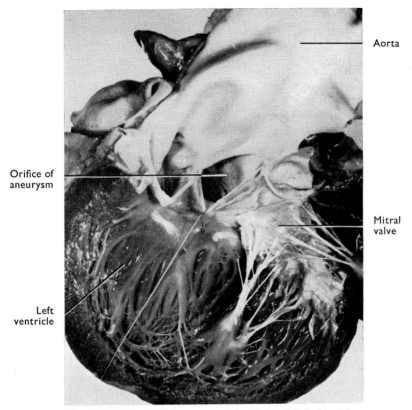

Aorta

Orifice of
aneurysm

Mitral
valve

Left
ventricle

Fig. 2.15B.§ Congenital aneurysm of a sinus of Valsalva. View
of orifice of the aneurysm in the non-coronary aortic sinus.

the blood flow to the aorta—the flow in the arch, ascending aorta and coronary arteries is therefore retrograde. The pulmonary venous return to the left atrium is led thence to the right atrium through an atrial septal defect or a valvular foramen ovale that has been forced open by the pressure of the blood flow.

This condition is probably the commonest form of fatal congenital heart disease in stillborn babies and neonates. In the latter, death usually occurs within five days;[131] despite this, palliative surgery has been successfully undertaken.[132] Cardiac catheterization may be dangerous, causing severe—even fatal—bradycardia if the catheter obstructs either the ductus or the hypoplastic ascending aorta itself.[133]

Anomalies of the Atrioventricular Valves.—At birth, the ventricular aspect of the atrioventricular valves may bear one or more small blood cysts, 1 to 2 mm in diameter, at the contact margin; it is probable that, ordinarily, they disappear in a few months. Rarely, a larger multilocular blood cyst develops at the base of a cusp: it may enlarge and even

cause obstruction, necessitating surgical removal. Blood cysts are common on the heart valves in cattle.[134]

Rarely, the tricuspid or mitral valve may have a double orifice. Both orifices have their own chordae tendineae: this distinguishes the condition from acquired perforation. One opening is usually smaller than the other ('accessory orifice').

In *mitral atresia* there is no mitral orifice: the outflow from the left atrium is into the right atrium through an atrial septal defect or a valvular foramen ovale forced open by the pressure of the blood. If these routes are not open the blood must pass by some other way—for instance, through mural sinusoids to the coronary arteries, veins and sinus and so to the right atrium. One classification of mitral atresia defines two main groups.[135] In Group I, the great vessels are normal, the left side of the heart is hypoplastic (see opposite), the aortic valve is atretic or hypoplastic and there may be a ventricular septal defect. In Group II, there is transposition of the great arteries with either a common ventricle, with or without infundibular inversion, or two ventricles. Other anomalies may accompany mitral atresia. Survival depends upon the adequacy of the aortic blood flow: usually it is measured in days to months.

Congenital mitral stenosis is rare and usually associated with other malformations.[136] The chordae tendineae are thickened and the spaces between them filled by fibrous tissue;[137] they may tether the cusps to a single papillary muscle (the so-called 'parachute mitral') and there may be a supravalvar shelf of left atrial tissue.[138]

'*Ballooning' of the mitral valve cusps* into the left atrium, causing regurgitation, is a well-known anomaly. The cusps are thick and fibrous. The condition is thought to be congenital in origin and not due to rheumatic endocarditis or other acquired diseases. It is sometimes referred to as prolapse of the posterior leaflet of the mitral valve,[139] this being the leaflet that is more noticeably affected radiologically. The same anatomical anomaly underlies the autosomal dominant familial '*syndrome of mid-late systolic click and late systolic murmur*'.[140] Sometimes the affected valve becomes infected.

Another fairly common abnormality is the '*floppy-valve syndrome*'[141] in which the mitral and aortic valves are enlarged, lax and regurgitant, and may contain an excess of mucopolysaccharide ('myxomatoid change'). Sometimes Marfan's syndrome is present (see page 82): for this reason the floppy valve syndrome is thought by some to be a *forme fruste* of this condition, and there is support for this view in the observation that there may be aortic medionecrosis in these cases.

In the ostium primum type of atrial septal defect, or when there is a common atrium, the mitral valve cusp is cleft by a deep inverted-V notch; in atrioventricularis communis there are no true septal cusps, for the mitral and tricuspid valves are continuous across the midline. In corrected transposition, the valve that guards the right atrium is bicuspid, and in appearance corresponds with the mitral valve.

The *tricuspid valve*, like the mitral valve, may have a deep notch in its medial cusp in association with ostium primum defect. In cases of corrected transposition, it is a tricuspid valve that guards the left atrium.

Tricuspid Atresia.[142]—In this condition the tricuspid valve is absent and the right ventricle is very small. Blood can reach the lungs only by passing from the right atrium through an atrial septal defect into the left atrium, and thence through the left ventricle and a patent ductus or ventricular septal defect to the pulmonary artery. This shunt causes much cyanosis, and the combination of severe cyanosis with an electrocardiograph of left ventricular preponderance is practically pathognomonic.

Instances of tricuspid atresia can be classed in two groups, corresponding to two main anatomical types;[143] in each group there are three subdivisions.[144] In Group I, survival to adulthood is possible because there is no transposition: the three subgroups are the cases with pulmonary atresia, those with pulmonary hypoplasia and a small ventricular septal defect, and those with a large ventricular septal defect alone. In Group II, the great arteries are transposed and the prognosis is poor, death being common in the first few weeks after birth, especially if aortic anomalies are also present:[145] the three subgroups are the cases with pulmonary atresia, those with pulmonary stenosis and those with a large pulmonary arterial trunk. Several types of palliative anastomotic operation have been undertaken to improve the poor pulmonary blood flow: one is the Glenn procedure,[146] which directs all superior vena caval blood into the right pulmonary artery near the hilum of the lung; another is 'balloon septostomy',[147] by which an inadequate interatrial shunt is increased. By contrast, an excessive pulmonary blood flow may require banding of the pulmonary trunk.

Aplasia of the Tricuspid Valve Leaflets.—Rarely, the tricuspid orifice may be present but quite unguarded because the entire valve is missing.[148]

Ebstein's Anomaly.[149]—The essential feature of Ebstein's anomaly is a malformation of the tricuspid valve. The tricuspid valve is derived not only from the atrioventricular endocardial cushions but also from the lower end of the right bulbar ridge; the unaffected parts of the valve in this anomaly are those derived from this ridge. The anterior cusp is large, and its attachment is in the normal site. The septal cusp and varying amounts of the posterior cusp are grossly abnormal, appearing as sacculate membranes held close to the wall by very small, and often aberrant, chordae tendineae. The papillary muscles related to these chordae are minute or absent.[150]

In a typical example (Fig. 2.16), the attachments of the septal and posterior cusps are displaced into the right ventricle: the portion of this chamber above the attachment of the cusps functions with the right atrium, while the remainder forms a diminutive right ventricle. The wall of the atrialized part of the ventricle is thin and may even be trans-

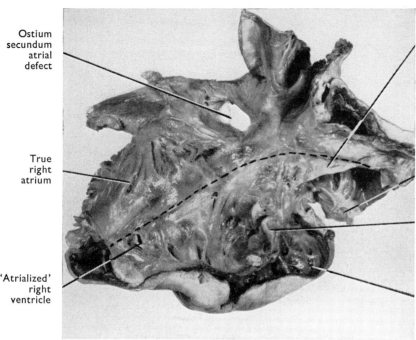

Ostium
secundum
atrial
defect

True
right
atrium

'Atrialized'
right
ventricle

Anterior
cusp of
tricuspid
valve

Pulmonary
valve

Malformed
medial and
posterior
cusps of
tricuspid
valve

Small right
ventricle

Fig. 2.16.§ Ebstein's anomaly with valve displacement. View of right atrium and ventricle. The dotted lines indicate the true atrioventricular junction: the posteromedial portion of the malformed tricuspid valve is displaced into the small right ventricle, with the result that the upper part of this chamber functions with the atrium. Note the ostium secundum atrial septal defect.

lucent. There is usually an ostium secundum defect in the atrial septum.

The deformed valve, although its cusps show the other defects characteristic of Ebstein's anomaly, is not always displaced into the ventricle. This has been called *dysplasia of the tricuspid valve*, the term '*Ebstein's malformation*' being restricted to the condition in which the valve is displaced, whether with or without dysplasia. When the displacement is minimal, the right ventricle may be dilated and hypertrophied. Other cardiac malformations, such as transposition, may be present.

Although the valve is so deformed, it may function well, and in such cases the expectancy of life is normal. In a personally studied case, the patient lived to the age of 79, never had any symptoms of heart disease, and died of a disease unrelated to the cardiovascular system.[151] Pregnancy may be accomplished successfully.[152] However, dysrhythmias are common and sudden death is known. Investigations such as cardiac catheterization may be hazardous: despite this, prosthetic or graft replacement of the valve has been accomplished successfully.

A closely similar picture is produced by the rare condition of '*dicuspid tricuspid valve*'. This

malformation may be associated with great enlargement of the right atrium and ventricle.

Another rarity in this group is *idiopathic enlargement of the right atrium*;[153] the chamber may be paper thin in places, but the valve is normal.[15] The condition may be related to 'parchment heart' (see page 81).

THE AORTA AND PULMONARY TRUNK

Development.—The process of fusion between the bilateral tubes (see page 77) is not limited to the heart but extends headward between the ventral aortae, which form a single dilated vessel, the aortic sac: the truncus arteriosus empties into this sac, and successive pairs of aortic arches radiate from it to the dorsal aortae. Fusion of the dorsal aortae occurs between the fourth thoracic and lumbar segments, to form a single descending aorta (Fig. 2.17A).

Since successive pairs of aortic arches connect the same structures—aortic sac and dorsal aortae— the first two pairs are largely redundant when the third pair is established, and they do not persist as main channels. The third arch persists and forms

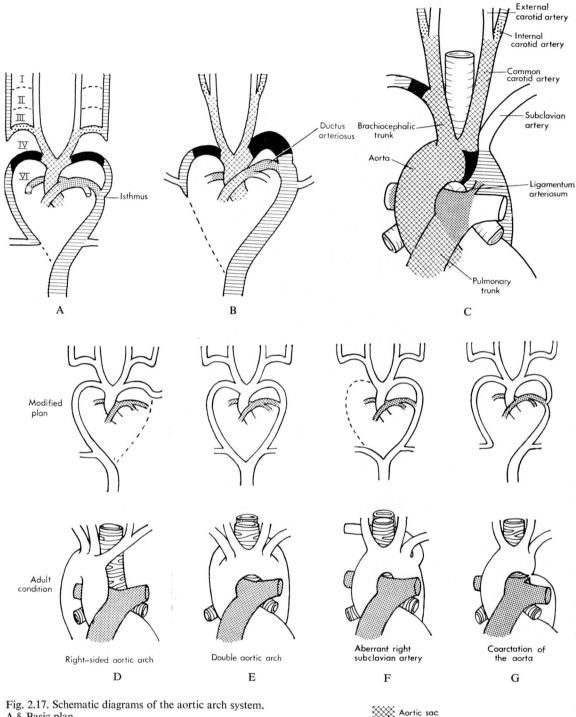

Fig. 2.17. Schematic diagrams of the aortic arch system.
A.§ Basic plan.
B.§ Condition in seventh week of embryonic development.
C.§ Normal adult derivatives.
D, E, F, G. Modifications in basic plan (upper row) and corresponding adult definitive forms of certain anomalies (lower row).

Key to shading:

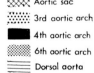

Aortic sac
3rd aortic arch
4th aortic arch
6th aortic arch
Dorsal aorta

the proximal part of the internal carotid artery (Figs 2.17B and 2.17C). As the neck elongates, the third and fourth arches draw out the aortic sac on each side, forming right and left horns. The root of the third arch further elongates to form the common carotid artery. The right horn forms the brachiocephalic trunk (innominate artery); the left horn forms that part of the arch of the aorta between the brachiocephalic trunk and the left common carotid artery. The fourth arches persist as channels connecting the horns of the aortic sacs, by way of the corresponding dorsal aorta, to the upper limb artery. The right fourth arch thus forms the proximal part of the right subclavian artery, extending from the brachiocephalic trunk; the left fourth arch forms that part of the arch of the aorta between the left common carotid and subclavian arteries. The fifth pair of arches is generally thought to be transient or absent in man; recently, however, persistence has been postulated as the explanation of a very rare anomaly, a double lumen localized to part of the arch of the aorta. The ventral ends of the sixth arches persist as the pulmonary arteries; connexion with the dorsal aortae is lost on the right side, but persists on the left side as the ductus arteriosus. Finally, the dorsal aortae disappear between the third and fourth arches, as does the unfused part of the right dorsal aorta distal to the limb artery.

The spiral ridges subdividing the truncus arteriosus lie left and right in the aortic sac, and extend on to its dorsal wall between the orifices of the fourth and sixth pairs of arches. When traced proximally, the ridges rotate through 180° so that, when they fuse, the channels lead from the ventral semilunar valve (pulmonary) to the dorsal part of the aortic sac and the sixth arches (pulmonary arteries) and from the dorsal semilunar valve (aortic) to the ventral part of the aortic sac (right and left horns). Thus are formed the pulmonary trunk and that part of the aorta proximal to the brachiocephalic trunk.

Anomalies of the spiral septum account for the varieties of transposition and the communications between the root of the aorta and the root of the pulmonary trunk.

Persistent Truncus Arteriosus.—If the whole spiral septum is absent, the truncus arteriosus persists as a single artery emerging from the heart to provide for the pulmonary, systemic and coronary circulations; the valve guarding its orifice usually has three cusps,[155] but the number varies, suggesting

that it may be determined haemodynamically rather than genetically; rarely, the valve is stenotic.[156] Since there is no bulbar septum to complete the ventricular septum, the interventricular foramen persists.

The blood supply to the lungs comes from this common trunk, either through pulmonary arteries, or, if these are inadequate, through enlarged bronchial arteries also. The origin of these pulmonary arteries varies: they may arise individually from the truncus, or they may arise from a single branch of the truncus.

Pulmonary hypertension develops early, cyanosis is usually severe, and life is short. The degree of disability depends largely on how well the systemic and pulmonary circuits function; only 15 per cent of the patients survive beyond 10 years. One woman bore a normal child at 22 and lived to 36, when she died of pulmonary hypertension with polycythaemia and multifocal thrombosis.[157]

Aortopulmonary Window.—When the two spiral ridges in the truncus arteriosus fail to join, an aperture—the aortopulmonary window—is left just above the semilunar valves. This defect ranges from a few millimetres across to almost total absence of the septum. The condition when the septum is almost totally absent differs anatomically from persistent truncus in that there are separate aortic and pulmonary valves; the two anomalies are indistinguishable clinically.

Aortopulmonary window is usually associated with a murmur, due to the left-to-right shunt. This sound is of greatest intensity about midway between the points where the murmurs of persistent ductus arteriosus and ventricular septal defect are usually heard best. Clinically, aortopulmonary window may also simulate a ruptured aneurysm of a sinus of Valsalva. The defect can be closed surgically.[158]

Transpositions

Transpositions are complicated anomalies in which the aorta and pulmonary trunk arise, wholly or partially, from the right and left ventricles respectively. In the ordinary, *uncorrected type* of transposition (sometimes referred to as the 'solitus'—that is, 'usual'—type), the aorta arises anteriorly from a right-sided right ventricle and therefore carries venous blood: an arteriovenous shunt is essential for survival. In the *corrected type* (inversus type), the aorta arises anteriorly from a left-sided right ventricle and carries arterial blood: a shunt is not necessary. Such 'correction' can also be the result of transplacement of the atria instead of the ventricles. Mirror-image counterparts of these various types add to the complexity of classification.

The factors responsible are probably haemodynamic. The plane in which the lower end of the bulbar septum approaches the primitive interventricular septum determines the relative positions of the orifices of the pulmonary trunk and aorta. The degree of rotation of the spiral septum in the truncus arteriosus determines which arches will be in communication with the anterior and posterior divisions of the bulbus.

Dextroposition of the Aorta.—It has already been seen that the aortic vestibule develops from the dorsal part of the bulbus cordis, so that in the normal heart the origin of the aorta is behind that of the pulmonary trunk. Dextroposition of the aorta results from increased rotation of the lower end of the bulbar septum, bringing the aorta farther to the right, although still in a posterior position. This is seen in Fallot's tetrad: in this condition the malalignment that causes the dextroposition is probably also the cause of the ventricular septal defect.

Double Outlet Right Ventricle.[159]—This condition is common in trisomy-18 (see page 75).[160] The aorta is completely transposed to the right ventricle and the pulmonary trunk also arises, completely or partially, from this chamber. Arterial blood can reach the aorta only by way of a ventricular septal defect (which therefore must not be closed surgically). When the pulmonary trunk is partly laevoposed, it overrides the septal defect, either anteriorly (Taussig–Bing type)[161] or posteriorly (Beuren type).[162]

Cyanosis from birth and progressive pulmonary hypertension are usual, unless there is pulmonary stenosis: in that case the clinical picture is like that of Fallot's tetrad except that some degree of heart block is common. Surgical alleviation is possible;[163, 164] in its absence, survival beyond the second decade is uncommon.[165]

Double outlet left ventricle, a condition that is not explicable on the basis of accepted embryological processes, has been reported.[166]

Complete Transposition.—When there is complete transposition the aorta arises wholly from the right ventricle and the pulmonary trunk wholly from the left ventricle (Figs 2.18A and 2.18B). This anomaly involves the whole process of bulbotruncal septation. The septum does not spiral but joins the aortic sac in such a way that the sixth arches, instead of the fourth, communicate with the posterior division of the truncus. The aorta and pulmonary trunk do not twist round one another but are parallel. The condition is incompatible with life, unless there is bidirectional shunting between the two circulations through a ventricular or atrial septal defect, or through a persistent ductus arteriosus.

The prognosis in cases of complete transposition is poor:[167] about 90 per cent of untreated babies die from heart failure or lung infection in their first year. Those with no effective shunt die soonest —within weeks or even days; those with a large ventricular septal defect may live into the second decade. Pulmonary stenosis usually improves the outlook; the bronchial arteries may enlarge and the clinical picture resembles that of Fallot's tetrad except that squatting and cyanotic attacks are much less common.[168]

Differential cyanosis—cyanosis that is intenser in the face and arms—occurs in transposition if there is a ductus arteriosus and pulmonary hypertension or if there is coarctation, hypoplasia or interruption of the aorta. In these circumstances the larger proportion of blood from the left ventricle reaches the descending aorta through the ductus, while the larger proportion of blood from the right ventricle reaches the branches of the aortic arch.

Pulmonary hypertension is usually present in cases of complete transposition. It is severest when there is a large ventricular septal defect, although survival is longer; in contrast, if the shunt is confined to a valvular foramen ovale, the changes in the lungs—dilatation of arteries and veins—resemble those of Fallot's tetrad although survival is usually briefer.[169] Even when pulmonary stenosis is present the development of obstructive vascular lesions in the lungs may not be precluded.[170] Rarely, the stenosis is subpulmonary and due to redundant tricuspid valve tissue.[171]

Associated anomalies are common and include hypoplasia of the right ventricle, Ebstein's anomaly (page 102) and anomalous pulmonary veins.

The development of surgical methods of alleviating transposition reflects the progress of cardiac surgery. Numerous ingenious palliative or corrective operations have been devised. Among the most popular palliative procedures are the creation or enlargement of an atrial septal defect (Blalock–Hanlon operation[172]) and balloon septostomy

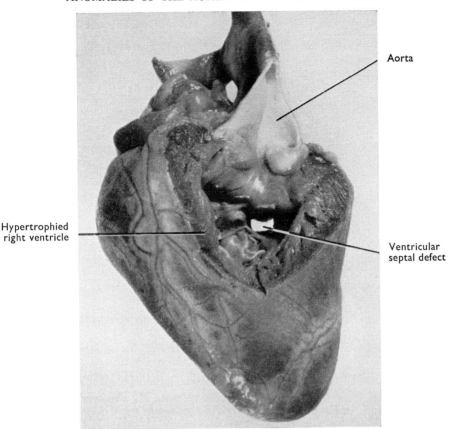

Fig. 2.18A.§ Complete transposition of the aorta and pulmonary trunk. View of right ventricle showing origin of aorta and ventricular septal defect.

(forcibly withdrawing a balloon-ended catheter through the valvular foramen ovale after inflating the balloon with mercury—the Rashkind operation[173]). These emergency procedures may permit survival to an age more suitable for corrective surgery, which has the purpose of redirecting the blood flow from each atrium into the appropriate great artery.[174] Excessive blood flow to the lungs can be limited by banding the main artery.

'Corrected' Transposition.—When the great arteries are transposed, the resulting abnormality may be 'corrected' anatomically or physiologically or in both ways. When correction is anatomical the aorta receives venous blood; when it is physiological, or anatomical and physiological together, the aorta receives arterial blood. Correction involves 'inversion' of the whole heart or of the atria alone or of the bulboventricular portion. As each of these three types has a mirror-image, there are six varieties of corrected transposition. The commonest is bulboventricular physiological correction (Fig. 2.19), in which the aorta is anterior but still arises from the left-sided (arterial) ventricle, the interior of which, however, has the architecture ordinarily found in the right ventricle; the left atrium communicates with this left ventricle by a tricuspid valve. The pulmonary trunk is posterior, and the right (venous) ventricle, from which it arises, has the internal architecture ordinarily found in the left ventricle, and communicates with the right atrium by a bicuspid ('mitral') valve. A ventricular septal defect is often present and complete heart block is common, the conducting system being disturbed by the altered anatomical situation. The left-sided tricuspid valve is usually incompetent at systemic pressures and there is often an additional anomaly such as single ventricle, pulmonary stenosis or atresia, Fallot's tetrad, Ebstein's anomaly or hypertrophic cardiomyopathy. Survival to adult life is possible—indeed, one man reached 73 years;[175] usually life is much

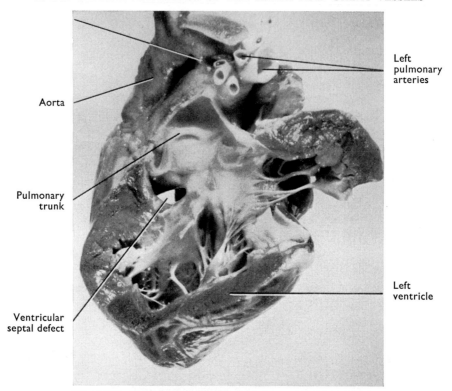

Aorta

Left pulmonary arteries

Pulmonary trunk

Left ventricle

Ventricular septal defect

Fig. 2.18B. Complete transposition of the aorta and pulmonary trunk. View of left ventricle with origin of pulmonary trunk and the high intramuscular ventricular septal defect.

shortened by the anomaly and the associated or additional defects, in spite of the correct circulation. Successful surgical relief of a complication is sometimes possible.

'Corrected' transposition is attributed to deflection of the bulboventricular loop. The bulbus comes off the left side of the common ventricle instead of the right, the bulbar septum therefore crossing the left margins of the fused atrioventricular cushions and so contributing to the left atrioventricular valve: the result is that the latter is tricuspid while the right atrioventricular valve is bicuspid (see page 102).

THE AORTIC ARCHES

Anomalies of the aortic arches are not uncommon. Numerous patterns are theoretically possible, and most of these variations have, in fact, been observed: the most frequent and important anomalies involve only the third, fourth and sixth pairs of arches and the corresponding portions of the aortae. Important in this group are anomalies causing some obstruction of the trachea and oesophagus, anomalous pulmonary arteries, aortic coarctation and persistent ductus arteriosus.

Anomalies Causing Dyspnoea or Dysphagia[176]

Right-Sided Aortic Arch (Fig. 2.17D).—Right-sided aortic arch, the normal condition in birds, is the reverse of the arrangement normally found in mammals. The left fourth arch forms the proximal part of the left subclavian artery. The ductus arteriosus may connect the left pulmonary artery with this subclavian artery, or with the right-sided aorta, by passing behind the oesophagus, thus forming a vascular ring that may compress the trachea and oesophagus.[177] Alternatively, the ductus may be on the right, connecting the aorta and the right pulmonary artery. The descending aorta may remain right-sided throughout, or it may cross to the midline to reach the normal aortic outlet from the thoracic cavity.

It is difficult to make a complete classification of the six main types and the subtypes of right-sided aorta. The anomaly is seldom isolated, the

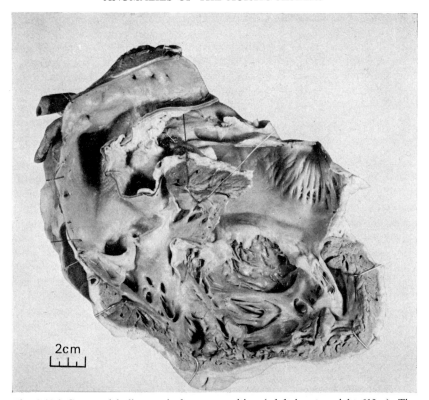

Fig. 2.19.§ Corrected bulboventricular transposition (adult heart, weight 610 g). The photograph shows the chambers of the left side. The atrium is normal, the atrioventricular valve is tricuspid, the ventricle has the appearance of a normal right ventricle (the crista supraventricularis is lifted by two hooks) and the aorta is anterior. There is only one coronary artery in this specimen. No other abnormalities, such as a septal defect, are present.

commonest associated abnormalities being—in descending order of frequency—ventricular septal defect, Fallot's tetrad, pulmonary stenosis, transposition, tricuspid atresia, laevocardia and dextrocardia.[178, 179]

Double Aortic Arch (Fig. 2.17E).—A double aortic arch is found normally in reptiles and frogs, both fourth arches persisting. When this occurs as an anomaly in the human, the two arches embrace the trachea and oesophagus and reunite to form the descending aorta—which may be on the left or the right. The arches are of different size, the anterior being usually the smaller. In this condition, the arteries that would arise from the single aortic arch usually arise from the arch that is more conveniently placed in relation to the normal course of the branches concerned. Most reported examples of double arch have been in patients with Fallot's tetrad; rarely, the condition is associated with a septal defect or transposition.[180]

Aberrant Right Subclavian Artery (Fig. 2.17F).— The first description of an aberrant right subclavian artery was by a London physician, Bayford,[181] in 1794. He referred to the symptoms that resulted from the anomaly as 'dysphagia lusoria', meaning a difficulty of swallowing associated with a sport, or freak. This term has since been applied to dysphagias due to other types of congenital anomaly. The anomalous subclavian artery is sometimes referred to as the lusorial artery. An aberrant right subclavian artery usually arises distal to the left subclavian artery and the ductus arteriosus—that is, beyond the sixth left arch—and its commencement probably represents persistence of the caudal part of the right dorsal aorta just before its union with the left dorsal aorta. In passing to the right, the aberrant artery runs behind the oesophagus, which it may therefore compress. A mirror image of the anomaly may be seen in an aberrant left subclavian artery associated with a right-sided aortic arch.

Anomalous Brachiocephalic Trunk and Left Common Carotid Artery.—If the brachiocephalic trunk arises from the arch of the aorta to the left of the midline, or if the left common carotid artery arises to the right of the midline, the trachea may be compressed as the vessel crosses to its proper side.

Anomalous Origin and Absence of the Pulmonary Arteries

The truncus arteriosus may fail to separate normally. The sixth arch may then remain connected to the aorta proximally as well as distally, the distal portion being the ductus arteriosus. If the proximal portion remains patent and the ductus involutes, the pulmonary artery will arise from the proximal part of the aorta; conversely, if the proximal portion involutes and the distal portion remains patent, the pulmonary artery will arise from the aortic arch by way of the ductus (a bilateral example is known[182]). If both portions, proximal and distal, involute, all those structures that develop from the sixth arches—the pulmonary trunk and its branches and the ductus arteriosus—will be absent, and the pulmonary valve will also fail to develop.[183, 184]

Anomalous development of the pulmonary arteries may be an isolated defect; usually, however, it is associated with other abnormalities, such as Fallot's tetrad, cystic lungs, or asplenia with laevocardia. Pulmonary hypertension is often an early consequence and death in infancy is common.

Coarctation of the Aorta

Coarctation means tightening or constriction. In coarctation of the aorta the constriction usually involves the region near the ductus arteriosus; exceptionally, it is near the diaphragm or even in the abdomen. The anomaly occurs twice as often in males as in females. It may accompany Turner's syndrome (see Chapter 26). It is commonly classified into infantile and adult types.[185]

In the *infantile type of coarctation* there is a localized eccentric narrowing of the aorta just beyond the origin of the left subclavian artery, usually proximal to but sometimes at the level of or distal to a persistent ductus arteriosus or, less commonly, the ligamentum arteriosum. Its development is probably unrelated to the process of closure of the ductus. Differential cyanosis—cyanosis of the feet in the absence of cyanosis of the hands and face—may occur if blood from the right ventricle is directed by the coarctation from the

ductus into the descending aorta. Other anomalies are often present, including bicuspid aortic valve, tubular hypoplasia of the aortic arch, ventricular septal defect, subaortic stenosis, left ventricular inflow obstruction, transposition, and anomalous pulmonary veins.[186] Babies with isolated coarctation fare much better than those with additional anomalies: the latter may require urgent surgery to combat progressive heart failure soon after birth.[187]

In the *adult type of coarctation* (Figs 2.17G and 2.20) the ductus arteriosus usually closes at birth. At first, the constriction is not so marked as to impede the blood flow significantly. Later, the rest of the aorta enlarges in the normal course of growth but the constricted part becomes progressively narrower, both relatively and absolutely, and the obstruction to the blood flow becomes progressively greater. The arterial circulation to the lower parts of the body is maintained by the opening of collateral channels between the prestenotic and poststenotic parts of the aorta. Although this anastomotic circulation is usually more than adequate for the needs of the organs and tissues thus supplied, the blood pressure and the strength of the pulses in the legs are much less than in the arms; indeed, there is usually hypertension in the upper part of the body, the reason for which is not certain—hyperplasia of the juxtaglomerular apparatus has been reported,[188] but the amount of renin in venous blood is generally within normal limits.[189] Progressive hypertrophy of the left ventricle usually develops. The mucopolysaccharides of the aortic wall undergo the same changes as occur in hypertension and in ageing.[190] There may be early atheroma of the coronary arteries.[191] There is no cyanosis, because there are no veno-arterial shunts and no part of the venous blood bypasses the lungs.

The anastomotic channels can be observed clinically in certain situations. They connect the subclavian and iliac arteries, and may be seen and felt to pulsate forcefully at the borders of the scapulae, in the supraclavicular fossae and in the axillae. Systolic murmurs may be heard over these vessels, and also over the line of the internal mammary and epigastric arteries, which are similarly dilated. Dilatation and tortuosity of the intercostal arteries result in the notching of the lower borders of the ribs that is such a characteristic and valuable diagnostic sign in radiographs. If thrombosis blocks the left subclavian artery, as happens occasionally, rib-notching will appear only on the right side. The change over a period of years

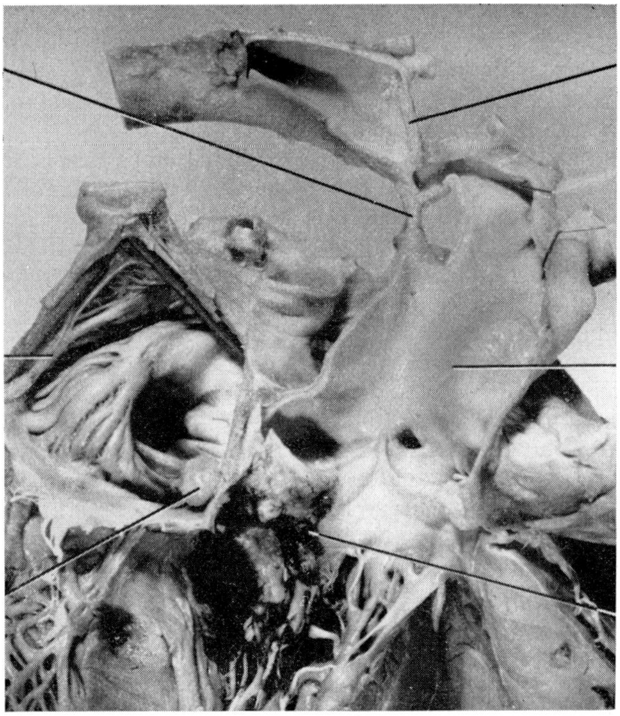

Fig. 2.20.§ Coarctation of the aorta. The stenosis lies at the site of the ligamentum arteriosum. There is also bacterial endocarditis of the aortic valve with involvement of the adjoining cusp of the tricuspid valve and consequent formation of an aneurysm of the cusp.

from a normal chest radiograph to the characteristic alteration in the outline of the heart and great vessels, with the development of notching of the ribs as the collateral channels enlarge, has been observed.[192] The combination of hypertension, small femoral pulses, pulsating anastomotic channels and absence of cyanosis makes a characteristic picture. Subaortic stenosis and aortic valve incompetence may be present.[193]

The outlook in most cases of the adult type of coarctation is quite good, the mortality being a little under 2 per cent in the first two decades and rising to almost 7 per cent in the sixth decade and beyond.[194] Those patients with considerable hypertension are constantly exposed to the risk of cerebral haemorrhage, rupture of the distended aorta, dissecting aneurysm of the aorta, and cardiac or renal failure. It is in such cases that surgical resection of the stenosed part of the aorta has been developed so successfully. The aorta distal to the coarctation may be greatly dilated and its wall very thin, and these changes may make the operation particularly difficult. In some cases resection of the stricture has been followed by acute necrosis of the small arteries

and arterioles of the abdominal viscera, the result of their exposure to a blood pressure much higher than before; this grave complication of the operation is comparable in pathogenesis to the necrotizing arterial lesions of malignant hypertension (see page 182 and Chapter 24).[195]

In the extreme form of coarctation, the ascending and descending segments of the aortic arch may be completely interrupted, the aorta beyond this level receiving its blood from the pulmonary trunk through a persistent ductus arteriosus; a ventricular septal defect is usual.[196] Rarely, there is no ductus, the distal aorta and axillary arteries then being fed retrogradely from the vertebral arteries; survival to adulthood and successful corrective surgery have been recorded in such cases.[197]

Pseudocoarctation. — The condition known as pseudocoarctation may be mentioned here: it is characterized by elongation of the aortic arch, which is kinked downward through the tethering action of the ligamentum arteriosum. There is no true obstruction. Secondary changes in the aortic wall, such as aneurysm or dissection, may make surgical treatment necessary.[198]

Persistent Ductus Arteriosus

The ductus arteriosus normally represents the connexion between the left sixth aortic arch and the left dorsal aorta. During fetal life, the blood in the inferior vena cava, enriched by blood joining it through the umbilical vein from the placenta, enters the right atrium, streams through the developing and still perforate interatrial septum to reach the left atrium, where it meets the pulmonary venous return with which it enters the left ventricle and thence the aorta and the branches of the aortic arch. This circulation ensures that the vital centres in the brain receive the best blood. In contrast, the fully venous blood in the superior vena cava crosses the inferior caval stream in the right atrium to enter the right ventricle and pulmonary trunk: about one-third enters the lungs and the rest traverses the ductus to reach the descending aorta whence, joined by the small residue from the arch and isthmus, it is distributed to the lower parts of the body and to the placenta.

At birth, the higher oxygenation of the blood following the onset of respiration, together with local secretion of catecholamines, causes constriction of the ductus[199] and therefore a characteristic murmur.[200] At the same time, expansion of the lungs unfurls the pulmonary vasculature and oxygenates the blood; the pulmonary vascular resist-ance falls precipitously. The great increase in the pulmonary venous flow to the left atrium closes the valve of the foramen ovale, so establishing the separation of the systemic and pulmonary circulations.

Obliteration of the ductus takes from several days to weeks to complete and is accomplished by intimal proliferation followed by mucoid degeneration and fibrosis of the wall, with the eventual formation of a fibrous cord, the ligamentum arteriosum.[201]

Why the ductus persists in some babies is not clear although known factors include high altitude (hypoxia)[202] and maternal rubella.[203] Spontaneous closure of a persistent ductus occurs in about 20 per cent of cases by the age of 60 years.[204]

If the ductus arteriosus persists (Fig. 2.21), blood continues to shunt from the aorta into the pulmonary trunk; the left ventricle therefore increases its output and becomes enlarged. This process cannot continue indefinitely, and the heart may eventually fail. The shunt is continuous, and is temporarily increased during each ventricular systole: there is thus a continuous murmur with systolic accentuation—the 'machinery murmur', or to-and-fro murmur, named after Gibson, who described it in 1900.[205]

The mortality of persistent ductus arteriosus is

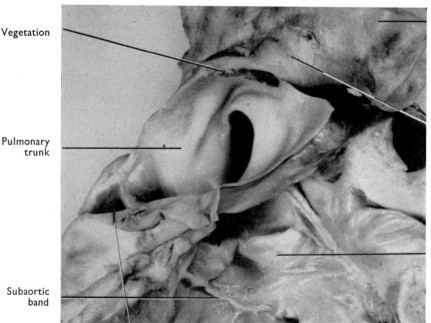

Fig. 2.21.§ Patent ductus arteriosus. View of the ductus with a bacterial vegetation at its pulmonary artery end. The aortic valve is thickened and there is a well-developed subvalvar aortic band.

greatest in the first year of life. In those who survive beyond the first year symptoms are rare for two decades; mortality then starts to rise, reaching 20 per cent at the age of 30 years and 60 per cent at 60 years.[204]

A persistent ductus arteriosus should be ligated in childhood, because of the risk of infective endarteritis.[206] This complication is comparable to infective endocarditis affecting the valves: when it develops, the vegetations usually appear in the pulmonary artery. A tubular ductus is relatively easy to ligate; often, however, the ductus is bowl-shaped, with an orifice in its floor opening directly into the pulmonary artery, or its wall may be weak because of atheroma—in such cases ligation may be difficult or hazardous.

Another important, but later, complication of persistent ductus arteriosus is pulmonary hypertension. At first this may be reversed by ligation of the ductus, but later there are secondary structural changes in the pulmonary arteries, and the condition becomes intractable. The pressure in the pulmonary artery may rise sufficiently to abolish the diastolic element of the murmur; occasionally, it equals or even exceeds the aortic pressure—the murmur then disappears and the patient becomes cyanosed. Reversal of the shunt in these cases may cause a plaque of thickening to form where the flow impinges on the wall of the aorta opposite the orifice of the ductus.

THE CORONARY ARTERIES

The coronary arteries are first seen as solid angioblastic buds growing out from the sinuses of Valsalva soon after aortopulmonary septation (Fig. 2.12E). They spread out under the epicardium and join the intramural vessels that have developed *in situ*.

There are considerable minor variations in their course and size. For example, the circumflex branch of the left coronary artery can sometimes extend to the back of the heart, although oftener its main portion goes no farther than the lateral border. The vessel that ordinarily is the first branch of a coronary artery may arise instead directly from the aorta: in this event there are two aortic ostia on the side concerned—a large one for the main trunk and a smaller one for the artery that is ordinarily the branch. The ostia of the coronary arteries may vary in position; they sometimes lie well above the level of the valve cusps.

Major anomalies include single coronary artery, arteriocameral or arteriovenous fistula, and origin from the pulmonary trunk.

Single Coronary Artery.—Both main coronary arteries may rise from a single stem from the aorta: when this is the case the blood supply to the myocardium may be adequate, but it is dependent upon the continued patency of the single artery. The consequent deviation of the main branches from their usual path may place them at risk in cardiac surgery; for example, the left anterior descending artery may cross the outflow of the right ventricle in the site of an approach incision. Rarely, the sole coronary artery may arise from one of the chambers of the heart.

Coronary Arteriocameral Fistula (Arterioluminal Fistula).—A coronary artery may communicate with a chamber of the heart or with the pulmonary trunk. There are two main types of this anomaly, that complicating pulmonary (or aortic) atresia and that occurring as an isolated abnormality. In *pulmonary atresia*, when the septum is intact and the tricuspid valve competent, the sole way for blood to leave the right ventricle is through persistent embryonic sinusoids in the chamber wall, forming a vessel that connects with a coronary artery (and that must not be ligated). A similar anomaly may develop in association with aortic atresia.

In the *isolated type* of coronary fistula, a coronary artery, commonly the right one, communicates directly or through an aneurysm or a complex of vessels with a chamber of the heart (commonly the right ventricle) or with the pulmonary trunk. The condition may cause palpitation, a thrill, Corrigan pulse, a 'machinery' murmur and enlargement of the heart: in contrast, and depending on the size of the shunt, there may be no symptoms until adulthood (and even until an advanced age— 80 years in one case[207]). Complications include heart failure, angina pectoris, pulmonary hypertension, infection and haemopericardium.[208] Surgical closure of the abnormal ostium may be possible and curative.

Coronary Aneurysms.—A coronary artery may be connected to the coronary sinus or one of its tributaries; the vessels involved become much dilated (arteriovenous aneurysm). Fistulous connexions between the left circumflex artery and the superior vena cava (or a persistent left superior vena cava) have been reported.[209] Surgical correction of these anomalies is possible.

Localized aneurysm of a coronary artery may be congenital but is usually the result of an arteritis. In one case an apparently congenital aneurysm of a coronary artery coexisted with a congenital aneurysm of a sinus of Valsalva.[210]

Anomalous Origin of Coronary Arteries from the Pulmonary Trunk.—A trivial abnormality of septation of the truncus may bring one or both coronary ostia into the pulmonary trunk. Origin of the *left coronary artery* from the pulmonary trunk was described by Abrikossoff;[211] the syndrome of cardiomegaly and ischaemic heart disease that may result is known as the Bland–White–Garland syndrome.[212] Damage to the papillary muscles may add mitral regurgitation to the disability. When atheroma develops, the anomalous left artery may show much less involvement than the normally derived right artery. Survival depends upon the efficiency of the collateral circulation: when the shunt is into the pulmonary trunk, or is balanced, the infant usually survives, but if the shunt is from the pulmonary trunk corrective surgery is necessary (and possible).[213] Survival to adulthood, even to 60 years, is well known, a continuous murmur being for long the main clinical finding; eventually, however, there is ischaemic heart disease, congestive failure, dysrhythmia and a liability to sudden death.[214] The case of an infant is on record in which the presence of an aortopulmonary 'window' ensured that aortic blood reached the anomalous artery.[215] Origin of the *right coronary artery* from the pulmonary trunk is a more benign condition. If *both coronary arteries* rise anomalously, survival is not possible unless there is a nearby arteriovenous shunt to supply the arteries with arterial blood.

THE CORONARY SINUS

Many anomalies of the coronary sinus have been reported.[216] Congenital enlargement is ordinarily due to its receiving a persistent left superior vena cava: the dilatation may be such as to form an 'accessory right atrium' (cor triatriatum dexter). The sinus may be absent when there is a left superior vena cava that enters the left atrium and there is an atrial septal defect. Its ostium may be atretic, the blood in the sinus entering the left atrium through Thebesian openings, one of which is known as Bochdalek's foramen. Hypoplasia of the sinus is relatively harmless, the venous drainage from the myocardium being assured by the Thebesian channels.

REFERENCES

DIAGNOSIS AND AETIOLOGY

1. Forssmann, W., *Klin. Wschr.*, 1929, **8**, 2085.
2. Cournand, A., Ranges, H. A., *Proc. Soc. exp. Biol. (N.Y.)*, 1941, **46**, 462.
3. Richards, D. W., Cournand, A., Darling, R. C., Gillespie, W. H., Baldwin, E. de F., *Amer. J. Physiol.*, 1942, **136**, 115.
4. McKusick, V. A., *Circulation*, 1955, **11**, 321.
5. Campbell, M., *Brit. Heart J.*, 1959, **21**, 65.
6. Campbell, M., Polani, P., *Lancet*, 1961, **1**, 463.
7. Emanuel, R., *Brit. Heart J.*, 1970, **32**, 28.
8. Gunning, J. F., Oakley, C. M., *Lancet*, 1971, **1**, 389.
9. Edwards, J. H., *Proc. roy. Soc. Med.*, 1968, **61**, 227.
10. Leachman, R. D., Latson, J. R., Kohlette, C. M., McNamara, D. G., *Circulation*, 1967, **35/36**, suppl. 2, 170.
11. Goerrtler, K., *Virchows Arch. path. Anat.*, 1956, **328**, 391.
12. Fales, D. E., *J. exp. Zool.*, 1946, **101**, 281.
13. Kalter, H., Warkany, J., *Physiol. Rev.*, 1959, **39**, 69.
14. Burnet, F. M., *Principles of Animal Virology*, 2nd edn, page 227. New York, 1960.
15. Gregg, N. M., *Trans. ophthal. Soc. Aust.*, 1941, **3**, 35.
16. Gregg, N. M., *Trans. ophthal. Soc. Aust.*, 1944, **4**, 119.
17. Dudgeon, J. A., *Proc. roy. Soc. Med.*, 1967, **67**, 642.
18. Leading Article, *Lancet*, 1962, **2**, 931.
19. Patten, B. M., *Pediatrics*, 1957, **19**, 734.

FUNCTIONAL DISTURBANCES

20. Callebaut, C., Denolin, H., Lequime, J., *Acta cardiol. (Brux.)*, 1949, **4**, 324.
21. Guntheroth, W. G., Morgan, B. C., Mullins, G. L., Baum, D., *Amer. Heart J.*, 1968, **75**, 313.
22. Cumming, G. R., Carr, W., *Lancet*, 1966, **1**, 519.
23. Wood, P. H., *Brit. med. J.*, 1958, **2**, 701, 755.
24. Chadd, M. A., Elwood, P. C., Gray, O. P., Muxworthy, S. M., *Brit. med. J.*, 1971, **4**, 516.
25. Brown, J. M., *Brit. Heart J.*, 1964, **26**, 778.
26. Krymsky, L. D., *Circulation*, 1965, **32**, 814.
27. Johnson, B. I., *J. clin. Path.*, 1951, **4**, 316.

ANOMALIES OF THE HEART AS A WHOLE

28. Sunderland, S., Wright-Smith, R. J., *Brit. Heart J.*, 1944, **6**, 167.
29. Nasser, W., Feigelbaum, H., Helmen, C., *Circulation*, 1966, **34**, 100.
30. Scott, G. W., *Guy's Hosp. Rep.*, 1955, **104**, 55.
31. Lev, M., Liberthson, R. R., Eckner, F. A. O., Arcilla, R. A., *Circulation*, 1968, **37**, 979.
32. Grant, R. P., *Circulation*, 1958, **18**, 25.
33. Kartagener, M., *Beitr. klin. Tuberk.*, 1933, **83**, 489.
34. Campbell, M., Deuchar, D. C., *Brit. Heart J.*, 1965, **27**, 69.
35. Chandra, R. K., Khetarpal, S. K., *Indian J. Pediat.*, 1963, **30**, 78.

36. Moller, J. H., Nakib, A., Anderson, R. C., Edwards, J. E., *Circulation*, 1967, **36**, 789.
37. Benson, P. F., Joseph, M. C., *Brit. med. J.*, 1961, **1**, 102.
38. Manning, G. W., *Amer. Heart J.*, 1950, **39**, 799.
39. Gordon, N., Hudson, R. E. B., *Brain*, 1959, **82**, 41.
40. Perloff, J. K., De Leon, A. C., Jr, O'Doherty, D., *Circulation*, 1966, **33**, 625.
41. De Wind, L. T., Jones, R. J., *J. Amer. med. Ass.*, 1950, **144**, 299.
42. Rosenbaum, H. D., Nadas, A. S., Neuhauser, E. B. D., *Amer. J. Dis. Child.*, 1953, **86**, 28.
43. Evans, W., *Brit. Heart J.*, 1949, **11**, 68.
44. Teare, D., *Brit. Heart J.*, 1958, **20**, 1.
45. Swan, D. A., Bell, B., Oakley, C. M., Goodwin, J., *Brit. Heart J.*, 1971, **33**, 671.
46. Braunwald, E., Lambrew, C. T., Rockoff, S. D., Ross, J., Jr, Morrow, A. G., *Circulation*, 1964, **30**, suppl. 4, 3.
47. Wigle, E. D., Trimble, A. S., Adelman, A. G., Bigelow, W. G., *Progr. cardiovasc. Dis.*, 1968, **51**, 83.
48. Emanuel, R., Withers, R., O'Brien, K., *Lancet*, 1971, **2**, 1065.
49. Moynahan, E. J., *Proc. roy. Soc. Med.*, 1970, **63**, 448.
50. Van Noorden, S., Olsen, E. G. T., Pearse, A. G. E., *Cardiovasc. Res.*, 1971, **5**, 118.
51. Still, W. J. S., Boult, E. H., *Lancet*, 1956, **2**, 117.
52. Żółtowska, A., *J. clin. Path.*, 1971, **24**, 263.
53. Geme, J. W. St., Noren, G. R., Adams, R., *New Engl. J. Med.*, 1966, **275**, 339.
54. Gersony, W. M., Katz, S. L., Nadas, A. S., *Pediatrics*, 1966, **37**, 430.
55. Kelly, J., Andersen, D. H., *Pediatrics*, 1956, **18**, 539.
56. Melhuish, B. P. P., Van Praagh, R. V., *Brit. Heart J.*, 1968, **30**, 269.
57. Osler, W., *Principles and Practice of Medicine*, 6th edn, page 820. London and New York, 1905.
58. Uhl, H. S. M., *Bull. Johns Hopk. Hosp.*, 1952, **91**, 197.
59. Prichard, R., *A.M.A. Arch. Path.*, 1951, **51**, 98.
60. Hudson, R. E. B., *Cardiovascular Pathology*, vol. 2, page 1584. London, 1965.
61. Hueper, W. C., *Amer. J. Path.*, 1941, **17**, 121.

THE SINUS VENOSUS

62. Powell, E. D. U., Mullaney, J. M., *Brit. Heart J.*, 1960, **22**, 579.
63. Jones, R. M., Niles, N. R., *Circulation*, 1968, **38**, 468.
64. Bennett, I. L., Jr, *Johns Hopk. Hosp. Bull.*, 1950, **87**, 290.
65. Watkins, E., Jr, Fortin, C. L., *Ann. Surg.*, 1964, **159**, 536.
66. Bedford, D. E., Hudson, R., *Actualités cardiol.*, 1961, **10**, 363.
67. Hudson, R., *Brit. Heart J.*, 1955, **17**, 489.
68. Ross, D. N., *Guy's Hosp. Rep.*, 1956, **105**, 376.
69. Johnson, A. L., Wigglesworth, F. W., Dunbar, J. S., Sidoo, S., Grajo, M., *Circulation*, 1958, **17**, 340.
70. Hickie, J. B., Gimlette, T. M., Bacon, A. P., *Brit. Heart J.*, 1956, **18**, 365.
71. Burchell, H. B., *Proc. Mayo Clin.*, 1956, **31**, 161.
72. Neill, C. A., Ferencz, C., Sabiston, D. C., Sheldon, H., *Bull. Johns Hopk. Hosp.*, 1960, **107**, 1.
73. Darling, R. C., Rothney, W. B., Craig, J. M., *Lab. Invest.*, 1957, **6**, 44.
74. Bonham Carter, R. E., Capriles, M., Noe, Y., *Brit. Heart J.*, 1969, **31**, 45.

75. Gathman, G. E., Nadas, A. S., *Circulation*, 1970, **42**, 143.
76. Loeffler, E., *Arch. Path.* (*Chic.*), 1949, **48**, 371.
77. Jorgensen, C. R., Ferlic, R. M., Varco, R. L., Lillehei, C. W., Eliot, R. S., *Circulation*, 1967, **36**, 101.
78. Winter, F. S., *Angiology*, 1954, **5**, 90.
79. Raghib, G., Ruttenberg, H. D., Anderson, R. C., Amplatz, K., Adams, P., Jr, Edwards, J. E., *Circulation*, 1965, **31**, 906.

THE INTERATRIAL SEPTUM

80. Raghib, G., Bloemendaal, R. D., Kanjuh, V. I., Edwards, J. E., *Amer. Heart J.*, 1965, **70**, 476.
81. Naeye, R. L., Blanc, W. A., *Circulation*, 1964, **30**, 736.
82. Feldt, R. H., Du Shane, J. W., Titus, J. L., *Circulation*, 1970, **42**, 437.
83. Campbell, M., Missen, G. A. K., *Brit. Heart J.*, 1957, **19**, 403.
84. Hickie, J. B., *Brit. Heart J.*, 1956, **18**, 320.
85. Hudson, R. E. B., *Cardiovascular Pathology*, vol. 3, page S.1023. London, 1970.
86. Campbell, M., *Brit. Heart J.*, 1970, **32**, 820.
87. Hudson, R. E. B., *Cardiovascular Pathology*, vol. 3, page S.1025. London, 1970.
88. Lutembacher, R., *Arch. Mal. Cœur*, 1916, **9**, 237.
89. Holt, M., Oram, S., *Brit. Heart J.*, 1960, **22**, 236.
90. Ellis, R. W. B., Creveld, S. van, *Arch. Dis. Childh.*, 1940, **15**, 16.
91. Giknis, F. L., *J. Pediat.*, 1963, **62**, 558.

THE VENTRICLES AND VALVES

92. Harley, H. R. S., *Guy's Hosp. Rep.*, 1958, **107**, 116.
93. Campbell, M., Reynolds, G., Trounce, J. R., *Guy's Hosp. Rep.*, 1953, **102**, 99.
94. Lev, M., Liberthson, R. R., Kirkpatrick, J. R., Eckner, F. A. O., Arcilla, R. A., *Circulation*, 1969, **39**, 577.
95. Roger, H., *Bull. Acad. Méd.* (*Paris*), 1879, **8**, 1074.
96. Campbell, M., *Brit. Heart J.*, 1971, **33**, 246.
97. Muller, W. H., Jr, Dammann, J. F., Jr, *Surg. Gynec. Obstet.*, 1952, **95**, 213.
98. Watson, H., McArthur, P., Somerville, J., Ross, D., *Lancet*, 1969, **2**, 1225.
99. Somerville, J., Brandao, A., Ross, D. N., *Circulation* 1970, **41**, 317.
100. Eisenmenger, V., *Z. klin. Med.*, 1897, **32**, suppl., 1.
101. Wood, P. H., *Brit. med. J.*, 1958, **2**, 701, 755.
102. Kobetzky, E. D., Moller, J. H., Korns, M. E., Schwartz, C. J., Edwards, J. E., *Circulation*, 1969, **40**, 43.
103. Fallot, A., *Marseille-méd.*, 1888, **25**, 418.
104. Marquis, R. M., *Brit. med. J.*, 1956, **1**, 819.
105. Steno [Stensen], N., *Acta med. phil. hafniae*, 1671–2, **1**, 200.
106. Peacock, T. B., *Malformations of the Heart*, 2nd edn. London, 1866.
107. Blalock, A., Taussig, H. B., *J. Amer. med. Ass.*, 1945, **128**, 189.
108. Ross, D. M., Somerville, J., *Lancet*, 1966, **2**, 1446.
109. Wagenvoort, C. A., Nauta, J., van der Schaar, P. J., Weeda, H. W. H., Wagenvoort, N., *Circulation*, 1967, **36**, 924.
110. Brock, R., *The Anatomy of Congenital Pulmonary Stenosis*. London, 1957.
111. Palois, *Bull. Fac. Méd. Paris*, 1809, **2**, 133.
112. White, P. D., Hurst, J. W., Fennell, R. H., *Circulation*, 1950, **2**, 558.

113. Gasual, B. M., Richmond, J. B., Krakower, C. A., *J. Pediat.*, 1949, **35**, 413.
114. Danilowicz, D., Ross, J., Jr, *Brit. Heart J.*, 1971, **33**, 138.
115. Somerville, J., *Brit. Heart J.*, 1970, **32**, 641.
116. Hartmann, A. F., Jr, Goldring, D., Carlsson, E., *Circulation*, 1964, **30**, 679.
117. Campbell, M., Kauntze, R., *Brit. Heart J.*, 1953, **15**, 179.
118. Peery, T. M., *J. Amer. med. Ass.*, 1958, **166**, 1123.
119. Ionescu, M. I., Ross, D. N., Wooler, G. H., *Biological Tissue in Heart Valve Replacement*. London, 1971.
120. Williams, J. C. P., Barratt-Boyes, B. G., Lowe, J. B., *Circulation*, 1961, **24**, 1311.
121. Black, J. A., Bonham Carter, R. E., *Lancet*, 1963, **2**, 745.
122. Morgan-Jones, A., Langley, F. A., *Brit. Heart J.*, 1949, **11**, 325.
123. Sakakibara, S., Konno, S., *Amer. Heart J.*, 1968, **75**, 595.
124. Page, D. L., Williams, G. M., *Circulation*, 1969, **39**, 841.
125. Levy, M. J., Lillehei, C. W., Anderson, R. C., Amplatz, K., Edwards, J. E., *Circulation*, 1963, **27**, 841.
126. Foxe, A. N., *Amer. J. Path.*, 1929, **5**, 179.
127. Campeau, L. A., Ruble, P. E., Cooksey, W. B., *Circulation*, 1957, **15**, 397.
128. Macartney, F. J., Miller, G. A. H., *Brit. Heart J.*, 1970, **32**, 483.
129. Koletsky, S., *Arch. intern. Med.*, 1941, **67**, 129.
130. Koletsky, S., *Arch. Path.* (*Chic.*), 1941, **31**, 338.
131. Krovetz, L. J., Rowe, R. D., Scheibler, G. L., *Circulation*, 1970, **42**, 953.
132. Cayler, G. G., Smeloff, E. A., Miller, G. E., Jr, *New Engl. J. Med.*, 1970, **282**, 780.
133. Miller, G. A. H., *Brit. Heart J.*, 1971, **33**, 367.
134. Smith, R. B., Taylor, I. M., *Cardiovasc. Res.*, 1971, **5**, 132.
135. Ehlers, K. H., Farnsworth, P. B., Ho, E., Levin, A. R., Engle, M. E., *Circulation*, 1967, **35/36**, suppl. 2, 102.
136. Ferencz, C., Johnson, A., Wigglesworth, F. W., *Circulation*, 1954, **9**, 161.
137. Tank, E. S., Bernhard, W. F., Gross, R. E., *Circulation*, 1967, **35/36**, suppl. 2, 246.
138. Shonc, J. D., Sellers, R. D., Anderson, R. C., Adams, P., Jr, Lillehei, C. W., Edwards, J. E., *Amer. J. Cardiol.*, 1963, **11**, 714.
139. Stannard, M., Sloman, J. G., Hare, W. S. C., Goble, A. J., *Brit. med. J.*, 1967, **3**, 71.
140. Shell, W. E., Walton, J. A., Clifford, M. E., Willis, P. W., III, *Circulation*, 1969, **39**, 327.
141. Read, R. C., Thal, A. P., Wendt, V. E., *Circulation*, 1965, **32**, 897.
142. Brown, J. W., Heath, D., Morris, T. L., Whitaker, W., *Brit. Heart J.*, 1956, **18**, 499.
143. Edwards, J. E., Burchell, H. B., *Med. Clin. N. Amer.*, 1949, **33**, 1177.
144. Keith, J. D., Rowe, R. D., Vlad, P., *Heart Disease in Infancy and Childhood*, pages 437, 571. New York, 1958.
145. Marcano, B. A., Riemenschneider, T. A., Ruttenberg, H. D., Goldberg, S. J., Gyepes, M., *Circulation*, 1969, **40**, 399.
146. Glenn, W. W. L., Gardner, T. H., Jr, Talner, N. S., Stansel, H. C., Jr, Matano, I., *Circulation*, 1967, **35/36**, suppl. 2, 122.

147. Rashkind, W., Friedman, S., Waldhausen, J. A., Miller, W. W., *Circulation*, 1967, **35/36**, suppl. 2, 217.
148. Kanjuh, V. I., Stevenson, J. E., Amplatz, K., Edwards, J. E., *Circulation*, 1964, **30**, 911.
149. Ebstein, W., *Arch. Anat. Physiol.*, 1866, 238.
150. Brown, J. W., Heath, D., Whitaker, W., *Amer. J. Med.*, 1956, **20**, 322.
151. Adams, J. C. L., Hudson, R., *Brit. Heart J.*, 1956, **18**, 129.
152. Littler, W. A., *Brit. Heart J.*, 1970, **32**, 711.
153. Pastor, B. H., Forte, A. L., *Amer. J. Cardiol.*, 1961, **8**, 513.
154. Tenckhoff, L., Stamm, S. J., Beckwith, J. B., *Circulation*, 1969, **40**, 227.

THE AORTA AND PULMONARY TRUNK

155. Collett, R. W., Edwards, J. E., *Surg. Clin. N. Amer.*, 1949, **29**, 1245.
156. Burnell, R. H., McEnery, G., Miller, G. A. H., *Brit. Heart J.*, 1971, **33**, 423.
157. Hicken, P., Evans, D., Heath, D., *Brit. Heart J.*, 1966, **28**, 284.
158. Cooley, D. A., McNamara, D. G., Latson, J. R., *Surgery*, 1957, **42**, 101.

TRANSPOSITIONS

159. Witham, A. C., *Amer. Heart J.*, 1957, **53**, 928.
160. Rogers, T. R., Hagstrom, J. W. C., Engle, M., *Circulation*, 1965, **32**, 802.
161. Taussig, H., Bing, R. J., *Amer. Heart J.*, 1949, **37**, 551.
162. Beuren, A., *Circulation*, 1960, **21**, 1071.
163. Gomes, M. M. R., Weidman, W. H., McGoon, D. C., Danielson, G. K., *Circulation*, 1971, **43**, 889.
164. Gomes, M. M. R., Weidman, W. H., McGoon, D. C., Danielson, G. K., *Circulation*, 1971, **43/44**, suppl. 1, 31.
165. Campbell, M., Hudson, R. E. B., *Guy's Hosp. Rep.*, 1958, **107**, 14.
166. Paul, M. H., Muster, A. J., Sinha, S. N., Cole, R. B., Van Praagh, R., *Circulation*, 1970, **41**, 129.
167. Liebman, J., Cullum, L., Belloc, N. B., *Circulation*, 1969, **40**, 237.
168. Rowe, R. D., Mehrizi, A., Hutchins, G. M., Folger, G. M., Jr, *Circulation*, 1965, **31/32**, suppl. 2, 182.
169. Wagenvoort, C. A., Nauta, J., van der Schaar, P. J., Weeda, H. W. H., Wagenvoort, N., *Circulation*, 1968, **38**, 746.
170. Viles, P. H., Ongley, P. A., Titus, J. L., *Circulation*, 1969, **40**, 31.
171. Riemenschneider, T. A., Goldberg, S. J., Ruttenberg, H. D., Gyepes, M. T., *Circulation*, 1969, **39**, 603.
172. Blalock, A., Hanlon, C. R., *Surg. Gynec. Obstet.*, 1950, **90**, 1.
173. Rashkind, W. J., Miller, W. W., *J. Amer. med. Ass.*, 1966, **196**, 991.
174. Mustard, W. T., *Surgery*, 1964, **55**, 469.
175. Lieberson, A. D., Schumaker, R. R., Childress, R. H., Genovese, P. D., *Circulation*, 1969, **39**, 96.

THE AORTIC ARCHES

176. Gross, R. E., *Circulation*, 1955, **11**, 124.
177. Neuhauser, E. B. D., *Amer. J. Roentgenol.*, 1949, **62**, 493.

178. Hastreiter, A. R., D'Cruz, I. A., Cantez, T., *Brit. Heart J.*, 1966, **28**, 722.

179. D'Cruz, I. A., Cantez, T., Namin, E. P., Licata, R., Hastreiter, A. R., *Brit. Heart J.*, 1966, **28**, 725.

180. Higashino, S. M., Ruttenberg, H. D., *Brit. Heart J.*, 1968, **30**, 579.

181. Bayford, D., *Mem. med. Soc. Lond.*, 1794, **2**, 275.

182. Kearney, M. S., *J. Path.*, 1969, **97**, 729.

183. Winship, W. S., Beck, W., Schrire, V., *Brit. Heart J.*, 1967, **29**, 34.

184. Stuckey, D., Bowdler, J. D., Reye, R. D. K., *Brit. Heart J.*, 1968, **30**, 258.

185. Bonnet, L. M., *Rev. Méd.*, 1903, **23**, 108.

186. Becker, A. E., Becker, M. J., Edwards, J. E., *Circulation*, 1970, **41**, 1067.

187. Sinha, S. N., Kardatke, M. L., Cole, R. B., Muster, A. J., Wessel, H. V., Paul, M. H., *Circulation*, 1969, **40**, 385.

188. Anderson, C., *J. Path.*, 1969, **97**, 671.

189. Werning, C., Schönberg, M., Weidmann, P., Baumann, K., Gysling, E., Wirz, P., Siegenthaler, W., *Circulation*, 1969, **40**, 73.

190. Berry, C. L., Tawes, R. L., Jr, *Cardiovasc. Res.*, 1970, **4**, 224.

191. Vlodaver, Z., Neufeld, H. N., *Circulation*, 1968, **37**, 449.

192. Symmers, W. St C. (quoted by Campbell, M., Suzman, S., *Brit. Heart J.*, 1947, **9**, 185).

193. Campbell, M., Baylis, J. H., *Brit. Heart J.*, 1956, **18**, 475.

194. Campbell, M., *Brit. Heart J.*, 1970, **32**, 633.

195. Benson, W. R., Sealy, W. C., *Lab. Invest.*, 1956, **5**, 359.

196. Roberts, W. C., Morrow, A. G., Braunwald, E., *Circulation*, 1962, **26**, 39.

197. Morgan, J. R., Forker, A. D., Fosburg, R. G., Neugebaur, M., Rogers, A. K., Bemiller, C. R., *Circulation*, 1970, **42**, 961.

198. Bruwer, A. J., Burchell, H. B., *J. Amer. med. Ass.*, 1956, **162**, 1445.

199. Born, G. V. R., Dawes, G. S., Mott, J. C., Rennick, B. R., *J. Physiol. (Lond.)*, 1956, **132**, 304.

200. Burnard, E., *Brit. med. J.*, 1958, **1**, 806.

201. Hoefsmit, E. C. M., *Het sluitingsproces van de ductus arteriosus bij de rat. Thesis:* Leiden, 1967.

202. Espino-Vela, J., Cardenas, N., Cruz, R., *Circulation*, 1968, **37/38**, suppl. 5, 45.

203. Gregg, N. M., *Trans. ophthal. Soc. Aust.*, 1941, **3**, 35.

204. Campbell, M., *Brit. Heart J.*, 1968, **30**, 4.

205. Gibson, G. A., *Edinb. med. J.*, 1900, **8**, 1.

206. Panagopoulos, P. G., Tatodes, C. J., Aberdeen, E., Waterston, D. J., Carter, R. E. B., *Thorax*, 1971, **26**, 137.

THE CORONARY ARTERIES

207. Colbeck, J. C., Shaw, J. M., *Amer. Heart J.*, 1954, **48**, 270.

208. Barnes, R. J., Cheung, A. C. S., Wu, R. W. Y., *Brit. Heart J.*, 1969, **31**, 299.

209. Gensini, G. G., Palacio, A., Buananno, C., *Circulation*, 1966, **33**, 217.

210. Hudson, R. E. B., *Cardiovascular Pathology*, vol. 3, page S.398. London, 1970.

211. Abrikossoff, A., *Virchows Arch. path. Anat.*, 1911, **203**, 413.

212. Bland, E. F., White, P. D., Garland, J., *Amer. Heart J.*, 1933, **8**, 787.

213. Perry, L. W., Scott, L. P., *Circulation*, 1970, **41**, 1043.

214. Wesselhoeft, H., Fawcett, J. S., Johnson, A. J., *Circulation*, 1968, **38**, 403.

215. Agius, P. V., Rushworth, A., Connolly, N., *Brit. Heart J.*, 1970, **32**, 708.

THE CORONARY SINUS

216. Mantini, E., Grondin, C. M., Lillehei, C. W., Edwards, J. E., *Circulation*, 1966, **33**, 317.

ACKNOWLEDGEMENTS FOR ILLUSTRATIONS

Figs 2.2, 5, 6A, 6B, 7, 9, 11, 13, 14B, 15A, 15B, 16, 18A, 19, 20 and 21. Reproduced by permission of the publishers, Messrs Edward Arnold, from: Hudson, R. E. B., *Cardiovascular Pathology*, vol. 2 (London, 1965) and vol. 3 (London, 1970).

Figs 2.3 and 4. Specimen provided by Dr R. R. Wilson, Stobhill Hospital, Glasgow. Photographs reproduced by permission of the publishers, Messrs Edward Arnold, from: Hudson, R. E. B., *Cardiovascular Pathology*, vol. 2; London, 1965.

Figs 2.8A and B. Specimen provided by Dr Jane Somerville, Cardiothoracic Institute, London. Photographs reproduced by permission of the publishers, Messrs Edward Arnold, from: Hudson, R. E. B., *Cardiovascular Pathology*, vol. 2; London, 1965.

Fig. 2.12B. Based on: Kramer, T. C., *Amer. J. Anat.*, 1942, **71**, 343.

Figs 2.17A, B and C. Based in part on: Barry, A., *Anat. Rec.*, 1951, **111**, 221.

E

3: *Arteries, Veins and Lymphatics; Hypertension*

CONTENTS

3A: *Arteries, Veins and Lymphatics*

by T. CRAWFORD

3B: *Hypertension*

by K. A. PORTER

3A: *Arteries, Veins and Lymphatics*

by T. CRAWFORD

ARTERIES AND ARTERIOLES

Normal Structure

The innermost layer of the arterial wall adjacent to the flowing blood is the *endothelium*, composed of a continuous sheath of flattened cells, often difficult to preserve in histological preparations. The integrity of this cell layer is of paramount importance, for damage to it is likely to initiate thrombus formation at the site. The endothelium is separated by a scanty zone of loose-mesh connective tissue (amongst which there may be a few longitudinally running visceral muscle fibres) from the *internal elastic lamina*—a fenestrated tube of elastic fibres. In fixed sections this appears as a continuous wavy line, but in life the membrane is taut, serving at once to limit distensibility and to restore the calibre of the lumen after limited distension. The internal elastic lamina, endothelium and intervening tissue constitute the *intima* or internal coat (Fig. 3.1).

The *media*, or middle coat, lies between the internal and external elastic laminae and, in all but the largest vessels, consists mainly of smooth muscle fibres running transversely round the artery. In large arteries, elastic fibres are mingled with the muscle, and in the largest arteries (the so-called 'elastic arteries') they predominate. The external elastic lamina, on the outside of the media, is less well defined than the internal lamina and is sometimes absent, notably in the cerebral arteries.

The *adventitia*, or outer coat, consists of loose-mesh fibrous tissue and merges with adjacent structures. It is rich in lymphatics and autonomic nerve fibres.

The arterial wall derives its oxygen and nutriment from two sources: the intima and the inner layers of the media are nourished by diffusion from the blood in the lumen and are normally without capillaries of their own, while the adventitia and outer layers of the media are supplied by the *vasa vasorum*—vessels arising from the parent artery or its branches or from adjacent vessels. Pathological increase in the thickness of the intima may, how-

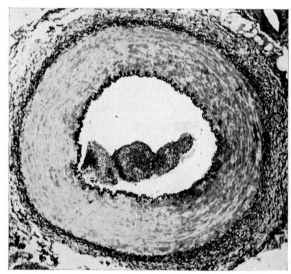

Fig. 3.1. Transverse section of wall of a radial artery from a young man. The dark convoluted line near the lumen is the internal elastic lamina and the similar, but thinner, line at the periphery is the external lamina. The bulk of the tissue, between these elastic laminae, is the muscular media. The intima is scarcely discernible at this magnification and consists of endothelial cells lying almost directly on the elastic lamina. *Weigert and Van Gieson stain.* × 20.

ever, disturb this arrangement and lead to the vascularization of layers that normally are avascular.

Age Changes in Arteries

The arterial structure outlined above is that normal in early life: on examining the arteries of middle-aged and elderly people, certain structural changes—not of a definitely pathological character—are regularly encountered. There is, indeed, no system in the body in which the borderline between normality and pathological states is so ill defined as in the vascular tree. The interpretation of a particular structural change as being a normal concomitant of advancing years on the one hand, or

120

the early manifestation of a pathological process on the other, will frequently be in doubt. Such changes may affect both intima and media.

Intimal Changes.—At birth the endothelium lies almost directly upon the internal elastic lamina, but even in childhood these layers come to be separated by loose-mesh connective tissue, which tends to increase in amount and density with the passage of the years.[1, 2] The coronary arteries and the arteries of the lower limbs are the most affected in this way and, in these vessels, the intima, by the age of 60, may equal or even exceed the media in thickness, without any definite pathological state existing (Fig. 3.2). Fatty droplets may appear amongst the connective tissue fibres: if these form significant

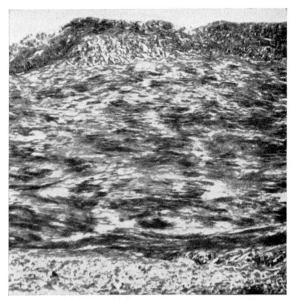

Fig. 3.3. Wall of brachial artery from a man aged 62 years. The darkly stained muscle fibres are widely separated by pale-staining collagen. *Picro–Mallory stain.* × 75.

are few in number and the collagen fibres that have replaced them may show hyaline degeneration. Chemical examination shows a rise in calcium content accompanying these changes, but this is not usually recognizable by histological methods.[3]

In medium-sized arteries (such as the vessels of the limbs) these changes may lead to dilatation and elongation, so that the artery pursues a tortuous course. In small arteries and arterioles some degree of narrowing may result from the intimal thickening.

This state of the arteries associated with advanced age is sometimes referred to as *senile arteriosclerosis*, though it is perhaps unfortunate to apply a term with pathological significance to a condition regarded as physiological. The term *presenile arteriosclerosis* may be applied to the occurrence of similar changes at an unusually early age and without apparent cause.

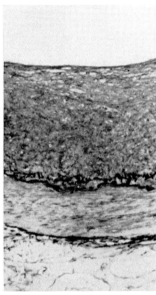

Fig. 3.2. Transverse section of the wall of an apparently normal coronary artery from a man of 62 years. The intima is now the bulkiest layer, and the internal elastic lamina is partly duplicated. *Weigert and Van Gieson stain.* × 50.

collections then the borderline to pathology has been crossed. The internal elastic lamina tends to thicken in later life and there may be patchy production of new fibres forming a second incomplete ring inside the original lamina; sometimes gaps of varying length develop in the elastic layer.

Medial Changes.—The media of the muscular arteries reaches its full development in early adult life. From middle age onward there is a progressive increase in collagen fibres at the expense of muscle cells (Fig. 3.3); at advanced ages the muscle fibres

'SCLEROTIC' CHANGES IN ARTERIES

Nomenclature

The nomenclature of this group of diseases is the cause of much confusion, which is heightened by different usages in different countries. The word *arteriosclerosis* was introduced as long ago as 1833 by Lobstein.[4] He employed it in a generic sense to indicate conditions with thickening and hardening of the vessel walls, and it has retained this sense in continental Europe and America; in Britain pathologists have tended to limit its use to conditions of medial sclerosis, excluding processes that mainly involve the intima. It is, perhaps, best to use the unqualified word only in a clinical sense for conditions of thickening and hardening of the arteries when the precise pathological state can only be guessed at. The pathologist, assessing all the evidence, will use the word only with appropriate qualification—examples from the clinical group may then finally be classified as one of the following:

(a) senile (or presenile) arteriosclerosis
(b) hypertensive arteriosclerosis
(c) Mönckeberg's sclerosis (calcification of the media)
(d) atherosclerosis.

The first of these conditions has been described above, and an account of the second is included in the discussion of hypertension (page 182).

Mönckeberg's Sclerosis

It was in 1903 that Mönckeberg[5] drew attention to cases in which calcification of the medial coat was the most conspicuous pathological feature, and, although the condition had been known long before this, Mönckeberg's name has since been regularly applied to it. Minor degrees of medial calcification are common but all grades of severity can be found, from a few scattered calcific granules up to rings and plates of calcified tissue, and indeed sometimes bony trabeculae, forming irregular bands round the artery or converting lengths of the vessel into rigid 'pipe-stems'. These fully developed examples are mostly seen at advanced ages but occasionally occur in younger people. The arteries of the lower limbs are most frequently and severely affected, those of the upper limbs next oftenest. The vessels tend to be dilated and, where superficial, can be palpated easily. The whole course of a vessel may show in an X-ray picture (Fig. 3.4).

Calcification of the media is in itself not a harmful condition and its incidental discovery in a limb X-rayed following an injury should not be regarded as a cause for alarm. On the other hand, the medial calcification may coexist with severe atherosclerosis (see below) and then the complications of the latter lesion may supervene.

It is doubtful if Mönckeberg's sclerosis is correctly regarded as a specific pathological entity; ordinarily, the calcium content of the media increases progressively with age and this increase may

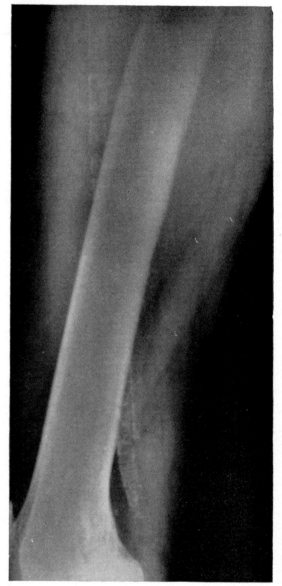

Fig. 3.4. Mönckeberg's sclerosis. Radiograph showing calcification in the femoral artery.

by intensified by abnormal stresses in hypertension, and in other unexplained ways. Microscopically, two varieties of change can be distinguished: in the first the sequence of events is fibrous replacement of muscle followed by hyaline degeneration of the collagen fibres, in which calcium salts are subsequently deposited; in the second, fatty changes occur in the muscle cells, which later fuse into an amorphous mass rich in fats and in which areas of calcification quickly develop (Fig. 3.5). Sometimes the calcified area is partially converted to

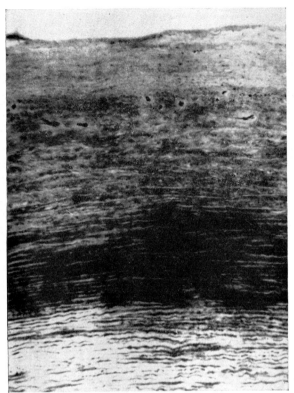

Fig. 3.5. Mönckeberg's sclerosis. Section of the wall of the brachial artery, showing marked calcification. Heavy deposits of calcium salts are present in the media, while the intima shows only a few granules. *Von Kossa stain.* × 75.

true bone and occasionally there may even be marrow spaces containing haemopoietic cells.

Metastatic calcification of the blood vessels occurring in hyperparathryoidism has little in common with the above conditions. It is patchy in distribution, may affect any vessel, including capillaries and veins, and is especially well seen in visceral arteries; the deposition may occur in the intima as well as the media.

Atherosclerosis

Atherosclerosis is at once the most important, the commonest, the most controversial, and the most paradoxical of arterial diseases. So universal is it that a case could be argued for regarding it as a normal concomitant of ageing, and yet it is the main pathogenetic factor in two of the commonest killing diseases of the middle-aged and elderly—ischaemic heart disease and cerebrovascular disease. It is not out of place to bracket atherosclerosis with cancer as the outstanding problems facing medical science today.

So little is known of the true nature of atherosclerosis that, for definition, we are forced back on a brief description. We may then say that atherosclerosis is a disease of the arterial intima, some degree of which is almost universal in the middle-aged and elderly; it is characterized by patchy accumulations of lipid, together with irregular fibrous thickening over and around the fatty patches, and by the frequent occurrence of calcification in the affected areas.

The disease affects, in a totally irregular manner, large and medium-sized arteries, and it tails away in the small arteries to disappear well above the pre-arteriolar segments. It thus extends not much beyond the first branches of the named cerebral and coronary arteries, and not as far as the arcuate arteries in the kidneys.

For convenience of description, three stages in the development of the lesions can be considered—fatty streaking, atheroma formation, and fully developed atherosclerosis—but it is important to realize that these stages regularly coexist in the same individual and indeed in adjacent segments of the same artery.

Fatty Streaking of the Intima

The earliest stage in this sequence of events may be seen even in young children and infants, especially when the final illness has been accompanied by some 'toxaemia', such as may occur in tuberculosis, gastroenteritis, pneumonia and other infective conditions. The lesions are best seen in the aorta, but may appear also in the carotid arteries and other branches of the aorta, including the coronaries. To display them, the vessel is split open longitudinally, when they appear as faintly yellow streaks, about a millimetre wide, running along the lining for some distance. In the aorta they often extend from the region of the arch down to the bifurcation, favouring the posterior wall and tending to divide and surround the orifices of branches. There may be as many as five or six streaks parallel to one another in parts of the aorta, but it is more usual to find one to three.

Under a hand lens the streak appears as a row of contiguous 'fatty dots' scarcely elevated above the general level of the intima.[6] Microscopical examination of frozen sections stained for fat with one of the Sudan stains shows the streak to be composed of a collection of large mononuclear cells stuffed with fat and lying immediately beneath the endothelium (Fig. 3.6). Studies with the electron microscope suggest that many of the lipid-containing

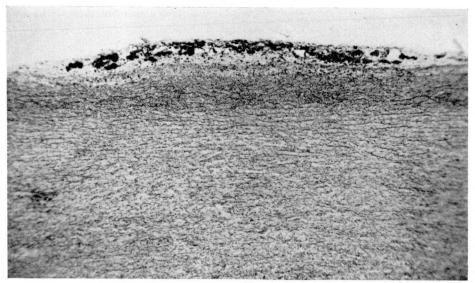

Fig. 3.6.§ Frozen section across a fatty streak in the aorta, stained for fat. The streak consists of smooth muscle cells, filled with darkly stained fat, lying under the endothelium. *Sudan III.* × 30.

cells are smooth muscle cells rather than histiocytes.[7] Inspection through crossed Nicol's prisms or polaroid filters shows much of the fat to be birefringent, and chemical tests confirm that there is a high proportion of cholesterol.

These lesions are not, of course, amenable to observation during life, and views on their natural history, regression or development must be of a speculative nature. It seems probable, however, that the relatively small amounts of lipid that form the streaks may be absorbed, dispersed or metabolized *in situ*, with disappearance of the streak in part or in whole. On the other hand, there may be a focal increase in the amount of lipid, so that more considerable accumulations form and the streak is replaced by a number of irregularly distributed atheromatous plaques. There are, however, differences of opinion as to whether or not the fatty streak acts in this way as the starting point for more advanced lesions.

The Atheromatous Plaque

Seen in the post-mortem room, when the empty vessel has been slit longitudinally with scissors, the uncomplicated plaque appears as a smooth, yellow or white, button-like lesion, circular in outline, 3 to 15 mm in diameter and slightly raised above the surrounding surface (Fig. 3.7).

A transverse section across an affected medium-

§ See *Acknowledgements*, page 169.

sized artery shows a characteristic signet-ring deformity of the lumen (Fig. 3.8); but this is in large part a post-mortem artefact, for if the vessel is fixed in distension at arterial pressure the lumen presents a more nearly circular outline.[8]

In slightly affected areas, the plaques may be widely separated by normal intima, or discrete plaques may be scattered in areas showing fatty streaking. More severely involved regions show clusters of plaques becoming confluent, and the most severely involved segments of the artery may be wholly lined by diseased intima.

Microscopical examination of one of the discrete yellow plaques (Fig. 3.9) shows a sizeable collection of fat—perhaps as much as a few millimetres in diameter—lying in and thickening the intima. The fat is still partly intracellular, but in the central parts of the collection the cells have often disintegrated to liberate a structureless fatty mass, among which are some acicular crystals and clefts. It is this material, which may accumulate in quite large amounts in large aortic plaques, that gives the condition its old name of atheroma, derived from the Greek word for a porridgy substance. As the lesions age, a thickening layer of hyaline fibres comes to separate the fat from the lumen, and the plaque loses its yellow colour and regains the whiteness of the adjacent intima (Fig. 3.10). At the base of the plaque the internal elastic lamina is often stretched and fragmented, while the media is regularly reduced in thickness, sometimes being almost completely lost.

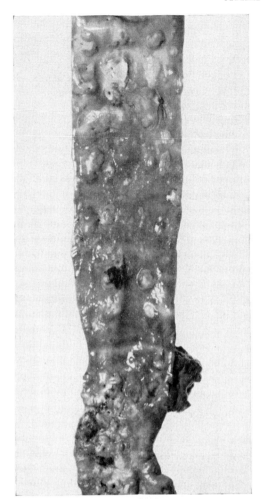

Fig. 3.7. Atheromatous aorta showing elevated plaques which tend to be localized round the orifices of the branches.

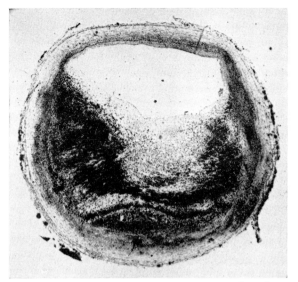

Fig. 3.8. Frozen section of a coronary artery through an atheromatous plaque. *Sudan III.* × 15.

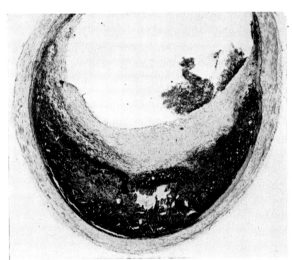

Fig. 3.9. Frozen section of a discrete lipid atheromatous plaque, stained for fat. The fatty material is deeply situated and some crystallization has occurred. *Sudan III.* × 20.

The Fully Developed Lesion

The condition may never advance beyond the stages outlined above, but all too often the development of fatty accumulations in the intima is accompanied by widespread proliferation of fibrous tissue round and between the plaques. In this way the entire intima becomes grossly but irregularly thickened along large stretches of the vessel (Fig. 3.11). It is no longer possible for this thick layer to be nourished throughout by diffusion from the lumen, and blood vessels extend into it through the media from the vasa vasorum. The intima, normally avascular, may thus become a highly vascular structure (Fig. 3.12).[9] The progressive thickening of the intima is likely, especially in smaller arteries, to reduce the calibre of the lumen, but this is not always so—a point that will be discussed later.

E*

Certain further developments are liable to ensue in severely affected vessels, namely calcification, ulceration, mural thrombosis and occlusive thrombosis. Calcification is an unpredictable occurrence but, as a generalization, it can be said to occur mainly in older people and in the most advanced lesions. The distal part of the aorta is especially prone to calcification, and may come to be lined by a rigid intima which fractures like an egg-shell when the vessel is incised and laid open. Coronary artery lesions also often become densely calcified.

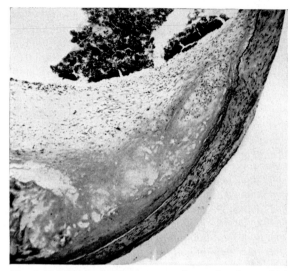

Fig. 3.10.§ Edge of atheromatous plaque showing a thick zone of fibrous tissue between the fatty debris and the lumen. Thinning of the media at the base of the plaque is also evident. *Weigert and Van Gieson stain.* × 25.

Microscopical examination shows the calcification to be sited mainly in the deepest part of the intima and at the sides of the fat collections (Fig. 3.13).

Ulceration of the plaques is also best observed in the distal part of the aorta though it may occur in smaller vessels too. It appears to result from softening in the hyaline fibrous tissue that separates the fatty debris from the lumen. When this layer gives way, the porridgy material may escape into the blood, with the possibility of embolic effects occurring peripherally. The atheromatous ulcer is quite shallow, with ragged edges and recognizable lipid debris in its base. It usually adsorbs pigments from the blood and becomes much darker than the surrounding intima. Not unexpectedly, mural thrombosis over the ulcerated area is of common occurrence (Fig. 3.14). The mural thrombus consists mainly of fibrin, with a varying admixture of blood cells; it soon becomes covered with endothelium and a slow process of organization converts it into a dense layer of hyaline fibrous tissue, thus leading to further thickening of the intima. The formation of small fibrin thrombi over and round atheromatous plaques, and their subsequent incorporation into the intima, are common occurrences, not limited to grossly ulcerated areas: the mechanism of their formation is not fully understood, though the abnormal state of the underlying vessel wall may be presumed to play some part. In the largest arteries these mural thrombi may have little effect, but in smaller vessels, particularly the coronary and carotid arteries, they are much likelier to reduce blood flow so that the risk of the thrombus extend-

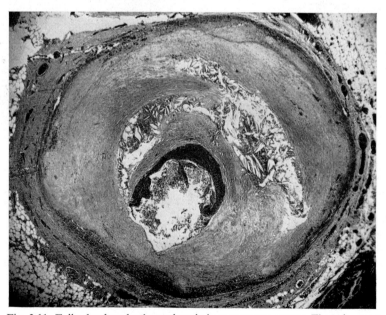

Fig. 3.11. Fully developed atherosclerosis in a coronary artery. There is great thickening of the intima by fibrous bands and fatty accumulations. The media is much thinned and the lumen is stenosed. A dark-staining fibrinous accretion is further encroaching on the lumen. *Picro–Mallory stain.* × 20.

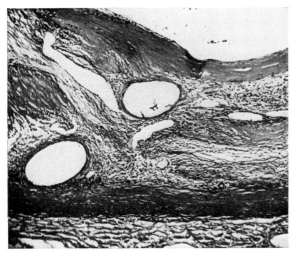

Fig. 3.12.§ Section of the wall of an atherosclerotic coronary artery, showing an extreme degree of vascularization of the thickened intima. *Haematoxylin–eosin.* × 150.

ing to become occlusive is a real and ever-present one and constitutes the common killing complication of atherosclerosis.

Effect on Arterial Calibre

The effect of atherosclerosis on the calibre of the affected artery is extraordinarily variable and unpredictable, and we are faced with the paradox that this single disease process may leave the affected vessel occluded, stenosed, unchanged, or dilated—even to the extent of aneurysm formation. The explanation seems to lie in the varying severity of the secondary degenerative changes that affect the media, and in the balance between this factor and the rate at which mural thrombosis and other processes build up the thickness of the intima. Blood pressure too must play its part, dilatation being more liable to occur in the largest vessels and in hypertensive subjects. The main site at which dilatation is encountered is the aorta: a severely atherosclerotic aorta may be dilated throughout its length, but the most characteristic (though relatively uncommon) lesion is a fusiform aneurysm in its distal part (see below). In the coronary arteries, on the other hand, stenosis is the typical effect, though diffuse dilatation is often seen in hypertensive subjects; in the cerebral arteries, too, both effects occur, with fusiform aneurysm of the basilar artery at one end of the scale, and stenosis of the middle cerebral artery at the other. Dilatation is particularly prone to occur in the larger cerebral arteries, as they have less muscle than other arteries, relative to the size of the lumen, and their elastic tissue is limited to a single internal elastic lamina; these anatomical peculiarities are also responsible for the fact that the cerebral arteries are virtually the only vessels that are liable to rupture when affected by atherosclerosis.

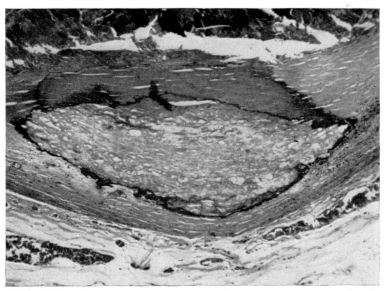

Fig. 3.13. Area of calcification in the thickened intima of an atherosclerotic femoral artery. The media, though much thinned, is not calcified. *Partially decalcified section; haematoxylin–eosin.* × 30.

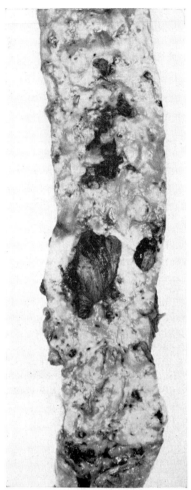

Fig. 3.14. Lower thoracic and abdominal aorta, showing confluent atherosclerosis with areas of ulceration and mural thrombosis.

Special Features in Particular Sites

In the *aorta* the lesions have a characteristic distribution. There may be a few plaques in the arch, but the lesions always increase in concentration and severity along the course of the aorta from the arch to the bifurcation. In severe examples they are commonly confluent below the level of the renal arteries and it is in this region that complications such as calcification, ulceration, mural thrombosis and aneurysm formation are likeliest to ensue. There is a strong tendency for plaques to form round or adjacent to the orifices of branches, so that there may be an almost symmetrical arrangement of two longitudinal rows of lesions round the mouths of the intercostal and lumbar arteries. On occasion the plaques may impair the entry of blood into the branches and lead to ischaemic changes in the areas supplied.

Mural thrombosis in the aorta is occasionally sufficient to impede significantly the flow of the blood, and sometimes complete occlusion occurs near the bifurcation. Oftener, there is narrowing or even occlusion of the orifice of a branch, and in this way infarction of a kidney or of much of the small intestine may occur.

The *carotid arteries* often show peculiarly well-developed fatty streaking in the proximal parts, and more advanced lesions are usually concentrated round the point of bifurcation and in the bulb, where calcification, ulceration, stenosis and thrombosis are most liable to occur. Beyond this, in severe cases, the lesions may be confluent up to the termination of the artery inside the skull.

The importance of atherosclerosis in the *vertebral arteries* was not fully realized until Hutchinson and Yates[10-12] showed how frequently atherosclerotic stenosis of the cervical portions of these arteries is a vital factor in the development of cerebral ischaemia. They used the term 'caroticovertebral stenosis' for those cases in which cerebral ischaemia results from atherosclerosis affecting both pairs of arteries. Narrowing or occlusion of the vertebral artery is most frequently located at its origin from the subclavian artery but may occur also where the vertebral artery passes over the arch of the atlas, or where it pierces the dura.

It is in the *coronary arteries* that atherosclerosis produces its most devastating effects, being the underlying structural lesion in most cases of sudden natural death and in a high proportion of sufferers from cardiac invalidism. It is a remarkable thing that atherosclerosis may have reached an advanced degree in the coronary arteries when other vessels are little if at all affected, though at other times the coronary lesions are part of a widespread arterial involvement. The lesions usually start at the orifices of the vessels, where an aortic plaque may surround and narrow the ostium itself. In general the disease is most advanced at the proximal ends of the arteries and diminishes in degree and concentration of lesions as the vessels diminish in size, fading away in the first branches of the main trunks. The left anterior descending (interventricular) artery is commonly the most severely affected, and it is particularly liable to be narrowed or occluded between 1 and 3 cm from its origin; but the circumflex and right coronary arteries are often just as severely affected and it is not uncommon in elderly people to find two or even all three main vessels much reduced in calibre in several segments. In the presence of hypertension the arteries may show even severer atherosclerosis; sometimes, however, there is a notable diffuse dilatation of the vessels instead of the more usual stenosis. Under the microscope atherosclerotic lesions in the coronary arteries are remarkable for the extent and advanced degree of the intimal fibrosis (Fig. 3.11), and in this connexion it is interesting to recall that even in young uninvolved vessels the intima of the coronary arteries is thicker than the intima of other vessels.[13]

The *cerebral arteries* are second only to the coronaries in importance as a site of atherosclerosis. Quite apart from the gross effects of cerebral artery thrombosis and cerebral haemorrhage—in both of which atherosclerosis is a major factor—a case can be argued for blaming the disease for the failure of mental powers that so often outweighs the benefits of survival to an advanced age. The tendency for atherosclerotic cerebral arteries to dilate and rupture in the presence of hypertension has been mentioned above and related to the anatomical peculiarities of the media. Major ischaemic episodes leading to infarction of the brain are most frequently due to atheromatous narrowing of the internal carotid or vertebral arteries. They may be precipitated by superimposed thrombosis and the detachment of thrombus, which gives rise to embolic obstruction in more distal cerebral arteries. A severely atherosclerotic basilar artery may dilate to form a fusiform aneurysm (Fig. 3.15). Atheroma plays a part also in the pathogenesis of the commoner berry aneurysms of the cerebral vessels (see page 148).

The *femoral, popliteal, and tibial arteries* are also commonly affected by severe atherosclerosis with thrombosis. Stenosis or occlusion resulting from the lesions in these sites is responsible for the third major clinical syndrome of atherosclerosis. This is the symptom-complex known as *intermittent claudication*, in which muscle pain develops after a fairly constant amount of activity and is promptly relieved by rest. With progression of the disease the amount of exercise that can be tolerated (measured by the distance walked) becomes less and less. In the late stages gangrene is liable to occur, commencing distally but tending to spread slowly upwards: ultimately a high amputation may be necessary. Examination of the vessels in the amputated limb usually shows the major obstruction to result from thrombosis in the popliteal or femoral artery[14] but there are often multiple occlusions in the tibial arteries as well. The older thrombi will be found partially organized and recanalized.

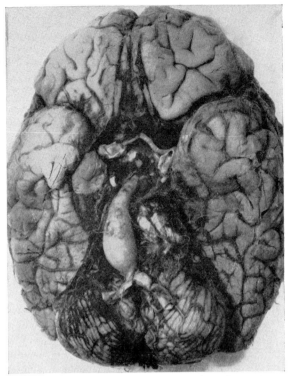

Fig. 3.15.§ Fusiform aneurysmal dilatation of an atheromatous basilar artery.

The Effects of Atherosclerosis

Many of the effects of atherosclerosis have been indicated in the preceding paragraphs: the list may now be summarized and completed.

(a) In the first place, it is important—in order to maintain a correct perspective of this disease—to remember that the majority of people who attain old age do so in spite of the presence of moderate, or even fairly severe, atherosclerosis. In other words, the disease often produces no effects whatever.

(b) Perhaps the commonest pathological effect is stenosis of the artery, with resultant ischaemic changes in the region supplied. This effect is observed principally in coronary, cerebral and renal arteries, and their branches, and results in atrophy of the specialized elements of the ischaemic part and overgrowth of the stroma.

(c) The most dramatic effect is occlusion of the affected artery, which may be brought about either by thrombosis or by prolapse of atheromatous debris into the lumen (Fig. 3.16). The result of the occlusion may be sudden death (when a major coronary or cerebral artery is involved), myocardial, cerebral or other infarction, or gan-

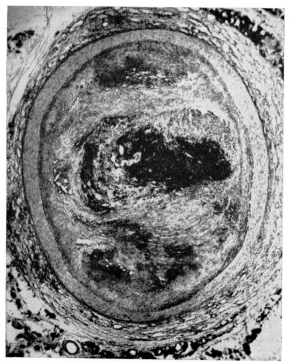

Fig. 3.16.§ Coronary artery occluded by a plug of athero-matous debris. Darkly stained fatty material occupies the narrowed lumen. *Sudan III.* × 15.

grene of an extremity; or—if there is an adequate collateral circulation—there may be no effect at all other than enlargement of the collateral vessels.

(d) Rupture of an artery as an effect of athero-sclerosis is almost limited to small branches of the cerebral arteries. It may also follow the development of an aneurysm, particularly of the aorta.

(e) Aneurysmal dilatation as a result of athero-sclerosis is seen mainly in the distal part of the aorta and now constitutes the commonest variety of aortic aneurysm in Britain. It also occurs occasionally in the basilar artery.

(f) Embolism may result from atherosclerosis in two ways. Thus, for example, atheromatous debris discharged from an ulcerated lesion may act as small emboli, although these are unlikely to produce clinical effects; alternatively, mural thrombus that has formed at a severely affected site may become detached. This latter effect is seen occasionally in the aorta, where a large embolus may lodge astride the bifurcation and impede the blood flow to both lower limbs—a so-called 'saddle embolus'.

Aetiology and Pathogenesis

Discussion of these important aspects is hindered by confusion between atherosclerosis itself and the main clinical syndromes associated with it, notably myocardial ischaemia. Nearly all the statistical studies contributed to the subject are based on myocardial ischaemia as the criterion of athero-sclerosis, but the assumption that that syndrome is not influenced by aetiological factors distinct from those concerned with atherosclerosis in general is by no means justifiable. Bearing this in mind, it is possible to state a few generalizations about the prevalence of atherosclerosis, based on the accumu-lated experience of generations of pathologists rather than on any recorded rates. The relationship with *age* is clear—fully developed lesions are un-common before the fourth decade, and prevalence and severity increase progressively in succeeding years. But here there is an important link with *sex*, for in women the development of the lesions lags one to two decades behind, or—to express it another way—women rarely show significant lesions until after the menopause; in the later decades the difference between the two sexes diminishes, and by the age of 70 it is no longer apparent. The roles of *race* and *heredity* are difficult to disentangle from those of *diet* and *environment*; there appears to be much less atherosclerosis—and there are certainly lower recorded death rates from the syndromes associated with it—in African and Asian countries than in Western Europe and North America, which have the highest rates:[15] but when the inhabitants of the former areas establish themselves in the latter they gradually acquire the higher rates of their new environment.[16]

It is not surprising that such important problems have attracted research workers in widely different disciplines. These studies require more extensive discussion.

Diet and Fat Metabolism

It was in 1847 that Vogel[17] demonstrated the presence of cholesterol in atheromatous plaques: much attention has been focused on the problem of how it gets there. Anitschkow[18] in 1913 described the production of atheroma-like lesions in rabbits kept on a diet to which cholesterol had been added: the significance of this experiment in relation to disease in man is clouded by several facts—the rabbit is normally herbivorous and unaccustomed to even small quantities of cholesterol in its diet; its normal blood cholesterol level is very low, and the levels attained on cholesterol feeding represent an elevation of many hundreds per cent; and the intimal cholesterolosis that results is part of a generalized loading of the tissues of many organs with cholesterol. In more recent years, atheroma-like lesions have been produced in other animals, including dogs[19] and chickens,[20] by procedures designed to maintain a high blood cholesterol over prolonged periods.[21] It is important to note that positive results are obtained in these experiments only when elevation of the cholesterol level is both marked and prolonged; and in considering the relation between these experimental lesions and human disease it is essential to answer two questions —(1) Are people whose blood cholesterol is raised as a result of other diseases especially prone to atherosclerosis? and (2) Do people with severe atherosclerosis have raised cholesterol levels?

The conditions most characteristically associated with hypercholesterolaemia are diabetes, hypo-thyroidism, the nephrotic syndrome and certain types of familial xanthomatosis. Of the frequency and severity of atherosclerosis in diabetics there can be no doubt,[22] and the same seems now to be well established in the case of the other conditions mentioned. Again, there may be particularly severe arterial lesions in cretins who survive without adequate treatment into adult life and also in patients with xanthomatosis.[23, 24] The converse question—that of the occurrence of hypercholes-terolaemia in patients with atherosclerosis—is more difficult to answer, their serum cholesterol usually falling within so-called 'normal' limits: but, as a group, they tend to show slightly but significantly raised levels on comparison with presumptively normal people of the same age.[25] Further work has attempted to link atherosclerotic manifesta-tions with specific blood lipids other than choles-terol, and particular significance has been claimed for beta-lipoproteins in this respect. Gofman and his associates[26, 27] have extended this concept and have classified lipoprotein complexes according to the rate—measured in Svedberg flotation (S_f) units —at which they migrate against centrifugal force. They found that lipoproteins with S_f values in the ranges 12–20 and 35–100 are significantly increased in the serum of patients with advanced athero-sclerosis, and indeed that this finding has prognostic significance.

It is not surprising that the cholesterol feeding experiments in animals led to the widespread assumption that diet plays an important part in the production of atherosclerosis in man. It has been shown, however, that the amounts of cholesterol in even the richest diet scarcely affect blood cholesterol levels;[28] on the other hand, the total fat content of the diet is directly related to the level of cholesterol and other lipids in the blood. Furthermore, popula-tions with a high fat intake show a higher incidence of the effects of atherosclerosis, though the relation is certainly not a linear one.[29] Certain fats, notably milk and meat fats, have been found specially blameworthy in raising the blood cholesterol: others—fats derived from vegetables and fish— actively depress it.[30] The latter action is associated with a high content of certain poly-unsaturated fatty acids in their natural form, chief among which are the so-called essential fatty acids, linoleic acid and arachidonic acid.[31, 32] The links between these observations and individual cases of athero-sclerosis or ischaemic disease are not yet forged: dietetic experiments on large enough groups of people are difficult to plan, but attempts are being made to achieve this.

The Thrombogenic Theory

More than a century ago von Rokitansky[33] main-tained that atheroma represented a settling out of debris from the blood to form encrustations on the wall of the arteries, but his views were overruled by those of Virchow, who taught that 'atheromas' were inflammatory and degenerative in origin with associated fatty changes. The encrustation hypo-thesis was thus forgotten by several generations of pathologists until Duguid revived it in a modified form in 1946.[34] Studying serial sections of coronary arteries in which thrombi had formed, he found transitions from thrombus to atheromatous plaque. He expressed his conclusion in these words, 'Many of the lesions we classify as atherosclerosis are arterial thrombi which, by the ordinary process of organization, have been transformed into fibrous thickenings', and he added that many of the 'atheromatous' fatty patches resulted from softening occurring in the thrombi (Fig. 3.17).

Duguid's observations have now been confirmed by many observers,[35] and the way in which fibrinous encrustations become incorporated as intimal thickenings has been studied.[36] A dual mechanism is involved in the organization of the deposits, the superficial parts, nearest the lumen, becoming permeated with endothelial cells, which, supported by oxygen and nutriments diffusing from the blood in the lumen, are responsible for organization of this layer into collagen-like fibres. The deepest parts of the deposit, however, are invaded by capillaries and fibroblasts extending into the intima from the vasa vasorum, and their organiza-tion follows the ordinary course. With thick deposits, or with successive deposits at the same site, these two zones of organization may fail to link up,

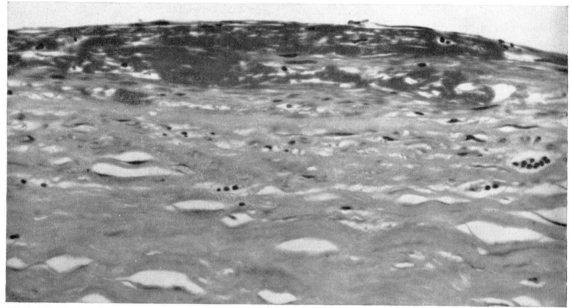

Fig. 3.17.§ Section of the aorta showing deeply stained layer of fibrin in the process of incorporation. A layer of endothelial cells can be seen extending over the surface. *Haematoxylin–eosin.* × 150.

leaving a band of unorganized debris, rich in fats, situated in the depths of the thickened intima and giving an appearance quite indistinguishable from atherosclerosis (Fig. 3.18). In these studies the authors were at pains to point out that, though fibrinous encrustations were easily and frequently found on the intima, they were never observed in a previously quite normal area. It now seems clear that the incorporation of fibrinous encrustations is an important element in the build-up of the fully developed atheromatous lesion,[37] although the earlier stages cannot be explained in this way. Use of a fluorescein-coupled anti-human-fibrin serum has enabled fibrin to be identified in fatty streaks:[38] it would seem that even in these early lesions the lipids passing from the plasma into the intima are accompanied by fibrinogen, which is deposited as fibrin in the vessel wall.

The source of the fat in the intimal plaques is a matter of some controversy. The orthodox view[39] is that the fat molecules diffuse into the intima from the circulating plasma—a process sometimes referred to as 'insudation' or imbition. Alternative views have been put forward: thus, fatty degeneration in incorporated thrombi is an integral part of the thrombogenic hypothesis; it has also been maintained[40] that the fat derives from the products of repeated intimal haemorrhage. Considerable accumulations of fat may, however, antedate the vascularization of the intima: the probability is

that fat first accumulates by 'insudation' and, in older lesions, may then be added to by the other mechanisms. Breakdown of elastic fibres has also been suggested as a source of lipid and as a focus for lipid accumulation.[41]

Disturbances of Blood Coagulation

Even qualified acceptance of the thrombogenic theory outlined above leads one to seek a cause for the fibrinous encrustation of the intima. Such a cause might lie in increased sensitivity of the blood coagulation mechanism on the one hand or in diminished fibrinolytic power of the blood on the other. Study of the former aspect has again shown an interesting link with the fat content of the diet, for fatty meals cause significant shortening of clotting time.[42, 43] This coagulation-accelerating activity appears to be particularly associated with ethanolamine phosphatide,[44] which is present in many animal and vegetable fats. Studies on the fibrinolytic activity of the blood—the capacity of the blood to dissolve fine fibrin deposits—have been handicapped by technical difficulties.[45] Improved, though still cumbersome, methods are now available,[46, 47] and some interesting findings are being reported. Fibrinolytic activity of the blood is found to be increased by exercise and inhibited by a fatty meal, while low levels of fibrinolytic activity have been reported in patients with inter-

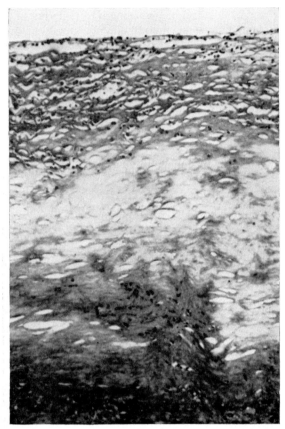

Fig. 3.18.§ Section of atherosclerotic aorta showing the zones of superficial and deep organization with an intervening zone of unorganized debris. Capillaries can be seen breaking through from the media into the base of the intima. *Haematoxylin–eosin.* × 180.

mittent claudication, presumably associated with atherosclerotic occlusion of the limb vessels.[48]

The Role of Endocrine Factors

The difference in sex incidence of atherosclerosis noted above suggests a protective action of oestrogens. Further, there is an impression that men receiving oestrogen treatment for prostatic carcinoma may also obtain some protection against atherosclerosis. The mechanism of this protection is indicated by the observation that depression of circulating cholesterol follows administration of the hormone to postmenopausal women[49] and to hypercholesterolaemic men.[50]

Epidemiological Studies

Studies in the fields of epidemiology and of social and geographical medicine have been directed more to ischaemic heart disease than to atherosclerosis itself. That the two, though obviously related, are subject to the consideration of independent factors, is clearly indicated by the work of Morris.[51] He examined the post-mortem records of the London Hospital (excluding cardiovascular deaths), comparing the amount and severity of atheroma recorded in the period 1908–1913 with similar observations made some 35 years later, when the same necropsy discipline was still in practice. He found that there had been no definable increase of atherosclerosis in the general necropsy material of the hospital over this period, although deaths due to ischaemic heart disease had, over the same period, risen by some 20 per cent.

More recently, analysis of a nation-wide necropsy survey[52] in Britain of men aged 45 to 70 years has shown a relatively lower prevalence of *myocardial scarring* in those who followed occupations of high physical activity than in those whose occupation was more sedentary; but when *severity of coronary artery disease* is considered, the 'protecting' influence of the physically more active occuptiaons is found to apply only to arterial disease associated with complete or near-complete occlusion of a main coronary artery. This work suggests the existence of some factor or process tending to convert the mural lesion of atherosclerosis into a stenosing or occlusive lesion, this factor or process being encouraged by a sedentary mode of life and inhibited by a habitually high level of physical activity.

It has been shown that there is an inverse relationship between hardness of water supply and death rates from ischaemic heart disease:[53, 54] this appears not to be explained by differences in severity of atherosclerosis in hard and soft water areas.[55] The evidence available suggests that the unknown water factor directly affects the sensitivity of the myocardium to ischaemia or other stresses.

Hypertension and Physical Factors

Elevation of the blood pressure is not necessary for the development of atherosclerosis, but there is no doubt that in the presence of hypertension the lesions tend to develop earlier and to become severer. These general impressions were confirmed and placed on a statistically firm basis as a result of a world-wide geographical and racial survey.[56] In this connexion it was concluded that hypertension and diabetes, though not primary causes of atherosclerosis, accelerated the natural progression of the lesions in all populations and regardless of sex, age, race and geographical location.[57] The participation of the blood pressure in the pathogenesis of atherosclerosis is further indicated by the limitation of lesions to those parts of the arterial tree subjected to the higher arterial pressures, by the occurrence of lesions in the pulmonary arteries only in the presence of pulmonary hypertension,[58] and by the occurrence of similar lesions in veins when trauma has established direct communication with an artery, allowing a high pressure to be transmitted into the veins. This pressure factor seems to act by inhibiting the organization of fibrin deposits,[59] or by exaggerating developmental weaknesses in the elastic lamina[60] and thereby localizing the disease process.

The grouping of atheromatous plaques round the orifices of branches and at points of bifurcation and anastomosis is a further pointer to localization of the lesion by some physical factor: for at these points the vessel wall may be subject to sheering strains and excessive stress as the blood flow is directed into a different course. These forces have received careful attention from Duguid,[61, 62] who described separation between the layers of the vessel wall, with resultant haemorrhage, and ascribed to these changes an important role in the development of the lesions.

Conclusions

It has been necessary to devote considerable space to the discussion of the aetiology and pathogenesis of atherosclerosis, for the problem is still at a stage at which, although much information and evidence have accumulated, one cannot be certain of what is significant. It seems established that the fatty lesions in the wall of the arteries are associated with subtle disturbances of lipid metabolism and that these are more liable to occur on a diet rich in animal fat than on a low-fat diet or a diet of vegetable fat. It seems clear, also, that incorporation of mural thrombus plays an important part in converting relatively benign atheroma to the fully developed disease in which stenosis and occlusion are liable to occur; and excessive dietary fat may again participate at this stage by increasing the coagulability of the blood.

Hyaline Arteriolosclerosis

This term is applied to a common pathological state, seen mainly in the visceral arterioles, in which the lumen is narrowed—sometimes to the point of obliteration—and the wall is correspondingly thickened by a layer of structureless eosinophile material immediately under the endothelium (Fig. 3.19). The condition is found almost constantly in the splenic arterioles in elderly people and is also well seen in the small vessels of the senile uterus and ovary. Its development is encouraged by the presence of hypertension, but this is by no means a necessary factor.

The sequence of events leading to hyaline arteriolosclerosis has usually been assumed to involve intimal fibrosis followed by hyaline degeneration in the collagen. However, an alternative

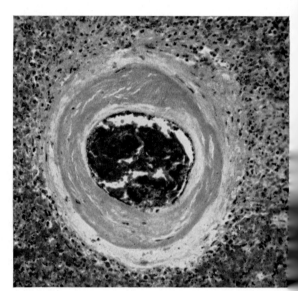

Fig. 3.19. Hyaline arteriolosclerosis affecting a splenic arteriole. *Haematoxylin–eosin.* × 100.

possibility is that the lesion, in the splenic vessels at least, results from a layer of fibrin on the intimal surface being subsequently incorporated by growth of the endothelium over it.[63] The persistence of this fibrin layer, perhaps in a modified form, is then responsible for the characteristic appearance. Studies making use of a fluorescein-labelled specific antibody for the identification of fibrin have supported this view.[64]

HYPERTENSION

The pathology of hypertension and of the associated changes in the blood vessels is dealt with later in this chapter (page 170). Fibromuscular arterial hyperplasia is described on page 178.

INFLAMMATORY CONDITIONS OF
THE ARTERIES

Endarteritis Obliterans

This term is applied to narrowing of small arteries
brought about by an increase in the amount of
fibrous tissue of the intima, sometimes proceeding
to complete obliteration of the lumen. The condition is in no sense a distinct pathological entity,
but apparently represents the reaction of the
arterial wall to a variety of noxious agents. It is
seen characteristically in small arteries adjacent to
chronic inflammatory foci, and especially good
examples are often found in the scar tissue at the
base of a chronic peptic ulcer of the stomach. It is
also well seen in association with tuberculous
cavities in the lung, varicose ulcers of the leg, and
bedsores. In tuberculous meningitis the arteries
traversing the subarachnoid space may become
much reduced in calibre by this process and some
sequelae of meningitis may be due to the ischaemia
so produced. Indistinguishable structural changes
occur in arteries when their physiological function
becomes diminished. It is, for example, by a similar
process that the ductus arteriosus becomes obliterated in the neonatal period; the same is true
of the arteries in the wall of the uterus during the
puerperium. Little is known of the mechanism by
which the intimal thickening is brought about, but
it is generally assumed that irritant substances

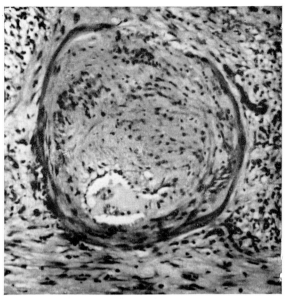

Fig. 3.21. Endarteritis obliterans. Eccentric narrowing of the
lumen of a small artery in the base of a chronic gastric ulcer.
Haematoxylin–eosin. × 150.

(bacterial toxins and tissue breakdown products)
diffusing from the inflammatory focus stimulate
fibroblastic activity in the intima. It is interesting
in this connexion that the intimal thickening, which
is usually concentric with the lumen (Fig. 3.20)
sometimes becomes markedly eccentric (Fig. 3.21),
with the thicker part toward the inflammatory
focus.

Little is known of the pathogenesis, but lesions
closely resembling endarteritis obliterans have been
found in segments of the femoral arteries of rabbits
after the injection of various irritants (for example,
30 per cent alcohol) into the lumen.[65] Thrombosis
may be observed sometimes as the mechanism of
the final closure of an affected vessel, and it may be
that organization of mural thrombi plays a part in
the progressive thickening of the intima. It is
tempting also to apply teleological arguments, for
there is no doubt that endarteritis obliterans serves a
protective function and frequently prevents the
occurrence of grave haemorrhage as a consequence
of ulcerative and excavating processes.

The Arteries in Tuberculosis

Arteries involved in a tuberculous focus usually
show the features of endarteritis obliterans, as
described above. Small vessels are likely to be
obliterated completely, and, as caseation spreads
through the area, their structural identity is lost.

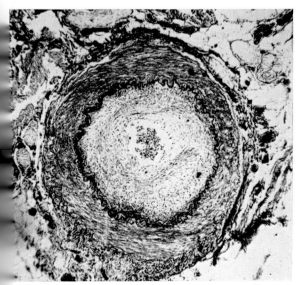

Fig. 3.20. Endarteritis obliterans affecting a small renal
artery in a chronically infected kidney. The intima is
thickened by concentric fibrous overgrowth. *Weigert and
Van Gieson stain.* × 100.

Occasionally infection spreading in from the adventitia may weaken the wall at a time when blood still flows under pressure through the lumen, and this may result in the formation of a small aneurysm which is likely to rupture and so lead to possibly severe haemorrhage. Such an occurrence, however, is rare except in relation to tuberculous cavities in the lungs: in this situation the lesion is known as Rasmussen's aneurysm. A tuberculous lymph node may become adherent to an adjacent artery or vein with direct extension of the disease process through the vessel wall. Matting of the structures by fibrous tissue usually prevents rupture of the vessel and the important result of this sequence of events—occurring usually in the hilum of the lung in the course of primary tuberculosis—is the discharge of tubercle bacilli into the blood stream, with resultant miliary tuberculosis. A true *tuberculous arteritis* with follicles forming in the media and adventitia—the organisms having reached these sites through the vasa vasorum—occurs in the course of miliary tuberculosis but is of little practical importance.

The Arteries in Syphilis

Arteritis is a constant feature of the lesions of all stages of syphilis. In common with other manifestations of this infection, syphilitic arteritis is much less frequent than formerly, and nothing can be added to the classic account of the pathology given by Turnbull in 1915.[66] In general terms, there is endarteritis obliterans, showing the same features as in non-specific infections; in addition, the cellular reaction that constitutes the lesion (chancre, secondary eruption, or gumma) radiates for some distance round the lesion in the form of a cuff within the periarterial tissues and the adventitia of the vessels. The terms *syphilitic endarteritis* and *syphilitic periarteritis* are customarily applied to these changes. Syphilitic arteritis also occurs apart from any association with other focal manifestations of the disease: this form of arteritis is of special importance in two situations—the aorta and the brain.

Syphilitic Aortitis.—This localization of syphilis is particularly important as it is, both clinically and pathologically, the commonest manifestation of the tertiary stage of infection. It has been said[67] that 80 per cent of all syphilitic patients have aortic lesions, but it must be added that in only a small proportion of these do clinical manifestations result. In attempting to explain the frequency of involvement of the aortic arch, Nichols[68] pointed

out that during the secondary (septicaemic) stage of the disease, large numbers of treponemes reach the lungs and are carried to the mediastinal lymph nodes. As secondary manifestations subside and the disease becomes latent, it is in these glands that treponemes survive, to emerge, perhaps many years later, when a changing balance of immunity and tissue sensitivity comes to favour their further activity. The adventitia of the aortic arch has a rich lymphatic network which is in close relationship to the mediastinal nodes, and it is in this way that the frequency of involvement of this site is accounted for. The anatomical connexions of the lymphatic vessels probably help to account for the distribution of syphilitic aortitis. Lesions are usually severest in the ascending part of the arch, become less obtrusive in the descending part and disappear completely—and sometimes abruptly—at the level of the diaphragm.

To the naked eye the severely affected aorta may be dilated and its wall slightly thickened and abnormally adherent to neighbouring structures. The most striking abnormalities are seen when the vessel is opened longitudinally and the intimal surface studied. The lesions, when present in a pure form, appear as greyish-white, rather gelatinous-looking thickenings of the intima, varying from a few millimetres up to a centimetre or more in diameter. The small plaques are circular in outline, but larger lesions, formed by fusion, may be quite irregular. The thickenings are separated by irregularly oriented grooves and the whole roughened surface has been compared to the bark of a tree. With progression of the lesions, depressed scars become more conspicuous, separating the elevated plaques; sometimes irregular pouching occurs. In older people, the lesions of atheroma become mixed with those of syphilis, and interpretation is then difficult. When a syphilitic plaque is cut into the tissue is found to be firm and fibrous throughout, whereas incision of an atheromatous lesion will usually reveal softened fatty debris a millimetre or so beneath the surface. The distribution of syphilitic and atheromatous lesions is also markedly different, for, as has been pointed out above, syphilitic lesions occur almost exclusively in the arch, while the lesions of atheroma, though they may be present in the arch, increase in severity and extent with increasing distance from the heart.

Microscopical examination shows that the essential feature is an endarteritis and periarteritis of the vasa vasorum. These vessels arise from the branches of the aorta, ramify in the adventitia and penetrate into the outer and middle thirds of the media. A the disease progresses they become encircled by increasing numbers of lymphocytes, plasma cells and macrophages, at first in their adventitial portions but later involving the greater part of the media also (Fig. 3.22). Sometimes the collections of cells become so bulky as to lose their obvious perivascular arrangement: the term *miliary gummas* may be applied to such larger foci. Obliterative

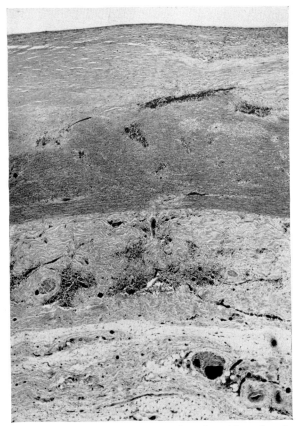

Fig. 3.22. Syphilitic aortitis. There is endarteritis and periarteritis of the adventitial vessels, and the vasa vasorum in the media are surrounded by lymphocytes and plasma cells. *Haematoxylin–eosin.* × 60.

changes progress synchronously in the vasa and may reach complete occlusion. These vascular and perivascular reactions are associated with important degenerative changes in the media: foci of necrosis appear, in the production of which syphilitic toxins and ischaemia may both play a part; later these foci are replaced by scar tissue, and sections stained to demonstrate elastic fibres show an astonishing degree of disruption of the normal close-woven pattern (Fig. 3.23). The intimal patches, which are the most conspicuous naked-eye features, are seen in sections to consist of dense bands of collagen fibres. This fibrous proliferation in the intima is perhaps analogous to the obliterative endarteritis of smaller vessels, but it is commonly explained teleologically as an attempt to buttress the weakened areas of the vessel wall. When, as so often happens, atherosclerosis and syphilis are present together, a complex microscopical picture results, with accumulations of fat in the thickened intima overlying syphilitic lesions of the media and adventitia.

The *effects* of syphilitic aortitis vary from the trivial to the catastrophic. Often there are no directly related signs or symptoms, and nothing more than slight dilatation of the arch is found on X-ray examination. However, the following major complications must be noted—

Aneurysm. This results from focal weakening of the media and is discussed below (page 146).

Stenosis of the Coronary Ostia. This complication occurs in about 20 per cent of cases of syphilitic aortitis and may lead to progressive myocardial fibrosis and occasionally to sudden death. It is particularly likely when the coronary ostia lie higher than usual, above the sinuses of Valsalva; in this situation the orifice is liable to be encircled by scar tissue in the aortic media, and intimal plaques may bulge into it.

Aortic Incompetence. In 1932 Campbell[69] found syphilis to be the cause of 38 per cent of his cases of pure aortic incompetence; today the figure is probably much lower. The incompetence results from two processes—stretching of the aortic ring from weakening of the contiguous aortic media; and contraction of the valve cusps as a sequel to the extension of fibrous tissue into them. The individual cusps become separated by widened commissures, and are thickened and shortened, showing a curious rolled appearance of their margins.

Before leaving the subject of syphilitic aortitis, it is appropriate to make a tabulated comparison between this disease and atheroma (Table 3.1).

Cerebral Syphilitic Arteritis.—Syphilitic arteritis may develop in the medium-sized and small cerebral arteries during the tertiary stage of the disease. Although the arterial lesion does not differ essentially from that occurring in other sites, it is sometimes designated Heubner's arteritis, in recognition of that author's early account of it in 1874.[70] The severest examples occur in association with syphilitic meningitis, but the arteries may be involved without overt meningeal inflammation. The vascular lesion follows the general pattern of

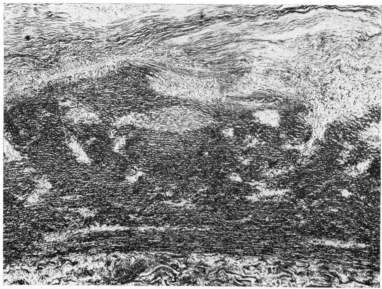

Fig. 3.23. Syphilitic aortitis. Section stained for elastic tissue, showing the interruption of elastic fibres. × 75.

Table 3.1 *Comparison of Syphilitic Aortitis and Aortic Atheroma*

	Syphilitic aortitis	Aortic atheroma
Site	Maximal in arch—absent below diaphragm	Lesions increase progressively from arch to bifurcation
Intimal lesion	Pearly white plaques	White and yellow plaques
	No fat in depths	Fat in depths
	No ulceration	Ulceration common
	Irregular depressed scars	No true scarring
	Calcification unusual	Calcification common
Effects	Often nil	Often nil
	Thoracic aneurysm	Abdominal aneurysm
	Aortic valve incompetence	Aortic valve stenosis
	Stenosis of coronary ostia	Stenosis of orifices of abdominal branches

endarteritis and periarteritis outlined above. Degenerative changes may occur in the medial muscle, and as the active phase subsides considerable fibrous replacement of muscle results. In the smaller arteries the endarteritis may progress to obliteration and this may result in areas of ischaemic atrophy in the brain. Macroscopically, the vessels may appear unusually white, rigid and thick-walled.

Rheumatic Arteritis

The focal lesions of acute rheumatism are usually found in close relationship to arteries: thus, in acute rheumatic myocarditis, the Aschoff bodies often occur in the adventitia of intramuscular branches of the coronary arteries (see page 25). The vessel wall becomes swollen, the endothelium prominent and the lumen narrowed; in the healing stage fibrous replacement of muscle is common. Similar changes may affect arterioles in the lungs, kidneys and other viscera.

Rheumatic aortitis was described by Pappenheimer and VonGlahn,[71] who found focal lesions analogous to Aschoff bodies in relation to the vasa vasorum in the adventitia and media. Although this may progress to patchy fibrosis, aneurysm formation is not a feature.

Rheumatoid (ankylosing) spondylitis has been observed[72] to have a particular association with aortic incompetence, the lesion being an aortitis, closely resembling syphilitic aortitis, with its main incidence at the origin of the aorta and with secondary dilatation of the aortic ring.

Thromboangitis Obliterans (Buerger's Disease)

This is a specific disease, of unknown cause but distinctive pathology, affecting the medium-sized arteries and veins, mainly of the limbs, and commonly resulting in peripheral gangrene. Though isolated cases had been described much earlier[73] it is mainly to the Austrian-American surgeon and pathologist, Leo Buerger, [74, 75] who died in 1943, that we owe our present knowledge of the disease that is commonly called by his name.

The disease affects young and middle-aged men. The symptoms usually start between the ages of 25 and 40 years and take the form of intermittent claudication (cramp-like pains in the muscles coming on after a fairly constant amount of activity and quickly relieved by rest). Women are very seldom affected. Formerly the disease was thought to occur mainly in Jews, but this view has been abandoned in the light of better knowledge of the condition: it is now known to occur in many races.

The vessels of the leg are affected most frequently, and often alone; the arm vessels are not uncommonly involved, usually following involvement of the legs. Other sites are rarely affected: involvement of cerebral, coronary and mesenteric arteries has been described. The largest arteries are not usually affected, and in the lower limb the lesions may be found in the arterial tree from the popliteal down to the dorsalis pedis and digital arteries; in the upper limbs, lesions are usually limited to the ulnar and radial arteries, but again may extend to the digital vessels. Arterioles do not become involved. The lesions are described as having an episodic and segmental character: this indicates that lesions of different age, and affecting a few centimetres of vessel, are separated by unaffected segments; in the final stages the unaffected segments may almost disappear. On dissecting an amputated limb—the pathologist's main source of material from this disease—the affected parts of the artery are found undilated, firm but pliable, and matted to the venae comitantes and adjacent structures. A cut across the segment will show the lumen of the artery and of its accompanying veins to be obliterated, and thrombus may be recognizable if the process is not too advanced.

Microscopical examination of specimens obtained in this way usually shows only the old burnt-out lesions, but occasionally an earlier stage is encountered and some indication of the sequence of events has been obtained by pooling the information derived from specimens showing these earlier changes. The process apparently commences as an inflammatory reaction involving the entire thickness of the vessel wall, and indeed extending to involve the neighbouring veins and nerves (Fig. 3.24). All these structures may be infiltrated with neutrophils at an early stage, and some swelling and proliferation of endothelial cells also occur. It has not been determined with any certainty whether the process originates in the lumen, spreading out through the wall of the vessel, or whether it first affects the adventitial coat.

This inflammatory reaction is soon complicated by the occurrence of thrombosis, which may affect both veins and arteries; and it is of course this event that leads to the clinical manifestations of

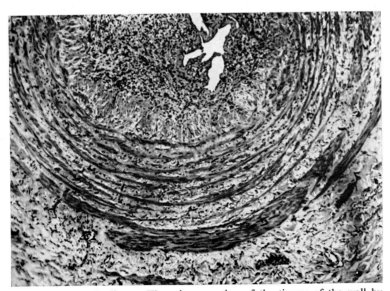

Fig. 3.24. Buerger's disease. There is separation of the tissues of the wall by inflammatory cells. The lumen is occupied by granulation tissue. *Haematoxylin–eosin.* × 120.

the disease. The thrombus is rapidly overrun by inflammatory cells and by endothelial cells and fibroblasts, while it is not uncommon to find a few giant cells of foreign body type. In the late stage— the stage usually found in amputation specimens— the thrombus is completely replaced by a highly cellular fibrous tissue, and recanalizing channels of varying size run through it and communicate with the patent sections of vessel above and below.[76, 77] The internal elastic lamina is usually remarkably well preserved, in contradistinction to its frequent disintegration in atherosclerosis.

Secondary changes in the affected limb follow the arterial occlusion and are non-specific in character. In the first place there will be an opening and remodelling of collateral and anastomotic arteries serving to bypass the occluded segments. This may attain a degree much greater than occurs following occlusion of atherosclerotic arteries: in the younger men with thromboangitis, the un-affected arteries are capable of greater hyper-trophic response to the altered conditions. Pro-gression of the disease, however, often leads to such extensive occlusion that adequate collateral blood flow becomes impossible. Ischaemic and trophic changes then make their appearance in the peripheral tissues and gangrene of the extremities is the likely outcome.

Aetiology

Age, sex and racial incidence have been mentioned above. Several examples of familial occurrence have been recorded,[78] but in the great majority of cases the family history is negative. Tobacco smoking has been blamed as either a causative or an aggra-vating factor: among 350 patients, 62 per cent were found to be heavy smokers and 1 per cent non-smokers, compared with 33 per cent heavy smokers and 26 per cent non-smokers among controls of the same age group.[79] Skin sensitivity to tobacco pro-teins was found in 87 per cent of patients compared with 16 per cent of controls;[80] other workers have reported variable results. In view of the well-known vasoconstrictive effect of tobacco smoking it is not surprising that it should have an aggravating effect in these cases, but any more direct causative relationship remains in doubt.

Search for a specific infective agent has been vigorously pursued but claims put forward incrimin-ating streptococci, viruses and fungi have all failed to find confirmation. An interesting suggestion was made by Goodman,[81] who noted a high incidence of the disease in patients from endemic typhus

regions and suggested that the arterial lesions might represent a chronic rickettsial infection. He claimed to find rickettsial bodies in sections of the arteries, but here again confirmation is lacking.

We must conclude that the cause of thrombo-angitis obliterans is undetermined. Though the clinical and pathological features are fairly dis-tinctive, they could follow from more than one triggering mechanism, and it may prove that Buerger's disease is not a single, specific entity. Some workers,[82] indeed, have doubted the very existence of Buerger's disease. Wessler and his colleagues[83] pointed out that the diagnosis is now being made much less frequently in vascular clinics: from study of their own material they concluded that the pathological condition described by Buerger could result from atherosclerosis or embolization, or from thrombosis from other causes, in a young and reactive vascular system. Dible,[84] however, re-emphasized the distinctive clinical and pathological features, and for the present, at least, the concept of thromboangitis obliterans as a cause of obliterative arterial disease, distinct from other known causes, is best retained.

Giant Cell (Temporal) Arteritis

In 1932, Horton, Magath and Brown [85,86] described cases of a chronic inflammatory disease affecting the temporal arteries in elderly people. Current knowledge of the condition dates from that descrip-tion, though in fact cases can be recognized in much earlier publications.[87] The disease was at first thought to be limited in its effects to the temporal arteries, but it is now appreciated that, although maximal incidence is in the cranial vessels, the lesions may involve the aorta and its branches.[88-90] Cases have been reported in which giant cell arteritis has led to dissecting aneurysm of the ascending aorta.[91] Patients with giant cell arteritis are usually over the age of 60 and there is a slight predominance of women. The onset is usually with headache and throbbing temporal pain. The disease often runs a benign course, the symptoms subsiding within 6 to 12 months. In a minority of cases visual disturbances occur and may progress to blindness, while occasionally cerebral arterial throm-bosis may lead to a fatal outcome.

The pathological features have been worked out from a study of temporal artery biopsies and from examination of the whole arterial tree in a number of fatal cases. The affected temporal artery is cord-like, with some nodular thickenings, and the lumen is irregularly reduced—usually to a mere slit—or may be obliterated by thrombus. Microscopy discloses a granuloma-like subacute or chronic inflammatory reaction situated at the junction of intima and media, involving both these coats and occasionally extending into the lumen or the adventitia (Figs 3.25 and 3.26). The lesion may involve the whole or only a segment of the circumference, and the lumen is commonly occupied by thrombus (mural or occlusive) in varying stages of organization. The lesion itself is an aggregation of histiocytes, lymphocytes and plasma cells with a varying admixture of eosinophils and perhaps a few neutrophils. Giant cells, though usually conspicuous, vary

elastic structure may be lost where it passes through the affected area; occasionally, fragments of the degenerate fibres may be recognized within the cytoplasm of a giant cell.

In the late stages reparative processes appear and fibrous tissue is somewhat irregularly laid down, separating the medial muscle fibres and thickening the intima. The disrupted internal elastic lamina is replaced by new, irregularly arranged, and usually multilayered, elastic fibres. The occurrence of thrombosis, with the subsequent organization of the thrombus, results in the ultimate conversion of segments of the vessel into a fibrous cord in which,

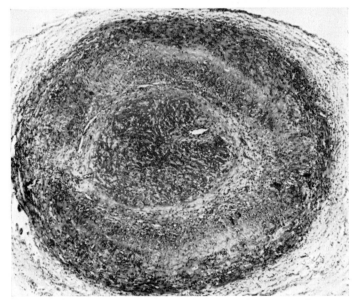

Fig. 3.25. Giant cell arteritis. Low-power view showing the granulomatous lesion in the arterial wall and occlusion of the lumen by organizing thrombus. *Elastic stain.* × 60.

greatly in number; sometimes they are very abundant, but again they may be so scanty as to be absent from an individual section. Both foreign-body-type giant cells (with numerous central nuclei) and the Langhans type (with peripheral nuclei) may be found. These giant cells tend to be distributed in a zone at the level of the internal elastic lamina, though they occur also more widely through the inflammatory area. Foci of necrosis may develop among both the tissue cells and the cells of the exudate. The internal elastic lamina shows striking changes; it becomes irregularly swollen and its characteristic staining properties are impaired though its highly refractile appearance is if anything exaggerated. Fragmentation occurs and in advanced lesions all trace of the original

however, there is usually a small residual blood channel.

Pathogenesis.—The cause of giant cell arteritis remains obscure. Searches for micro-organisms have been unsuccessful. Compression of the temporal arteries by tight-fitting headwear was at first suggested, but the demonstration that the lesions are frequently of wider distribution has shown that this is not the explanation.

Some resemblance between the lesions of giant cell arteritis and polyarteritis (see below) has raised speculation as to a possible allergic mechanism in the disease, but no sensitizing agent or provoking stimulus has been recognized, and this hypothesis— like the hypothesis of a specific viral infection—

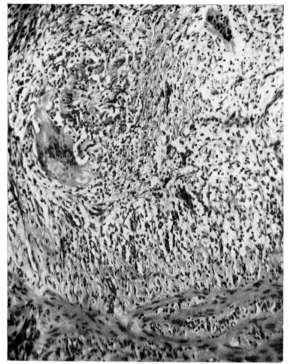

Fig. 3.26. Giant cell arteritis. High-power view showing the granulomatous type of reaction with giant cell formation, centred on the fragmented internal elastic lamina. *Haematoxylin–eosin.* × 300.

remains unsupported by evidence. To the histopathologist the focusing of the reaction round the internal elastic lamina and the resemblance of the process to a foreign body reaction suggests that some alteration has occurred in the lamina to make the tissues react to it as if it were a foreign substance.[92] It may be that some form of autosensitization to elastic tissue has developed—but this hypothesis too lacks supporting evidence.

'Pulseless Disease'

This somewhat unsatisfactory name has come to be used for a syndrome characterized by absence of the pulse in both arms (and perhaps in other sites), associated with ischaemic changes. Cases of this type were described in 1908 by Takayashu[93] and sometimes his name is given to the condition, but, in fact, at least one case had been reported very much earlier.[94] Many of the first case reports came from Japan, but similar cases have now been recognized in India,[95, 96] Europe,[97–99] America[100] and Africa.[101] Many of the patients are young women and the syndrome presents with manifestations of ischaemia in the arms, face, eyes or brain. It has been stressed that the syndrome may result from obstruction to the arteries arising from the arch of the aorta brought about by a variety of causes, including syphilis, trauma, dissecting aneurysm, atheroma and congenital vascular anomalies.[102] Nevertheless, in a proportion of the reported cases the underlying pathological process has been an arteritis affecting the aortic arch and its branches and characterized by cellular infiltration of the adventitia and media, destruction of elastic tissue, intimal fibrosis, and thrombosis: in some of these cases the other causes listed above have been carefully excluded. Nothing is known of the causation of this form of local arteritis, and whether it constitutes a specific disease entity remains undetermined.

Polyarteritis

Polyarteritis nodosa (periarteritis nodosa) is the pathological basis of one of the most intriguing and elusive clinical syndromes. The condition is neither rare nor common and there is some evidence that its incidence has waxed and waned in recent decades. It may affect those of any age and either sex, but the majority of patients are men in middle life. Depending on the apparent chance of involvement of different anatomical regions, the presenting symptoms and clinical course show an astonishing variability. The signs and symptoms may be cardiac, renal, muscular, cutaneous, alimentary, neural, cerebral or respiratory, or any combination of these, and it is usually the bizarre admixture of clinical features that suggests the diagnosis. Intermittent fever and leucocytosis (perhaps with eosinophilia) are common. Formerly, the diagnosis was usually made in the post-mortem room and the disease was regarded as inevitably fatal; but with increased clinical awareness the diagnosis can be confirmed by biopsy of skin, muscle or other tissues and it is now recognized that milder forms occur that subside without fatal results.

Early descriptions of the pathology of polyarteritis nodosa were given by von Rokitansky[10] and by Kussmaul and Maier.[104] These early workers stressed the occurrence of multiple small aneurysms on the affected vessels, though it is now clear that these are the exception rather than the rule, and that the majority of cases run their course without developing anything more than microscopical arterial dilatations.[105]

The pathology of polyarteritis can be summarized under the following headings, each of which merits separate discussion—

(a) fibrinoid necrosis in the arterial wall
(b) inflammatory reaction in and around the artery
(c) thrombosis
(d) aneurysm formation
(e) renal glomerular lesions
(f) healing
(g) secondary effects: i. haemorrhage
                  ii. ischaemic lesions
                iii. hypertension.

Though any medium-sized or small artery in the body may be affected, some regions are much more regularly involved than others. The following are named in approximate descending order of frequency of involvement: kidneys, heart, skeletal muscle, skin, mesentery, alimentary canal, spleen, pancreas, lungs, liver, nerves, meninges, brain and spinal cord. Endocrine and sex glands are also frequently involved. The size of artery affected varies somewhat from case to case, the lesions in some involving mainly medium-sized vessels, such as the radial artery or primary branches of the mesenteric or renal arteries, while in others smaller and more distal branches within the substance of the viscera bear the brunt of the disease.

The term *fibrinoid necrosis* is applied to a characteristic disruption of the vessel wall that seems to constitute the initial pathological lesion. The elements forming the media fuse into an amorphous eosinophile mass in which all structural detail is lost. The material gives the empirical staining reactions associated with fibrin, and for this reason has been designated 'fibrinoid', but studies employing fluorescein-labelled specific anti-fibrin antibodies indicate that the material is in fact largely fibrin.[106] In the light of these observations, the concept of a particular fibrin-like protein (fibrinoid) can be abandoned. It appears that as a result of some harmful reaction the tissue proteins are altered in such a way that fibrinogen diffuses into the area and is subsequently deposited as fibrin. Other serum proteins, notably globulins, may also contribute to the fibrinoid mass.

Patches of fibrinoid necrosis occur in an unpredictable distribution along the course of the vessels: usually only part of the circumference is affected, but elsewhere a complete ring of necrosis may develop. The media seems first and most severely affected, but fibrinoid may extend into both the intima and the adventitia and it is usual for the internal elastic lamina to be destroyed at the site of the lesions.

The *inflammatory reaction* is maximal round the areas of fibrinoid necrosis, but spreads to involve larger segments of the artery. Cellular exudate is particularly abundant in the adventitia and circumvascular tissues (periarteritis) but extends through all the coats of the wall, so that the condition is in fact a panarteritis. In early lesions neutrophils predominate, but later lymphocytes, plasma cells and macrophages are more conspicuous. Eosinophils are a variable element, present sometimes in enormous numbers but oftener only scanty. Fluid exudate also accumulates between and around the tissue elements, which therefore may appear to be abnormally separated.

Thrombosis is liable to occur in any severely affected segment of artery. In larger vessels the thrombus may occupy only part of the lumen, but often, and especially in small arteries, it becomes occlusive. The inflammatory cells spread into the thrombus in the later stages: ultimately, organization occurs.

Aneurysm formation is most frequent when lesions affect larger vessels. Interlobular arteries in the kidneys and comparable branches of the mesenteric, splenic and coronary arteries are often affected. Weakening of the media and loss of the elastic laminae, at a time when the lumen still contains blood under arterial pressure, allow localized aneurysmal dilatation to occur (Fig. 3.27). The dilatation is usually checked by the occurrence of thrombosis within the developing aneurysm or in the vessel as a whole. For this reason aneurysms

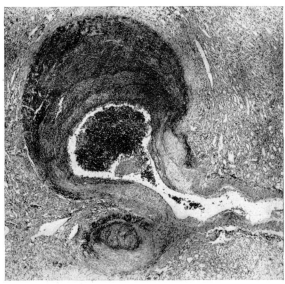

Fig. 3.27. Polyarteritis nodosa. Aneurysm formation on a small renal artery. The aneurysm is partially filled with laminated thrombus. *Haematoxylin–eosin.* × 40.

more than a centimetre in diameter are unusual, while the majority are only a few millimetres across. They form nodose swellings irregularly spaced along the vessel and may become extremely numerous: in one recorded case more than 500 were counted at necropsy.[107]

Characteristic *renal glomerular lesions* occur in about 65 per cent of cases.[108] They take the form of a florid patchy fibrinoid necrosis of glomerular tufts accompanied by a circumglomerular inflammatory infiltration similar to that occurring round the affected arteries (see above). This lesion has to be distinguished from the glomerular lesion of malignant hypertension, to which it bears a close resemblance. In the latter condition, however, the fibrinoid change rarely extends so widely through the glomerular tuft, and inflammatory cells are inconspicuous, while in polyarteritis the glomerular lesion is accompanied by the typical lesions in the renal and other vessels. Haematuria is one of the most constant clinical findings in polyarteritis, even when renal involvement is relatively slight. In those cases with severe renal lesions, renal failure with uraemia may be the final phase.

In most necropsy material arteries showing evidence of *healing* are to be found side by side with those showing active lesions. Healing is manifested by resorption of the inflammatory exudate, fibrous replacement of the fibrinoid area, organization of the thrombus in the lumen, and some degree of recanalization of occluded segments. Cases treated with corticotrophin may show advanced healing in a remarkably high proportion of affected vessels.[107] A comparable degree of healing is seen in cases treated with cortisone and analogous steroid hormones. Healed vessels are usually markedly narrowed, if not obliterated; there is much fibrous replacement of their muscle, and gaps in the internal elastic lamina are a conspicuous feature (Fig. 3.28).

From the pathological point of view, many of the important clinical features of polyarteritis are *secondary effects*. Ischaemic lesions, varying from areas of fibrous replacement to frank infarcts, are common in the heart, kidneys, skeletal muscles, lungs, nerves and other sites. Haemorrhage may result from rupture of an aneurysm in any situation: cerebral haemorrhage, and intraperitoneal, retroperitoneal and pulmonary haemorrhages are perhaps the most frequent. Hypertension is a common clinical finding in polyarteritis, sometimes present at the time when the patient is first seen, in other cases developing during the later course of the disease. Though allowance must be made for the occasional chance occurrence of polyarteritis in a hypertensive subject, there can be little doubt that in most instances the hypertension is of renal origin and is initiated by ischaemic lesions in the kidney.

Aetiology and Pathogenesis.—The age and sex incidence of polyarteritis has been discussed above. The causation must now be considered. Negative results followed attempts to incriminate direct infection, and it is now widely accepted that the lesions represent a hypersensitivity reaction in the vessel wall. The evidence for this comes from both

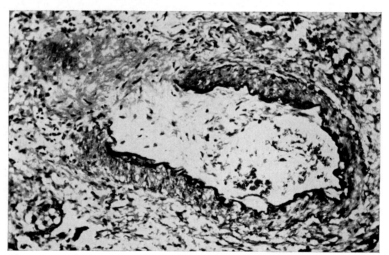

Fig. 3.28. Healed lesion of polyarteritis. The necrotic segment has been replaced by fibrous tissue, and a gap in the internal elastic lamina remains. *Weigert and Van Gieson elastic stain.* × 250.

clinical and experimental observations. An association between polyarteritis and allergic asthma was noted in 1939.[109] A few years later attention was drawn to the occurrence of polyarteritis as a complication of serum sickness and of the administration of sulphonamides.[110] Since then a considerable variety of other drugs has been suspected in individual cases, including iodides, aspirin, arsenicals, mercurials, hydantoins, thiouracils, promazines and some antibiotics.[111, 112] It must be admitted, however, that in many cases of the disease it proves impossible to recognize any sensitizing agent.

On the experimental side, it had earlier been shown[113] that rabbits given repeated injections of foreign serum occasionally developed arterial lesions indistinguishable from polyarteritis, and this has now been abundantly confirmed.[114, 115] The experimental work is, however, somewhat confused by the fact that lesions indistinguishable from polyarteritis nodosa may be produced in rats rendered hypertensive by the application of a renal artery clip.[116, 117] The nature of the pathological changes is in keeping with the concept of an antigen-antibody reaction localized in the tissues of the vessel wall. Such reactions are known to be associated with histamine liberation, which could be expected to increase the permeability of the tissues and permit protein-rich fluids to diffuse into the damaged area. Fibrinogen gaining access in this way would then be deposited diffusely in the damaged tissues as fibrin, giving the histological picture of 'fibrinoid'. There appear to be basic similarities in the pathological lesions of polyarteritis and rheumatism.[118]

Natural History and Prognosis.—Formerly an established case of polyarteritis ran a relapsing downhill course with death occurring within a period of six months to three years. The introduction of treatment with corticosteroids, however, has improved the outlook for these patients, in many of whom the manifestations of the disease can be controlled for long periods.[119]

Related Conditions.—*Wegener's granulomatosis* (see pages 213 and 371) is the name applied to a condition in which a vascular lesion of the polyarteritis type is associated with extensive granulomas involving mainly the nasopharyngeal area and upper respiratory tract. Wegener[120] believed the condition to be a distinct pathological entity, but it may be essentially similar to polyarteritis, with special localizing factors because the allergen or sensitizing agent gains entry by the respiratory tract.[121] The

prognosis is uniformly bad, and widespread lesions are usually present at necropsy.

Allergic vasculitis is a term sometimes applied to lesions resembling those of polyarteritis but confined to one organ (*localized visceral arteritis*), or to the skin (see Chapter 39),[122] and occurring in association with relatively minor inflammatory processes. The organ affected may be the appendix,[123] gall bladder,[124] urinary bladder,[125] or breast.[126] It is important to bear in mind that the unexpected discovery of lesions of this sort in a surgical specimen does not necessarily imply the existence of generalized polyarteritis: the significance of their presence must be carefully considered in each case in relation to the whole clinicopathological picture (Fig. 3.29).

In *systemic lupus erythematosus* (see Chapters 24 and 39) vascular lesions closely resembling those of polyarteritis may be found.[127, 128] There is similar fibrinoid necrosis with destruction of media and elastica, but the inflammatory exudate is less marked, and thrombosis and aneurysm formation rarely develop. Concentric circumvascular fibrosis (the 'onion skin' lesion) is often found in the spleen and lymph nodes in this disease.

Arterial lesions also occur in *scleroderma* (see Chapter 39). In the acute phase, fibrinoid necrosis may occur in the walls of small arteries, or an abundance of mucoid ground-substance may

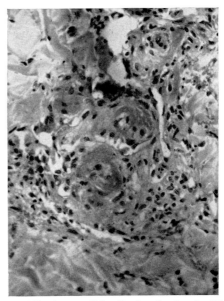

Fig. 3.29. Allergic vasculitis affecting the dermis. Fibrinoid change has occurred in the dermal arterioles and cellular exudate has formed round the vessels. *Haematoxylin–eosin.* × 110.

accumulate in the intima; fibrous thickening of the vessel wall is the usual finding. The characteristic lesions in the renal vasculature are described in Chapter 24.

ANEURYSMS

An aneurysm of an artery is a swelling formed by localized dilatation of the lumen. The wall of a true aneurysm (as distinct from false and dissecting aneurysms) is therefore formed by the stretched remnants of the arterial wall. The general shape of an aneurysm will depend on whether the stretching process affects the whole circumference of the artery or only a small part. In the former case, a *fusiform aneurysm* results, forming an ovoid swelling with its long axis parallel to the long axis of the adjacent unaffected segments of the artery; in the latter case, the result is a *saccular aneurysm*, protruding from the wall of the vessel and communicating with the lumen through an ostium of varying calibre.

While the pathogenesis of aneurysms varies widely in different sites, it is possible to formulate certain generalizations. In the first place, it may be taken as axiomatic that dilatation can only occur when there is some localized weakening of the vessel wall. In large arteries, the main strength of the wall resides in the medial coat, and in such vessels aneurysms are always associated with some process that has weakened the media in a patchy manner. In smaller arteries, however, the internal elastic lamina and possibly also the adventitia contribute significantly to the strength of the wall and localized damage to these elements may play a part in the development of aneurysms.

The second requirement for the occurrence of aneurysmal dilatation is a distending force: this, of course, is provided by the blood pressure. Clearly, therefore, hypertension must be a contributory factor in the causation of aneurysms, for it is to be expected that a weakening of the vessel wall insufficient to permit yielding to a normal blood pressure might well allow the vessel to stretch before a pathologically elevated pressure.

Once aneurysmal dilatation has commenced it is likely to continue at a progressively increasing rate, for the strain on the wall of the vessel increases as the diameter increases. The tendency is, therefore, for an aneurysm to go on enlarging until rupture occurs. There is, however, the possibility of this progression being checked by the occurrence of thrombosis within the aneurysmal sac. Some degree of mural thrombus deposition is a constant feature of aneurysms of a centimetre or more in diameter. Sometimes the thrombosis extends to obliterate much or even the whole of the sac, resulting at times in a virtual cure of the condition; it may even extend beyond the aneurysm and occlude the parent vessel. There is the further possibility of thrombus formed in the aneurysm becoming detached and giving rise to embolism.

The wall of a true aneurysm is by definition formed of the stretched elements of the wall of the artery itself. In practice, however, the structures of the vessel wall can usually be traced only a short way into the sac, soon merging in ill-defined fibrous tissue rich in histiocytes and blood pigments and formed partly from the original vessel wall, partly from compressed adjacent structures, and often largely from incompletely organized mural thrombus.

Syphilitic Aneurysms

The way in which syphilis damages the media of the aorta and its large branches has been described on page 136. Until recently this was the most frequent cause of aneurysms and, indeed, there was a tendency to assume a syphilitic basis for all lesions of this sort. Today, however, with the falling incidence of tertiary syphilis and the rising proportion of elderly people in the population, atherosclerosis has usurped the place of syphilis as the most frequent cause of aneurysm.

Syphilitic aneurysms affect mainly the arch of the aorta, which bears the brunt of syphilitic aortitis, and (except for dissecting aneurysms—see page 149) they are virtually the only form of aneurysm occurring in this region. They may be fusiform or saccular and often arise just above the aortic valve, extending to involve the major part of the arch. The expansile pulsating mass may attain an enormous size and may be responsible for a wide range of signs and symptoms: a swelling may present in the suprasternal notch, or in the back; there may be pressure effects involving trachea and bronchi, oesophagus, nerves and veins; a remarkable erosion of vertebral bodies (with sparing of the intervertebral discs) and thoracic cage may be a cause of intractable pain (Fig. 3.30). The end may come with rupture and haemorrhage, either externally or, oftener, into the pericardial or pleural sac or a hollow viscus. The clinical features may be further diversified by concomitant disease of the aortic valve, which is present in the majority of cases, and by the occurrence of embolic phenomena due to separation of either developmental (see page 99) or syphilitic.[129] Any or all of the sinuses may be affected.

The special interest of these aneurysms arises from the fact that as they enlarge they bulge into one of the cardiac chambers—usually the right atrium or ventricle—and when rupture occurs a cardio-aortic fistula results which may lead to profound disturbances of pressure in the chambers of the right side of the heart. Cardiac failure may ensue, but if the condition can be recognized during life it may prove amenable to surgical repair.[130, 131]

Atherosclerotic Aneurysms

The weakening of the media that may occur in severe atherosclerosis has been described on page 127, and today is regarded as the commonest pathological basis for aneurysm. This is a disease of the elderly, being seldom seen under the age of 60 years and having its main incidence in the eighth and ninth decades. The abdominal aorta is the typical site but atherosclerotic aneurysms are common also on the iliac, femoral and popliteal arteries. In these situations they are often multiple. Their occurrence on smaller arteries is less common, but they are encountered from time to time on such vessels as the basilar artery and the coronary arteries.[132]

Atherosclerotic aneurysms are usually fusiform or even cylindrical, but saccular forms may occur. Confluent ulcerated atheromatous plaques are likely to be present on the adjacent arterial intima and to extend into the aneurysmal sac, where they are obscured by thrombus. Thrombus formation is particularly abundant in these aneurysms, and it is not uncommon for the greater part of even a large aneurysm to be occupied by a firm mass of thrombus around which the blood percolates (Fig. 3.31). Occasionally complete obstruction, even of the aorta, may occur.

The hazards discussed in connexion with syphilitic aneurysms are equally important here: thrombus may be detached and give rise to embolic closure of an artery, usually in a lower limb; an important branch (for example, renal or mesenteric) may be occluded at its origin; there may be pressure effects on adjacent viscera, vessels, nerves or bones; or the aneurysm may rupture—usually into the peritoneal cavity or the retroperitoneal tissues.

'Mycotic Aneurysms'

A 'mycotic aneurysm' is infective in origin, resulting from weakening of the vessel wall by bacterial

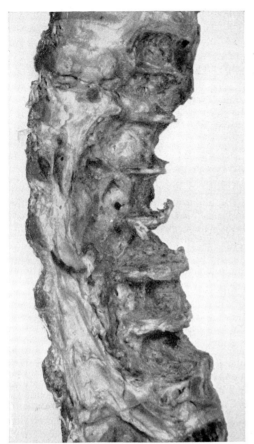

Fig. 3.30. Dorsal spine, showing erosion of the vertebral bodies by an aortic aneurysm. The intervertebral discs are relatively spared.

fragments of thrombus from the wall of the sac. It is surprising how seldom the blood flow into the vessels of the head and upper limbs is impaired, though this is a further possibility. The commonest cause of death is congestive cardiac failure as a consequence of aortic incompetence.

Syphilis is of minor importance as a cause of aneurysms in other sites, but examples sometimes occur in the large branches of the aortic arch, and, more rarely, in arteries of the abdominal viscera.

Aneurysms of the Aortic Sinuses

Aneurysms arising in the aortic sinuses of Valsalva—the three small pouches at the root of the aorta lying behind the three cusps of the aortic valve—constitute a rare but distinct group that presents features of special interest to both the pathologist and the cardiologist. The lesion, which permits increasing dilatation of the pouch to occur, may be

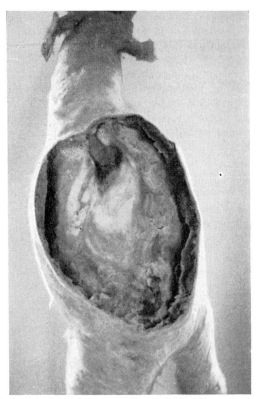

Fig. 3.31. Atherosclerotic aneurysm of the abdominal aorta. The aneurysm is almost filled by bulky thrombus.

invasion from within. This occurs in the course of pyaemic infections, the organisms reaching the intima in the substance of an infected embolus. It is seen oftenest as a complication of acute bacterial endocarditis. The lesions develop most frequently on the cerebral vessels though such visceral arteries as the mesenteric, splenic and renal arteries are not uncommon sites. These aneurysms have a considerable tendency to rupture while they are still quite small. They rarely attain a diameter of more than a centimetre.

Microaneurysms

Aneurysms of microscopical dimensions are a characteristic feature of the vascular lesions of *thrombotic thrombocytopenic purpura* (see Chapter 8). In this disease dilatation of the smallest calibre blood vessels, particularly the smallest arterioles and the capillaries, is accompanied by the formation of granular thrombi that partly occlude the affected vessels. The nature of these thrombi is still uncertain; they probably consist largely of platelets, and this has been held to account for the thrombocytopenia

that is one of the constituent features of the characteristic tetrad of the syndrome (acute febrile illness; haemolytic anaemia; thrombocytopenic purpura; bizarre, fluctuating neurological disturbances).[133] The microaneurysms, which may be fusiform or saccular, develop particularly at the arteriolocapillary junction.[134]

The microaneurysms of diabetic retinopathy are described in Chapter 40.

Aneurysms of the Cerebral Arteries

Aneurysms of the cerebral arteries occupy a place of particular importance because of their frequency —they now form the largest group of aneurysms —and because of the challenge that their treatment presents.[135]

Several varieties of aneurysm may develop on the cerebral arteries, but much the most frequent and important is that usually (though inaccurately) designated as *congenital aneurysm*. The common descriptive name, *berry aneurysm*, likening the lesions to berries on the twigs of the arterial tree, is perhaps preferable and is particularly applicable when they are multiple, as occurs in some 12 to 15 per cent of cases.

The berry aneurysm develops from any of the angles of branching and anastomosis in the circle of Willis, or on any of the branches of the circle (and then seldom more than 3 cm from the origin of the branch). The commonest sites, in order of frequency, are—the angle between the anterior cerebral artery and the anterior communicating artery and that between the internal carotid and the posterior communicating artery; the first main division of the middle cerebral artery; and the bifurcation of the internal carotid. Once aneurysmal dilatation has commenced, it tends to progress. The aneurysm as it enlarges may become embedded in the brain substance or may wrap itself round adjacent nerves, arteries or veins. It often becomes irregularly lobulate. Its thin wall becomes partially transparent.[136]

Microscopical study of the neck of such an aneurysm shows an abrupt cessation of the medial muscle at the point of origin. The internal elastic lamina extends a short way into the wall of the aneurysm, but is soon lost, and the wall of the aneurysm at its fundus consists merely of a thinned-out layer of fibrous tissue merging with the varying amount of thrombus in the cavity.

The effects of these aneurysms are inconstant. Occasionally an aneurysm is an incidental post-mortem finding, having produced no clinical sign of its presence. The main effect is intracranial haemorrhage as a result of rupture, and this may vary clinically from a rapidly fatal stroke to a relatively minor neurological disturbance, depending on the extent and situation of the actual burst. The blood may enter the subarachnoid space, or may pass directly into the substance of the brain. At the time of rupture the aneurysm is usually 0·5 to 1·5 cm in diameter; the rupture is situated in the fundus in some 75 per cent of the cases—a point of some importance to the neurosurgeon seeking to clip the aneurysm. Occasionally an aneurysm attains a larger size and produces pressure effects comparable to those of a benign intracranial tumour.

Three factors are operative in the pathogenesis of berry aneurysm—developmental faults in the medial muscle, the blood pressure, and atherosclerosis. The developmental faults, to which attention was drawn by Forbus,[137] consist of gaps in the medial muscle at the points of junction and branching (Fig. 3.32). These gaps are much more

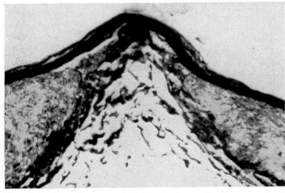

Fig. 3.32. Developmental fault of the media in a cerebral artery. The section is cut longitudinally through the spur at the point of bifurcation of the middle cerebral artery of a child. The lumen is above. The internal elastic lamina is intact, but the media is absent for a short distance in the angle between the branches. *Elastic stain.* × 80.

frequent than the aneurysms we are discussing,[138] but they vary greatly in size. Large developmental faults of this type are the main pathogenetic factor in the rare instances of berry aneurysms occurring in children. The developmental basis for these aneurysms gains support also from the fact that they may be associated with other developmental lesions, including polycystic kidneys,[139] aortic coarctation and arteriovenous malformation.[140] The distending force required to produce the aneurysms is the blood pressure, and it is obvious that a small medial fault, capable of withstanding a normal blood pressure, might yield before the elevated

pressure of hypertension—and hypertension is present in more than half the adult cases.

Atherosclerosis is an important contributing factor in the older patients,[141] the coincidence of an atheromatous plaque at the site of a medial fault leading to further weakening of the wall, often with loss of the internal elastic lamina.

Other forms of aneurysm found on the cerebral arteries are the so-called mycotic aneurysms (page 147), which are seen oftenest on the middle cerebral arteries as a complication of acute bacterial endocarditis, and the fusiform atherosclerotic aneurysm, which is virtually confined to the basilar artery (see Fig. 3.15). Following fracture of the base of the skull a traumatic varicose aneurysm may result from communication between the internal carotid artery and the cavernous sinus.

Traumatic, False and Varicose Aneurysms

Traumatic aneurysms result from physical damage to the wall of an artery, usually by a stab wound or gun-shot wound, or by a fragment of bone when the lesion develops in association with a fracture. Traumatic aneurysms have also sometimes followed surgical dissections in such areas as the groin, axilla or neck, especially for removal of neoplastic lymph nodes. Aneurysms resulting from trauma are likely to be *false aneurysms*, this term implying that the extension of the arterial lumen is enclosed not by the stretched vessel wall but by blood clot (more or less organized) and compressed adjacent tissues. The formation of such a lesion involves leakage from the damaged vessel into a confined space, with subsequent excavation of the haematoma; with the passage of time the limiting layer may become lined by vascular endothelium. Damage to an artery is frequently associated with damage to the accompanying vein, and when this happens a communication may form so that arterial blood passes into the veins, which become distended and tortuous as a result of the transmission of the arterial blood pressure into them. Such a lesion is referred to as a *varicose aneurysm* when an aneurysmal sac connects the two structures, or as an *aneurysmal varix* when no such sac develops. Arteriovenous anastomoses of this type, if involving large vessels such as a subclavian or carotid, may embarrass the heart and lead to high-output cardiac failure.

Dissecting Aneurysm and Mucoid Medionecrosis

The term dissecting aneurysm implies an extension of blood within the substance of the wall of an artery, where it occupies an intramural cavity. The most important and frequent examples occur in the aorta.

Dissecting aneurysm of the aorta has been observed for many centuries, but attention was focused on it in modern times by the classic monograph of Shennan.[142] It cannot be described as common, but with the falling incidence of syphilis it is now the most frequent variety of aneurysm to involve the thoracic aorta; the post-mortem incidence has been estimated at one in 363 necropsies.[143] No age is exempt, but over half the cases occur in the sixth and seventh decades. Men are affected about three times as often as women. The onset is usually associated with some physical exertion and is often characterized by sudden stabbing or tearing pain in the chest. A few patients recover completely, but oftener death results, either suddenly from rupture or more slowly from impairment of the blood flow to vital areas.

At necropsy a remarkable picture is commonly disclosed (Fig. 3.33). The trouble usually starts in the ascending aorta, 1 to 2 cm above the aortic ring, where a transverse slit in the intima (usually quite small) marks the point at which blood passes into the wall. The inner layers of the wall are displaced centrally to narrow the natural lumen of the vessel. A transverse section across the area will display the haematoma within the layers of the wall and will show it either as a ring, or, oftener, when only part of the circumference is affected, as a crescent. It can usually be made out, even with the naked eye, that the blood lies in the substance of the media and microscopy will confirm that about two-thirds of the media then lie central to the new cavity with the outer third of the media and the adventitia lying externally (Fig. 3.34).

The extent of dissection in the long axis of the aorta is the most variable element in these lesions. Often it reaches proximally to the root of the aorta and distally into the abdominal portion, and from time to time examples are encountered in which the lesion has extended through iliac and femoral vessels, and perhaps even as far as the popliteal. The major branches of the aortic arch and the renal and mesenteric vessels are also sometimes dissected in this manner.

Subsequent events are also variable. *Rupture through the outer wall* is the commonest outcome and is usually quickly fatal. The haemorrhage is into the pericardial sac, pleural cavity, mediastinum or retroperitoneal tissues, in descending order of frequency. *Rupture through the inner wall* is less frequent and may occur at any level. This is con-

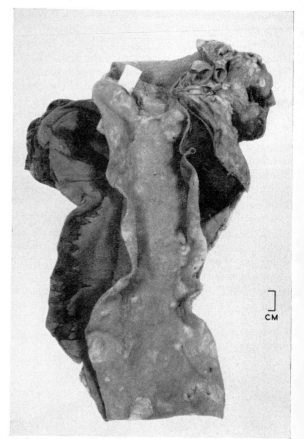

Fig. 3.33. Dissecting aneurysm of the aorta. The blood has been washed away but the separation of the aortic wall into two layers can be seen. A white marker has been passed through the breach in the inner layer.

sistent with long survival and the false channel may then undergo adaptive changes and become lined by a well-formed 'intima', so that ultimately an appearance suggesting a double aorta results. *Healing* has occurred when the dissection has stopped without having ruptured in either direction: the contained blood then clots and subsequently becomes organized to form a fibrous scar in the aortic wall.[144] *Narrowing of branches* may result from extension of the dissection into them or from compression by the haematoma. Results will vary from loss of peripheral pulses (perhaps progressing to gangrene) to signs of renal, myocardial or cerebral ischaemia or intestinal infarction.

Pathogenesis

The main factor in the pathogenesis of dissecting aneurysm is its association with a degenerative

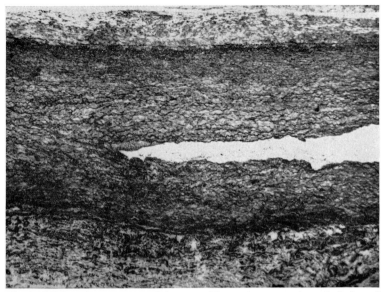

Fig. 3.34. Dissecting aneurysm of the aorta. The section passes through the lateral edge of the false channel in the wall, which can be seen to lie approximately between the middle and outer thirds of the media. *Elastic stain.* × 80.

lesion involving the media. While it may be that other forms of degenerative process play a part, there is now no doubt that most dissecting aneurysms arise as a result of *mucoid 'medio-necrosis.'* This condition was first recognized in 1928 by Gsell,[145] while Erdheim[146] in 1930 described it in detail and coined the name *medio-necrosis aortae idiopathica cystica.* Necrosis, however, is not a conspicuous feature and *mucoid medial degeneration* is a better name. The characteristic features of this condition are loss of elastic and muscle fibres in the aortic media and the accumulation of large amounts of metachromatic material between the widely separated surviving tissue elements (Fig. 3.35). This material gives the histochemical reactions of a mucopolysaccharide and is sometimes so abundant that it leads to the formation of cyst-like spaces that interrupt the fibres. At necropsy the wall of an aorta with severe involvement separates very readily into inner and outer layers, in a manner reminiscent of the separation of two layers of wet filter paper.

Having incriminated mucoid medial degeneration as a basic cause of dissecting aneurysm, we must consider the causation of the medial lesion itself, and it may be said at once that this is unknown. A few interesting observations have nevertheless been made. In the first place, the degenerative change affects first and most severely the middle zone of the media, which represents the farthest limit of the wall to be supplied with blood by the vasa vasorum. Any impairment of blood flow in the vasa might be expected to have its effect here. Second, there is some suggestion that the lesion may have a hereditary or developmental basis: it has occasionally been observed in brothers or in father and son; it is sometimes associated with congenital cardiovascular disease, notably coarctation of the aorta, bicuspid aortic valves and hypoplasia of the aorta; and the lesion is of frequent occurrence in *Marfan's syndrome*,[147] in which an inherited defect of mesodermal tissues is manifested by multiple skeletal lesions (including arachnodactyly, or 'spider fingers') and ocular defects. Third, a possibly toxic or dietetic element in the causation of the medial degeneration is suggested by experimental work, although its relevance to the human disease is uncertain. It was found that rats fed a diet rich in sweet-pea (*Lathyrus odoratus*) meal develop both skeletal deformities and dissecting aneurysms;[148] further studies incriminated beta-aminoproprionitrile, a water-soluble constituent of sweet-pea meal, as the toxic factor. The action of this substance in rats is inhibited by a high protein diet.[149]

That hypertension plays some part in the pathogenesis of dissecting aneurysm is indicated by its presence in well over half the reported cases.[150] It probably acts by increasing the strain on the inner

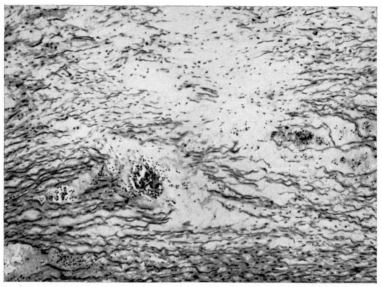

Fig. 3.35. Mucoid medionecrosis of the aorta. Section of the media showing accumulations of mucoid material separating and disrupting the elastic fibres. *Elastic stain.* × 150.

wall of the aorta and thereby increasing the liability to dissection if medial degeneration is present; however, the possibility that it may itself aggravate the medial lesion cannot be ruled out.

Dissecting aneurysm occurring as a complication of coarctation of the aorta[151, 152] illustrates well the possible interplay of mechanical and developmental factors in the pathogenesis, for the aortic segment proximal to a coarctation is commonly the seat of mucoid medial degeneration and is exposed to local hypertension.

Dissecting Aneurysms of Smaller Arteries

These have attracted much less attention than the aortic lesions, but examples have been recorded affecting coronary, renal, cerebral,[153] carotid, pulmonary and other arteries.[154] In these smaller vessels the plane of dissection is more variable, sometimes forming between media and adventitia, sometimes between media and intima. Mucoid degeneration of the media is a less constant aetiological factor, while trauma plays a greater part, at least in initiating dissection.

VEINS

Normal Structure

The structure of the veins follows the same pattern as we have seen in the arteries, the wall being divisible into intima, media and adventitia, but these three coats are much less sharply demarcated from one another. The media in particular is poorly developed: muscle fibres are few in number and widely separated by collagen fibres, while elastic tissue is also scanty and is not organized into the well defined internal and external laminae seen in the arteries.

These relative weaknesses of the walls of veins in comparison with arteries clearly reflect the much lower pressures to which veins are subjected. It is interesting to note that the pulmonary and portal veins, in which pressures are somewhat higher than in the systemic veins, approach more closely the structure of an artery.

An important and distinctive structural feature of the veins is the system of valves, which is best developed in the lower limbs. The venous valve cusps consist of folds of intima—a double layer of endothelium separated by scanty fibrous and elastic tissue—arising usually in pairs and often attached just distal to the point of entry of a tributary. These valves serve an important dual function, limiting the extent to which retrograde flow can occur from fluctuations in pressure at different levels, and also breaking the blood column up into segments and thus reducing the hydrostatic pressure to which the distal parts of the veins of the lower limb may be subjected. This latter aspect is of particular importance to man, who, in the upright posture, would, without the venous valves, subject the veins round his ankles to the full pressure exerted by a column of blood some 4 ft (120 cm) in height.

Varicose Veins

This term implies a condition of permanent dilatation and tortuosity affecting segments or groups of veins. The veins of the lower extremity are involved very much more frequently than those of other parts of the body, and indeed varicose veins in the leg constitute one of the commonest ailments of man. In this situation the lesion varies in degree from a trivial and symptomless knot of distended vessels, to grave and disabling distension of the whole venous system of the limb, with secondary trophic disturbances.

Aetiology and Pathogenesis

It is convenient to consider examples of varicose veins as divisible into primary and secondary groups, the primary group comprising those cases in which the essential fault resides in the veins themselves, whereas in the secondary group the venous dilatation results from some underlying pathological process that leads to local elevation of venous pressure.

It has been estimated that as many as 10 to 17 per cent of the population have some degree of varicosity of the leg veins,[155] though only a fraction of these people develop symptoms. Most patients present for treatment between the ages of 30 and 50 years, and two-thirds of them are women.[156] The great majority of cases of varicose veins in the legs appear to be of the primary type, and it has been postulated that an inherited structural weakness of either the vein walls or the valves is the basic lesion. It might be regarded as evidence of incomplete adaptation to the erect posture, for the condition does not occur in quadripeds. A positive family history has been reported in 43 per cent of cases.[156] In some instances the familial lesion has involved the same segment of the same vein.

Although there can be little doubt that the main factor in most cases is constitutional, other factors may play a part. Pressure in the leg veins is normally some five to ten times greater in the erect position than when recumbent, and it is even further increased in certain forms of physical exertion.

These facts may link with a high incidence of varicose veins in athletes and in those following occupations requiring long periods of standing, such as guardsmen, policemen, nurses and surgeons. In many instances the varicosities originate or increase during pregnancy: it may be that a hormonal factor responsible for generalized relaxation of smooth muscle is operative, but a more obvious cause could be pressure of the gravid uterus on the iliac veins. Congestive cardiac failure with its associated elevation of systemic venous pressure may also play an aggravating, or perhaps sometimes precipitating, role.

In only a small proportion of cases of varicose veins of the leg is the condition clearly secondary to a thrombotic episode involving the main trunks in the thigh or pelvis, or to destruction of these trunks by tumour or some other process.

Structural Changes

Whether incompetence of valves or dilatation of the lumen comes first has never been determined: the one will inevitably lead to the other and the net result is a segment of vein in which pressure and strain on the wall are both increased. The vein increases in both length and diameter so that tortuosity develops (Fig. 3.36), and the dilatation is always irregular so that pouching rather than cylindrical distension is the result. Once started, the varicosity is likely to extend progressively throughout the length of the affected vein, for as each valve becomes incompetent a progressively increasing strain is thrown on the one below.

The microscopical changes in the wall of the vein are analogous to those observed in arteries in states of arterial hypertension, and the term *phlebosclerosis* is sometimes used to describe them. A strictly limited amount of proliferation of muscular and elastic tissue may occur in the early stages, but soon fibrous replacement of these elements occurs, and ultimately the wall comes to consist mainly of hyaline fibrous tissue with some patchy calcification. Some degree of mural thrombosis is a constant feature and incorporation of these thrombi into the wall by a process of organization leads to irregular thickening of the intima. The thickened plaques usually contain some fatty droplets, but fat is never as conspicuous as in arterial intimal thickenings. Widespread occlusive thrombosis is an exceptional event in varicose veins, but when it occurs the obliteration of veins and cutting off of pressure which it effects may be accompanied by marked relief of symptoms. It is

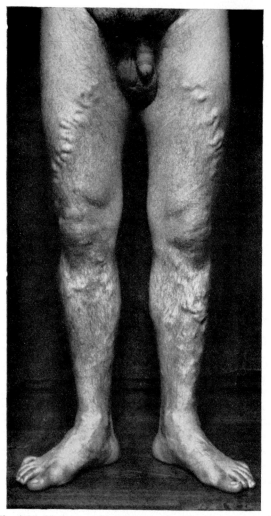

Fig. 3.36. Varicose veins. There is irregular pouching and tortuosity affecting the tributaries of the saphenous systems on both sides.

to this end that the injection treatment of varicose veins is directed.

The lesser degrees of varicose veins commonly have no effects at all, but with severer lesions signs of impaired nutrition of the tissues develop. Oedema occurs and becomes persistent, and the skin becomes atrophic and abnormally sensitive to minor trauma and infection; all too often ulceration develops and fails to heal, so that ultimately extensive *varicose or 'gravitational' ulcers*[157] may cover the tibial region and present a very difficult therapeutic problem. Haemorrhage from varicose veins in the legs is unusual except following trauma. The risk of embolism from thrombosed varicose veins is fortunately very slight.

Varicose Veins in Other Sites

Haemorrhoids are varicose dilatations of the veins of the rectum and anal canal and may occur either inside or outside the anal sphincter. Again there may be a hereditary basis to this localization of varicosity. The condition is aggravated by constipation and pregnancy; it rarely results from portal obstruction, as in cirrhosis of the liver; occasionally it is a complication of rectal tumours. Bleeding is an almost invariable feature and may be so persistent as to lead to chronic iron-deficiency anaemia. Thrombosis is common, while prolapse of the mucosa and distended veins through the sphincter may cause strangulation of the tissue, with sloughing and possibly spreading infection. Chronic infection and the organization following successive thrombotic episodes may result in much scarring and distortion with associated anal discomfort.

Oesophageal varices occur almost entirely as a complication of cirrhosis of the liver. The high portal pressure leads to opening up of venous anastomoses between radicles of portal and systemic veins at the lower end of the oesophagus. The distended veins, covered with oeseophageal epithelium, bulge into the lumen and can often be demonstrated radiographically (Fig. 3.37). In the post-mortem room, however, they are singularly unimpressive, for they collapse completely at death and all that remains to be seen is a little bluish discoloration of the area, though it may be possible to recognize a point through which haemorrhage has occurred. Bleeding from these varices is a common and often fatal event in patients with cirrhosis.

Varicocele is the condition of varicosity of the veins forming the pampiniform plexus (Fig. 3.38), with the production of a characteristic pendulous swelling in the scrotum. It is much commoner on the left side, for the left testicular vein enters the left renal vein while the right testicular vein opens directly into the inferior vena cava. In most cases no underlying cause can be found, but occasionally, and particularly when the condition is of sudden onset, obstruction to the main veins by thrombosis or tumour may be responsible.

Phlebitis

Some degree of involvement of the small veins must occur in the course of any bacterial inflammation. At the periphery of a carbuncle, for instance, the adventitial coats of the small veins are permeated with leucocytes and these may extend throughout the wall. An involved vein may then be

veins, and if the thrombus becomes invaded by pyogenic bacteria, grave sequelae may ensue. Softening of the thrombus may liberate septic emboli into the circulation with the establishment of a generalized pyaemia—a sequence of events

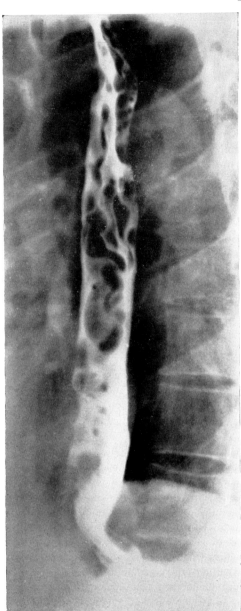

Fig. 3.37. Oesophageal varices. X-ray examination following a barium swallow shows the varices as filling defects outlined by the opaque medium.

narrowed and finally obliterated by a process of endophlebitis, analogous to the endarteritis obliterans occurring in arteries; more frequently, however, the vein becomes occluded by thrombus which is subsequently organized—a process that may be designated as *thrombophlebitis*. Such a process serves a protective function, limiting the risk of bacteria gaining access to the blood stream; but if the thrombotic process extends to involve larger

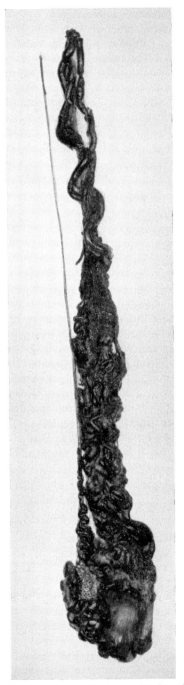

Fig. 3.38. Dried specimen showing varicosity of the veins of the pampiniform plexus (varicocele).

particularly associated with thrombophlebitis of the lateral sinus and jugular vein complicating middle ear and mastoid infection. Portal pyaemia arises in a similar way as a complication of appendicitis, just as puerperal and post-abortion pyaemia follow involvement of uterine veins in a septic process spreading from the endometrium.

Non-bacterial phlebitis is a somewhat doubtful entity, apart from the inflammation of small veins that occurs in the course of typhus fever, in which the rickettsiae actually multiply within the endothelial cells.

The acute phlebitis that accompanies the arterial lesion in thromboangitis obliterans is mentioned on page 138 and does not differ significantly from the arteritis. This venous lesion occurs in only about 40 per cent of cases; the giant cell character of the reaction is often conspicuous in affected veins.

Thrombophlebitis migrans (recurrent idiopathic thrombophlebitis) is a condition in which episodes of venous thrombosis occur without discoverable cause, affecting first one and then another region, and recurring over a number of years. Usually only superficial veins are affected, but occasionally there is involvement of visceral or cerebral veins, with serious results. Biopsy of an affected vessel shows a lesion not definitely distinguishable from the venous lesion in thromboangitis obliterans, and a close aetiological relationship between the two conditions has been postulated.[158, 159] Only rarely, however, is the migrating superficial phlebitis associated with occlusive arterial disease.

A closely similar migrating thrombophlebitis occurs as an unexplained manifestation of malignant disease (Trousseau's sign). It is seen oftenest in the course of carcinoma of the pancreas (see Chapter 23); other tumours with which it has been associated include carcinoma of lung, ovary and alimentary tract.[160] It has been suggested in relation to the occurrence of the condition in cases of pancreatic carcinoma that tryptic enzymes liberated from the pancreas sensitize the coagulation mechanism of the blood,[161] but it must be admitted that we have no satisfactory explanation for its development.

Mondor's disease is a peculiar, localized form of phlebitis affecting subcutaneous veins in the thoracoabdominal wall, particularly in the region of the breast. The lesions present as cord-like thickenings, which histologically show a chronic, sclerosing, inflammatory reaction with concentric constriction of the lumen of the vessel. Some authors have considered the lesion to be in fact a lymphangitis,[162] but most recognize that the affected vessels are veins.[163] The disease has a benign course, although many months may pass before the cords cease to be palpable.

Venous Thrombosis

The inflammatory lesions of the veins discussed above are all characterized by the occurrence of thrombosis; but thrombosis may also develop in veins in the absence of definitely inflammatory features, and it is to describe such an event that the term *phlebothrombosis* (contrasting with thrombophlebitis) was coined. It must be conceded that once thrombosis has occurred the subsequent reaction in the vein wall, concerned with the organization of the thrombus, may render it impossible to ascertain whether or not an inflammatory reaction preceded thrombosis; nevertheless, the term phlebothrombosis is of value in serving to remind us of the important fact that inflammation *per se* plays no part in pathogenesis in many examples of venous thrombosis.

The factors concerned in the development of thrombi, the mechanism of their growth and their fate, are discussed in detail in works on general pathology[164, 165] and do not require repetition here. However, certain specific thrombotic syndromes call for comment.

Widespread thrombosis affecting the veins of the lower extremity is of common occurrence and may be designated as *postoperative* or *puerperal* when following operations or childbirth. It is not infrequently seen also in elderly or debilitated people who are confined to bed, even apart from operative procedures. When venous thrombosis has arisen as a complication of confinement to bed, dissection of the venous system reveals, in a large proportion of the cases, that the thrombotic process has commenced in the veins within the substance of the gastrocnemius and soleus muscles (Fig. 3.39). Once thrombosis has been initiated in these veins it is all too liable to propagate and involve larger and larger vessels, until perhaps the main femoral vein is occluded; sometimes it may extend even farther, to the iliac veins and perhaps to the inferior vena cava itself. In only a minority of cases does the process originate in other sites, such as a superficial varicose vein or the veins of the plantar muscles.[166] The factors responsible for the initiation of thrombosis vary from case to case, but in general terms they can be listed as—

Immobilization, particularly the complete immobility associated with anaesthesia or paralysis.

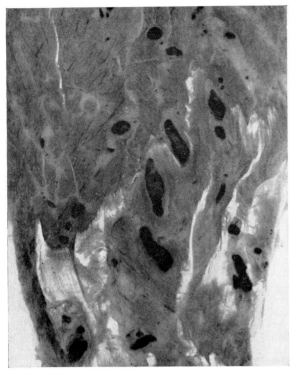

Fig. 3.39. Thrombosis of veins in the substance of a soleus muscle. The specimen comes from the leg of a man who died of massive pulmonary embolism on the sixth day following an abdominal operation.

This robs the venous return of assistance by the milking action of skeletal muscular contraction.

Inhibition of abdominal respiration, by pain, abdominal wounds and the like. This abolishes the waxing and waning of pressure in the inferior vena cava that normally assists venous return.

Low cardiac output associated with many disease states, which is further lowered by inactivity, and is associated with a reduced rate of venous flow.

Pressure trauma to venous endothelium. In an immobile patient the greater part of the weight of the lower limb may bear on the calf muscles, which may therefore be compressed against a firm mattress, or perhaps a harder surface such as an operating table or trolley. It is not difficult to believe that this may lead to loss of endothelial cells.

Changes in the blood that increase its intrinsic coagulability. A rise in platelet count[167] and increased platelet adhesiveness[168] have been shown to develop in the days following an injury to the tissues, such as a surgical operation.

In most instances several of these factors will be operative, each in quite minor degree, but each

reinforcing the others; sometimes, perhaps, infection also plays a part. Anything interfering with free venous drainage from the legs, such as external pressure on the thigh or pressure from a pelvic mass, will further encourage the thrombotic process.

Effects and Sequelae of Thrombosis

It is fortunate that evolution has provided man with some reserve of veins in those areas of the body that are oftenest the site of venous thrombosis. Even quite extensive thrombosis of the superficial veins of the legs or arms may occur without causing any functional disturbance, the deep veins being capable of taking over the entire venous return from the limb; but if the thrombosis becomes very extensive, and particularly if it extends to involve the junction of superficial and deep veins, clinical evidence of local chronic venous congestion, with swelling and cyanosis, will result. Overt oedema is usually limited to dependent parts but sometimes becomes more extensive, though in such cases it is believed that some obstruction to the lymphatic drainage from the area is also concerned. The term *phlegmasia alba dolens* is applied to the painful, white, swollen state of the lower limb that is associated with thrombosis involving the iliac veins and thus obstructing both the superficial and deep venous flow from the limb. This condition occurs oftenest in the puerperium, and pelvic infection undoubtedly plays a part in most cases, producing some element of lymphatic obstruction in addition to the venous thrombosis. With the passage of time the offending thrombus becomes organized, and restoration of a lumen in the vein may be brought about; but there is no restoration of the system of valves, and some degree of venous insufficiency together with varicosity of surrounding veins often remains as a permanent legacy of the event.

It must be mentioned that in certain areas thrombosis of the main veins is incompatible with survival of the tissue concerned, and haemorrhagic infarction of the area will ensue; in other sites, though the tissue may survive there will be major functional disturbances. Thus, infarction is likely to follow thrombosis of a major intracranial venous sinus, or of an adrenal vein, while the usual result of renal vein thrombosis is gross impairment of renal function, though without actual infarction.

Obstruction of the Venae Cavae

The inferior vena cava is occluded oftener than the superior vena cava. The commoner causes are

F*

obstruction by thrombosis extending into it from below, and pressure by tumours, aneurysms or effusions; the superior vena cava is liable to compression by mediastinal tumours, aneurysms and constrictive pericarditis. In either case, if the patient survives for some time a remarkable opening up of collateral veins joining the two main drainage areas occurs. These veins are abundant in the subcutaneous tissues of the chest and abdominal wall. They may be easily detectable on clinical examination; they are particularly well visualized by infrared photography (Fig. 3.40).

The most dreaded sequel of venous thrombosis is *pulmonary embolism* (see also page 277). Though the risk of this complication is ever present it is relatively slight in those cases in which thrombosis arises in varicose veins or is clearly linked with some inflammatory process. In thrombophlebitis migrans and thromboangitis obliterans, embolism is a very exceptional event, for the inflammation rapidly obliterates the plane between intima and thrombus. Conversely, embolism is likeliest in those instances in which thrombosis complicates confinement to bed (postoperative or otherwise), as inflammation plays no part in the process. Small emboli entering the pulmonary arteries may have no effect, but in the presence of pulmonary venous congestion or when larger emboli are concerned, infarction of lung tissue occurs. Massive pulmonary embolism with sudden death occurs when such lengths of propagated thrombus—perhaps as much as 25 to 40 cm long—become detached from the saphenous, femoral or iliac veins that they lodge in the trunk of the pulmonary artery, often plugging both left and right main branches.

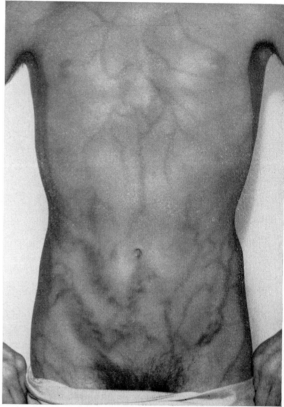

Fig. 3.40. Dilatation of the anastomotic veins following thrombosis of the inferior vena cava. The tortuous veins have been rendered more conspicuous by infrared photography.

LYMPHATIC VESSELS

Although the lymphatic vessels are of paramount importance in pathology as routes for the spread of two major pathological processes—inflammation and neoplasia—they are seldom the seat of primary disease, and the paragraphs that follow describe mainly their secondary involvement by disease in the area which they drain.

In structure the larger lymphatics approximate to veins and like them are supplied with valves to direct the flow centrally. The capillary lymphatics from which they originate are of irregular calibre, branch and anastomose freely, and terminate in slightly expanded blind ends. The walls of these capillary vessels are very permeable, so that tissue

fluids, proteins and, in pathological states, even particulate matter can pass through freely.

Lymphangitis

In the course of many bacterial infections the multiplying bacteria gain entry to the lymphatics, which convey them to the regional lymph nodes. This is seen in most acute infections but especially when the invading organism is a beta-haemolytic streptococcus. Infection with such an organism—in the tissues of a finger, for example—may soon be associated with painful swelling of lymph nodes in the axilla. Sometimes the lymphatic channels conveying the bacteria remain unaffected themselves; in other cases the inflammation spreads through their wall, and their course comes to be marked by ominous red streaks in the skin. Sections taken from the periphery of an inflammatory focus show the lymphatics dilated up to many times their resting calibre and filled with fluid exudate and cellular and bacterial debris (Fig. 3.41). The

tuberculosis and syphilis, may also spread in the lymphatics. For example, this is seen in primary tuberculosis, in which the initial focus in a lung is invariably accompanied by involvement of the corresponding hilar lymph nodes; usually the intervening lymph channels remain normal, but sometimes tubercles develop along their course. Lymphatic involvement is seen also in relation to

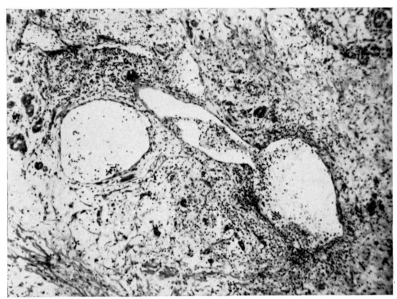

Fig. 3.41. Dilated lymphatics in inflamed tissue. The section comes from the mesentery of an acutely inflamed appendix. *Haematoxylin–eosin.* × 60.

mechanism of this lymphatic dilatation is of some interest, for one might expect these low-pressure channels to be collapsed as a result of the rise of pressure in the tissue spaces, which are distended by inflammatory exudate. It has been shown, however, that the walls of the lymph channels are attached by fine fibres to surrounding tissues so that distension of the tissues results in comparable distension of the channels, which the fluid then readily enters, so to be drained away.[169] The pressure in the lymphatics and the amount of lymph drained from the area are both greatly increased in inflammation. The fluid entering the lymphatics may contain high concentrations of fibrinogen: it may coagulate, lymphatic thrombi resulting. It has been said that this so-called fibrin barrier, by occluding the lymphatic drainage of the area, is an important mechanism in the localization of infection;[170] in contrast, others have found little evidence for the existence of such a barrier round experimental streptococcal and staphylococcal abscesses.[171]

The organisms of chronic infections, notably

tuberculous ulceration of the intestine; the circumferential course of the lymphatics determines the circumferential spread of the lesions.

Actinomycotic infection is an interesting exception to the general rule in that it rarely extends by the lymphatic route.

Lymphatic Spread of Tumours

The lymphatic vessels form what is perhaps the most important route of spread for carcinomas;[172, 173] sarcomas are less likely to spread in this way. Two modes of lymphatic spread are recognized: *lymphatic embolism*, when fragments of tumour are transported in the lymph stream to the related lymph nodes; and *lymphatic permeation*, in which the tumour cells grow as solid columns, forming a core within the lymphatic capillaries (Fig. 3.42) and extending sometimes to involve major lymph trunks. It is this latter mode of involvement that concerns us here, for lymphatic permeation may result in widespread obliteration

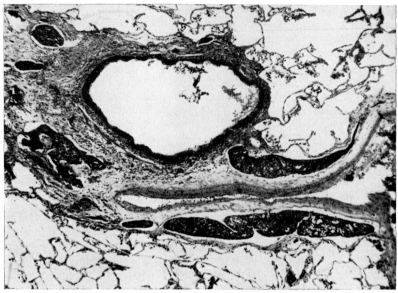

Fig. 3.42. Lymphatic spread of carcinoma. In this section of lung, columns of darkly stained carcinoma cells can be seen permeating the bronchial lymphatics. *Haematoxylin–eosin.* × 50.

of lymphatics with important secondary effects. Sometimes the permeation of the lymphatics leads to oedema of the area, and at the same time the presence of the tumour cells excites a proliferation of fibrous tissue round the vessels, and for this pseudo-inflammatory lesion the term *lymphangitis carcinomatosa* was coined. It is seen particularly in the skin in connexion with carcinoma of the breast and in the lungs when the lymphatics are diffusely infiltrated either by a primary bronchial carcinoma or by a tumour that has metastasized to the lung from some other site.

Lymphatic Obstruction

Lymphatic obstruction may result from strangulation of the channels by scar tissue, permeation or pressure by tumour tissue, plugging by parasites or severance by trauma. Unless major trunks are involved or the obliteration is unusually extensive there will be no ill effect, for collateral routes are abundant in most areas, and in addition the vessels are capable of vigorous reparative proliferation.[174] Obstruction of main trunks, or widespread obliteration of smaller vessels, especially when this occurs in a key situation such as a groin or axilla, is likely to lead to oedema in the area of drainage: this is particularly prone to develop when there is associated venous obstruction, for then venous pressure will be raised and

there will be an increased rate of tissue fluid formation, throwing a further demand on the lymphatic drainage.

Prolonged lymphatic obstruction with oedema leads to progressive dilatation of the lymph vessels —*lymphangiectasis*—and this is accompanied by progressive overgrowth of the fibrous tissue of the area. In this way gross permanent enlargement of the affected part—usually a limb or the external genitalia—results, the condition known as '*elephantiasis*'.

Filariasis.[175]—This is an important cause of elephantiasis. The parasite concerned is *Wuchereria bancrofti* (*Filaria bancrofti*), which is widespread in the tropics and subtropics, including India, West and Central Africa, South America, the north of Australia and the Pacific islands. Many species of mosquito (members of the genera *Culex*, *Anopheles* and *Aedes*) can transmit the parasite. The larvae, deposited on the skin by the feeding mosquito, penetrate the puncture, enter the lymphatics, and grow into adult worms, which are hair-like, transparent nematodes. The male is 2 to 4 cm long and only 0·1 mm thick; the female grows to a length of 8 to 10 cm and is some 0·3 mm thick. They settle in groups, having a predilection for the lymphatics of the groin, scrotum and abdominal wall; there the females produce countless microfilarias, which enter the blood stream and appear in the peripheral blood at night. Heavy infestation with these parasites may lead to lymphatic obstruction, partly because of the presence of dead worms in the lumen, but more as a result of recurrent low-grade inflammatory episodes, probably allergic in character, that lead to fibrosis in and around the vessels. Lymphoedema, lymphangiectasis and elephantiasis follow in the worst cases.

Milroy's Disease.—In 1892 and 1928, Milroy[176, 177] described an interesting form of congenital and familial oedema that has become known as *Milroy's disease.* The oedema affects usually only one limb, but is sometimes more extensive and may involve the eyelids and lips. Examination of the affected tissues[178] shows enormously dilated lymph channels, and the whole area has a honeycomb or spongy character. The abnormal tissue is susceptible to infection, and recurrent episodes of cellulitis may lead to increasing fibrosis round the cavernous lymphatics. The pathogenesis of the condition, apart from the genetic factor, is quite unknown; it might perhaps be better described as a congenital lymphangiectasis than as lymphoedema. A similar condition is sometimes seen without a family history, occasionally developing in adolescence intsead of being truly congenital.

Any of these conditions in which the lymphatics are dilated may be complicated by rupture of the distended vessels, either externally, producing a troublesome 'lymphorrhage', or internally, leading to such conditions as chylothorax, chylous ascites and chyluria. The loss of fluid, protein and fat that follows may endanger life.

VASCULAR HAMARTOMAS AND NEOPLASMS

Albrecht[179] in 1904 introduced the term hamartoma to distinguish tumour-like malformations from true neoplasms. The whole subject has been fully discussed by Willis.[180] A hamartoma is made up of a mixture of the tissues that normally occur in the affected part, but often with one element predominating. The mass does not show the progressive and uncontrolled proliferation that is the essential feature of neoplasia: in general, it no longer increases in size after the body as a whole has attained adult proportions. The distinction between hamartomas and true tumours is, however, somewhat blurred by the fact that the cells of a hamartoma are at least as liable as the cells of other tissues to take on neoplastic growth. There are, therefore, many instances of true tumours developing from pre-existing hamartomas.

Hamartomas

The following are the main examples of hamartomas in which blood or lymphatic vessels are the most conspicuous feature.

Capillary Haemangiomas.—These are the well known capillary naevi, or birthmarks, formed of aggregations of blood-containing channels approximating to capillaries in size and structure. They are most frequently found in the skin or mucosae, where they form flat or slightly elevated (rarely pedunculated) lesions ranging in size from a few millimetres to several centimetres in diameter and occasionally covering large areas of the face, trunk or limbs. The margins of the lesion are ill defined, and a pseudo-invasive appearance may be produced by extension of the abnormal capillaries into underlying tissue planes: however, true neoplasia probably never occurs. The histological picture is often distorted by the occurrence of thrombosis and organization in groups of vessels. When this change is widespread, the vascular spaces become compressed and separated by a dense stroma in which groups of histiocytes containing lipid and haemosiderin occur. The term *sclerosing haemangioma* is then sometimes applied (see Chapter 39).

Capillary Lymphangioma.—This is precisely similar to the haemangioma, except that the connexions are with the lymphatic system and clear lymph occupies the vascular channels. It is an uncommon lesion, occurring mainly in the skin (often about the head and neck) and in the buccal and lingual mucosa.

Cavernous Haemangioma.—The cavernous haemangioma (Fig. 3.43) is a circumscribed aggregation of dilated blood-containing spaces, lined by well-formed endothelium and often with a few muscle and elastic fibres in the walls. It approximates to the structure of erectile tissue such as is seen, for instance, in the corpora cavernosa of the penis. Here again the occurrence of thrombosis

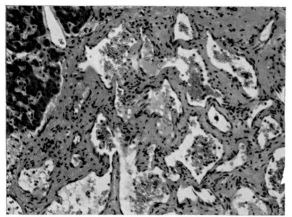

Fig. 3.43. Cavernous haemangioma of the liver. The lesion comprises an aggregation of large blood-containing sinusoids. There is no evidence of neoplastic proliferation of the endothelium. *Haematoxylin–eosin.* × 60.

and organization may confuse the basic picture. These lesions occur in the skin and mucosae; they are also not uncommon incidental findings in the liver and spleen at necropsy. In the brain and cerebellum they may lead to haemorrhage. Occasionally they affect bones, particularly the frontal bone of the skull.

Cavernous Lymphangioma.—The lymphatic counterpart of the cavernous haemangioma occurs oftenest in the angle between shoulder and neck, or in the axilla. In these sites it commonly attains a very large size, and the name *cystic hygroma* is often used for it (Fig. 3.44). It is composed of distended lymphatic spaces, often in close communication with the upper end of the thoracic duct, and damage to it may lead to serious leakage of lymph. Abnormal veins may also enter into the make-up of the mass. Similar, though smaller, lesions are not uncommon in mucous membranes, retroperitoneal tissues and abdominal viscera.

Arteriovenous Malformation.—This is the most appropriate term for irregular masses comprising dilated and convoluted channels of both arterial and venous structure, though they are often called cirsoid aneurysms, or vaguely referred to as 'angiomas'. They occur most typically in the leptomeninges, but may also develop deep in the substance of the brain. They also occur in the soft tissues of the scalp, and more rarely in other parts of the body. Abnormal anastomoses develop between arteries and veins so that the veins draining the region become dilated and tortuous and haemorrhage may occur. Similar but purely venous

malformations are less common; they affect mainly the meninges, especially of the spinal cord.[181]

Glomus Tumour (Glomangioma)

Masson[182, 183] described the glomus as a highly organized structure forming a short-circuit between arterioles and veins in the skin and serving to control blood flow and skin temperature in the area. The arteriole breaks up into numerous distensible channels that are surrounded by layers of cells of epithelioid appearance. These channels are collected into a short efferent vein that links with the veins of the part. The whole structure is minute. It is richly supplied with nerve fibres, derived mainly from the plexus in the wall of the artery. The nature of the epithelioid glomus cells has been the subject of controversy: the presence of short myofibrils within their cytoplasm suggests origin from the muscle of the vessel walls,[184] but other workers,[185] following tissue culture studies, have equated them with Zimmermann's pericytes. The latter somewhat resemble endothelial cells, but are situated external to the reticulin basement membrane of the capillary wall; they are themselves the cell of origin of the haemangiopericytoma (see below).

Glomus tumours are comparatively rare. They

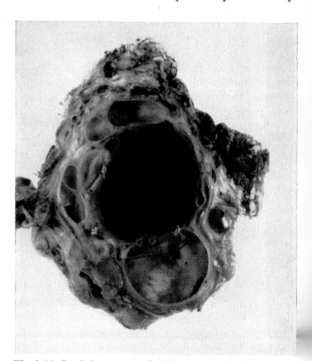

Fig. 3.44. Cystic hygroma excised from the neck of an infant. Haemorrhage has occurred into one of the larger cysts.

develop in either sex and at any age. In the female they usually occur beneath or adjacent to the finger nails; in the male they often affect other parts of the body surface. Exquisite tenderness and attacks of lancinating pain are the characteristic clinical features, and may be so extreme as to drive the victim to suicidal attempts, or occasionally to local assaults on the tumour itself. There is often a clear history of local trauma, and the status of glomus tumour as true tumour, hamartoma or traumatic reparative proliferation remains in doubt. The diameter of the lesion is usually only a few millimetres and rarely exceeds a centimetre. It is poorly demarcated from the surrounding tissues, pink or bluish in colour, and on section is composed of endothelium-lined channels of varying calibre, surrounded by rows and sheets of regular polygonal cells with uniform nuclei, resembling closely the cells of the normal glomus (Fig. 3.45). Transition between these cell forms and smooth-muscle cells has been observed. The lesion is static or slow-growing; metastatic spread has rarely been described (see Chapter 39).

Other True Neoplasms

The nomenclature of true neoplasms taking origin from blood vessels is at present most confused. A profusion of names, of doubtful differential significance, is employed in current texts and papers on the subject and no widely used system can be discerned amongst them. The nomenclature under which the tumours are described below, while possibly representing an oversimplification, nevertheless provides for all the well-recognized varieties.

Benign Haemangioendothelioma.—This term is employed for a benign neoplasm of blood-vessel endothelium. It is necessary to include the word benign, for without this epithet some authors have implied a malignant tumour by the term haemangioendothelioma,[186] while others have implied a benign one.[187] Many practising pathologists would refer to these tumours as haemangiomas, but a different term is required in order to differentiate them from the much commoner hamartomatous vascular naevi usually called by that name.

Undoubted neoplasms coming within this definition are not common. They occur mainly in the skin and subcutaneous tissues, but also sometimes in the spleen, liver and other viscera. Their distinctive features are that they are not congenital (though they may complicate a congenital naevus), and that they show progressive though usually slow growth, forming poorly demarcated, firm, pinkish masses, which in the skin tend to become polypoid. Microscopically, they are distinguishable from capillary naevi by evidence of more active growth, involving definite proliferation of endothelial cells rather than budding of formed capillaries. Some-

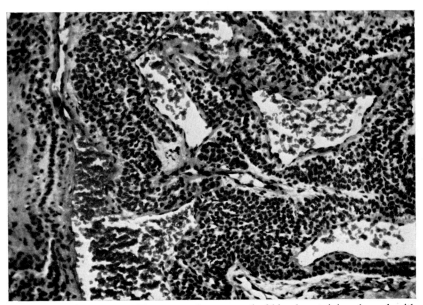

Fig. 3.45. Glomus tumour. The tumour is composed of blood-containing channels with well-defined endothelial lining and surrounded by rows of glomus cells. *Haematoxylin–eosin.* × 120.

times this leads to the formation of solid sheets of cells without the development of vascular lumina, but silver impregnation of the reticulin fibres will reveal the grouping of the cells into the characteristic vascular pattern.

There is some tendency for these tumours to become locally invasive, and occasionally true malignancy may supervene. This is particularly true of haemangioendotheliomas occurring in the region of the breast (see Chapter 28).

Haemangioblastoma.—This name, sanctioned through usage,[188] is now reserved for the rather characteristic tumours of blood-vessel origin occurring in the cerebellum and, less frequently, the cerebrum. The commonest variety is the cystic haemangioblastoma, which appears in a cerebellar hemisphere as a neoplastic nodule in the wall of a cyst containing clear, faintly yellow fluid. Solid varieties also occur. In a minority of cases these tumours are associated with vascular tumours of the retina and liver, cysts of the pancreas, kidneys and liver, and adenomas of the kidneys and adrenals, constituting the so-called Lindau–von Hippel disease: it is this occasional association which is held to justify the term haemangioblastoma, with its implication of origin from embryonic cells. Under the microscope the tumour shows proliferating endothelial cells, often with many atypical forms and

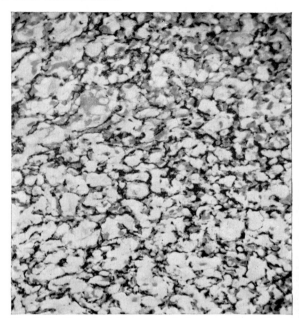

Fig. 3.47. Haemangioblastoma of the cerebellum. Silver impregnation reveals the reticulin network that represents the endothelial basement membrane. × 200.

'foam cells'—histiocytes distended with lipid material (Figs 3.46 and 3.47). The aberrant cells and frequent mitotic figures suggest a tumour of malignant potentialities, but in practice these tumours are slow growing, seldom recur after surgical removal, and never metastasize.

Haemangiopericytoma.—The uterus is the main site for tumours arising from the pericytes of Zimmermann.[189] Normally these cells are arranged concentrically outside the basement membrane of the endothelium, and this arrangement is maintained in the tumours to which they give rise. The structure is therefore one of compressed capillaries surrounded by a zone of proliferating spindle-shaped pericytes (Fig. 3.48). These tumours have a wide range of behaviour, varying from the slowly growing circumscribed lesion (resembling a fibromyoma), through the locally invasive forms to rare examples in which distant metastasis occurs.[190] Microscopically the degree of differentiation shows a corresponding range. The qualifications benign and malignant are used, but it may be difficult to determine which is the more appropriate in individual cases.

Haemangiosarcoma (Malignant Haemangioendothelioma).—True malignant tumours of proliferating vascular endothelium are rarities. Two diagnostic hazards have tended to lead to their overdiagnosis.

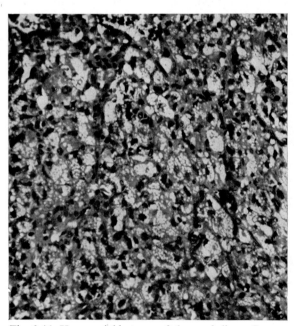

Fig. 3.46. Haemangioblastoma of the cerebellum. Groups of foam cells are conspicuous among the endothelial cells. *Haematoxylin–eosin.* × 200.

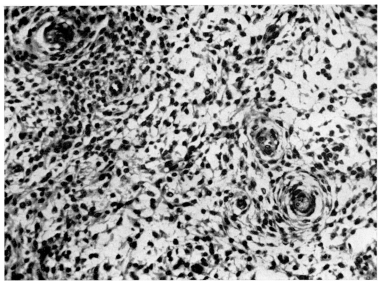

Fig. 3.48. Haemangiopericytoma of the uterus. The tumour is composed of spindle cells that in places are arranged in whorls round the small blood vessels. *Haematoxylin–eosin.* × 200.

First, benign haemangioendotheliomas may be multiple and rapidly growing, and this may give a false impression of a primary tumour with metastasis; second, other types of sarcoma may develop so rich a vascular network (so-called telangiectatic sarcomas) that the endothelial cells are mistaken for the neoplastic element.

A true haemangiosarcoma may arise *de novo* or from a pre-existing vascular malformation or a benign haemangioendothelioma. Breast, liver and spleen are among the commoner sites, but the soft tissues of any part of the body may be the source. The tumour forms a white or pink lobulated mass; there are often areas of haemorrhage into its substance. Microscopical diagnosis depends on the unequivocal demonstration that the tumour cells themselves are forming vascular channels. Often the greater part of the tumour is too undifferentiated for this to be evident and the condition then merges with other varieties of undifferentiated soft-tissue sarcomas.

It has been recognized recently that there is a high incidence of haemangiosarcoma of the liver among workers in the plastics industry in the United States of America[190a] and elsewhere (see Chapter 21). Exposure to vinyl chloride monomer, used in the manufacture of polyvinyl chloride, has been incriminated.

Kaposi's Sarcoma.[191–193]—This condition (Fig. 3.49), which is also known as multiple idiopathic haemorrhagic sarcoma, is customarily classed with the angiosarcomas, but it is doubtful if this represents a correct assessment of its nature.[194] The condition affects coloured more than white races and men more than women. It usually starts in middle life with multiple red swellings of the skin of the legs and arms (see Chapter 39). The lesions enlarge and increase in number. In the late stages visceral involvement may occur. Microscopically, the tumours resemble haemangiomas, but have a spindle-cell stroma often infiltrated with leucocytes and macrophages; it is this stroma that, in the later stages, appears to take on sarcomatous features.

Neoplasms of Veins.—Tumours arising in the walls of veins are very uncommon. A review in 1960 could cite only 23 reported examples.[195] The inferior vena cava and the large veins of the lower limbs are the usual sites of origin, and most of the tumours are leiomyomas or leiomyosarcomas. Venous obstruction resulting from such a tumour is a rare cause of the Budd–Chiari syndrome (see Chapter 21).[196]

Lymphangioma and *Lymphangiosarcoma.* — These lymphatic counterparts of the benign and malignant tumours of blood vessels are rarities and do not require separate description. They are seen most frequently as complications developing in the

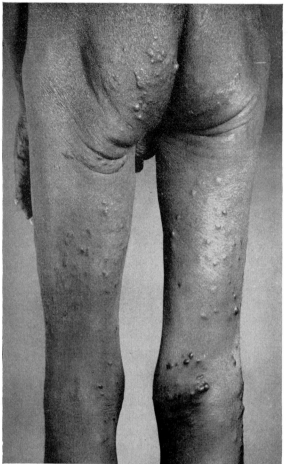

Fig. 3.49. Kaposi's sarcoma. Typical appearance of lesions in a Ugandan man, aged about 40 years.

presence of lymphoedema, whether congenital or acquired (see Chapter 28).[197]

Telangiectases

A telangiectasis is a localized dilatation of capillaries and venules, occurring oftenest in the skin, where it forms a characteristic red macule, fading when the vessels are emptied by pressure and slowly regaining colour as they fill when pressure is released. The most important variety occurs in *hereditary haemorrhagic telangiectasia* (Osler's disease), in which multiple small lesions develop in the skin and mucous membranes. There is a strong tendency to haemorrhage, especially from alimentary lesions, and this may prove fatal as the lesions are too widespread to permit of cure by surgical resection. The condition appears to be due to a genetic weakness of the capillaries, inherited as a dominant characteristic (see Chapter 39 also).

Other varieties of telangiectasis are the so-called *spider naevi* that develop—often on the face—in the course of chronic diseases, notably cirrhosis of the liver, and *Campbell de Morgan's spots*—tiny capillary dilatations forming bright red dots about the trunk and shoulders of middle-aged and elderly people. Though once thought to point to malignant disease, de Morgan's spots are in fact of no particular significance.

REFERENCES (CHAPTER 3A)

ARTERIES AND ARTERIOLES—AGEING
1. Levene, C. I., *J. Path. Bact.*, 1956, **72**, 79.
2. Movat, H. Z., More, R. H., Haust, M. D., *Amer. J. Path.*, 1958, **34**, 1023.
3. Lansing, A. I., Blumenthal, H. T., Gray, S. H., *J. Geront.*, 1948, **3**, 87.

'SCLEROTIC' CHANGES IN ARTERIES
4. Lobstein, J. G. C. F. M., *Traités d'anatomie pathologique*. Paris, 1833.
5. Mönckeberg, J. G., *Virchows Arch. path. Anat.*, 1903, **171**, 141.
6. Movat, H. A., Haust, M. D., More, R. H., *Amer. J. Path.*, 1959, **35**, 93.
7. Geer, J. C., McGill, H. C., Strong, J. P., *Amer. J. Path.*, 1961, **38**, 263.
8. Crawford, T., Levene, C. I., *J. Path. Bact.*, 1953, **35**, 93.
9. Winternitz, M. C., Thomas, R. M., Le Compte,

P. M., *The Biology of Arteriosclerosis*. Springfield, Illinois, 1938.
10. Hutchinson, E. C., Yates, P. O., *Brain*, 1956, **79**, 319.
11. Hutchinson, E. C., Yates, P. O., *Lancet*, 1957, **1**, 2.
12. Yates, P. O., Hutchinson, E. C., *Spec. Rep. Ser. med. Res. Coun. (Lond.)*, No. 300, 1961.
13. Levene, C. I., *J. Path. Bact.*, 1956, **72**, 83.
14. Dible, J. H., *The Pathology of Limb Ischaemia*. Edinburgh, 1966.
15. Keys, A., *J. chron. Dis.*, 1956, **4**, 364.
16. Larsen, N. P., *Arch. intern. Med.*, 1957, **100**, 436.
17. Vogel, J., *The Pathological Anatomy of the Human Body*. Philadelphia, 1847.
18. Anitschkow, N., *Beitr. path. Anat.*, 1913, **56**, 379.
19. Steiner, A., Kendall, F. E., *Arch. Path. (Chic.)*, 1946, **42**, 433.
20. Dauber, D. V., Katz, L. N., *Arch. Path. (Chic.)*, 1942, **34**, 937.

21. Katz, L. N., Stamler, J., *Experimental Atherosclerosis*. Springfield, Illinois, 1953.
22. Warren, S., *The Pathology of Diabetes Mellitus*, 2nd edn. Philadelphia, 1938.
23. Hueper, W. C., *Arch. Path. (Chic.)*, 1944, **38**, 162, 245, 350.
24. Hueper, W. C., *Arch. Path. (Chic.)*, 1945, **39**, 51, 117, 187.
25. Oliver, M. F., Boyd, G. S., *Brit. Heart J.*, 1953, **15**, 387.
26. Gofman, J. W., Jones, H. B., Lindgren, F. T., Lyon, T. P., Elliott, H. A., Strisower, B., *Circulation*, 1950, **2**, 161.
27. Gofman, J. W., Glazier, F., Tamplin, A., Strisower, B., De Lalla, O., *Physiol. Rev.*, 1954, **34**, 589.
28. Keys, A., *Circulation*, 1952, **5**, 115.
29. Brontë-Stewart, B., *Brit. med. Bull.*, 1958, **14**, 243.
30. Ahrens, E. H., Blankenhorn, D. H., Tsaltas, T. T., *Proc. Soc. exp. Biol. (N.Y.)*, 1954, **86**, 872.
31. Sinclair, H. M., *Lancet*, 1956, **1**, 381.
32. Sinclair, H. M., *Lancet*, 1956, **2**, 101.
33. Rokitansky, C. von, *A Manual of Pathological Anatomy*, trans. by G. E. Day, vol. 4, page 272. London, 1852.
34. Duguid, J. B., *J. Path. Bact.*, 1946, **58**, 207.
35. Morgan, A. D., *The Pathogenesis of Coronary Occlusion*. Oxford, 1956.
36. Crawford, T., Levene, C. I., *J. Path. Bact.*, 1952, **64**, 523.
37. Woolf, N., Carstairs, K. C., *Amer. J. Path.*, 1967, **51**, 373.
38. Woolf, N., Crawford, T., *J. Path. Bact.*, 1960, **80**, 405.
39. Aschoff, L., *Lectures on Pathology*, page 131. New York, 1924.
40. Morgan, A. D., *The Pathogenesis of Coronary Occlusion*, page 87. Oxford, 1956.
41. Adams, C. W. M., Tuqan, N. A., *J. Path. Bact.*, 1961, **82**, 131.
42. Fullerton, H. W., Anastasopoulos, G., *Brit. med. J.*, 1949, **2**, 1492.
43. Fullerton, H. W., Davie, W. J. A., Anastasopoulos, G., *Brit. med. J.*, 1953, **2**, 250.
44. Robinson, D. S., Pool, J. C. F., *Quart. J. exp. Physiol.*, 1956, **41**, 36.
45. Astrup, T., *Lancet*, 1956, **2**, 565.
46. Billimoria, J. D., Drysdale, J., James, D. C. O., Maclagan, N. F., *Lancet*, 1959, **2**, 471.
47. Chakrabarti, R., Bielawiec, M., Evans, J. F., Fearnley, G. R., *J. clin. Path.*, 1968, **21**, 698.
48. Nestel, P. J., *Lancet*, 1959, **2**, 373.
49. Eilert, M. L., *Metabolism*, 1953, **2**, 137.
50. Oliver, M. F., Boyd, G. S., *Circulation*, 1956, **13**, 82.
51. Morris, J. N., *Lancet*, 1951, **1**, 69.
52. Morris, J. N., Crawford, M. D., *Brit. med. J.*, 1958, **2**, 1485.
53. Morris, J. N., Crawford, M. D., Heady, J. A., *Lancet*, 1961, **1**, 860.
54. Crawford, M. D., Gardner, M. J., Morris, J. N., *Brit. med. Bull.*, 1971, **27**, 21.
55. Crawford, T., Crawford, M. D., *Lancet*, 1967, **1**, 229.
56. *The Geographic Pathology of Atherosclerosis*, edited by H. C. McGill, Jr. Supplement to: *Lab. Invest.*, 1968, **18**, 463(–653).
57. Robertson, W. B., Strong, J. P., *Lab. Invest.*, 1968, **18**, 538.

58. Heath, D., Wood, E. H., DuShane, J. W., Edwards J. E., *Lab. Invest.*, 1960, **9**, 259.
59. Crawford, T., Levene, C. I., *J. Path. Bact.*, 1952, **64**, 523.
60. Levene, C. I., *J. Path. Bact.*, 1956, **72**, 79.
61. Duguid, J. B., *J. Path. Bact.*, 1926, **29**, 371.
62. Duguid, J. B., Robertson, W. B., *Lancet*, 1957, **1**, 1205.
63. Duguid, J. B., Anderson, G. S., *J. Path. Bact.*, 1952, **64**, 519.
64. Crawford, T., Woolf, N., *J. Path. Bact.*, 1960, **79**, 221.

ARTERITIS
65. Williams, A. W., Montgomery, G. L., *J. Path. Bact.*, 1959, **77**, 63.
66. Turnbull, H. M., *Quart. J. Med.*, 1915, **8**, 201.
67. Beck, H., *Amer. Heart J.*, 1943, **25**, 307.
68. Nichols, C. F., *Ann. intern. Med.*, 1940, **14**, 960.
69. Campbell, M., *Brit. med. J.*, 1932, **1**, 328.
70. Heubner, O., *Die luetische Erkrankung der Hirnarterien*. Leipzig, 1874.
71. Pappenheimer, A. M., VonGlahn, W. C., *J. med. Res.*, 1924, **44**, 489.
72. Toone, E. C., Pierce, E. L., Hennigar, G., *Amer. J. Med.*, 1959, **26**, 255.
73. Winiwarter, F. von, *Arch. klin. Chir.*, 1879, **23**, 202.
74. Buerger, L., *Amer. J. med. Sci.*, 1908, **136**, 567.
75. Buerger, L., *The Circulatory Disturbances of the Extremities*. Philadelphia, 1924.
76. Dible, J. H., *J. Path. Bact.*, 1958, **75**, 1.
77. Dible, J. H., *The Pathology of Limb Ischaemia*, page 79. Edinburgh, 1966.
78. Samuels, S. S., *Amer. J. med. Sci.*, 1932, **183**, 465.
79. Barker, N. W., *Proc. Mayo Clin.*, 1931, **6**, 65.
80. Harkavy, J., *Bull. N.Y. Acad. Med.*, 1933, **9**, 318.
81. Goodman, C., *Arch. Surg. (Chic.)*, 1937, **35**, 1126.
82. Fisher, C. M., *Medicine (Baltimore)*, 1957, **36**, 169.
83. Wessler, S., Ming, S., Gurewick, V., Freiman, D. G., *New Engl. J. Med.*, 1960, **263**, 412.
84. Dible, J. H., *Lancet*, 1960, **2**, 1138.
85. Horton, B. T., Magath, T. B., Brown, G. E., *Proc. Mayo Clin.*, 1932, **7**, 700.
86. Horton, B. T., Magath, T. B., Brown, G. E., *Proc. Mayo Clin.*, 1937, **12**, 548.
87. Hutchinson, J., *Arch. Surg. (Lond.)*, 1890, **1**, 323.
88. Gilmour, J. R., *J. Path. Bact.*, 1941, **53**, 263.
89. Cooke, W. T., Cloake, P. C. P., Govan, A. D. T., Colbeck, J. C., *Quart. J. Med.*, 1946, N.S. **15**, 47.
90. Heptinstall, R. H., Porter, K. A., Barkley, H., *J. Path. Bact.*, 1954, **67**, 507.
91. Harris, M., *Brit. Heart J.*, 1968, **30**, 840.
92. Kimmelstiel, P., Gilmour, M. T., Hodges, H. H., *A.M.A. Arch. Path.*, 1952, **54**, 157.
93. Takayashu, M., *Acta Soc. ophthal. jap.*, 1908, **12**, 554.
94. Broadbent, W. H., *Trans. clin. Soc. Lond.*, 1875, **2**, 165.
95. Misra, S. S., Prakash, S., Agrawal, P. L., *Amer. Heart J.*, 1959, **57**, 177.
96. Pahwa, J. M., Pamdey, M. P. N., Gupta, D. P., *Brit. med. J.*, 1959, **2**, 1439.
97. Lessof, M. H., Glynn, L. E., *Lancet*, 1959, **1**, 799.
98. Martorell, F., Fabré-Tersol, J., *Med. clín. (Barcelona)*, 1944, **2**, 26.
99. Caldwell, R. A., Skipper, E. W., *Brit. Heart J.*, 1961, **23**, 53.

100. Kalmansohn, R. B., Kalmansohn, R. W., *Circulation*, 1957, **15**, 237.
101. Isaacson, C., Klachko, D. M., Wayburne, S., Simson, I. W., *Lancet*, 1959, **2**, 542.
102. Lessof, M. H., Glynn, L. E., *Lancet*, 1959, **1**, 799.
103. Rokitansky, C. von, *Denkschr. Akad. Wiss. Wien*, 1852, **4**, 49.
104. Kussmaul, A., Maier, R., *Dtsch. Arch. klin. Med.*, 1866, **1**, 484.
105. Rose, C. A., Spencer, H., *Quart. J. Med.*, 1957, N.S. **26**, 43.
106. Gitlin, D., Craig, J. M., Janeway, C. A., *Amer. J. Path.*, 1957, **33**, 55.
107. Symmers, W. St C., *J. Path. Bact.*, 1953, **66**, 109.
108. Davson, J., Ball, J., Platt, R., *Quart. J. Med.*, 1948, N.S. **17**, 175.
109. Rackemann, F. M., Greene, J. E., *Trans. Ass. Amer. Phycns*, 1939, **54**, 112.
110. Rich, A. R., *Bull. Johns Hopk. Hosp.*, 1942, **71**, 375.
111. Rich, A. R., in *Sensitivity Reactions to Drugs*, edited by M. L. Rosenheim, R. Moulton, S. Moeschlin and W. St C. Symmers, page 196. Oxford, 1958.
112. Symmers, W. St C., in *Sensitivity Reactions to Drugs*, edited by M. L. Rosenheim, R. Moulton, S. Moeschlin and W. St C. Symmers, page 209. Oxford, 1958.
113. Klinge, F., *Beitr. path. Anat.*, 1929–30, **83**, 185.
114. Rich, A. R., Gregory, J. E., *Bull. Johns Hopk. Hosp.*, 1943, **72**, 65.
115. Crawford, T., Nassim, J. R., *J. Path. Bact.*, 1951, **63**, 619.
116. Wilson, C., Byrom, F. B., *Quart. J. Med.*, 1941, N.S. **10**, 65
117. Smith, C. C., Zeek, P. M., McGuire, J., *Amer. J. Path.*, 1944, **20**, 721.
118. Pagel, W., *J. clin. Path.*, 1951, **4**, 137.
119. Frohnert, P. P., Sheps, S. G., *Amer. J. Med.*, 1967, **43**, 8.
120. Wegener, F., *Beitr. path. Anat.*, 1939, **102**, 36.
121. Walton, E. W., Leggat, P. O., *J. clin. Path.*, 1956, **9**, 31.
122. Ruiter, M., Hadders, H. N., *J. Path. Bact.*, 1959, **77**, 71.
123. Cottier, H., Vogt, W., *Schweiz. med. Wschr.*, 1957, **87**, 43.
124. Lindgren, Å. G. H., *Acta path. microbiol. scand.*, 1957, **41**, 281.
125. Engel, W. J., McCormack, L. J., *J. Urol. (Baltimore)*, 1958, **79**, 230.
126. Waugh, T. R., *Amer. J. Path.*, 1950, **26**, 851.
127. Gold, S. C., Gowing, N. F. C., *Quart. J. Med.*, 1953, N.S. **22**, 457.
128. Symmers, W. St C., in *Eight Colloquia on Clinical Pathology*, edited by M. Welsch, P. Dustin and J. Dagnelie, chap. 29, page 749. Brussels, 1958.

ANEURYSMS

129. Merten, C. W., Finby, N., Sternberg, I., *Amer. J. Med.*, 1956, **20**, 345.
130. Oram, S., East, T., *Brit. Heart J.*, 1955, **17**, 541.
131. Abrams, L. D., Evans, D. W., *Quart. J. Med.*, 1964, N.S. **33**, 285.
132. Munscheck, H., *Zbl. allg. Path. path. Anat.*, 1958, **98**, 172.
133. Symmers, W. St C., *Brain*, 1956, **79**, 511.
134. Orbison, J. L., *Amer. J. Path.*, 1952, **28**, 129.
135. McKissock, W., Paine, K., Walsh, L., *J. Neurol. Neurosurg. Psychiat.*, 1958, **21**, 239.
136. Crawford, T., *J. Neurol. Neurosurg. Psychiat.*, 1959, **22**, 259.
137. Forbus, W. D., *Johns Hopk. Hosp. Bull.*, 1930, **47**, 239.
138. Glynn, L. E., *J. Path. Bact.*, 1940, **51**, 213.
139. Bigelow, N. H., *Amer. J. med. Sci.*, 1953, **225**, 485.
140. Anderson, R. McD., Blackwood, W., *J. Path. Bact.*, 1959, **77**, 101.
141. Carmichael, R., *J. Path. Bact.*, 1950, **62**, 1.
142. Shennan, T., *Spec. Rep. Ser. med. Res. Coun. (Lond.)*, No. 193, 1934.
143. Hirst, A. E., Varner, J. J., Kime, S. W., *Medicine (Baltimore)*, 1958, **37**, 217.
144. Shennan, T., *J. Path. Bact.*, 1932, **35**, 161.
145. Gsell, O., *Virchows Arch. path. Anat.*, 1928, **270**, 1.
146. Erdheim, J., *Virchows Arch. path. Anat.*, 1930, **276**, 187.
147. Pygott, F., *Brit. J. Radiol.*, 1955, **28**, 26.
148. Ponseti, I. V., Baird, W. A., *Amer. J. Path.*, 1952, **28**, 1059.
149. Lalich, J. J., Barnett, B. D., Bird, H. R., *A.M.A. Arch. Path.*, 1957, **64**, 643.
150. Hirst, A. E., Varner, J. J., Kime, S. W., *Medicine (Baltimore)*, 1958, **37**, 217.
151. Reifenstein, G. H., Levine, S. A., Gross, R. E., *Amer. Heart J.*, 1947, **33**, 146.
152. Dunnill, M. S., *J. Path. Bact.*, 1959, **78**, 203.
153. Wolman, L., *Brain*, 1959, **82**, 276.
154. Watson, A. J., *J. Path. Bact.*, 1956, **72**, 439.

VEINS

155. Franklin, K. J., *A Monograph on Veins*. Springfield, Illinois, 1937.
156. Larson, R. A., Smith, F. L., *Proc. Mayo Clin.*, 1943, **18**, 400.
157. Rivlin, S., *Lancet*, 1958, **1**, 1363.
158. Buerger, L., *Int. Clin.*, 1909, **19**, 84.
159. Barker, N. W., *Proc. Mayo Clin.*, 1936, **11**, 513.
160. Perlow, S., Daniels, J. L., *A.M.A. Arch. intern. Med.*, 1956, **97**, 184.
161. Gore, I., *Amer. J. Path.*, 1953, **29**, 1093.
162. Jönsson, G., Linell, F., Sandblom, P., *Acta chir. scand.*, 1955, **108**, 351.
163. Lunn, G. M., Potter, J. M., *Brit. med. J.*, 1954, **1**, 1074.
164. Wright, G. Payling, *An Introduction to Pathology*, 3rd edn, pages 317–318. London, 1958.
165. French, J. E., Macfarlane, R. G., in *General Pathology*, edited by H. W. Florey; 4th edn, chap. 9. London, 1970.
166. Barker, N. W., Nygaard, K. K., Walters, W., Priestley, J. T., *Proc. Mayo Clin.*, 1941, **16**, 33.
167. Dawbarn, R. Y., Earlam, F., Evans, W. H., *J. Path. Bact.*, 1928, **31**, 833.
168. Wright, H. Payling, *J. Path. Bact.*, 1942, **54**, 461.

LYMPHATIC VESSELS

169. Pullinger, B. D., Florey, H. W., *Brit. J. exp. Path.*, 1935, **16**, 49.
170. Menkin, V., *Biochemical Mechanisms in Inflammation*, 2nd edn. Springfield, Illinois, 1956.

171. Miles, A. A., *Lectures on the Scientific Basis of Medicine*, vol. 3, page 235. London, 1955.
172. Willis, R. A., *The Spread of Tumours in the Human Body*, 2nd edn. London, 1952.
173. Handley, W. S., *Cancer of the Breast and its Treatment*. London, 1922.
174. Reichert, F. L., *Arch. Surg. (Chic.)*, 1930, **20**, 543.
175. Galindo, L., in *Pathology of Protozoal and Helminthic Diseases with Clinical Correlation*, edited by R. A. Marcial-Rojas and E. Moreno, chap. 53. Baltimore, 1971.
176. Milroy, W. F., *N.Y. med. J.*, 1892, **56**, 505.
177. Milroy, W. F., *J. Amer. med. Ass.*, 1928, **91**, 1172.
178. Mason, P. B., Allen, E. V., *Amer. J. Dis. Child.*, 1935, **50**, 945.

VASCULAR HAMARTOMAS AND NEOPLASMS

179. Albrecht, E., *Verh. dtsch. path. Ges.*, 1904, **7**, 153.
180. Willis, R. A., *The Borderland of Embryology and Pathology*, 2nd edn, page 351. London, 1962.
181. Wyburn-Mason, R., *The Vascular Abnormalities and Tumours of the Spinal Cord and its Membranes*. London, 1943.
182. Masson, P., *Lyon chir.*, 1924, **21**, 257.
183. Masson, P., *Bull. Soc. franç. Derm. Syph.*, 1935, **42**, 1174.
184. Bailey, O. T., *Amer. J. Path.*, 1935, **11**, 915.
185. Murray, M. R., Stout, A. P., *Amer. J. Path.*, 1942, **18**, 183.
186. Cappell, D. F., Anderson, J. R., *Muir's Textbook of Pathology*, 9th edn, page 252. London, 1971.
187. Landing, B. H., Farber, S., *Tumors of the Cardiovascular System* (Atlas of Tumor Pathology, sect. 3. fasc. 7), page 47. Washington, D.C., 1956.
188. Lindau, A., *Acta path. microbiol. scand.*, 1926, suppl. 1.
189. Charles, A. H., *J. Obstet. Gynaec. Brit. Cwlth*, 1961, **68**, 648.
190. Pedowitz, P., Felmus, L. B., Grayzel, D. M., *Amer. J. Obstet. Gynec.*, 1955, **69**, 1291, 1309.
190a. Falk, H., Creech, J. L., Heath, C. W., Johnson, M. N., Key, M. M., *J. Amer. med. Ass.*, 1974, **230**, 59.
191. Bluefarb, S. M., *Kaposi's Sarcoma; Multiple Idiopathic Hemorrhagic Sarcoma*. Springfield, Illinois, 1957.
192. Dutz, W., Stout, A. P., *Cancer (Philad.)*, 1960, **13**, 684.
193. *Symposium on Kaposi's Sarcoma*, edited by L. V. Ackerman and J. F. Murray. Basel and New York, 1963.
194. Aegerter, E. E., Peale, A. R., *Arch. Path. (Chic.)*, 1942, **34**, 413.
195. Light, H. G., Peskin, G. W., Ravdin, I. S., *Cancer (Philad.)*, 1960, **13**, 818.
196. Cardell, B. S., McGill, D. A. F., Williams, R., *J. Path.*, 1971, **104**, 283.
197. Stewart, F. W., Treves, N., *Cancer (Philad.)*, 1948, **1**, 64.

ACKNOWLEDGEMENTS FOR ILLUSTRATIONS (CHAPTER 3A)

Figs 3.6, 10, 12, 17, 18. Reproduced by permission of the editors from: *J. Atheroscler. Res.*, 1961, **1**, 3; *Recenti Progr. Med.*, 1960, **29**, 549.

Fig. 3.15. Reproduced by permission of the editor from: Crawford, T., *J. Neurol. Neurosurg. Psychiat.*, 1959, **22**, 259.

Fig. 3.16. Reproduced by permission of the editor from: *Pathogenesis and Treatment of Arterial Disease*, edited by L. McDonald; London, 1960.

3B: *Hypertension*

by K. A. PORTER

INTRODUCTION

The term hypertension, used without qualification, implies persistent elevation of systolic and diastolic pressure in the systemic arteries—*systemic hypertension*. Systolic hypertension, in which the systolic pressure only is raised, may also occur.

Significant elevation of the pressure in the pulmonary arteries constitutes *pulmonary hypertension* and occurs in a variety of conditions in which there is resistance to the flow of blood through the lungs. Pulmonary hypertension is considered in Chapter 7 (page 282).

Increased resistance to blood flow within the liver leads to a rise in pressure in the portal venous system—*portal hypertension*: this is considered in Chapter 21.

Systemic blood pressure normally tends to rise with age; the rise is different in the two sexes. In childhood and youth the pressure is higher in the male, but between the ages of 35 and 45 years the blood pressure of women rises to equal that of men and thereafter rises more steeply. In the younger age groups the range of blood pressure is small; as age advances the pressure tends to rise faster in some individuals than in others. For this reason, the limits of what constitutes normal blood pressure are wide, and a pressure that would be regarded as high in a young person might be considered normal in an elderly person. The dividing line between normal and abnormal for each sex at any age is arbitrary and varies from observer to observer.

Mortality rises steadily and markedly with increasing elevation of blood pressure over the whole range of arterial pressure. The excessive mortality among those with higher than average blood pressure is primarily due to heart failure, stroke, and renal failure: analysis shows that these result from a variety of lesions that are consequences of several factors, of which hypertension is one.

High blood pressure frequently accompanies certain diseases, particularly those of the kidneys (*secondary hypertension*). No more than 10 to 15 per cent of cases of hypertension are secondary to some demonstrable cause. When cases of secondary hypertension are excluded there remains a large group of patients whose hypertension has no apparent cause: this is the condition known as primary hypertension or, oftener, *essential hypertension*.

When the gradient of the progressive rise in blood pressure in either primary or secondary hypertension is slow the patient is said to be in the *benign phase of hypertension*. Benign phase hypertension may go on for many years with few symptoms and little deterioration. The pressure rises are usually modest, although high levels may eventually occur and be sustained for long periods, particularly in women. The condition usually terminates in cardiac failure or a cerebrovascular accident; only rarely is death due to renal failure.

When the gradient of the rise in blood pressure in either primary or secondary hypertension is very steep, the condition—if untreated—has a rapidly downhill course to a fatal outcome within a period of about six months to two years. This accelerated or *malignant phase of hypertension* is usually accompanied by papilloedema and commonly leads to renal failure. Malignant hypertension is often preceded by a variable period of benign phase hypertension.

It is often suggested that cardiovascular morbidity and mortality are more closely linked to the diastolic pressure than to the systolic pressure and that systolic elevations are innocuous. This contention is not borne out by prospective epidemiological data obtained in the town of Framingham, in Massachusetts, where 5290 people have been followed for 20 years and the evolution of cardiovascular disease studied in relation to their blood pressure.[198] Also, the large collection of data in the Build and Pressure Study of the Chicago Society of Actuaries showed that at any level of diastolic pressure cardiovascular mortality increases in proportion to the associated systolic pressure.[199]

Pregnancy and Hypertension

A woman who has essential hypertension or secondary hypertension may become pregnant.

About 4 per cent of women who become pregnant have essential hypertension. Their blood pressure is raised from the beginning of the pregnancy, whereas in pre-eclampsia hypertension does not occur until about the thirtieth week (see Chapter 24). The fertility of women with essential hypertension is low and there is an increased incidence of abortion, premature birth and perinatal death. These complications have been attributed to poor decidual development as a consequence of endometrial deficiency caused by vascular disease. Premature separation of the placenta and accompanying accidental haemorrhage occur more commonly in these patients than in patients who are normotensive. In most cases the blood pressure remains stable during pregnancy; in about 8 per cent there is a rise in the last trimester.[200] Pre-eclampsia is much commoner in women with essential hypertension (see Chapter 24).

Pregnancy occurring in association with hypertension secondary to chronic glomerulonephritis or pyelonephritis often leads to deterioration of renal function and increased fetal morbidity and mortality, unless there is proper therapeutic control of the blood pressure, which may improve the outlook greatly. Pregnancy is seldom seen in the presence of secondary hypertension due to other causes. Women who have Cushing's syndrome rarely become pregnant; when they do, the pregnancy usually terminates in spontaneous abortion. Pregnancy in patients who have a phaeochromocytoma is dangerous to both mother and child.

Coarctation of the aorta may be first discovered during pregnancy.

Systolic Hypertension

Hypertension in which only the systolic pressure is raised may be due to an increase in the stroke output of the heart or to increased rigidity of the aorta and its larger branches in atherosclerosis. Conditions in which there is an increase in the stroke output of the heart include bradycardia (for instance, due to complete heart block), aortic regurgitation, arteriovenous fistula, patent ductus arteriosus, severe anaemia, Paget's disease of bone, thyrotoxicosis, fever and pregnancy.

The importance of systolic hypertension is difficult to assess. Prospective studies in the elderly have shown it to be associated with increased morbidity and mortality from cardiovascular disease, but whether this is related specifically to the systolic pressure or whether the latter is a sign of inelasticity of vessels that are prone later to develop atheroma is not clear.[201]

ESSENTIAL HYPERTENSION
(Primary Hypertension)

It has been argued by Pickering that essential hypertension is not a disease but simply represents that section of the population having an arterial pressure above an arbitrary value and without disease to which the high pressure can be attributed.[202] He suggested that arterial pressure is inherited polygenically as a graded character throughout the ranges conventionally described as normal blood pressure and hypertension.

Another view, however, is that there are two groups in the population: one in which, as a result of a single incompletely dominant gene, blood pressure rises significantly in middle age (essential hypertension) and one in which pressure rises very little with increasing age. According to this view, homozygotes develop a severe form of hypertension and heterozygotes only a moderate rise in pressure.[203]

It has long been recognized that essential hypertension tends to occur in families. Observations on identical twins with hypertension suggest that this is due to genetic rather than environmental influences: although they have lived apart for many years, similar elevations in blood pressure are generally found in both.[203] The case for inheritance of essential hypertension is supported by other evidence, but the exact mode of inheritance is not clear.[204]

Environmental factors, particularly those operating through the mind, may play a part in the genesis of high blood pressure, but none has yet been clearly identified.

Essential hypertension begins in middle life. Individuals whose blood pressure is going to rise little in the course of their life develop only a small elevation of pressure between the ages of 20 and 60 years; those who eventually become hypertensive show a considerable rise between 30 and 50 years.[205] This is in contrast to the secondary forms of hypertension, which may appear even during childhood.

Those who are obese are likelier to develop high blood pressure than those who are lean.

Essential hypertension is commoner in women than in men; its prognosis is better in women. It is common in blacks in the United States of America and in the population of the West Indies, West Africa and Papua, New Guinea.

The incidence of essential hypertension in the general population of the United States of America, as indicated by a systolic blood pressure of 160 mmHg or higher or by a diastolic pressure of 95 mmHg or higher, is about 14 per cent among white adults and about 27 per cent among black adults.[206] Less comprehensive surveys indicate that the incidence in Britain is probably comparable.

Prognosis

The experience of life insurance companies shows that in men aged 40 years and older a blood pressure of 150/100 mmHg is associated with an additional mortality of about 125 per cent. In women the corresponding increase is about 85 per cent.[207] Men with a systolic blood pressure of 178 mmHg or higher in combination with a diastolic pressure of 108 mmHg or higher have an increase in mortality rate of about 600 per cent.[208] The excess mortality associated with hypertension is chiefly due to cardiac and other circulatory diseases and to cerebral haemorrhage.

Benign Phase of Essential Hypertension

Clinical Features

The benign phase of essential hypertension is usually symptomless until the pressure becomes very high, when the patient experiences cardiac asthma, hypertensive headache or symptoms of some vascular complication. The raised blood pressure is often detected when the patient visits his doctor about some other matter. There may be changes in the fundus of the eyes; these do not include papilloedema. The urine may be normal, or proteinuria and some hyaline or granular casts may be found. Renal function tests are usually normal at first: as the disease progresses the renal plasma flow, maximum tubular excretory capacity and glomerular filtration rate become lowered.

When the amount of renin in the plasma is measured these patients fall into three groups— those whose plasma renin is low (about 25 per cent), those whose plasma renin is normal (about 60 per cent) and those whose plasma renin is high (about 15 per cent). The low renin group is of interest because it has been claimed, although not yet confirmed, that such patients have a low incidence of vascular complications, and show an unusually favourable response to diuretics. The low concentration of renin in the plasma is not associated with an increase in the amount of aldosterone.[209] The role of renin, the angiotensins and aldosterone in relation to the development of hypertension is referred to on page 186.

Most patients with benign phase essential hypertension die from congestive heart failure, myocardial infarction, cerebral haemorrhage or cerebral infarction, or intercurrent disease. About 5 per cent develop the malignant phase of essential hypertension and die from renal failure.[210] A very small number of patients aged over 60 years die from renal failure because of progressive obliteration of the vascular bed by arteriolosclerosis and atherosclerosis.[211]

Pathological Changes in the Kidneys

Gross Appearances.—Both kidneys are usually smaller than normal and equally affected. The reduction in size is moderate and it is rare for either kidney to weigh less than 100 g. The subcapsular surface is finely granular (Fig. 3.50). If there is much atherosclerosis there may also be some coarser scars, the outcome of local ischaemia. There is thinning of the cortex of those kidneys that are decreased in size. The arcuate arteries are prominent and appear thick-walled. Because of the reduction in renal mass there is an apparent increase in the amount of fat in the hilum.

If the hypertension is of short duration the kidneys may appear normal.

Light Microscopy.[212]—A variable number of glomeruli show wrinkling and thickening of the capillary basement membrane. In some, this process is accompanied by collapse and shrinkage of the tuft, loss of tuft cellularity, obliteration of the capillary lumen, and thickening of Bowman's capsule, with accumulation on its inner aspect of a material with many of the staining characteristics of collagen. Continuation of this process leads to shrinkage and sclerosis of glomeruli. These glomerular changes are focal and even in small kidneys many glomeruli are normal.

The tubules are atrophic in the depressions between the macroscopical granules. The granules are formed of hypertrophied and dilated tubules. The atrophic tubules have a thickened basement

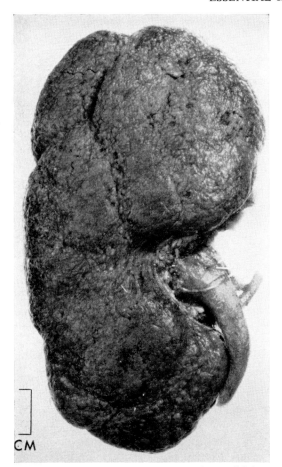

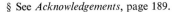

Fig. 3.50.§ Kidney in the benign phase of essential hypertension, showing the granular subcapsular surface.

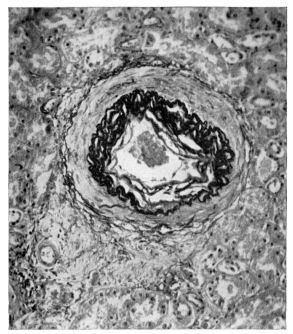

Fig. 3.51.§ Benign phase of essential hypertension. Elastosis of an interlobular artery in a kidney. The intima is thickened and contains an excess of elastic fibres. *Elastic stain.* × 140.

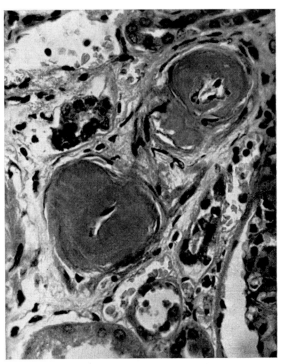

Fig. 3.52.§ Benign phase of essential hypertension. Renal arterioles showing hyaline thickening of the wall and reduction of the lumen. *Haematoxylin–eosin.* × 400.

membrane and are usually related to ischaemic glomeruli. Homogeneous eosinophile casts are sometimes seen in the tubules.

The intima of the interlobular arteries is thickened by collagenous fibrous tissue and the presence of multiple, roughly concentric, layers of elastic fibres (*elastosis*) (Fig. 3.51). The media is usually normal. The wall of some of the afferent glomerular arterioles may be thickened and largely replaced by a homogeneous material that stains palely with eosin and may contain very fine droplets of lipid. This process, which is described as *hyalinization*, characterizes the condition of *arteriolosclerosis* and occurs focally along the length of the arterioles (Fig. 3.52). It is not pathognomonic of the benign phase of hypertension: it may occur in patients with normal blood pressure; it is particularly marked in diabetes mellitus. The efferent glomerular arterioles may be involved, but not with

§ See *Acknowledgements*, page 189.

the frequency or to the degree that is observed in diabetes. The arcuate and larger arteries may show some fibrous intimal thickening, fraying and splitting of the internal elastic lamina and, sometimes, an increase in the thickness of the media.

The juxtaglomerular apparatus is usually normal in size (see Chapter 24). The granularity of its cells is normal or decreased.

There is usually some focal fibrosis in the areas of tubular atrophy. Groups of chronic inflammatory cells may also be present, particularly in relation to sclerotic glomeruli.

The pelvis of the ureter is usually normal, in contrast to the changes that affect it in cases of chronic pyelonephritis (see Chapter 24).

Electron Microscopy.—The thickened intima of those interlobular arteries that show elastosis consists of smooth muscle cells, myointimal cells and fine collagen fibrils. Thickened basement membrane and bundles of elastic fibrils separate the intimal cells. Lipofuscin is common in the smooth muscle and myointimal cells.[213]

The hyalinized arterioles contain collections of uniformly finely granular, weakly electron-dense material (hyalin) that often includes small, osmiophile droplets of fat and membrane-bound vesicles. The collections of hyalin are predominantly intimal and subendothelial; small deposits are also commonly seen between the smooth muscle cells of the media, and sometimes most of the vessel wall consists of this material.[214]

The capillary basement membrane of the ischaemic glomeruli is often thickened by 50 per cent or more. Reticulin fibres, matrix and spindle-shaped epithelial cells accumulate between Bowman's capsule and a new basement membrane that is laid down by the parietal epithelial cells.[215]

The amount of matrix between the juxtaglomerular cells is increased and their cytoplasm contains more lipofuscin.[216]

Pathological Changes in Other Organs

Heart.[217]—The heart responds to the sustained pressure overload in hypertension by gradually increasing its muscle mass (see page 42). Almost all of this increase is by hypertrophy of the existing cells, but when the heart becomes very large some hyperplasia occurs also, as is shown by a rise in the myocardial cell count.[218, 219] After many years of hypertension it is common for the heart to weigh about 500 g; the greater part of the increase is in the left ventricle. The increase in the weight of the heart and in the thickness of the wall of the left ventricle correlates well with the systolic blood pressure.[220]

Quantitative ultrastructural studies of the hypertrophied heart in cases of hypertension have shown that the enlarged muscle fibres contain many myofibrils but fewer mitochondria than would be expected from the size of the cell. This discrepancy between the energy-consuming and energy-generating organelles may account, in part, for the inefficiency of energy utilization in these enlarged hearts.[221] The increased myocardial mass at first maintains left ventricular stroke volume, but dilatation of the left ventricle and, eventually, congestive cardiac failure may occur. A factor that precipitates heart failure is progressive atherosclerosis in the coronary arteries; hypertension accelerates and intensifies the atherosclerotic state.[222] While the coronary arteries are normal the blood flow through them increases in direct proportion to the increase in left ventricular mass; when they become narrowed by atherosclerosis the oxygen requirements of the myocardium are not adequately met, myocardial contractility is reduced and the stroke volume falls.

Brain.[223]—High blood pressure is detrimental to the brain (see Chapter 34). It exerts its effect directly, by accelerating cerebral atherosclerosis and by initiating a series of pathological changes in small arteries and arterioles, or indirectly, by causing cardiac failure, which results in a lowering of cerebral performance.

The relative frequency and severity of atherosclerosis of the intracranial arteries are increased in patients with hypertension.[224] Atherosclerosis also appears in vessels of a calibre smaller than those that generally are affected among normotensive people. These changes predispose to cerebral infarction.

Hyalinization and fibrinoid necrosis ('lipohyalinosis'),[225] followed by microaneurysm formation,[226] are found in the small arteries and arterioles in the putamen, thalamus, pons, cerebellum and cerebral subcortex. An affected vessel may rupture, causing intracerebral haemorrhage, or segmental arterial occlusion may cause small infarcts that, as they resolve, leave lacunae. The severity of the damage inflicted on these vessels by sustained benign phase hypertension may be related to the fact that the small cerebral arteries have relatively thin walls and are the least muscular arteries in the body.

Hypertension probably has a contributory role

in the expansion and rupture of 'berry' aneurysms of the circle of Willis (see page 148 and Chapter 34).

Other Organs.—Hyalinization of the wall of arterioles is seen commonly in the pancreas, less frequently in the adrenals, brain and liver, and rarely in other organs. Hyaline arteriolosclerosis is common in the spleen, but this is also true of normotensive individuals (see page 134).

It is said that nodular adrenal cortical hyperplasia is present in many of those cases of the benign phase of essential hypertension in which the amount of renin in the plasma is low (see Chapter 30).[227]

The eyes show the changes of arteriosclerotic and hypertensive retinopathy (see Chapter 40).

Malignant Phase of Essential Hypertension

Clinical Features

The malignant phase of essential hypertension usually follows a period of the benign phase, the mean duration of which is about eight years.[228] A few patients appear to be in the malignant phase from the beginning of the illness. This phase usually presents between the ages of 35 and 50 years; black patients may develop malignant phase hypertension in their late twenties. Men are affected oftener than women.

The initial symptoms are commonly visual impairment, acute headache and haematuria. Occasionally, the patient presents with anuria. The diastolic blood pressure is almost always more than 130 mmHg. The main feature that distinguishes the malignant phase of essential hypertension from the benign phase is the presence of bilateral papilloedema, accompanied by retinal haemorrhages and exudates.

The urine contains protein and, usually, red cells. Renal function rapidly deteriorates during the course of the illness. There may be haemolytic anaemia with deformed red cells and a decrease in the number of platelets (haemolytic-uraemic syndrome—see Chapter 8).[229]

The level of renin and of angiotensin II in the plasma is high.[230] In contrast to the benign phase of hypertension, there is marked oversecretion of aldosterone and this is accompanied by hypokalaemia.[231] As the hypertension is not usually corrected by adrenalectomy, the occurrence of aldosteronism is considered to be a secondary phenomenon.

If untreated, about 70 per cent of patients in the malignant phase of essential hypertension die in uraemia within about a year of the onset of symptoms. The course of the malignant phase is faster in cases of essential hypertension than when it complicates secondary hypertension.[232]

Pathological Changes in the Kidneys

Gross Appearances.—The size of the kidneys varies greatly from case to case and depends upon the occurrence and duration of a pre-existing benign phase of hypertension. The subcapsular surface of those kidneys that are of normal size is smooth; that of the shrunken ones is finely granular. Petechial haemorrhages are usually present. The cut surface of the cortex is mottled red and yellow.

Light Microscopy.[233]—The most important change is *fibrinoid necrosis* of some of the arterioles (Fig. 3.53). The wall of the affected part of the vessels is replaced by eosinophile granular material that

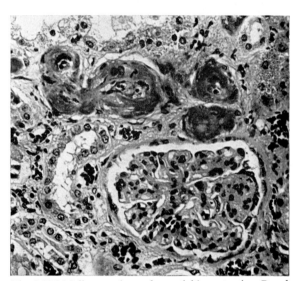

Fig. 3.53.§ Malignant phase of essential hypertension. Renal arterioles showing fibrinoid necrosis of their wall. There are a few red blood cells in the fibrinoid material. *Haematoxylin-eosin.* × 200.

gives the staining reactions of fibrin. Red blood cells are often seen in the necrotic tissue and there may be small periarteriolar haemorrhages. The arteriolar lumen is reduced or obliterated by thrombus. Occasionally, neutrophile polymorphonuclear leucocytes and mononuclear cells are present in and around the wall; the term *necrotizing arteriolitis* is frequently used to describe this change (Fig. 3.54).

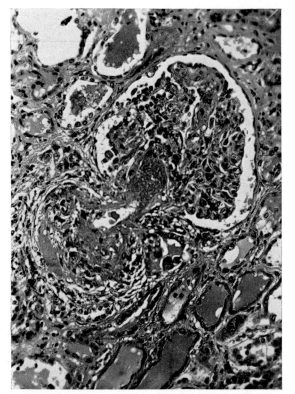

Fig. 3.54.§ Malignant phase of essential hypertension. Afferent glomerular arteriole showing fibrinoid necrosis, which extends into the glomerular tuft, with infiltration of neutrophils and mononuclear cells in and around the wall of the vessel (necrotizing arteriolitis). *Haematoxylin–eosin.* × 240.

The interlobular arteries are narrowed or obliterated by marked intimal thickening in the form of concentric layers of elongated cells and collagen. Sometimes there is relatively little collagen and the cells are embedded in a basiphile material. The amount of collagen is greatest in the kidneys of patients who have been treated with antihypertensive drugs. Lipid is sometimes present in the thickened intima. The media is thinner than normal. The term *endarteritis fibrosa* has been used to describe these obliterative changes in the interlobular arteries (Fig. 3.55). Very similar changes occur in the renal vasculature in cases of radiation nephritis, the haemolytic-uraemic syndrome of childhood, systemic sclerosis, and chronic rejection after renal transplantation (see Chapter 24). In contrast to polyarteritis, necrosis is not seen in the arcuate and larger arteries in the malignant phase of hypertension.

Up to 30 per cent of the glomeruli show segmental fibrinoid necrosis of the glomerular tuft, usually in continuity with a necrotic afferent arteriole (Fig. 3.54). There is often increased cellularity of the tuft, including the presence of neutrophils and some proliferation of the parietal epithelial cells in relation to the foci of necrosis in the glomeruli. Epithelial crescents may be present, but seldom in large numbers. Lipid and hyaline droplets are common in the visceral epithelial cells and, to a smaller extent, in the parietal epithelial cells. Glomerular necrosis is less widespread in the kidneys of patients treated with antihypertensive drugs: focal and segmental glomerular scars may be present in these cases and may represent old, healed, necrotic lesions.

In addition, there are often some sclerotic glomeruli. These are commonest in shrunken kidneys and are probably an effect of a preceding phase of benign hypertension. The size of the juxtaglomerular apparatus and the granularity of its cells are usually normal. In most cases at least half the glomeruli are normal. This fact is helpful in differentiating cases of primary malignant phase hypertension from proliferative glomerulonephritis with secondary malignant phase hypertension.

Atrophy and disappearance of groups of tubules are pronounced features of this disease. The atrophic tubules may contain homogeneous eosino-

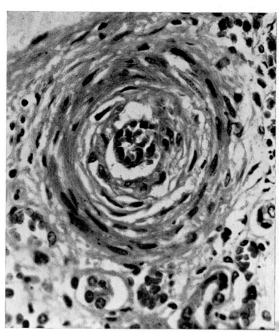

Fig. 3.55.§ Malignant phase of essential hypertension. Inter lobular artery showing 'endarteritis fibrosa'. There is ᵃ considerable reduction of the lumen. *Haematoxylin–eosin.* × 240.

phile casts and red cell casts. Occasionally there are very small cortical infarcts. Chronic inflammatory cells and some polymorphonuclear leucocytes may be scattered through the parenchyma.

These changes may be superimposed upon those of the benign phase of hypertension in patients whose acute illness was preceded by a period of slowly rising blood pressure.

Immunofluorescence.[234] — Fibrinogen is usually present in the wall of necrotic arterioles and in the necrotic foci in glomeruli. Immunoglobulins, complement and albumen are also usually present, suggesting that there has been a non-specific seepage of constituents of the plasma into the wall of the damaged vessels.

Electron Microscopy.[215]—The thickened intima in the vessels that show endarteritis fibrosa consists of a loose laminar arrangement of basement membrane, reticulin fibres, elastic fibres, smooth muscle cells and myointimal cells. The wall of arterioles affected by fibrinoid necrosis contains collections of granular, electron-dense material, red cells and red cell fragments. Many of the muscle cells of the media are necrotic. Mural or obstructive thrombi, formed of fibrin and platelets, are commonly present. In the glomeruli the focal necrotic lesions are characterized by plugging of the capillaries by platelets, fibrin and necrotic debris, and there is rupture of the capillary basement membrane, with extravasation of red cells and neutrophils into the mesangium and into Bowman's space and deposition there of fibrin.

Pathological Changes in Other Viscera

Heart.—The changes that occur in the benign phase of hypertension are present (see page 174). Their severity will depend on the duration and severity of the hypertension, particularly during the benign phase.

Brain.—In addition to the changes that accompany the benign phase of hypertension, diffuse cerebral oedema, confirmed by measurement of the water content of the brain, occasionally develops in patients in the malignant phase of hypertension who are not in cardiac failure.[235] Present evidence suggests that a sudden increase in blood pressure during the malignant phase of hypertension can break down the normal regulatory mechanisms and result in an abnormally high cerebral blood flow. This overperfusion of the brain leads to exudation of plasma through the wall of arterioles and capillaries, cerebral oedema resulting, with a marked rise in intracranial pressure and the clinical picture of acute hypertensive encephalopathy (see Chapter 34).[236]

Adrenals.—The adrenals are almost always larger than normal and show either cortical hyperplasia or cortical adenomas (see Chapter 30).[237] Fibrinoid necrosis is common in the wall of the small adrenal arteries and arterioles.

Other Organs.—Fibrinoid necrosis of the arterioles occurs, in order of descending frequency, in the pancreas, adrenals, gastrointestinal tract, brain, eyes, heart and liver. It is not found in the vessels of muscles and skin. In the intestines the arteriolar lesions may cause small foci of haemorrhagic necrosis.

The eyes show the changes of hypertensive retinopathy (see Chapter 40).

SECONDARY HYPERTENSION

High blood pressure in either the benign or the malignant phase may occur as a manifestation of a recognized disease. In such cases it is described as secondary hypertension. Most of the conditions that may lead to secondary hypertension are diseases of the kidneys or urinary tract, adrenal diseases, coarctation of the aorta, complications of pregnancy and diseases of the central nervous system. Secondary hypertension will be discussed in this sequence.

Hypertension Secondary to Diseases of the Kidneys and Urinary Tract

The renal diseases likeliest to be complicated by hypertension are glomerulonephritis, chronic pyelonephritis and polycystic disease. Hypertension is occasionally due to stenosis of a renal artery, and to the renal lesions of diabetes mellitus, systemic lupus erythematosus, systemic sclerosis, polyarteritis, the haemolytic-uraemic syndrome of childhood, amyloidosis, obstruction of the urinary tract, certain tumours (in particular juxtaglomerular cell tumours and nephroblastomas), radiation nephritis, analgesic nephropathy and pseudohyperaldosteronism. Most of these conditions are described in Chapter 24. Renal artery stenosis will be discussed here.

Stenosis of a Renal Artery

High blood pressure may result from stenosis of a main renal artery or of one of its larger branches. About 5 per cent of cases of hypertension are said to be due to this cause.

Causes of Obstruction

Atherosclerosis.[238]—In men over the age of 45 years atherosclerosis is the commonest cause of obstruction of a renal artery. Most frequently, the origin of the artery is occluded by an atheromatous plaque; less often, the lesion is elsewhere in the renal artery or in one of its segmental branches. In about 40 per cent of cases the lesion is bilateral. Atheromatous plaques seen in the renal arteries at necropsy, and narrowed arteries revealed by angiography, are not necessarily causes of functional stenosis. *Functional stenosis* can be said to be present only when there is a reduction in the volume of urine excreted by the affected kidney and in the concentration of sodium on that side: it is only in such cases of effective stenosis that high blood pressure may develop.

Fibromuscular Arterial Hyperplasia (Arterial Dysplasia).[238]—This condition occurs predominantly in young people, particularly young women. It is not confined to the renal arteries: the involvement of other vessels is sometimes a cause of obstructive symptoms.[239] The three most frequently found variants of this condition are medial fibroplasia with aneurysm formation, perimedial fibroplasia and medial hyperplasia.

Medial fibroplasia with aneurysms. This is the commonest variety. It is characterized by alternating changes that take the form respectively of stenosis (associated with increase in the amount of muscle and fibrous tissue in the media) and areas of great thinning of the vessel wall (where the internal elastic lamina is lost and bulging develops). This lesion shows on angiography as a 'sausage-string' or 'string of beads' deformity. It is commonly bilateral, usually affects the distal two-thirds of the renal artery, and may extend into the segmental arteries.

Perimedial fibroplasia. This is the second commonest variant. A dense rim of fibrous tissue replaces the outer half to two-thirds of the media of the renal artery.

Medial hyperplasia. This variant takes the form of a segmental stenosis of the renal artery due to hyperplasia of the muscle fibres in the media.

Rarer variants. These include *primary intimal fibroplasia*, in which there is marked thickening of the intima by moderately cellular, laminated tissue; *periarterial fibroplasia*, in which collagen ensheaths the adventitia; and *medial dissection*, in which a new channel forms in the outer third of the media.

Aortic Arteritis.—Arteritis of the type found in Takayashu's syndrome ('pulseless disease'—see page 142) may cause hypertension if the origin of a renal artery is involved.[240]

Other Conditions.—A congenital aneurysm of a renal artery and pressure on a renal artery by a tumour or by external fibrous or muscular bands are occasional causes of functional obstruction.

Clinical Features[241]

The only clinical ground for suspecting the presence of stenosis of a renal artery is the discovery of an epigastric bruit. Bruits of continuous or systolic-diastolic duration are heard in about half the cases. The hypertension is often severe: it averaged 210/125 mmHg in one series. Renal arteriography and comparative renal function studies will usually localize the site of stenosis and determine whether the lesion is a functional one. The level of renin and of angiotensin II in the plasma is high in a proportion of patients with stenosis of a main renal artery, particularly if the narrowing is marked. In such cases the hypertension may be in the malignant phase. These changes are accompanied by secondary aldosteronism, with an increase in the concentration of aldosterone in the plasma and a reduction in the concentration of sodium and of potassium. Measurement of the renin activity in blood from the renal veins shows that there is suppression of renin secretion by the kidney that has the intact arterial circulation and an abnormal increase in the renin content of the venous blood from the kidney on the side of the stenotic artery. Competitive inhibitors of angiotensin II can be used to identify those patients with renal artery stenosis whose hypertension is due to increased renin secretion.[242]

Pathological Changes in the Kidney with the Obstructive Arterial Lesion

Gross Appearances.—In those cases in which the obstructive lesion is confined to one artery in a kidney supplied by several arteries, or in which the lesion is in a segmental artery, the affected part of the kidney is depressed and the cortex in the affected area is reduced in width. When the single, main renal artery is affected the kidney is usually slightly and uniformly decreased in size and there is some fairly uniform reduction in cortical thickness.

Microscopical Findings.—In those kidneys in which shrinkage is visible grossly there is striking tubular atrophy, most marked in the superficial part of the cortex (Fig. 3.56). The diameter of the tubules is greatly reduced and they are lined by cubical epithelial cells. As a consequence of this atrophy the glomeruli are crowded together but structurally may appear surprisingly normal. Some show collagen formation internal to Bowman's capsule and collapse of the tuft. The interlobular and larger arteries may show some fibrous intimal thickening; the arterioles are normal. The interstitium is often fibrotic; there is no cellular infiltration. Hyperplasia of the juxtaglomerular apparatus is rarely found in such kidneys.

In other cases there is much less tubular atrophy. In these cases there is enlargement of the juxtaglomerular apparatus (Fig. 3.57), especially in the deeper, more normal parts of the cortex. The enlargement of the juxtaglomerular apparatus can be very marked, particularly when stenosis of a renal artery is associated not only with high blood pressure but also with a potassium-losing syndrome. Although the number of cells in the juxtaglomerular apparatus is increased, most of them lack granules; occasionally, in contrast, their granularity is increased.

In kidneys in which there is no tubular atrophy the hyperplasia of the cells of the juxtaglomerular apparatus is greatest in the superficial third of the cortex.[243]

When only one branch of a renal artery is stenotic the parts of the kidney that are not ischaemic may show hypertensive vascular changes that in cases of stenosis of the main artery are confined to the kidney of the opposite side (see below).

Pathological Changes in the Opposite (Non-Ischaemic) Kidney

Hypertensive vascular changes may be seen in the opposite, non-ischaemic, kidney if the stenosis of the renal artery is unilateral. Depending upon the duration of the hypertension and the gradient of

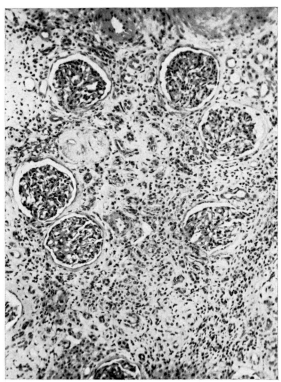

Fig. 3.56. § The artery to this kidney was stenotic: as a result, there is much atrophy of the tubules, although the glomeruli are relatively little affected. This change has been referred to as incomplete infarction. *Haematoxylin–eosin.* × 100.

blood pressure rise the changes will be those associated with either the benign or the malignant phase of hypertension (see pages 173 and 175). The juxtaglomerular bodies are normal.

Prognosis.—Atherosclerosis has a much worse prognosis than fibromuscular hyperplasia, probably because it affects older patients: even if the hypertension is relieved by operation, there is an appreciable risk of morbidity or mortality from atheromatous lesions in the vasculature elsewhere.

Treatment.[241]—Reconstructive operations, such as splenorenal arterial anastomosis in the case of stenosis of the left renal artery and a saphenous vein bypass graft from the aorta when the right renal artery is involved, cure the hypertension in over 50 per cent of young patients with fibromuscular arterial hyperplasia.

If the obstructive lesion is confined to the origin of a renal artery, autotransplantation of the affected kidney may be curative.

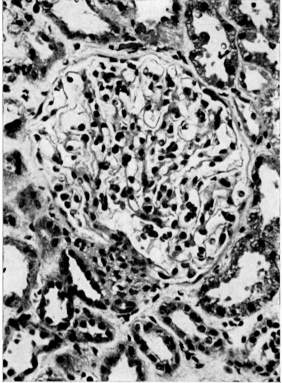

Fig. 3.57. Hyperplastic juxtaglomerular apparatus. There was stenosis of the artery to the kidney. *Haematoxylin–eosin.* × 240.

Hypertension Secondary to Diseases of the Adrenal Glands

Recognized diseases of the adrenals are responsible for less than 2 per cent of cases of hypertension.

Phaeochromocytoma[244]

The phaeochromocytoma is a neoplasm of the chromaffin cells of the adrenal medulla or, rarely, of chromaffin tissue elsewhere in the body (see Chapter 30). In a high proportion of cases the tumour cells elaborate both adrenaline and nor-adrenaline, which are liberated into the blood in abnormal amounts. The release of these substances is commonly episodic, resulting in paroxysmal attacks of headache, sweating, palpitation, pallor and hypertension. Paroxysms occur spontaneously; they may also be provoked by exercise, local pressure on the tumour or eating citrus fruits (which contain synephrine, an aromatic amine that releases noradrenaline). Not all patients suffer attacks of this type: in some cases there is sustained hypertension. Many patients whose hypertension is associated with a phaeochromocytoma become normotensive if the tumour is removed; in others there is either no fall in the blood pressure or hypertension recurs.

The kidneys usually show some degree of arteriolar hyalinization and arterial intimal thickening, sometimes with glomerular sclerosis. It is rare to find fibrinoid necrosis of the arterioles or endarteritis fibrosa, both indicative of the malignant phase of hypertension (see page 175).

Primary Aldosteronism (Primary Hyperaldosteronism; Conn's Syndrome[245])

Primary aldosteronism is a useful designation for a rare group of primary or apparently primary diseases of the adrenals that are characterized by the secretion of an excess of the mineralocorticoid aldosterone (see Chapter 30). This causes increased retention of sodium in the distal portion of the renal tubules. The total volume of body water, including the volume of extracellular fluid and of plasma, is expanded, causing hypertension of mild or moderate severity and suppression of renin release.[246] Potassium is exchanged, and lost in the urine, resulting in hypokalaemia and a metabolic acidosis. The kidneys usually show some arteriolar hyalinization, fibrous intimal thickening of the arteries and a few sclerotic glomeruli. Vacuolation of the epithelial cells of the proximal convoluted tubules has also been described.

Primary aldosteronism is associated with three types of adrenal lesion.

Adrenal cortical adenoma. This is the usual cause of primary aldosteronism. A benign, usually solitary, adenoma of the adrenal cortex secretes an excess of aldosterone. Removal of the tumour is followed in about 70 per cent of cases by the eventual return of the blood pressure to normal levels. The fall in blood pressure may not begin for several months after operation.[247]

Nodular hyperplasia of the adrenal cortex. This accounts for about a quarter of all cases of primary aldosteronism. A discrete adenoma is not found; instead, the cortex of one or both adrenal glands shows micronodular hyperplasia or hypertrophy of the zona glomerulosa. The biochemical abnormalities are generally less severe than in cases of aldosterone-secreting adenoma. Surgical removal of sufficient adrenal tissue to correct the oversecretion of aldosterone usually controls the condition.

Aldosterone-secreting carcinoma. Aldosterone secreting carcinomas are particularly rare. They may arise in the adrenal cortex or, exceptionally, in the ovary.

Congenital Adrenal Hyperplasia[244]

In this very rare condition of infants an enzymatic defect in the synthesis of cortisol leads to compensatory hyperplasia of the adrenal cortex and incidental secretion of large amounts of mineralocorticoid hormones that cause hypertension. Two forms of defect have been recognized: 11-hydroxylase and 17-hydroxylase deficiencies.

11-Hydroxylase Deficiency.—This blocks both the formation of cortisol from its precursor, 11-deoxycortisol, and the conversion of deoxycorticosterone to corticosterone. The decrease in cortisol synthesis activates the release of corticotrophin, which stimulates the secretion of adrenal androgens, causing virilization (see Chapter 30). The output of aldosterone is reduced. The excess of deoxycorticosterone induces hypertension and hypokalaemia.

17-Hydroxylase Deficiency.—This blocks the synthesis of cortisol and of adrenal androgens and oestrogens. Aldosterone secretion is reduced. There is no virilization: instead, in affected girls there is failure of secondary sexual development at puberty, with hypogonadism and amenorrhoea, and in boys the genitals are ambiguous. Hypocortisolaemia results in overproduction of corticotrophin by the pituitary: this stimulates adrenal synthesis of deoxycorticosterone, which causes hypertension and hypokalaemia.

Pseudohyperaldosteronism (Liddle's Disease).—Pseudohyperaldosteronism is an inherited disorder of sodium transport in which the kidneys conserve sodium excessively; it is characterized by hypertension associated with a reduction in the output of aldosterone (see Chapter 24). It should not be confused with congenital adrenal hyperplasia or other syndromes associated with corticosteroid overproduction (see Chapter 30).

Cushing's Syndrome

Cushing's syndrome results from overproduction of glucocorticoids as an accompaniment either of adrenal cortical hyperplasia or of an adrenal cortical tumour (see Chapter 30).

Hypertension occurs in about 85 per cent of patients with the syndrome, and may be severe.[248] The rise in blood pressure is probably caused by the increase in the level of circulating cortisol, which commonly is present in an amount that ranges from twice to four times the normal figure. The excess of cortisol leads to retention of salt and expansion of the volume of extracellular fluid, and consequently to a sustained rise in the blood pressure. In some cases the presence of other adrenal steroids, such as deoxycorticosterone and corticosterone B, may play an important part in raising the blood pressure. There is no increase in the output of aldosterone in cases of Cushing's syndrome. The level of renin in the plasma is usually normal. If the arterial hypertension has been present for a long time, it may persist despite removal of the source of excess cortisol and recovery from other manifestations of the syndrome.[249]

The renal changes are those seen in the benign phase or in the malignant phase of essential hypertension (see pages 173 and 175), depending on the severity of the rise in pressure accompanying the hormonal disturbance.

Oversecretion of 18-Hydroxydeoxycorticosterone[250]

Increased secretion of 18-hydroxydeoxycorticosterone has been found in certain cases of hypertension in which there is suppression of plasma renin and normal or diminished secretion of aldosterone. The condition is rare.

Coarctation of the Aorta

In this congenital abnormality the aorta is greatly narrowed or completely occluded, usually near the site of the ductus arteriosus (see page 110). In the 'adult' form of coarctation the blood pressure is high in the parts of the body (head and arms) that receive their arterial supply from the aorta proximal to the stenosis; it is normal, subnormal or, at most, slightly raised in those parts supplied from the aorta distal to the stenosis. Plasma renin levels are within normal limits.[251] The kidneys show no characteristic pathological changes.

Surgical correction of the coarctation results in a substantial reduction in the arterial blood pressure but usually leaves it above the norm for the patient's age. In some cases resection of the coarctation has been followed by fibrinoid necrosis of the small arteries and arterioles distal to the block (see page 111).

Hypertensive Complications of Pregnancy

Pre-Eclamptic Toxaemia

In this condition secondary hypertension develops at about the 30th to the 36th week of pregnancy. There is usually a dramatic recovery within a short

G

time of the delivery of the child although in a few cases the blood pressure remains elevated (see Chapter 24).

In about 30 per cent of women who have had pre-eclampsia the blood pressure rises some years later. It is still not clear whether this is the result of the pre-eclamptic toxaemia[252] or whether pre-eclampsia no more than hastens the onset of essential hypertension in women who otherwise would acquire it at a later date.[253]

Irreversible Post-Partum Renal Failure

This disease is sometimes accompanied by severe hypertension. The fact that hypertension is not invariably present suggests that it is the consequence of the renal lesions rather than their cause (see Chapter 24).

Hypertension Complicating Diseases of the Central Nervous System

The systemic arterial blood pressure rises in cases of increased intracranial pressure. This is presumably a compensatory response to the increasing resistance to the flow of blood through the brain.

Thrombosis of the basilar artery may lead to sudden development of arterial hypertension:[254] it is debatable whether this is compensatory or due to direct disturbance of centres rendered relatively ischaemic by the circulatory disturbance resulting from the thrombosis. There is little evidence, however, that primary organic changes in the central nervous system produce persistent high blood pressure.[255]

ARTERIAL AND ARTERIOLAR CHANGES IN HYPERTENSION

Although the changes in the arteries and arterioles in hypertension have been noted in the accounts of the vasculature of the kidneys and other organs on pages 172 and 175, it is appropriate to summarize their main features here. The changes fall into two categories—those that do not occur in normotensive people but are initiated by the raised blood pressure, and those that occur in normotensive people but are aggravated by hypertension. Both groups of lesions are sometimes included under the term 'hypertensive arteriosclerosis' (see page 122).

Arterial and Arteriolar Changes Initiated by Hypertension

The changes that are initiated by hypertension are of the same general nature whether the hypertension is primary (essential hypertension) or secondary. Their severity varies greatly in relation to the rate of development of the rise in blood pressure.

Changes in the Benign Phase of Hypertension

Large and Medium-Sized Muscular Arteries.—Large and medium-sized muscular arteries throughout the body may show hypertrophy of the smooth muscle of the media (*medial hypertrophy*). The degree of medial hypertrophy runs parallel with the degree of hypertrophy of the left ventricle of the heart.[255a] Medial hypertrophy is not found in the arteries of normal people; its cause is raised blood pressure, and the evidence suggests that it is a work hypertrophy.

Small Arteries.—In small arteries, medial hypertrophy is often inconspicuous or absent, and the predominant change is elastosis (see below).

Arterioles.—Hypertrophy of the media of arterioles has not been shown. The ratio of the thickness of the wall of arterioles to the diameter of their lumen is increased although the cross-sectional area of the wall is not enlarged. The diameter of the arteriolar lumen is consistently smaller in hypertensive patients than in others. A possible explanation of this decrease in diameter is that there is a persistent shortening of their circular muscle as a consequence of their prolonged constriction.[255b]

Changes in the Malignant Phase of Hypertension

Small Arteries.—The small arteries in cases of the malignant phase of hypertension show concentric 'onion skin' thickening of the intima by smooth muscle cells and fibroblasts (Fig. 3.55). This process is often marked, and it may obliterate the lumen. Lipid-containing cells are sometimes present, and there may be basiphilia of the intima. The terms *endarteritis fibrosa*, 'productive endarteritis' and 'hyperplastic arteriolosclerosis' are used to describe this change. It is commonest and most developed in the interlobular arteries of the kidneys. It occasionally affects small arteries elsewhere: in the small branches of the coronary arteries it is sometimes accompanied by the development of glomus-like or plexiform lesions, identical to those that occur in the pulmonary vasculature in association with severe pulmonary hypertension (see page 282).[255c]

Arterioles.—There may be focal replacement of the wall of arterioles by deeply eosinophile, granular material, the process known as *fibrinoid necrosis* (Fig. 3.53). When polymorphonuclear leucocytes and mononuclear cells are also present the term 'necrotizing arteriolitis' is frequently applied to the condition (Fig. 3.54). Fibrinoid necrosis occurs in the wall of the arterioles of the kidneys, pancreas, adrenals, gastrointestinal tract, brain, eyes, heart and liver, but very rarely elsewhere.

Pathogenesis.—The rapidly rising blood pressure of the malignant phase of hypertension damages the endothelium of the arterioles and small arteries.[255d] This allows blood cells and plasma to leak into the vessel wall, with consequent precipitation there of fibrin and the formation in the lumen of thrombi. The presence of angiotensin and renin, which are known to circulate in excess in cases of malignant hypertension, may also play a part in increasing the permeability of the wall of the vessels.[255e] At one time it was thought that fibrinoid necrosis of arterioles was caused by persistent arteriolar spasm, and the consequent occurrence of foci of ischaemic damage in the vessel wall. Intense focal spasm, associated with segmental dilatation, certainly occurs in the smaller arteries and in the arterioles of patients with hypertension in the malignant phase, but it is now known that fibrinoid necrosis occurs only in the dilated segments and not in the constricted ones.[255e]

Endarteritis fibrosa is probably the result of organization of mural thrombi that form in consequence of endothelial damage.[255f]

Arterial and Arteriolar Changes Aggravated by Hypertension

Large and Medium-Sized Arteries.—In cases of long-standing hypertension, which usually are cases of hypertension in the benign phase, there is acceleration and intensification of the changes that occur with increasing frequency in the large and medium-sized arteries throughout the body as age advances sometimes referred to as 'senile arteriosclerosis'—page 121). Atherosclerosis also tends to be particularly severe in the vessels of this range of size in patients with prolonged hypertension: experimental evidence shows that elevation of the blood pressure aggravates this condition.

Small Arteries.—The small arteries often show an increase in the amount of elastic and fibrous tissue in the intima. Several concentric rings of elastic fibres may be seen adjacent to the internal elastic lamina (Fig. 3.51). The terms *elastosis* and 'reduplication of the internal elastic lamina' are used to describe this process. Elastosis affects the vessels in many organs but occurs most frequently and severely in the interlobular arteries of the kidneys. Although it is commoner and more marked in patients who have been subject to prolonged benign phase hypertension, it also occurs with increasing frequency as age advances in people whose blood pressure is normal.

Arterioles.—The arterioles may show thickening of the wall by a layer of palely eosinophile, structureless ('hyaline') material, often situated immediately beneath the endothelium and sometimes more peripherally (Fig. 3.52). This material may contain finely dispersed lipid. The process, which is patchy in distribution, can cause narrowing and even obliteration of the lumen. It is referred to as *arteriolar hyalinization*, 'arteriolar hyalinosis', 'fatty hyaline intimal thickening' and 'hyaline arteriolosclerosis'. Hyalinization is most commonly seen in the wall of splenic arterioles; it is also common in renal arterioles. The arterioles of the pancreas, adrenals, brain, liver and eyes may also be affected; those elsewhere are seldom involved.[255g]

Pathogenesis.—The pathogenesis of elastosis and of arteriolar hyalinization is unknown. Both conditions seem to be ageing processes that are accentuated by hypertension.

EXPERIMENTAL HYPERTENSION

A confusingly large number of experimental procedures will produce hypertension in animals. Only some of the more significant are considered here.

Infusion of Pressor Substances Normally Present in the Body

Infusion of Renin

It is possible to produce a sustained hypertension if rabbit renin is infused intravenously into rabbits over a period of as long as 18 days. The severest hypertension that can be produced in the rabbit by infusing renin is well below that produced by renal artery constriction (see below).[256]

Renin is a proteolytic enzyme formed by the granular cells of the juxtaglomerular apparatus in the kidneys (see Chapter 24). It splits a decapeptide, angiotensin I, from a glycoprotein of the alpha$_2$-globulin fraction of plasma. Its release is mainly controlled by two mechanisms—a receptor in the afferent arteriole that responds to changes in tension in the wall, and a sodium-sensitive receptor in the macula densa.[257]

Infusion of Angiotensin

Intravenous infusion of rabbit angiotensin into rabbits produces a sustained hypertension that remains constant with dose for up to a hundred days.[258]

Angiotensin consists of two fractions. The decapeptide, angiotensin I, is converted into an octapeptide, angiotensin II, by an enzyme in plasma. Both fractions have pressor activity, but angiotensin II is much the more active and is believed to be the important fraction in the circulation, under normal conditions. Indeed, it is the most powerful vasopressor known. It raises arterial pressure by its vasoconstrictive action on the small systemic arteries and arterioles. It is broken down into inactive peptides and amino acids by a group of enzymes collectively called angiotensinases.

Infusion of Adrenaline and Noradrenaline

Noradrenaline is a very potent vasoconstrictor substance. Its infusion at low dosage into animals has been shown to produce a substantial elevation of pressure for as long as seven weeks.[259]

Overdosage with Salt and Adrenal Cortical Hormones

Salt

The presence of an excess of salt in the diet produces substantial hypertension in rats. Some strains are particularly susceptible.[260] Neither adrenalectomy nor nephrectomy relieves the hypertension that is produced in this way. A high intake of salt does not cause hypertension in rabbits or dogs.

Deoxycorticosterone Acetate[261]

Sustained hypertension is regularly produced by the administration of deoxycorticosterone acetate (DOCA) to rats that have been maintained on a diet with a high salt content or that have had one kidney removed. Deoxycorticosterone acetate is much less effective as a cause of hypertension in dogs and rabbits.

In rats made hypertensive by these means the size and granularity of the juxtaglomerular bodies are reduced.

Interference with the Kidneys

Renal Artery Constriction

Constriction of one or both renal arteries by a small adjustable silver clamp produces hypertension.[262]

Constriction of One Renal Artery, the Other Kidney Being Intact.—In most animals this operation produces a small rise of arterial pressure that lasts a few weeks only. The rat, however, responds with prolonged, severe hypertension.[263] Man appears to behave like the rat in that stenosis of one renal artery may produce sustained hypertension (see page 178).

In the rat, the cells of the juxtaglomerular bodies of the ischaemic kidney increase in number and become larger and more granular. The enlargement is pronounced in the week following renal artery constriction and then subsides.[264] The amount of renin that can be extracted from the clamped kidney increases,[265] and the concentration of renin in the venous blood from that kidney rises.[266] Reabsorption of sodium by the proximal tubules increases in the ischaemic kidney. As a result, sodium and water may be retained initially; however, as the opposite, intact kidney excretes the excess sodium, the salt and water balance returns to normal. The tubules in the ischaemic kidney gradually atrophy, but the arterioles and arteries remain normal. Dependent upon the level of blood pressure attained, the changes of the benign phase or of the malignant phase of hypertension eventually appear in the vasculature of the intact kidney. The output of aldosterone by the adrenals increases[267] and the concentration of potassium in the plasma falls.

The hypertension can usually be abolished by excising the ischaemic kidney,[268] or by injection of antibodies against angiotensin II,[269] or by giving the animal a pentapeptide that inhibits the conversion of angiotensin I to angiotensin II.[270] Removal of the ischaemic kidney may fail to reduce the blood pressure if there is much vascular disease in the other kidney.[268]

Induction of hypertension by this procedure is not prevented by prior active immunization against angiotensin II, even though antibodies are produced that are capable of neutralizing the pressor effects of large quantities of infused angiotensin II or renin.[271] These findings seem to show that circulating angiotensin is not essential for the initiation of hypertension following constriction of one renal artery when the contralateral kidney is intact, but that it may have a role in the maintenance of hypertension.

Constriction of One Renal Artery after Excision of the Other Kidney.—This operation produces a greater rise of pressure than the procedure described above and hypertension tends to persist.[272] Sometimes, after some months, the pressure starts to fall: in these cases it may be restored to its high level by severing collateral vessels that have grown into the kidney from the pericapsular tissues.

The renin content of the ischaemic kidney falls[273] and the juxtaglomerular bodies decrease in size and granularity.[274] However, the output of renin by the kidney is normal. The output of aldosterone by the adrenals and the concentration of potassium and sodium in the plasma are also normal.

The high blood pressure is not reduced by injection of antibodies against angiotensin II,[269] or by administering a pentapeptide that inhibits the conversion of angiotensin I to angiotensin II.[270] It is abolished only by removing the constricting clamp.[275] If the animal has been hypertensive for months or years, removal of the clamp may not be followed by return of the blood pressure to normal levels.[268]

In the rabbit, active immunization with angiotensin II inhibits the pressor effects of infused renin and angiotensin II but will neither prevent the onset of hypertension after renal artery constriction and contralateral nephrectomy nor modify its course or severity.[276, 277] Such results make it difficult to sustain the possibility that circulating angiotensin or renin have a pathogenetic role in this form of hypertension.

Compression of the Kidneys

One of the most effective ways of producing hypertension is by inducing an inflammatory reaction round a kidney by wrapping it in cellophane, silk or latex.[278] Whether this acts by compression of the kidney or of its pedicle is disputed. The hypertension that results behaves in all ways like that due to renal artery constriction.

X-Irradiation of the Kidneys

X-irradiation of the kidneys produces hypertension.[279] When the irradiation is confined to one kidney, excision of that kidney soon after the arterial pressure has begun to rise reverses the effect; later nephrectomy does not do so.

Removal of Both Kidneys

The excision of both kidneys produces hypertension in animals after a latent period of a few days.[280] However, if sodium balance and hydration are carefully controlled the blood pressure does not rise.[281] Experience of bilateral nephrectomy in man confirms this.[282]

Constriction of the Aorta

Partial occlusion of the abdominal aorta above the level of the origin of the renal arteries produces hypertension.[283] A constriction of the thoracic part of the aorta may not have this effect because the collateral vessels effectively maintain the circulation. Partial occlusion of the aorta below the origin of the renal arteries has no effect.

Section of the Nerves of the Carotid Sinus and of the Depressor Nerves

In the rabbit, hypertension is caused by section of the carotid sinus nerves on both sides, followed 14 days later by section of the depressor nerves.[284] The arterial pressure is very unstable in animals that have been submitted to this procedure: it reaches very high levels during excitement or when the animal is under anaesthesia, and is then accompanied by tachycardia; it is normal during sleep and when the animal is quiet. In these respects it differs from most cases of high blood pressure in man.

Interference with the Brain

Intracisternal Injection of Kaolin.—Injection of kaolin into the cisterna magna of dogs leads to a rise in blood pressure that is sustained for many months.[285]

Cerebral Ischaemia.—Successive ligature of the carotid, vertebral and anterior spinal arteries is said to produce hypertension.[286]

Selective Breeding

Selective breeding has produced strains of rats and rabbits that develop spontaneous hypertension.[287, 288] The level of renin activity in the blood from the renal vein of these rats is normal or subnormal, even when the blood pressure is rising.[289] The granularity of the cells of the juxtaglomerular bodies is less than normal. Genetically hypertensive rats aged three months or less show no histological abnormality in the kidneys: this indicates that the hypertension does not stem from intrarenal vascular disease.[290]

PATHOGENESIS OF HYPERTENSION IN MAN

Hypertension Secondary to Renal Diseases

Two, or possibly three, processes appear to be involved in the pathogenesis of hypertension as a complication of renal disease.[291]

Overproduction of Renin

Renin may be released in excess from a diseased kidney, with a resultant rise in the level of renin and angiotensin II in the plasma, which causes widespread vasoconstriction, including profound effects in the splanchnic and renal vessels. Angiotensin II stimulates secretion of aldosterone, which causes a reduction in the excretion of sodium by the kidneys. The secondary hyperaldosteronism also accentuates the hypertension by leading to expansion of the volume of plasma and of extracellular fluid.[292] Release of renin is wholly responsible for the hypertension that accompanies the very rare juxtaglomerular cell tumour (see Chapter 24); it is probably responsible in part for the hypertension that accompanies acute proliferative glomerulonephritis (see Chapter 24) and for the hypertension that occurs in some cases of terminal renal failure. The hypertension that accompanies advanced renal failure can usually be controlled by withholding sodium and water; in a small proportion of cases, in which the level of renin in the plasma is high, restriction of sodium and water intake is ineffective and the hypertension is relieved only by nephrectomy. In these cases the output of renin from the failing kidneys appears to be inappropriate to the state of sodium and water balance.[293]

Sodium Retention

Retention of sodium by the kidneys leads to an expansion of the volume of plasma and of extracellular fluid, causing hypertension. The production of renin and angiotensin II is depressed, perhaps through the activity of a sodium-sensitive mechanism in the macula densa of the juxtaglomerular apparatus: this mechanism responds to a fall in the concentration of sodium in the tubular fluid by inhibiting the release of renin by the granular cells.[294] In experiments on animals this process operates in the period shortly after constriction of the artery to the remaining kidney, following unilateral nephrectomy. The same mechanism probably operates in some cases of chronic renal failure in man. Retention of sodium and water is at least partly responsible for the hypertension that follows bilateral nephrectomy in animals[295] and, sometimes, in man.[296]

Deficiency of Blood-Pressure-Lowering Substances

It is possible that a reduction or absence of certain blood-pressure-lowering substances that are found in the normal renal medulla may be partly responsible for the hypertension that occurs after experimental bilateral nephrectomy and, sometimes, in cases of renal diseases that greatly reduce the amount of functioning renal parenchyma.[297] Some of these substances are prostaglandins; they may be produced by the interstitial cells of the medulla.[298]

Hypertension Secondary to Adrenal Disorders

Primary Aldosteronism

In primary aldosteronism (see Chapter 30) the uncontrolled release of aldosterone from the adrenals induces retention of sodium by the kidneys, which causes expansion of the volume of the plasma and of the extracellular fluid, and consequent hypertension. The output of renin and, therefore, the production of angiotensin II are depressed and these substances have no apparent role in producing or maintaining the hypertension.[299]

Extracts of liquorice contain glycyrrhizinic acid, a substance with an aldosterone-like action, and the drug carbenoxolone contains a derivative of glycyrrhizinic acid that shares this action: both these substances are sometimes used in the treatment of peptic ulcer and may produce hypertension in consequence of the retention of sodium that they cause.[300]

Cushing's Syndrome

The hypertension of other conditions characterized by overproduction of corticosteroids, including Cushing's syndrome, is probably of a similar nature, although in some cases mechanisms other than those of sodium homoeostasis may be involved.

Phaeochromocytoma

In cases of phaeochromocytoma the release of adrenaline and noradrenaline produces a rise in blood pressure by their action on the peripheral vessels and renal vasculature. The constriction of the renal vasculature prevents sodium diuresis.

Persistence of Hypertension after Removal of the Primary Cause

When the primary cause of hypertension— a phaeochromocytoma, an aldosterone-secreting tumour, or a kidney with a stenotic renal artery— has been removed, the blood pressure does not always fall to normal. Occasionally, this is because of coincidental existence of essential hypertension; in most cases, however, the likely explanation is that renal damage, caused by the hypertension, maintains the blood pressure at unduly high levels after removal of the primary cause.

Benign Phase of Essential Hypertension

Very little is known about the mechanisms operating in essential hypertension. In the benign phase the level of renin in the plasma is within the normal range, or is lower than normal, and therefore it is unlikely that the raised blood pressure is due to exaggeration of the peripheral effects of the renin-angiotensin system.

It has been tentatively suggested[301, 302] that essential hypertension may be initiated by the autonomic response to emotional stress in certain genetically susceptible individuals.[303] This response, mediated by the sympathetic nervous system, causes severe vasoconstriction in the kidneys and transient hypertension. The vasoconstriction is most marked in the efferent arterioles and results in transient sodium retention, with consequent expansion of the volume of plasma and of extracellular fluid. The expansion of the fluid volume leads to an increase in cardiac filling pressure and cardiac output and causes an inappropriately high rate of tissue perfusion. This stimulates an autoregulatory vasoconstrictive response in the peripheral and renal vasculature that results in a further elevation of blood pressure. At this early ('labile') stage the blood pressure can be restored to normal by drugs—such as reserpine—that deplete the sympathetic nerve endings of noradrenaline. The second stage of benign hypertension is brought about by irreversible narrowing of renal vessels, which results in a permanent rise in the renal pressure threshold for sodium excretion. The blood pressure then becomes stabilized at a higher level. Increased peripheral vasoconstriction proceeds, while cardiac output and the volume of extracellular fluid return to near normal.

Malignant Phase of Essential Hypertension

A severe and steep rise in intravascular pressure is thought to cause physical damage to the walls of the afferent arterioles.[304] Injury to the endothelium and muscle enables plasma proteins and red cells to seep into the wall and stimulates the formation of platelet and fibrin thrombus over the damaged area. The intravascular fibrin strands may cause fragmentation of red cells and produce a 'microangiopathic haemolytic anaemia' (see Chapters 8 and 24). Organization of mural fibrin deposits is the probable cause of the intimal thickening that is referred to as endarteritis fibrosa (see page 176). Fibrinoid necrosis of the wall of afferent arterioles stimulates the juxtaglomerular apparatus, with consequent release of renin. The amount of renin in the peripheral blood rises and the resulting increase in the concentration of angiotensin II directly contributes to the hypertension. In some patients with malignant phase hypertension the level of angiotensin II in the plasma is disproportionately high in relation to the total amount of exchangeable sodium: this abnormality could well be largely responsible for the hypertension.[293]

REFERENCES (CHAPTER 3B)

INTRODUCTION

198. Kannell, W. B., Castelli, W. P., McNamara, P. M., McKee, A., Feinleib, M., *New Engl. J. Med.*, 1972, **287**, 781.

199. Gubner, R. S., *Amer. J. Cardiol.*, 1962, **9**, 773.

200. Morris, W. I. C., in *Symposium on Non-Toxaemic Hypertension in Pregnancy*, edited by N. F. Morris and J. C. McC. Browne, page 44. Boston, 1958.

201. Colamdrea, M. A., Friedman, G. D., Nichaman, M. Z., Lynd, C. N., *Circulation*, 1970, **41**, 239.

ESSENTIAL HYPERTENSION

202. Pickering, G. W., *High Blood Pressure*, 2nd edn. London, 1968.
203. Platt, R., *Lancet*, 1963, **1**, 899.
204. Thomas, C. B., Onesti, G., Kim, K. E., Moyer, J. H., *High Blood Pressure*. New York, 1973.
205. Cruz-Coke, R., *Lancet*, 1959, **2**, 853.
206. *National Health Survey: Hypertension and Hypertensive Heart Disease in Adults, U.S. 1960–62.* Washington, D.C., 1966.
207. Society of Actuaries, *Build and Pressure Study*, vols 1 and 2. Chicago, 1959.
208. Bolt, W., Bell, M. F., Harnes, J. F., *Trans. Ass. Life Insur. med. Dir. Amer.*, 1957, **41**, 61.
209. Brunner, H. R., Laragh, J. H., Baer, L., Newton, M. A., Goodwin, F. T., Krakoff, L. R., Bard, R. H., Buhler, F. R., *New Engl. J. Med.*, 1972, **286**, 441.
210. Perera, G. A., *J. chron. Dis.*, 1955, **1**, 33.
211. Freis, E. D., *J. Amer. med. Ass.*, 1970, **213**, 1143
212. Heptinstall, R. H., *Brit. Heart J.*, 1954, **16**, 133.
213. Jones, D. B., *Lab. Invest.*, 1970, **22**, 502.
214. Biava, C. G., Dyrda, I., Gencot, J., Bencosme, S. A., *Amer. J. Path.*, 1964, **44**, 349.
215. Jones, D. B., *Lab. Invest.*, 1974, **31**, 303.
216. Biava, C., West, M., *Amer. J. Path.*, 1965, **47**, 287.
217. Cohn, J. N., Limas, F. J., Guiha, N. H., *Arch. intern. Med.*, 1974, **133**, 969.
218. Sasaki, R., Lehikawa, S., *Jap. Heart J.*, 1971, **12**, 325.
219. Astorri, E., Chizzola, A., Visiol, O., *J. molec. cell. Cardiol.*, 1971, **2**, 99.
220. Kannel, W. B., Castelli, W. P., McNamara, P. M., McKee, A., Feinleib, M., *New Engl. J. Med.*, 1972, **287**, 781.
221. Straver, E. B., Tauchert, M., *Klin. Wschr.*, 1973, **51**, 322.
222. Heptinstall, R. H., Porter, K. A., *Brit. J. exp. Path.*, 1957, **38**, 55.
223. Sandok, B. A., Whisnant, J. P., *Arch. intern. Med.*, 1974, **133**, 947.
224. Baker, A. B., Resch, J. A., Loewenson, R. B., *Circulation*, 1969, **39**, 701.
225. Rothemund, E., Frische, M., *Arch. Psychiat. Nervenkr.*, 1973, **217**, 195.
226. Ross Russell, R. W., *Brain*, 1963, **86**, 425.
227. Gunnells, J. G., McGuffin, W. L., Robinson, R. R., Grim, C. E., Wells, S., Silver, D., Glenn, J. F., *Ann. intern. Med.*, 1970, **73**, 901.
228. Milliez, P., Tcherdakoff, P., Samarcq, P., Ray, L. P., in *Essential Hypertension: An International Symposium*, edited by K. D. Bock and P. T. Cottier, page 214. Berlin, 1960.
229. Linton, A. L., Gavras, H., Gleadle, R. I., Hutchinson, H. E., Lawson, D. H., Lever, A. F., Macadam, R. F., McNicol, G. P., Robertson, J. I. S., *Lancet*, 1969, **1**, 1277.
230. Hollenberg, H. K., Epstein, M., Basch, R. I., Couch, N. P., Hickler, R. B., Merrill, J. P., *Amer. J. Med.*, 1969, **47**, 855.
231. Laragh, J. H., Ulick, S., Januszewicz, V., Kelly, W. G., Lieberman, S., *Ann. intern. Med.*, 1960, **53**, 259.
232. Kincaid-Smith, P., McMichael, J., Murphy, E. A., *Quart. J. Med.*, 1958, N.S. **27**, 117.
233. Heptinstall, R. H., *J. Path. Bact.*, 1953, **65**, 423.
234. Paronetto, F., *Amer. J. Path.*, 1965, **46**, 901.
235. Adachi, M., Rosenblum, W. I., Feigin, I., *J. Neurol. Neurosurg. Psychiat.*, 1966, **29**, 451.

236. Skinhoj, E., Strandgaard, S., *Lancet*, 1973, **1**, 461.
237. Russell, R. P., Masi, A. T., Richter, E. D., *Medicine (Baltimore)*, 1972, **51**, 211.

SECONDARY HYPERTENSION

238. Harrison, E. G., McCormack, L. J., *Mayo Clin. Proc.*, 1971, **46**, 161.
239. Claiborne, T. S., *Amer. J. Med.*, 1970, **49**, 103.
240. Danaraj, T. J., Wong, H. O., Thomas, M. A., *Brit. Heart J.*, 1963, **25**, 153.
241. Hunt, J. C., Strong, C. G., *Amer. J. Cardiol.*, 1973, **32**, 562.
242. Brenner, H. R., Laragh, J. H., Gavras, H., Keenan, R., *Lancet*, 1973, **2**, 1045.
243. Parker, R. A., *Nephron*, 1967, **4**, 315.
244. Kaplan, N. N., *Arch. intern. Med.*, 1974, **133**, 1001.
245. Conn, J. W., *J. Lab. clin. Med.*, 1955, **45**, 6.
246. Conn, J. W., Cohen, E. L., Rovner, D. R., *J. Amer. med. Ass.*, 1964, **190**, 213.
247. Conn, J. W., *J. Amer. med. Ass.*, 1963, **183**, 871.
248. Ross, E. J., Marshall-Jones, P., Friedman, M., *Quart. J. Med.*, 1966, N.S. **35**, 149.
249. O'Neal, L. W., Kissane, J. M., Hartroft, P. M., *Arch. Surg.*, 1970, **100**, 498.
250. Melby, J. C., Dale, S. L., Wilson, T. E., *Circulat. Res.*, 1971, **28**, suppl. 2, 143.
251. Brown, J. J., Davies, D. L., Lever, A. F., Robertson, J. I. S., *Brit. med. J.*, 1965, **2**, 1215.
252. Epstein, F. H., *New Engl. J. Med.*, 1964, **271**, 391.
253. Browne, F. J., Sheumack, D. R., *J. Obstet. Gynaec. Brit. Emp.*, 1956, **63**, 677.
254. Montgomery, B. M., *Arch. intern. Med.*, 1961, **108**, 559.
255. Tyler, H. R., Dawson, D., *Ann. intern. Med.*, 1961, **55**, 681.

ARTERIAL AND ARTERIOLAR CHANGES IN HYPERTENSION

255a. Barrett, A. M., *J. Path. Bact.*, 1963, **86**, 9.
255b. Short, D., *Brit. Heart J.*, 1966, **28**, 184.
255c. Salyer, W. R., Hutchins, G. M., *Arch. Path.*, 1974, **97**, 104.
255d. Byrom, F. B., *The Hypertensive Vascular Crisis: An Experimental Study*. London, 1969.
255e. Giese, J., *Amer. J. Med.*, 1973, **55**, 315.
255f. Kincaid-Smith, P., *Lancet*, 1969, **2**, 266.
255g. Dustin, P., *Int. Rev. exp. Path.*, 1962, **1**, 73.

EXPERIMENTAL HYPERTENSION

256. Blacket, R. B., Pickering, G. W., Wilson, G. M., *Clin. Sci.*, 1950, **9**, 247.
257. Davis, J. O., *Amer. J. Med.*, 1973, **55**, 333.
258. Brown, J. J., Chapuis, G., Robertson, J. I. S., *Clin. Sci.*, 1964, **26**, 165.
259. Dickinson, C. J., De Swiet, M., *Lancet*, 1967, **1**, 986.
260. Dahl, L. K., Heine, M., Tassinari, L., *J. exp. Med.*, 1962, **115**, 1173.
261. Sturtevant, F. M., *Ann. intern. Med.*, 1958, **49**, 1281.
262. Goldblatt, H., Lynch, J., Hanzal, R. F., Summerville, W. W., *J. exp. Med.*, 1934, **59**, 347.
263. Wilson, C., Byrom, F. B., *Lancet*, 1939, **1**, 136.
264. Tobian, L., Thompson, J., Twedt, R., Janecek, J., *J. clin. Invest.*, 1958, **37**, 660.
265. Tobian, L., Janecek, J., Tombulian, A., *Proc. Soc. exp. Biol. (N.Y.)*, 1959, **100**, 94.

266. Koletsky, S., Rivera-Velez, J. M., Marsh, D. G., Pritchard, W. H., *Proc. Soc. exp. Biol. (N.Y.)*, 1967, **125**, 96.

267. Singer, B., Losito, C., Salmon, S., *Acta endocr. (Kbh.)*, 1963, **44**, 505.

268. Wilson, C., Byrom, F. B., *Quart. J. Med.*, 1941, N.S. **10**, 65.

269. Brunner, H. R., Kirshman, J. D., Sealey, J. E., Laragh, J. H., *Science*, 1971, **174**, 1344.

270. Krieger, E. M., Salgado, H. C., Assan, C. J., Greene, L. L. J., Ferreira, S. H., *Lancet*, 1971, **1**, 269.

271. Eide, I., *Circulat. Res.*, 1972, **30**, 149.

272. Pickering, G. W., Prinzmetal, M., *Clin. Sci.*, 1938, **3**, 357.

273. Regoli, D., Brunner, H., Peters, G., Gross, F., *Proc. Soc. exp. Biol. (N.Y.)*, 1962, **109**, 142.

274. Heptinstall, R. H., *Lab. Invest.*, 1965, **14**, 2150.

275. Goldblatt, H., *Ann. intern. Med.*, 1937, **11**, 69.

276. Eide, I., Aars, H., *Nature (Lond.)*, 1969, **222**, 571.

277. Louis, W. J., MacDonald, G. J., Renzini, V., Boyd, G. W., Peart, W. S., *Lancet*, 1970, **1**, 333.

278. Page, I. H., *J. Amer. med. Ass.*, 1939, **113**, 2046.

279. Wilson, C., Ledingham, J. M., Cohen, M., *Lancet*, 1958, **1**, 9.

280. Grollman, A., Muirhead, E. E., Vanatta, J., *Amer. J. Physiol.*, 1949, **157**, 21.

281. Leonards, J. R., Heisler, C. R., *Amer. J. Physiol.*, 1951, **167**, 553.

282. Merrill, J. P., Giordano, C., Hertderks, D. R., *Amer. J. Med.*, 1961, **31**, 931.

283. Goldblatt, H., Kahn, J. R., *J. Amer. med. Ass.*, 1938, **110**, 686.

284. Koch, E., Mies, H., Nordmann, M., *Z. Kreisl.-Forsch.*, 1927, **19**, 585.

285. Hamperl, H., Heller, H., *Naunyn-Schmiedeberg's Arch. exp. Path. Pharmak.*, 1934, **174**, 517.

286. Taylor, R. D., Page, I. H., *Circulation*, 1951, **3**, 551.

287. Okamoto, K., Aoki, K., *Jap. Circulat. J. (En.)*, 1963, **27**, 282.

288. Alexander, N., Hinshaw, L. B., Drury, D. R., *Proc. Soc. exp. Biol. (N.Y.)*, 1954, **86**, 855.

289. Koletsky, S., Shook, P., Rivera-Velez, J. M., *Proc. Soc. exp. Biol. (N.Y.)*, 1970, **134**, 1187.

290. Smirk, F. H., Phelan, E. L., *J. Path. Bact.*, 1965, **89**, 57.

PATHOGENESIS OF HYPERTENSION IN MAN

291. Ledingham, J. M., *J. roy. Coll. Phycns Lond.*, 1971, **5**, 103.

292. Bianchi, G., Brown, J. J., Lever, A. F., Robertson, J. I. S., Roth, N., *Clin. Sci.*, 1968, **34**, 303.

293. Schalekamp, M. A., Beevers, D. G., Briggs, J. D., Brown, J. J., Davies, D. L., Fraser, R., Lebel, M., Lever, A. F., Medina, A., Morton, J. J., Robertson, J. I. S., Tree, M., *Amer. J. Med.*, 1973, **55**, 379.

294. Nash, F. D., Rostorfer, H. H., Bailie, M. D., Wathen, R. L., Schneider, E. G., *Circulat. Res.*, 1968, **22**, 473.

295. Ledingham, J. M., Pelling, D., *J. Physiol. (Lond.)*, 1970, **210**, 233.

296. Coleman, T. G., Bower, J. D., Langford, H. G., Guyton, A. C., *Circulation*, 1970, **42**, 509.

297. Muirhead, E. E., Brown, G. B., Germain, G. S., Leach, B. E., *J. Lab. clin. Med.*, 1970, **76**, 641.

298. Muirhead, E. E., Germain, G. S., Leach, B. E., Brooks, B., Pitcock, J. A., Stephenson, P., Brosius, W. L., Hinman, J. W., Daniels, E. G., *Clin. Res.*, 1972, **20**, 69.

299. Biglieri, E. G., Forsham, P. H., *Amer. J. Med.*, 1961, **30**, 564.

300. Borst, J. G. G., Borst-de-Geus, A., *Lancet*, 1963, **1**, 677.

301. Ledingham, J. M., *Practitioner*, 1971, **207**, 5.

302. Brown, J. J., Lever, A. F., Robertson, J. I. S., Schalekamp, M. A., *Lancet*, 1974, **2**, 320.

303. Brod, J., Fencl, V., Hejl, Z., Jirka, J., *Clin. Sci.*, 1959, **18**, 269.

304. Byrom, F. B., *The Hypertensive Vascular Crisis: An Experimental Study*. London, 1969.

ACKNOWLEDGEMENTS FOR ILLUSTRATIONS (CHAPTER 3B)

Figs 3.50–52, 54–56. Reproduced by permission of Professor R. H. Heptinstall, The Johns Hopkins University School of Medicine, Baltimore, Maryland, United States of America, from his chapter, 'The Kidneys', in: *Systemic Pathology*, 1st edn, edited by G. Payling Wright and W. St C. Symmers, chap. 24, pages 709–768. London, 1966.

Fig. 3.53. Reproduced by permission of Sir Theo Crawford, St George's Hospital Medical School, London, from his chapter, 'Arteries, Veins and Lymphatics', in: *Systemic Pathology*, 1st edn, edited by G. Payling Wright and W. St C. Symmers, chap. 3, pages 91–140. London, 1966.

4: *The Nose and Nasal Sinuses*

by I. Friedmann *and* D. A. Osborn

CONTENTS

4: *The Nose and Nasal Sinuses*

by I. FRIEDMANN *and* D. A. OSBORN

The nose and sinuses form a complex system of airways and cavities. The anterior half to two-thirds of the vestibular part of the lateral wall of the nose (the inner aspect of the ala) is lined by an extension of the epidermis: this is provided with sebaceous and sweat glands and carries a number of short hairs (the vibrissae, which may offer some protection against the access of foreign bodies, particularly the larger of these, such as insects). The posterior part of the vestibule is lined by non-keratinized, stratified squamous epithelium: this merges a little farther back with the respiratory tract type of epithelium that lines the rest of the nose except for the olfactory area (see below). The nasal columella—the movable structure that separates the nostrils—is covered with skin, which merges through a narrow, non-keratinized zone of stratified squamous epithelium into the respiratory tract epithelium of the septum.

The Respiratory Passages of the Nose

The mucosa of the respiratory passages of the nose is sometimes known as the Schneiderian membrane. Its surface is pseudostratified, columnar, ciliate epithelium, which rests on a basement membrane. The latter is often unusually thick and may include mature collagen and elastic fibres in addition to reticulin. Varying numbers of goblet cells are scattered among the ciliate cells. The Golgi apparatus of the goblet cells participates in the production of a secretion formed mainly of mucopolysaccharide or mucoprotein: this is stored as granules, which are eventually discharged. The secretory sequence is partly controlled by lysosomal hydrolytic enzymes.[1] It has been suggested that the ciliate epithelial cells may be transformed into goblet cells:[1] this has not been supported by studies of the effects of osmium tetroxide vapour on the structurally similar tracheal epithelium of rats.[2]

Under inflammatory or toxic influences, the ciliate cells may undergo profound changes, although the cilia themselves may be retained under even quite extreme conditions (see below).

Ultrastructure and Function of Cilia.[3]—Electron microscopy shows the cilium to have nine peripheral microtubules or filaments surrounding a central pair of microtubules—the basic $9+2$ pattern of the axoneme.[4] Where the axoneme reaches the cell body the two central microtubules end in a plate (the basal body). The extracellular part of the cilium is thus anchored within the cell through its continuity with the basal body, which is intracellular. A rootlet extends from the basal body deep into the cell and is composed of longitudinally arranged fibres that interdigitate with transverse striations. Blind processes—the basal feet—have been mistaken under the light microscope for connecting strands. A structure known as the alar sheet is attached to the basal body and gradually unfolds from its point of origin.[5] These various accessory structures—rootlet, basal feet and alar sheet—anchor the basal body and through it the cilium itself. The rootlets and alar sheets probably assist in maintaining the vertical position of the basal body; its lateral position is influenced by the basal feet.

Cilia are mobile organelles that, when stimulated, beat in one direction and so induce a unidirectional movement of the secretion that bathes them and of particles such as dust suspended within it. Laminate or striate structures in the neighbourhood of the basal body and rootlets are linked with these and probably with one another: their organization suggests that they have a contractile function, and it is possible that they are responsible for ciliary movement. Mucus is a necessary intermediary in the transport system and must be present if the cilia are to function properly.[6] The failure of the ciliary system in such conditions as chronic bronchitis, sinusitis, asthma, mucoviscidosis and secretory otitis media represents an inability of the mucosa to meet the transport demands under pathological conditions.[6]

Inflammation of the mucosa of the upper respiratory tract may result in loss of its cilia. Epithelium that is destroyed may be replaced through proliferation and differentiation of surviving basal cells that abut on the basement membrane. Ciliogenesis is an important feature of the regenerating epithelium: the formation of new cilia is associated with intense activity of the surviving or replicated basal bodies. Giant and otherwise atypical cilia are variations that are probably attributable to precocious regeneration. Such atypical cilia are usually multiple, two or more forming a complex enveloped by the bulging outer membrane of the cell. They are commoner in inflamed or otherwise diseased mucosae. It seems likely that they would impede the regular rhythmic action of the mucociliary apparatus.

The Nasal Lamina Propria and Vascular System.— The lamina propria of the mucosa of the respiratory passages of the nose is a vascular tissue that blends with the periosteum and perichondrium of the nasal skeleton. It contains a considerable amount of elastic tissue as well as abundant collagen. It encloses the nasal mucous and seromucous glands.

The vascular system of the nose is supplied by arteries that enter the mucosa through the bony walls of the nasal cavities and terminate in dense capillary networks in the lamina propria. The capillaries drain into veins that form part of a system of plexuses in the deeper parts of the mucosa. The walls of the veins forming the plexuses contain smooth muscle that is arranged in a spiral manner round their lumen. The outlets from the plexuses are surrounded by muscular sphincters that lie close to the bone. Studies of the development of the nasal vasculature in many species have shown it to be very complex.[7] Three strata of vessels develop and are connected by venous, arterial and arteriovenous anastomosis. After birth, the deepest stratum ordinarily atrophies, leaving the more superficial strata, which gradually lose their identity as distinguishable layers. The vein-like arteries of the superficial strata have been regarded as arterial anastomoses. The plexuses are best developed in the mucoperiosteum of the middle and inferior conchae, and particularly the posterior part of the latter and the choanal region generally; they are also to be found in the mucosa of the septum, particularly posteriorly, and in the nasopharynx and nasal sinuses, but in these situa-

tions they are not developed to the same extent. They form an erectile tissue that can rapidly become so engorged with blood that it may partly or completely obliterate the nasal cavities.

The musculature of this tissue is controlled by the autonomic nervous system, and it also reacts to various pharmacologically active agents, including some hormones. Its function is probably to bring about rapid changes in the local blood flow, with consequent variation in the temperature of the inspired air. Disturbances in hormonal balance may account for the rhinitis and sinusitis that sometimes occur at the menopause, and the hormonal changes accompanying pregnancy are probably the cause of the swelling of the nasal mucosa that is occasionally observed then. It is relevant that some women are troubled by swelling of the nasal mucosa during the premenstrual phase of the menstrual cycle, and the accompanying engorgement and tendency to epistaxis are the cause of at least some instances of the so-called 'vicarious nasal menstruation'. The erectile parts of the nasal lining may become swollen in some individuals, of either sex, during sexual excitement.[8] The swelling may be accompanied by excessive secretion of watery mucus, and a comparable state may develop during emotional disturbances: the nasal obstruction that accompanies crying is a familiar example, the effects of the mucosal engorgement being then aggravated by the drainage of tears through the lacrimal ducts. It is clear that these responses must be mediated through the autonomic nerves. It has been suggested that the association between the nasal mucosa and sexual stimulation is a vestigial reflection of the role of the sense of smell in the mating activity of animals.

The *nasal sinuses* are lined by a mucoperiosteum that differs only slightly from that of the nasal cavities themselves. The epithelium is of the same type, but thinner, and with fewer goblet cells. The lamina propria is thin and there are relatively few glands.

It may be noted that both the nasal mucosa and that of the sinuses often contain scattered lymphocytes, plasma cells and macrophages; sometimes, even when apparently healthy, an occasional neutrophil or eosinophil may be present. Lymphoid follicles may be found in the mucosa towards the choanae, where the nasal cavities merge into the nasopharynx.

The structure of the nose is admirably adapted for the protection of the lower and more vulnerable parts of the respiratory tract.[9, 10] The arrangement of the septum and the conchae ensures that the current of inhaled air is directed against the mucous membrane, with the result that most of the finer particles, among them bacteria, become trapped in the surface mucus and later removed by ciliary action. Not only does the nose serve as an effective filter but it also warms and moistens the inhaled air, so that even with great variations in the temperature and humidity of the external atmosphere, the inspired air is nearly saturated with water vapour and raised to body heat before it passes the larynx. When this warming and humidification fail, as may happen in some forms of rhinitis, ciliary action and mucus secretion in the trachea and bronchi are adversely affected and a most effective means of protecting the lungs against infection is correspondingly handicapped.

The Olfactory Area of the Nose

The mucosa of the olfactory area has a highly specialized microscopical structure, in keeping with its function as the end-organ of one of the special senses. It includes not more than the upper one-third of the mucosa of the septum, in the region opposite to the superior concha, the corresponding part of the very narrow roof of the nasal cavity, and the mucosa above and on the upper and medial aspects of the superior concha itself. The cell bodies of the afferent olfactory neurons are situated immediately deep to the single layer of columnar sustentacular cells that form the surface of the olfactory mucosa: the terminal processes of the sensory cells project on the surface between the sustentacular cells and end in expanded structures surmounted by cilia and microvilli. It may be noted that the olfactory organ is the only part of the body in which the cell bodies of neurons are at the surface, directly in contact with the external environment: this accounts for the frequency with which the sense of smell may be permanently impaired or destroyed by inflammatory diseases of the nasal lining. The olfactory mucosa contains the tubulo-acinar glands of Bowman, which are peculiar to this region: they lie deep to the basement membrane and their ducts traverse this and the olfactory epithelium to reach the surface. It is their function to bathe the surface with the thin fluid in which odoriferous substances are thought to become dissolved before their presence can effectively stimulate the processes of the sensory cells. The demonstration of Bowman's glands in what in other respects is simple respiratory mucosa in non-olfactory areas of the roof of the nose may be regarded as evidence that the areas concerned were part of the olfactory mucosa and have lost their sensory function as a result of local disease.

Pigmentation of the olfactory mucosa is referred to on page 222.

MALFORMATIONS

Malformations of the external nose range from slight deformity to bizarre anomalies.[11] They are less frequent than congenital anomalies of the external ear. Least rare are involvement of the nose in defects of closure of the facial clefts (cleft lip), atresia of the anterior naris on one or both sides, and stenosis ('collapse') of the anterior parts of the nasal passages. The bridge of the nose is characteristically widened ('saddle nose') in association with hypertelorism (abnormally wide separation of the eyes), which may occur with or without other defects as a genetically determined condition: some of these cases are instances of what has been called the 'first arch' syndrome, which is sometimes attributed to premature involution of the artery of the first branchial arch.[12]

Internal malformations of the nose include involvement in cleft palate and unilateral or bilateral choanal stenosis or atresia.

Congenital malformations must be distinguished from deformities caused by acquired disease, including trauma, specific infections—particularly tuberculosis, leprosy and syphilis—and other destructive conditions, especially neoplasms, involving the nose or nasal sinuses.

INFLAMMATORY CONDITIONS

Rhinitis and Sinusitis

Acute Rhinitis

By far the commonest form of acute inflammation of the nasal passages is the common cold (see below), which is primarily a viral infection, familiar to everybody from personal experience. Acute rhinitis may also occur as a prodromal or symptomatic manifestation of the acute infectious fevers, particularly measles, and it may be the result of specific bacterial infections, such as diphtheria (see opposite) and, exceptionally, gonococcal infection. In some cases, acute rhinitis is caused by exposure to irritant chemical substances or is due to working in a dusty environment. Acute allergic rhinitis is a common clinical problem, particularly as a symptom of hay fever (see page 201).

In any of these conditions the disease may be confined to the nasal cavities or it may also involve the nasal sinuses. Acute rhinitis, especially when due to infection, is very likely to be accompanied by acute nasopharyngitis as a natural consequence of the continuity of the nasal passages and naso-pharynx: it must be stressed that the conventional distinction between these parts of the upper respira-tory tract is a purely arbitrary, topographical one, with no functional basis.

The Common Cold

The common cold (acute coryza) is caused by a virus,[13-15] the viral infection usually being followed within two or three days by secondary bacterial infection. The bacteria usually involved include organisms that are ordinarily part of the nasal and pharyngeal flora, such as *Streptococcus pneumoniae*, *Staphylococcus aureus* and *Streptococcus pyogenes*, and, possibly, *Neisseria catarrhalis*, *Klebsiella pneumoniae* and *Haemophilus influenzae*. Immunity to the common cold is very transient, perhaps partly because of the occurrence of numerous immunologically distinct strains of the virus. The virus has been isolated in tissue cultures and can be grown on the chorioallantoic membrane of eggs, and the infection can be transmitted to human volunteers, although not to any animals. No means of immunization has been discovered, and there is no specific treatment. Although the disease usually runs a short course, it is the cause of a serious annual loss of productivity wherever it occurs, for it is very infectious, and in most urban communities in temperate climates it is endemic throughout much of the year, and particularly frequent in the cold, damp periods. Exposure to wet and cold predispose to the infection, and local disease—such as deflection of the nasal septum sufficient to cause partial obstruction of one airway, or the presence of adenoids—is also a predisposing factor.

Except in very young or weakly babies, whose feeding and sleeping are interfered with by the nasal obstruction, an uncomplicated common cold is a minor malady as far as the individual patient's health is concerned. The potential severity of the disease is, in fact, wholly determined by the effects of the secondary bacterial invaders, and these effects, in their turn, are largely determined by the potential pathogenicity of the bacteria themselves. In the average case the bacterial infection has no effect other than to convert the abundant, serous nasal discharge that characterizes the first two or three days of the viral infection into a scantier, mucopurulent or, sometimes, purulent discharge that is occasionally flecked with blood: this stage lasts only a further two or three days, recovery then following rapidly. If, however, the sinuses become involved during the stage of bacterial rhinitis the resulting infection may linger for many weeks, and may pass into a chronic phase.

In some cases, especially in debilitated people, or at the extremes of age, the bacterial phase of the common cold leads to tracheobronchitis and bronchopneumonia.

Histopathology of Acute Rhinitis.—The mucosal blood vessels are engorged, and the mucosa in general is oedematous and rather sparsely infiltrated by neutrophils. There is considerable overactivity of the mucous and seromucous glands. With the development of the bacterial phase the number of neutrophils in the inflammatory exudate increases quickly, and these cells migrate through the surface epithelium in considerable numbers. There may be considerable loss of the ciliated cells of the surface epithelium, but this necrobiotic process is super-ficial, and the cells regenerate rapidly once the infection subsides.

Nasal Diphtheria

Diphtheria of the nose, in common with other forms of diphtheria, has become a rare disease in most parts of the world. It seems always to have occurred mainly in childhood. The characteristic diphtheritic membrane forms mainly on the middle and inferior conchae or on the septum. In the great majority of cases the strain of *Corynebacterium diphtheriae* is of the mitis type. The patients are highly infective.

Toxaemia is strikingly uncommon in cases of nasal diphtheria, and the usual presenting manifestation is unilateral or bilateral nasal obstruction, some-times with epistaxis, and often of several weeks' duration. The infection clears up without sequelae in almost all cases, although some patients become chronic nasal carriers of the organisms.

The suggestion that the ozaena type of chronic atrophic rhinitis may be the outcome of infection by a non-toxigenic strain of *Corynebacterium diphtheriae* is mentioned on page 196.

Chronic Non-Specific Rhinitis
Chronic Hypertrophic Rhinitis*

Repeated attacks of acute rhinitis may be followed by chronic hypertrophic rhinitis.* It is possible that

* The term 'chronic hypertrophic rhinitis' has sometimes been misapplied to cases of the transitional type of papilloma of the nasal cavity (see page 218).

unhealthy conditions of work, such as dusty or damp surroundings, or frequent exposure to nasal irritants, are predisposing factors.

Marked displacement of the septum, chronic sinusitis and adenoids are often accompanied by hypertrophic rhinitis.

Histopathology.—The condition is characterized by hyperplasia of the mucosal glands and thickening of the mucous membrane, much of which is due to the persistent engorgement of the vascular plexuses. The engorgement is to some extent explained by rigid fibrous thickening of the walls of the vessels, with replacement of muscle fibres by collagen. The thickening is further increased by the considerable infiltration of the lamina propria by lymphocytes, often with the development of many well-formed lymphoid follicles with conspicuous germinal centres. Plasma cells and macrophages also collect, but are less numerous. There is considerable thickening, and often hyalinization, of the basement membrane, and there may be a general increase in the fibrous tissue throughout the mucosa.

Chronic Atrophic Rhinitis

Clinically, two varieties of chronic atrophic rhinitis are generally distinguished—*simple atrophic rhinitis* and *ozaena* (atrophic rhinitis associated with fetor). In addition, a special clinical variety, *rhinitis sicca*, is sometimes described: rhinitis sicca has been regarded as an occupational disease of those who work in a hot, dry, dusty atmosphere—for example, in smelting works, steel mills, foundries, vulcanizing shops, glass-working shops, bakeries and stokeholds.

Ozaena.—The characteristic fetor of ozaena comes from the presence of dry crusts formed from viscid secretion: these crusts collect in the meatuses under the conchae, and elsewhere in the nasal cavities, causing considerable obstruction of the airways. The patient is usually quite unable to detect the smell, and in fact the condition is almost always associated with complete anosmia. The disease is much commoner in women than in men, and it often begins at about the time of puberty. It was formerly seen most frequently among the poor, often in association with undernourishment and anaemia, and there seems to be no doubt that its incidence has fallen appreciably with the general rise in the standard of living. It remains predominantly a disease of town-dwellers, and particularly of indoor workers.

The causes of ozaena are obscure. The sex incidence suggests that there may be a hormonal factor: in this context it may be significant that both the intensity of the smell and the amount of crusting may be markedly increased during menstruation. However, most authorities consider ozaena to be the result of infection. There are two main theories of infection—that the disease is the end-result of various non-specific forms of infective rhinitis, and that it is a specific infection. In the past, ozaena was sometimes attributed to tuberculosis or syphilis, but in the few cases in which healing of these infections was followed by atrophic rhinitis, fetor was not a feature, unless due to persistent foci of necrosis and ulceration. In some cases of ozaena, however, there is good evidence that the atrophic state is the outcome of inadequately treated chronic suppurative rhinitis, of the type that may be a sequel to the acute rhinitis of measles or scarlet fever, or that may accompany chronic suppurative sinusitis.

It may be that the causation of ozaena is most nearly explained by combining these two views: rhinitis as a sequel to another disease may predispose to secondary infection of the diseased mucosa by an organism that leads to the establishment of this peculiar form of atrophy. Certain anomalies of the vessels in the nasal mucosa may also contribute to its pathogenesis.[16]

Bacteriology of Ozaena.—Many different types of bacteria have been isolated from cases of ozaena and supposedly identified as its immediate cause. They include organisms of three main types—klebsiellae, corynebacteria, and an ill-defined group of coccobacilli of which the so-called *Coccobacillus fetidus* of Perez is the only one that has some claim to consideration. The klebsiellae include particularly *Klebsiella ozaenae*, the classic ozaena bacillus of Loewenberg and Abel, which can be isolated from between 70 and 100 per cent of cases of the disease: it is noteworthy that *Klebsiella ozaenae* has only exceptionally been isolated in the absence of atrophic rhinitis. This organism is a serologically distinct species—serotype 4(D)—of the capsulate Gram-negative bacilli. Other klebsiellae, including *Klebsiella pneumoniae* (Friedländer's bacillus), have been isolated from the nose in cases of ozaena.

More recently, corynebacteria have been described by a number of bacteriologists as possible causes of ozaena: these include a non-toxigenic organism, *Corynebacterium belfantii*, which has been isolated in a high proportion of cases when selective culture media have been used. It is believed that *Corynebacterium belfantii* is, in fact, a non-toxigenic form of the mitis type of *Corynebacterium diphtheriae*:[17] it can be converted *in vitro* into a toxigenic and lysogenic form by phage *beta*. It is known that toxigenic strains of *Corynebacterium diphtheriae* can be transformed to a non-toxigenic, non-lysogenic state by cultivation in broth containing anti-phage-*beta* antiserum, and it has been assumed that this might occur *in vivo* as a result of the natural production of antiphage antibodies in cases of infection by these organisms. Henriksen and Gundersen suggested, therefore, that ozaena is a late result of nasal diphtheria.[17] They suggested that diphtheria might cause irreparable damage to the nasal mucosa, leading to atrophy, a reduction in the blood supply, and lessened resistance to infection: these conditions would favour persistence of the diphtheria bacilli, which in the course of time could become transformed into non-toxigenic variants, the continuing infection ultimately manifesting itself as ozaena.[18, 19]

Histopathology of Ozaena.—There is marked atrophy of the mucous membrane throughout the nose and also of the bone of the conchae: when the characteristic, dry, greenish, sickeningly fetid crusts are removed, the nasal cavities and the sub-conchal meatuses appear strikingly roomier than in the normal nose. Microscopical examination shows changes that are sometimes considerably less remarkable than the clinical impression of severe atrophy leads one to expect. Usually, however, the surface epithelium is thinner than normal, with replacement of the ciliate columnar cells by simple columnar or cuboidal cells, and there is a marked reduction in the proportion of goblet cells, or they may have disappeared completely. In many cases there is some squamous metaplasia, and this may be very widespread; keratinization does not occur, or, at most, is of very limited extent. The basement membrane may be thickened and hyaline, or it may be normal. The mucosal glands are atrophic, and the lamina propria is often very thin and fibrous.

Acute and Chronic Sinusitis

Acute Sinusitis

Acute inflammation of the nasal sinuses is almost always the result of extension of infection from the nose itself. The common cold, influenza and the acute infectious fevers are the usual precipitating causes. Occasionally, acute sinusitis is the direct consequence of the entry of fluid into the nose, for instance while bathing or diving, or in injudicious attempts at nasal medication, particularly by lavage: in such cases the presence of an excess of fluid in a sinus may encourage bacterial growth, especially if the opening of the sinus does not allow its ready escape. Occasionally, infection may spread directly into the maxillary sinus (antrum of Highmore) from the roots of the teeth, especially the first and second molars. Again, infection may pass from one sinus to another as a result of the gravitation of infected secretion. Anomalies of the position and size of the openings between the sinuses and the nasal cavities may also predispose to infection, mainly by hindering free drainage.

Most cases of acute sinusitis are due to infection by Gram-positive cocci—*Streptococcus pyogenes*, *Streptococcus pneumoniae* and sometimes *Staphylococcus aureus*. Rarer causes are *Klebsiella pneumoniae*, *Haemophilus influenzae* and *Escherichia coli*. In cases arising as a complication of dental sepsis, such organisms as *Treponema vincentii* and its companion, *Fusobacterium fusiforme*, may be present, contributing a characteristic fetor to the purulent exudate filling the maxillary sinus. It may be noted that anaerobic organisms may be associated with these infections, particularly maxillary sinusitis, taking the place of the aerobic pathogens as the local conditions alter during the progress of the inflammatory changes. It ought to be mentioned that in about one-quarter of our cases no organisms could be isolated.

Chronic Sinusitis

Chronic sinusitis follows the acute disease, except in a small proportion of cases in which it possibly develops as a consequence of some other pathological process, including structural anomalies.

Histopathology of Acute and Chronic Sinusitis.[20]—The earliest change in the mucous membrane in a case of acute sinusitis is intense hyperaemia, accompanied by moderate oedema, a slight infiltration by neutrophile leucocytes, and active secretion by the goblet cells and mucosal glands. Complete resolution is possible if the inflammatory reaction does not progress beyond this stage. In severer cases there is an increasingly heavy accumulation of neutrophils, with the formation of seropurulent or mucopurulent exudate on the surface of the mucosa: at this stage there may be some erosion of the epithelial lining, although recovery may still be accompanied by a virtually complete return to normal.

The outcome of an attack of acute sinusitis

depends on the virulence of the infecting organisms and, particularly, on the adequacy of drainage through the natural openings. If inflammatory oedema leads to persistent blockage of the ostium, the exudate accumulates within the sinus and, if the infection is a pyogenic one, an acute empyema results, with extensive destruction of the mucosal epithelium. If drainage is established at this stage the inflammatory changes will usually subside, but in a proportion of cases chronic suppurative sinusitis results, or even a chronic closed empyema.

As the acute stages of sinusitis subside the neutrophils in the exudate are replaced by a variably heavy accumulation of lymphocytes, often with a conspicuous admixture of plasma cells. Histiocytes and, in some cases, eosinophils may also be present. Fibroblastic proliferation leads to fibrosis, and there is eventually much mucosal atrophy, although the ciliated epithelium is often well preserved. There may be widespread squamous metaplasia of the epithelium.

Complications of Sinusitis

In some cases of acute sinusitis the infection extends into the bony wall of the sinus, causing *acute suppurative osteitis*. This may lead, for instance, to an acute, spreading osteomyelitis of the maxilla, but more usually the destruction of bone is followed by spread of the infection directly into the adjacent tissues, with the formation of a *subcutaneous abscess* or the development of *orbital cellulitis* or of *intracranial suppuration*. The intracranial complications include suppurative leptomeningitis, extradural or intracerebral abscesses, and septic thrombosis of the cavernous venous sinus. In other cases, these complications may develop without destruction of the bony wall of the sinus, presumably as a result of lymphatic spread or, possibly, of septic thrombosis of the blood vessels of the sinus mucosa.

Infection of any of the nasal sinuses may be complicated by orbital cellulitis and abscess formation, for all of them abut on the orbit. Infection of the orbit may, in its turn, be the immediate source of infection of the intracranial structures, but by far the commonest source of the intracranial complications is frontal sinusitis, with direct extension of the infection from the sinus into the meninges and brain. Cavernous sinus thrombosis, however, is almost always the result of sphenoidal sinusitis.

Any of the complications mentioned above may occur either in the course of acute sinusitis or as a result of chronic sinusitis. There are some other complications of chronic sinusitis that deserve to be noted. In some cases of chronic sinusitis there is a well-marked *polypoid hypertrophy of the mucosa*, which may become very considerably thickened: much of the thickening may be due to oedema, the accompanying cellular accumulation being largely confined to the zone immediately underlying the epithelium. This type of mucosal change may be the origin of some *nasal polyps*, particularly those that arise in the maxillary sinus (antronasal polyps) or in the ethmoidal air cells. A *mucocele* results when the mucus secretion of the lining of a sinus accumulates as a consequence of obstruction of its ostium. It is found most frequently in the anterior ethmoidal air cells or in the frontal sinuses, and, exceptionally, in the posterior ethmoidal air cells or the sphenoidal sinus: it also occurs in the maxillary sinus. The accumulation of mucus eventually leads to pressure atrophy of the bone round the sinus, and in the case of anterior ethmoidal and frontal mucoceles this gives rise to a painless swelling that may displace the contents of the orbit. Mucoceles develop very slowly. If they become infected they are transformed into abscesses (the so-called *pyoceles*): the consequences are then likely to be very grave.

Chronic fibrosing osteitis is the sequel of low-grade inflammatory changes in the interlamellar spaces of the bone forming the wall of chronically infected sinuses. It is commonly observed in the chips of bone removed during operations on the sinuses, but has little or no practical significance. There may also be marked new bone formation, amounting even to the development of cancellous osteomatoid masses that are sometimes misinterpreted as osteomas.

Nasal Polyps

Nasal polyps are essentially rounded projections of oedematous mucous membrane. They may develop in association with chronic hypertrophic rhinitis, chronic sinusitis and allergic diseases of the nose. They are common lesions. In our material, 75 per cent of the specimens are from patients of 40 to 70 years of age, and men outnumber women by three to one.

Polyps may be unilateral or, usually, bilateral. They arise most commonly in the ethmoidal region and particularly from the mucosa of the semilunar hiatus and of the middle concha: the ethmoidal air cells themselves may be filled by sessile polyps whereas the polyps that arise from the surface mucosa are likely to become pedunculate. As they enlarge they come to fill the nasal cavity, which may become appreciably dilated, with the result that the external nose itself is broadened and enlarged in a characteristic fashion.

As seen clinically, polyps are smooth, shiny, movable swellings, usually bluish-grey in colour, although occasionally traversed superficially by sparse, fine, ramifying blood vessels. Exceptionally, they are more vascular, appearing pink or red, and such polyps may be mistaken for swollen conchae, until probing reveals their mobility, uniform softness, and lack of sensitivity.

Classification.—Nasal polyps may best be described in two categories, non-allergic and allergic. This grouping is adopted in the following account of their pathology. The relative importance of the two groups is indicated by the experience of our laboratories: in a representative year's material there were almost 700 specimens of nasal polyps—over 600 of these were of the allergic type.

Non-Allergic Polyps

Histology.—Like the allergic polyps (see below), non-allergic nasal polyps consist of very oedematous fibrous tissue, the sparse fibres of which are often so widely separated by the accumulation of fluid that they are difficult to demonstrate. Reticulin staining reveals a characteristic alveolar pattern. A consistent feature is a hyaline condensation of the basement membrane (Fig. 4.1), generally referred to as a thickening of that structure although in fact probably a product of the interstitial material in its vicinity. The surface of the polyp is covered by well-ciliated epithelium of respiratory tract type, often showing goblet cell hyperplasia, and only rarely becoming ulcerated. Squamous metaplasia is not unusual on the exposed surface of a polyp that has long presented at the nostril. There is a variable, but usually rather scanty, lymphocytic infiltration of the tissue immediately under the epithelium; the lymphocytes may be accompanied by some plasma cells and neutrophils. In some instances plasma cells are exceptionally numerous and may even give rise to a suspicion of myeloma (see page 231).

Antronasal Polyps (Choanal Polyps)

Antronasal polyps differ from the usual non-allergic nasal polyps in two respects—they arise in the maxillary sinus, and they occur predominantly in children and young adults. They are solitary, as a rule, although one may be present on each side. The polyp grows through the ostium of the sinus into the middle meatus, extending forward toward the front of the nose or, more characteristically, backward to present at the choana (hence the alternative names, *choanal polyp* and *antrochoanal polyp*). Their pathological appearances are similar to those of ethmoidal polyps, except that they are liable to pseudocystic degeneration: a considerable amount of serous fluid may escape from these pseudocystic foci when they are ruptured during removal of the lesion or on probing it. Haemorrhage may occur into the degenerating tissue. In some cases cholesterol granulomas form: these are quite similar to the familiar cholesterol granulomas of the middle ear (see Chapter 41).

Similar polyps occasionally arise within the sphenoidal and ethmoidal sinuses.

Allergic Polyps

Pathogenesis and Histology.—The essential feature in the pathogenesis of the allergic type of nasal polyp is the presence of oedema. The fluid has the characteristics of an inflammatory exudate, particularly a high content of protein. Its accumulation is the direct consequence of increased capillary permeability, mediated by vasodilator substances that have been liberated in the course of antigen–antibody reactions at cell surfaces. When such antigen–antibody reactions occur repeatedly, the oedema that thus results tends to become persistent: polyps form because the accumulation of fluid leads to progressive distension of the lamina propria of the mucosa and consequent protrusion of the epithelial covering, which may show patchy atrophy (Fig. 4.1). Once polyps have developed in this manner, their histological appearances are often characteristic to the point of being pathognomonic. There is extensive replacement of the ciliate cells of the surface epithelium by large goblet cells. The mucous glands in the stroma become hyperplastic and distended (Figs 4.1 and 4.2): cyst formation may result if their outlet is obstructed by stretching or kinking or by the surrounding oedema. The cysts are filled with fluid that may be mucous or proteinaceous.

Infiltration of the stroma by eosinophils is characteristic (Fig. 4.3): their number varies greatly, and whenever such an infiltrate is found in any biopsy specimen from this region its presence should raise the question of an allergic process. Their distribution may be uniformly diffuse, or they

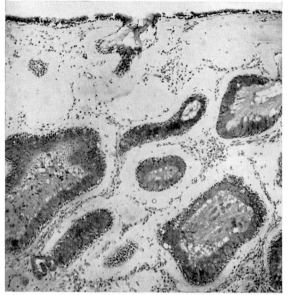

Fig. 4.1. Allergic type of nasal polyp, with atrophy of surface epithelium although there is hyperplasia of the glands. The basement membrane and stroma are extensively hyalinized: they appear as homogeneous clear areas in the photograph —for instance, outlining the glands. *Haematoxylin–eosin.* × 55.

lymphocytes predominate in the lesions only in the presence of secondary infection. Their presence in smaller numbers does not necessarily indicate infection: it may indicate a reaction to an allergen, and the possibility that antibodies are being produced locally. Before the dangers inherent in the method were known, the Prausnitz–Küstner technique was used on volunteers to demonstrate that the titres of reaginic antibodies in the oedema fluid of the allergic type of nasal polyp are higher than those in the serum of the same patient collected at the same time.[21] More recently, it has been found that IgE, including the fraction believed to be responsible for reaginic activity, is present in polyp fluid in a concentration higher than can be accounted for by simple filtration:[22] this suggests its local production.

Allergic polyps are often a part of the clinico-pathological picture of allergic rhinitis, particularly vasomotor rhinitis (see below). The spectrum of conditions included under such diagnostic terms as allergic rhinitis, vasomotor rhinitis, allergic polyps and simple polyps is continuous: none of the varieties is an entity, for there is overlap in clinical picture and pathological findings between them all.

may be confined to the subepithelial zone, or they may occur only in scattered foci. A frequent feature is the presence of sharply defined granuloma-like accumulations of eosinophils and plasma cells together, maybe with lymphocytes. Plasma cells and

Differential Diagnosis of Nasal Polyps

It may be quite impossible to distinguish clinically between simple nasal polyps, polypoid lesions due to specific granulomatous diseases, and polypoid neoplasms, including cancers. For this reason *it is*

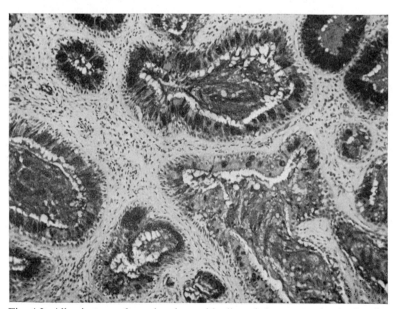

Fig. 4.2. Allergic type of nasal polyp, with distended mucous glands showing increased secretory activity. *Haematoxylin–eosin.* × 85.

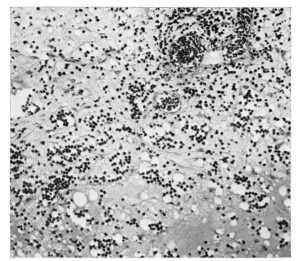

Fig. 4.3. Allergic type of nasal polyp, with oedematous stroma and heavy infiltration by eosinophils. *Haematoxylin–eosin.* × 115.

essential that all polyps removed from the nose and nasal sinuses should be fully examined histologically.

Allergic Rhinitis

The importance of allergy in the causation of various diseases affecting the nose is well known. These diseases include hay fever, vasomotor rhinitis and a proportion of cases of nasal polyposis. The pathogenetic mechanism and the essential histopathological changes that characterize these conditions are, in general, similar. They differ in such details as the circumstances and time of occurrence of the attacks, and the extent to which other tissues are also affected.

Hay Fever

Hay fever, or pollen allergy, is a distressing complaint in which the patient suffers from severe rhinitis and, usually, conjunctivitis as a result of allergic sensitization to the pollens of certain plants. In Britain, the commonest allergen is the pollen of Timothy grass (*Phleum pratense*): the pollination season (April to July) is a time of much discomfort, and even incapacity, to those who are severely sensitive. In other parts of the world other plants may be responsible, although it seems to be the pollens of grasses or trees that account for most cases. In parts of the United States of America, for instance, there are two distinct hay fever seasons—the Timothy grass season, and then, in

August and September, the ragweed season:* some patients suffer from the disease during only one or the other of these seasons, but some are unfortunate enough to be allergic to the pollen of both types of plant.

The pollens that are responsible for hay fever have certain characteristics in common: the grains are very light and therefore readily airborne, they are produced in large quantities, they are widespread in the countryside, and they are allergenic. Once a person becomes sensitized, an attack of hay fever will be precipitated by inhalation of the pollen concerned. The specific pollen responsible can be identified by intradermal inoculation of pollen extracts, a local urticarial response, sometimes with vesiculation, indicating a positive reaction: it may be noted, however, that cross-reactions sometimes occur between pollens of similar or even dissimilar species of plants. A positive Prausnitz–Küstner reaction can be obtained, but *this test is now known to be too dangerous to use*—the subject to whom the intradermal injection of the patient's serum is given is exposed to the twofold risk of homologous serum jaundice (see Chapter 21) and of an acute, systemic anaphylactic reaction, which may prove fatal.

The discovery that hay fever is causally related to the pollens of certain trees, grasses and other plants was made in 1873 by Charles Harrison Blackley, himself a sufferer from the disease.[23, 24] He found that there was an immediate local reaction when he inoculated an extract of grass pollen into his skin.

Hay fever is rather commoner in men than in women. Its onset is usually in the latter part of childhood. It recurs year after year until the attacks begin to become less frequent and less severe in late middle age, after which the liability to the disease may gradually disappear. There is not uncommonly a well-marked familial predisposition to hay fever, or to other allergic conditions, such as infantile eczema and bronchial asthma. About half of those who suffer from hay fever also suffer from asthma.

Hay fever differs from vasomotor rhinitis (see below) in its seasonal incidence, and in the occur-

* 'Ragweed', in America, is the name given to various species of *Ambrosia*, whereas in Britain ragweed is synonymous with ragwort, which is a popular term for a number of species of *Senecio*. Species of *Ambrosia* are important causes of pollen allergy in America: in contrast, none of the British species of *Senecio* has been incriminated with any certainty as a cause of any form of respiratory tract allergy, although some species, such as groundsel and marsh ragwort, are occasional causes of allergic contact dermatitis.

rence of symptoms due to an associated conjunctival sensitization: these symptoms include hyperaemia and oedema of the conjunctival mucosa and eyelids, and are accompanied by troublesome lacrimation.

Vasomotor Rhinitis

Vasomotor rhinitis (paroxysmal rhinorrhoea) is aetiologically a less clearly defined manifestation of allergy in the upper respiratory tract. In its usual form it presents as sudden attacks of sneezing, associated with swelling of the nasal mucosa, particularly on the conchae, and a sudden, profuse flow of seromucous secretion. The episode may last no more than a minute or two, or it may continue for considerably longer, and even until the patient is prostrated by exhaustion. A wide range of specific allergens has been incriminated, including constituents of house dust, animal dander (dandruff), the orris-root base of face powders, feathers, moulds and many others.

The allergen or allergens responsible in any case may often be identified by skin tests. However, investigation of the allergic state in individual patients is a highly specialized study and a good deal more complex and time-consuming than is sometimes realized. A careful evaluation of the history and habits of the patient is the first step. It is necessary to elicit in the minutest detail the circumstances that surround the occurrence of each of the attacks of rhinitis, and any clues thus obtained can be followed up with the help of skin tests to determine whether there is evidence of sensitization to suspected materials. The skin testing may be carried out either by impregnating a small patch of absorbent paper or fabric with an extract of the suspected material (patch test), or by intradermal inoculation of a minute quantity of the extract. The latter method is more sensitive and more reliable; a favourite means of carrying out the test inoculation is to put a drop of the extract on the skin, and gently prick or scratch the epidermis through it. Unfortunately, these tests are often difficult to interpret, for the reactions to the substances responsible are not always well marked, while substances that are harmless to the patient may give reactions that are no less intense than the reaction to the substance that eventually proves to be the cause of the patient's condition. Confusion may also result from the occurrence of cross-reactions with materials of similar antigenic structure: once a person has become so sensitized against one foreign substance that it provokes a positive skin reaction, there is a considerable

likelihood that cutaneous cross-reactions will develop, even though natural exposure to the cross-reacting material does not cause symptoms of any kind.

Identical symptoms can have a purely psychogenic basis, and attacks of vasomotor rhinitis may, therefore, be precipitated by events quite unrelated to allergy. Thus, one patient who had initially been sensitized to a pollen also had attacks whenever the telephone bell rang: this was, in effect, a form of conditioned reflex following the earlier coincidence of important telephone calls with the beginning of acute attacks of pollen-induced rhinorrhoea.

In addition to the cases that appear undoubtedly to be manifestations of allergic sensitization to substances in the patient's environment, there are many cases of vasomotor rhinitis that occur in association with infections of the nose or sinuses. Infection may, of course, occur as a complication of an allergic rhinitis caused by sensitization to an exogenous allergen: in some cases, however, no exogenous allergen can be identified, and it is believed that sensitization in such cases may be evoked by a bacterial allergen in the course of chronic nasal infections, including sinusitis. However, the aetiological role of bacterial allergens is certainly not clear: this is readily appreciated from the fact that a considerable proportion of these cases of 'allergic-infective' rhinitis do not respond to therapeutic measures that might have been expected to relieve symptoms due to allergy associated with infection (antibiotics, efficient drainage and antihistaminics).

Histopathology of Vasomotor Rhinitis.—Oedema with consequent polypoid thickening of the mucosa is the predominant pathological change. Its immediate cause is presumed to be an increase in the permeability of the vascular endothelium, the result of injury in the course of the local antigen–antibody reaction, and probably mediated by histamine. The loose texture of the tissues encourages accumulation of fluid, and this eventually leads to the formation of *polyps* (see above, and Figs 4.1 to 4.3).

Inevitably, sooner or later, secondary infection becomes established in the course of persistent allergic rhinitis. Fibrosis of the mucosa eventually begins to develop, and the mucosal thickening then tends to become less marked, although there is unlikely to be any spontaneous regression of the more conspicuously polypoid changes. There is usually considerable thickening of the basement membrane. The oedematous stroma may contain more or less extensive foci of inflammatory granulation tissue.

It is difficult to be sure how large a part allergy plays in the development of these 'mixed' types of infective-allergic rhinitis, but its importance is probably considerable. It is not possible by clinical examination alone to distinguish between the cases in which allergy plays a part and those that are instances of simple, non-allergic, polypoid rhinitis and sinusitis. In the former, eosinophils may be present in the lumen of the mucosal glands and reach the surface of the mucosa in their secretion; they may also pass directly through the surface epithelium into the secretion that covers it. For these reasons it is sometimes of diagnostic help to prepare films of the nasal secretion in cases of suspected nasal allergy and examine them for the presence of these cells. Biopsy—not infrequently in the form of polypectomy—is also valuable in the investigation of these conditions, but the microscopical interpretation must always be closely correlated with the clinical picture.

Chronic Specific Infective Rhinitis

The chronic specific infections of the nose include a considerable variety of diseases, many of which are rare. Some of them have a special geographical distribution, for example scleroma, leprosy and some of the fungal infections, but in these days of greatly increased travel for business or pleasure, and of voluntary and involuntary migration, cases of diseases that ordinarily would be regarded as exotic may be encountered anywhere in the world. Moreover, the relative frequency and importance of some of the hitherto less common nasal granulomas have been enhanced by the fall in the incidence of such formerly pre-eminent diseases as tuberculosis and syphilis. It is important, however, to realize that in spite of their much lower incidence nowadays, both tuberculosis and syphilis must still always be considered in the differential diagnosis of ulcerative granulomatous and neoplastic diseases of the nose.

Tuberculosis

There are two clinical forms of tuberculosis of the nose—lupus vulgaris and the so-called granulomatous tuberculosis of the nasal cavity. There is no difference in the microscopical picture. Both are now infrequent. Lupus was commoner in women than in men, and its incidence was greater than that of the other form of tuberculosis of the nose.

Lupus vulgaris of the nose usually begins at the mucocutaneous junction of the vestibule: the initial lesion is the development of typical lupus foci in the adjacent skin (see Chapter 39).

The so-called granulomatous tuberculosis starts on the anterior part of the septum and does not involve the skin. It sometimes presents in the form of a sessile nodule, ranging from 0·5 to 1·0 cm in diameter, but although this lesion slowly breaks down it never involves the bony septum and there is no collapse of the bridge of the nose. If the vestibule and columella are affected, scarring and retraction follow the ulcerative process and result in the tip of the nose being drawn inward and downward toward the upper lip, with stenosis and even complete occlusion of the nostrils. Granulomatous tuberculosis is least rare in the elderly, in whom it is particularly liable to be confused with malignant neoplasms.

Nasal tuberculosis may involve the lacrimal duct and spread along it to give rise to dacryocystitis and, occasionally, tuberculous ulceration in the region of the inner canthus of the eye.

Atrophic rhinitis is an occasional sequel, particularly when the conchae have been involved (page 196).

Leprosy

The nose is frequently involved in leprosy.[25] Granulomatous nodules, ulceration or perforations may be found, particularly on the septum and the inferior conchae. The course of the disease is often marked by the occurrence of spontaneous remissions, and atrophic rhinitis develops as the granulomatous lesions heal. Nasal involvement is commonly the first manifestation of leprosy: it is important to bear this in mind when children who may have been exposed to the infection begin to have nose-bleeding. The diagnosis is made by finding the causative mycobacteria in Ziehl–Neelsen preparations of scrapings or biopsy specimens from the mucosal lesions. Histological preparations are preferable, because they greatly facilitate recognition of the characteristic lepra cells with their clustered intracytoplasmic masses of the bacilli (see Figs 4.38A and B, page 233).

Care must be taken not to mistake scleroma (page 204) for leprosy, particularly in those parts of the world where both infections occur.

Leprosy must be distinguished also from tuberculous rhinitis.

Syphilis

The nose is always involved in congenital syphilis, and it may be affected at any stage in the course of the acquired disease. A *primary chancre* of the nose is usually the result of an accidental inoculation, for instance scratching or picking the nose with a freshly contaminated finger after attending to an infected patient, or scratching the nose with a pencil that has just been licked by a patient with oral lesions, or using a contaminated handkerchief, powder-puff or snuff box. Nasal chancres are usually in the vestibule or on the anterior part of the septum, and they are associated with enlargement of the pre-auricular or submandibular lymph nodes on the same side.

The nasal lesions of *secondary syphilis* are essentially of the same type as those in the mucous membrane of other orifices, particularly the mouth.

Tertiary syphilis of the nose may present as a gummatous mass, with or without ulceration, or as perichondritis with necrosis of the cartilage, or as an atrophic rhinitis with ozaena. These lesions may appear at any time following the secondary stage, and their onset may even be recognizable before the symptoms of the latter have fully subsided. In most cases, however, they present at about the fifth year of the disease, although they may be delayed for up to 20 years or more. The sites most frequently affected are the septum, the inferior conchae, the floor of the nose and the alae. Involvement of the alae may take the form of an indolent, brawny, ulcerating granulation tissue, and the appearances of this lesion may easily be mistaken for lupus vulgaris, malignant granuloma, rodent ulcer or squamous carcinoma. Perforation of the septum may occur in the anterior, cartilaginous part, usually near the floor of the nose: if this is accompanied by destruction of the columella, the subsequent retraction of the tip of the nose produces a peculiarly ugly deformity. Much more commonly, the perforation is situated far back, in the vomerine part of the septum. A posterior septal perforation is, in fact, usually due to syphilis; an anterior perforation, on the contrary, is rarely syphilitic, the more usual causes being trauma, lupus vulgaris, the use of chromic acid as a cauterizing agent, or industrial exposure[26] to chromium or arsenical compounds.

The inflammatory process in the cases of tertiary syphilitic rhinitis may be very extensive. In untreated cases, contraction of the resulting scar tissue leads to the disfigurement that is so characteristic of syphilis of the nose. The falling in of the bridge is not the outcome of destruction of the

septum for, like all bridges, that of the nose is supported by its buttress on each side, and not merely at the centre of the arch: the arch gradually founders, in fact, because of the traction by the shrinking scar tissue. Syphilitic caries of the lateral nasal wall may lead to erosion of the maxillary sinus, or destruction of the lacrimal canal, or even invasion of the cranial cavity. It is important to note that the presence of necrotic bone in the nose should always raise the suspicion of syphilis.

The nasal lesions of *congenital syphilis* may correspond in type to those of the secondary or tertiary stages of the acquired infection. Lesions of secondary type may be present at the time of birth, but oftener they first appear between one and six weeks afterwards, and they may be delayed until the third to the sixth month. The lesions are erythematous or mucous patches, and attention is usually drawn to them by the persistent catarrhal signs that are known as 'snuffles'. The discharge is often thick, yellow and blood-streaked: crusts form when it dries and increase the obstruction. It is the chronicity of the condition that distinguishes it from a simple coryza. The tertiary type of congenital lesion, which accounts for the characteristic nasal deformity, may follow immediately on the secondary symptoms: oftener, however, they begin to become manifest either at about the age of three or four years or at the time of the second dentition, when the other late stigmas of the infection become apparent. Collapse of the bridge, perforation of the septum and of the hard palate, and ulceration of the vestibule or of the outer surface of the alae are the commonest manifestations.

Scleroma

Scleroma, or rhinoscleroma, is a very chronic progressive granulomatous disease that begins in the nose and eventually extends into the nasopharynx and oropharynx, the larynx, and sometimes the trachea and bronchi. It was originally described by Hebra, in 1870:[27] his name for it, rhinoscleroma, is nowadays generally replaced by the term scleroma, which is more appropriate for a disease that is not necessarily confined to the nose.

Aetiology.—Scleroma occurs at any age and in both sexes. It is endemic in Eastern Europe, including parts of Hungary, Slovakia, Poland, and the Ukraine, in some countries on the Mediterranean (particularly in North Africa), in Pakistan and Indonesia, and in parts of Central America and

Central Africa. Occasional cases are seen in other parts of the world.[28] It has been observed in immigrant families in the British Isles. An indigenous case was recognized in County Fermanagh, in the North of Ireland, in 1940, and another in Edinburgh in 1942 (the Scottish patient was the wife of a Polish soldier, who was free from evidence of the disease).[29] People of any race may be affected. The factor common to most patients, but not all, is a poor standard of domestic hygiene. It is significant that in the countries in which the disease is endemic it is frequent only in some areas, and practically unknown elsewhere, even in the same region—thus, there may constantly be cases in one village and none in the neighbouring villages. Oomen[30] found scleroma in some 20 of the inhabitants of an Indonesian village with a population of about 1000: most of the patients were relatives, and he regarded a household relationship as the decisive aetiological factor. This suggests that the disease results from the exposure of the members of an affected household to a common source of infection, although it does not imply that infection is necessarily conveyed by person-to-person contact.

Attempts to reproduce the disease experimentally in animals and man have had conflicting results. There is general agreement that it is due to infection by *Klebsiella rhinoscleromatis*, the organism described by von Frisch in 1882. This bacillus, which is serologically related to *Klebsiella pneumoniae* of serotype C, can always be found in the lesions of scleroma (Fig. 4.6), and specific antibodies are found in a considerable proportion of patients with the disease. Serological investigations are, in fact, valuable in establishing the diagnosis of scleroma. Further evidence that *Klebsiella rhinoscleromatis* is causally concerned has been provided by the successful treatment of the disease by various antibiotics to which this organism is sensitive *in vitro*, particularly streptomycin and terramycin. However, it is possible that scleroma is one of those diseases that are caused by two organisms in symbiosis, and some authorities believe that a virus is concerned in association with the von Frisch bacillus.

Histopathology (Figs 4.4 to 4.6).—Scleroma is characterized by the growth of nodular masses of sclerotic, granulomatous tissue that has a strikingly cartilaginous consistency. Ulceration and foul discharge are typically present. The initial sites of involvement are usually the septum, the floor of the nose or a concha: the process slowly extends throughout the interior of the nasal cavities, although ordinarily sparing the superior meatus. The sinuses become involved, and the disease eventually spreads to the rest of the respiratory passages. In some cases the skin of the upper lip is involved.

Microscopically, the only specific feature of the inflammatory reaction is the presence of the intracellular klebsiellae (see below). The mucosa is greatly thickened by an accumulation of plasma cells, lymphocytes and macrophages (Fig. 4.4). The most characteristic aspect of the picture is the Mikulicz cell (Fig. 4.5): this is a large macrophage with foamy-looking cytoplasm in which the bacilli are loosely clustered. The mucous capsule that the bacilli produce gives a positive periodic-acid/Schiff reaction, and this is helpful in demonstrating their presence (Fig. 4.6). They are also well seen in Warthin–Starry and similar silver preparations. The Mikulicz cells are to be found anywhere in the affected tissue, although most frequently in the

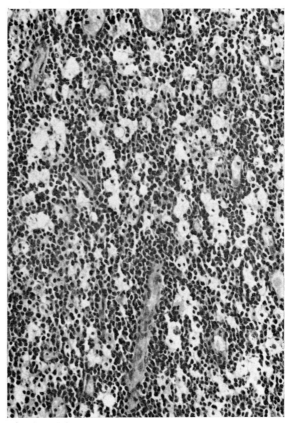

Fig. 4.4.§ Scleroma. Biopsy of thickened nasal mucosa. The pale areas among the densely packed plasma cells represent the clear cytoplasm of the infected macrophages (Mikulicz cells). See Figs 4.5 and 4.6. *Haematoxylin–eosin.* × 160.

§ See *Acknowledgements*, page 235.

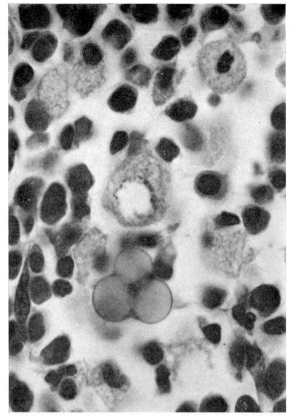

Fig. 4.5.§ Scleroma. Same specimen as in Fig. 4.4. Several macrophages with foamy-looking cytoplasm are seen, the one just above the centre of the field containing a large vacuole that has several klebsiellae at its periphery, where they appear as dark particles. There is a group of three typical Russell bodies below that cell. *Haematoxylin–eosin.* × 1000.

globules results in the formation of the Russell body.[33, 34] The electron microscopical study of the formation of Russell bodies has been greatly facilitated by the investigation of material from cases of scleroma because of their particular frequency in this disease.

There is frequently squamous metaplasia of the surface epithelium. 'Pseudocarcinomatous hyperplasia' of the squamous epithelium may develop, probably as a reactive change due to chronic infection and irritation. This may lead to histological confusion with cancer.[35]

Fungal Infections

There is no fungal infection that will not occasionally affect the nose and nasal sinuses. Some, like actinomycosis and nocardiosis, are very rare in these parts; others are relatively frequent, and some seem even to have a predisposition to occur here. Those that occur with special frequency include candidosis, phycomycosis, aspergillosis and rhinosporidiosis, all of which will be dealt with below. South American blastomycosis (paracoccidioidomycosis) also has a particular tendency to

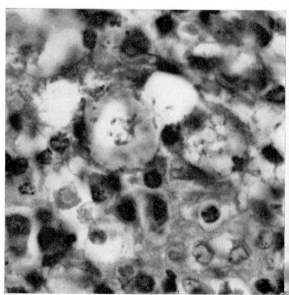

Fig. 4.6.§ Scleroma. Same specimen as in Figs 4.4 and 4.5. The klebsiellae are more clearly seen in several of the macrophages in this field: their mucous capsule has given a positive periodic-acid/Schiff reaction. The patient was a white mining engineer who apparently acquired his infection in Central Africa. The initial biopsy diagnosis was myeloma (plasmacytoma) and he was treated for this for many months before the true nature of the disease was recognized (see page 231). *Periodic-acid/Schiff; haemalum.* × 1000.

subepithelial zone. They may be so numerous as to be very readily seen, or many sections may have to be searched, field by field, under the high powers of the microscope, before one is recognized.

There is often some degree of ulceration of the lesions, and secondary infection by other organisms may result in infiltration by neutrophils. Extensive fibrosis is found in the older lesions.

As is frequently the case in conditions in which plasma cells are numerous, Russell bodies are present in scleromatous lesions. Indeed, they are particularly numerous and conspicuous in many cases (Fig. 4.5). The name Mott cell[31] has been suggested for the type of plasma cell that is the origin of the Russell body.[32] This cell is also known as the thesaurocyte, because the cisternae of its endoplasmic reticulum are distended with stored globules of secretory matter. Coalescence of these involve the nose, spreading from the mouth. Cryptococcosis, histoplasmosis, North American blastomycosis, coccidioidomycosis, chromomycosis, and sporotrichosis are occasional causes of cutaneous or mucocutaneous ulceration of the nose. The specific nature of such lesions can be established only by identifying the fungus in histological sections or, preferably, by culture. The cutaneous lesions of some of these infections are often difficult to tell clinically from ulcerated basal cell carcinomas (Figs 4.7 and 4.8).

It is noteworthy that examples of nasal involvement in all the fungal infections named above, including those that are not indigenous, have been seen in Britain since the first edition of this book appeared at the end of 1966.[36] This reflects again the importance of considering rare and exotic diseases in an increasingly international environment.

Candidosis.—It is generally said that candidosis is the commonest fungal infection of the nose. In most cases the organism is *Candida albicans* and the nasal involvement accompanies superficial mucosal candidosis of the mouth and throat (thrush). Nasal thrush is much less frequent than oral thrush.

Granuloma formation is very seldom the result of infection by species of candida: supposed examples in the nose are particularly rare.[37] The diagnosis demands isolation of the fungus in pure culture as well as its identification in the granulomatous tissue; in this context it is important to

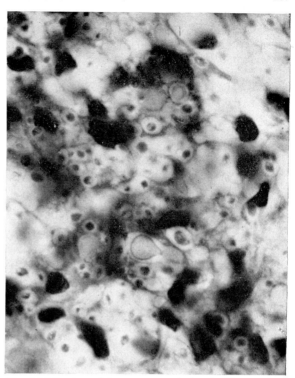

Fig. 4.8.§ Section of the cryptococcal ulcer in Fig. 4.7. The fungal cells are considerably smaller than is commonly the case in this infection (compare with Fig. 7.48, page 354, which is at the same magnification). The clear capsule surrounds the palely stained cell body of the fungus. One of the larger fungal cells, just below the centre of the field, has budded: the bud, indistinctly stained and to the right of the parent cell, is connected to the latter by a narrow process. The darkly stained structures are the nuclei of macrophages: many of them are out of focus in this photograph of a thick section. *Haematoxylin–eosin.* × 750.

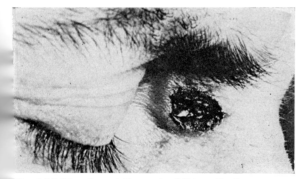

Fig. 4.7.§ The ulcer at the root of this patient's nose was thought clinically to be a primary basal cell carcinoma of the skin. A biopsy was taken with the object of confirming the diagnosis before treatment was given, the patient being already under treatment for longstanding Hodgkin's disease and the possibility that the ulcer was due to cutaneous involvement by the latter requiring consideration. In fact, the sections showed the lesion to be a cryptococcal ulcer (see Fig. 4.8). The patient developed cryptococcal meningoencephalitis and died.

note that other fungi that may cause granulomas in the respiratory tract may be overgrown by candidas when the latter are also present in the cultures, as they may well be in specimens from these parts. Histologically, the candida granuloma is said to be a straightforward tuberculoid lesion, with multinucleate giant cells and foci of suppurative or caseous necrosis. The fungal elements are present both within the giant cells and free in the tissues, especially in the microabscesses. The differentiation from similar granulomas caused by, for instance, species of aspergillus is often impossible by conventional histological means, for the appearances of the fungi in the sections are not always distinctive.

Phycomycosis (Rhinophycomycosis).—There are two clinically, aetiologically and mycologically distinct forms of phycomycosis of the nose and sinuses. Fungi of the order Entomophthorales cause very chronic infections that develop without recognized predisposing causes. In contrast, fungi of the order Mucorales cause rather rapidly progressive infections, originating in the sinuses, in patients whose resistance is lowered by other diseases or their treatment. Both forms of phycomycosis are important and will be considered in more detail.

Entomophthorosis.[38] This mycosis was first described in 1961, as a nasal granuloma of horses in Texas, in the United States of America,[39] and in 1965 as the cause of a comparable condition in a boy in the West Indies.[40] The disease had been defined clinically in Nigeria in 1963 and was mycologically confirmed there in 1967:[41] most of the published cases have been from West Africa. It has been recognized in Brazil[42] and probably in India[43] and Malaysia.[44] It seems thus to be a disease of hot climates. Most of the patients have been adults, men predominating. The source and method of infection are unknown. The earliest lesions are commonly on the inferior concha on one side, the infection spreading widely to involve the rest of the nasal passages, the sinuses, the orbits and the subcutaneous tissue of the face. Pain is unusual and secondary infection rare. Little is known about the outcome; it is doubtful whether the infection regresses spontaneously, as is sometimes the case in the very similar condition of the skin of other parts of the body caused by *Basidiobolus meristophorus* (subcutaneous phycomycosis—see Chapter 39). Extension to the lungs has been noted in a fatal case.[45]

The histological picture is like that of subcutaneous phycomycosis.[45, 46] The broad hyphae are usually surrounded by an eosinophile deposit that has been attributed to an antigen–antibody reaction. The eosinophile material attracts a histiocytic response and the hyphae are often at the centre of a broad sleeve of radially oriented macrophages (Fig. 4.9). Eosinophils are usually numerous.

'Opportunistic rhinophycomycosis'.[47] Infection by species of *Rhizopus*, *Absidia*, *Mucor* or other phycomycetes is the cause of a rapidly fatal infection that originates in the sinuses and spreads to the orbit and brain.[48] These fungi are ubiquitous saprophytic moulds that seem incapable of causing disease unless the patient's resistance to their invasion is broken by the effects on the body's defences of other diseases or of drugs and other therapeutic procedures: the mycoses that they cause are, in fact, classic examples of so-called opportunistic

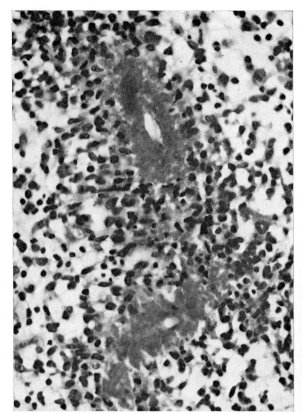

Fig. 4.9.§ Entomophthorosis. The illustration is from a pulmonary granuloma in a case of nasal infection by *Entomophthora coronata* with secondary involvement of the lungs. The broad, amorphous or rather granular, eosinophile deposit round the hyphae (the clear, sharply outlined structures) is conspicuous. Many of the cells in the exudate are eosinophils. *Haematoxylin–eosin.* × 340.

infection.[49] The fungi belong to the order Mucorales and the infections that they cause are sometimes given the name mucormycosis. Usually the portal of infection is the maxillary antrum or the ethmoidal air cells; usually one side only is affected. In most cases the infection is a complication of some severe metabolic disorder characterized by persistent acidosis, particularly uncontrolled diabetes mellitus. The association of severe diabetes mellitus, orbital cellulitis with ophthalmoplegia, and signs of meningoencephalitis makes up a syndrome that is diagnostic of phycomycosis. Clinical evidence of the underlying sinus involvement is rarely apparent. In the absence of effective antifungal treatment the disease is inevitably fatal.

The opportunistic phycomycetes have a special affinity for blood vessels, thrombosis resulting with infarction of the tissues supplied by the affected vessels. The fungus colonizes the thrombu and the dead tissue: it is readily recognized by its very broad, ribbon-like hyphae, which range from 3 to 35 µm in diameter and are largely without septa (Figs 4.10 and 4.11).

Aspergillosis.—Aspergillosis presents in two main forms in the nasal region. As so often, the facts have been unnecessarily complicated by careless abuse of terminology. It is a pity that those interested in the nasal infections have described the granulomatous aspergillous infections of the sinuses by the name aspergilloma, which in terms of bronchopulmonary disease is used exclusively to denote the common intracavitary fungal ball colony, a condition that ordinarily is not accompanied by

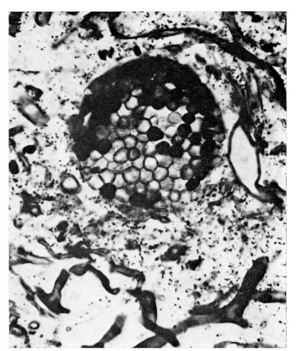

Fig. 4.11.§ Hyphae and sporangium of *Rhizopus* species in a biopsy specimen in a case of acute leukaemia complicated by extensive phycomycotic infection of ulcers involving the posterior parts of the nasal passages, the postnasal space and the pharynx. There was widespread haematogenous dissemination of the infection. Sporangia are very rarely seen in these infections: when they are present they are confined to ulcerated lesions that are exposed to the air. *Hexamine (methenamine) silver.* × 630.

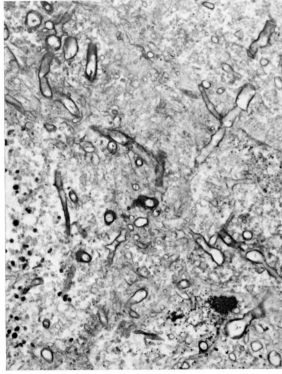

Fig. 4.10.§ Field in an infarct of a kidney, in a case of naso-orbitocerebral phycomycosis caused by a species of *Mucor.* The patient was a young adult with severe, ill-controlled diabetes mellitus. Generalized dissemination of the infection in the blood stream occurred. The appearances of the fungal elements illustrated are typical of those in all the lesions, including the mucosa and wall of the maxillary and ethmoid sinuses. The variable width of the hyphae is characteristic, as are the very thin wall, tendency to right-angle branching, and scarceness of septa (most of the septum-like structures are folds due to shrinkage of the hyphae during histological processing). Phycomycetes are not often so readily seen in haematoxylin–eosin preparations. *Haematoxylin–eosin.* × 215.

fungal invasion of the tissues (see page 350). It would be in the interests of everybody if this misuse of conventionally accepted terminology might end.

Aspergillus fungal ball. A ball colony of aspergillus, usually—as in the lungs—*Aspergillus fumigatus*, is a rare finding in a nasal sinus. In most cases it occurs in a maxillary antrum or frontal sinus, particularly the former. The colony is free within the lumen of the sinus, and in some cases its mobility can be demonstrated radiologically. Although it predisposes to secondary infection by pyogenic bacteria and may therefore be associated with erosion or ulceration of the lining of the sinus, it is exceptionally rare for the tissues to be invaded by the fungus. Nevertheless, as in the case of the pulmonary aspergilloma, if the patient's resistance to invasion is lowered by other disease or by drugs such as corticosteroids and cytotoxic agents, the fungus may invade the blood stream and establish a fatal septicaemia.

Aspergillous granuloma. This is the condition that

has been mistermed 'aspergilloma' in recent publications. It is a granulomatous infection, usually confined to one of the sinuses but occasionally more widespread. It is particularly frequent in hot, dry climates, and most of the reported cases have been in the Sudan.[50, 51] The fungus most frequently identified as its cause has been *Aspergillus flavus*. The lesion is a sclerosing giant cell granuloma (Fig. 4.12), often with foci of necrosis and suppuration. The hyphae are widespread, but they are often surprisingly hard to see in sections stained with haematoxylin and eosin: the hexamine–silver (methenamine–silver) method is the best of the fungal stains for showing the organisms in the granulomas, and its use should be a regular practice in the investigation of all giant cell granulomas of the nasal region.

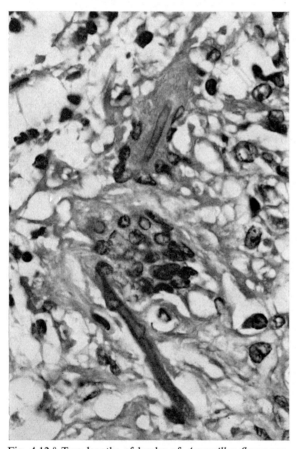

Fig. 4.12.§ Two lengths of hypha of *Aspergillus flavus* are seen, one within a multinucleate giant cell and the other lying free. From a biopsy specimen in the case of a diabetic Chinese woman with bilateral naso-orbital aspergillosis. The infection spread to the meninges. The patient recovered on treatment with amphotericin and flucytosine. *Periodic-acid/Schiff; haemalum.* × 630.

Rhinocerebral aspergillosis. Although very rare in comparison with the two varieties of nasal aspergillosis described above, this form of infection is important because of its high mortality. It is comparable in aetiology and course to the opportunistic form of rhinophycomycosis (see above), occurring as a complication usually of persistent severe metabolic disturbances, such as uncontrolled diabetes mellitus, and spreading from the sinuses to the orbit and thence to the meninges and brain. It tends to be less rapidly progressive than the corresponding phycomycosis, perhaps because the aspergilli have less affinity for the blood vessels, tending to spread through the tissue spaces. As in the case of the aspergillous granuloma, this type of aspergillosis is usually caused by *Aspergillus flavus*.[52]

Rhinosporidiosis.[53, 54] — Rhinosporidiosis is a chronic infection caused by *Rhinosporidium seeberi*, an endosporulating organism that is nowadays generally classified among the fungi, although it has not been isolated in culture and nothing is known about its occurrence outside infected tissues. The disease also occurs in some animals, particularly horses, but neither the route of infection nor its source has been discovered.

The lesions are vascular, polypoid masses that develop on the nasal mucosa and occasionally in the conjunctiva or on the skin. They ultimately obstruct the airway and predispose to bacterial infection. Occasionally, rhinosporidial lesions develop at a distance from the initial site of the infection in the nose, the characteristic, polypoid masses growing from the mucosa of the trachea or bronchi. The microscopical appearances are distinctive, for the spherical sporangia, which range from about 50 to 350 μm in diameter, are unmistakable (Fig. 4.13). The sporangium has a thick, structureless wall, and it contains innumerable spores that, when mature, are about the size of a red blood cell. The tissue reaction is a nondescript chronic inflammation, in which lymphocytes and plasma cells predominate rather than macrophages and giant cells, although these may be conspicuous in some specimens, while virtually absent in the majority.

Rhinosporidiosis is seen most frequently in Sri Lanka and in parts of India and of Central and South America, and is comparatively uncommon elsewhere, although the disease has been recognized as an exceptional rarity in patients who have never been out of Europe. Occasional cases are seen in Britain among visitors or immigrants from lands where the disease is endemic.[55]

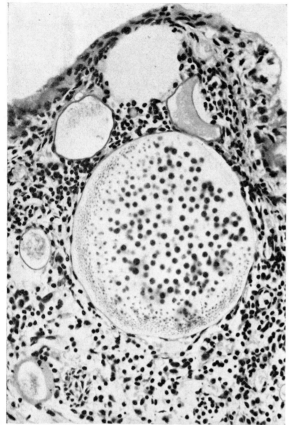

Fig. 4.13.§ *Rhinosporidium seeberi* in nasal mucosa. A large, maturing sporangium is in the centre of the field; the spores vary in size, those that are not fully grown remaining closest to the thick, homogeneous wall of the cyst-like structure. Several effete, small rhinosporidial spherules are also present. The inflammatory infiltrate in the mucosa consists mainly of lymphocytes and plasma cells. *Haematoxylin–eosin.* ×210.

Leishmaniasis[56]

Both Old World and New World cutaneous leishmaniasis may involve the nose. The lesions of the former, which is due to *Leishmania tropica*, seldom extend to the mucous membrane. In contrast, the nose is the commonest site of the mucocutaneous form of New World leishmaniasis, which is caused by *Leishmania brasiliensis*.

Mucocutaneous Leishmaniasis.—Involvement of the skin and mucous membrane at body orifices is a characteristic feature of the form of New World cutaneous leishmaniasis that is known as *espundia*. Espundia occurs in Central and South America, particularly in the Amazon basin and in the northern parts of the basin of the River Paraguay and the Gran Chaco. The reservoirs of infection are various rodents, particularly forest rats, and the vectors are *Lutzomyia* sandflies.

The initial lesion of infection with *Leishmania brasiliensis* is a cutaneous sore, usually on a foot or leg. This is quite comparable to the Old World leishmanial ulcer caused by *Leishmania tropica* (see Chapter 39). Mucocutaneous lesions develop in a proportion of cases that ranges from about 1 per cent in parts of Central America to over 20 per cent in parts of Brazil and considerably higher in some endemic areas of Paraguay. They may appear within a few months of the development of the initial sore, or the interval may be many years. The nose and upper lip are by far the most frequent site of mucocutaneous involvement. The occurrence of these lesions at a distance from the primary sore is conventionally attributed to 'metastasis'. There is doubt about the means of such metastatic spread: rather than being haematogenous it may well be effected merely by digital transfer of the organisms from the initial lesion to the nose or other mucocutaneous site, with their implantation there through 'picking' and the resulting damage to the mucosa by the contaminated finger nail. While the sore at the site of the primary inoculation usually heals within a matter of months, or at most a couple of years, leaving a distinctive scar, the mucocutaneous lesions tend to be chronic and may not heal without treatment.

The affected mucocutaneous tissues are thickened by oedema, inflammatory cellular infiltrate and fibrosis. Within the nose the lesions may resemble polyps.[57] Superficial ulceration and secondary bacterial infection contribute to the picture. Gross distortion and destruction of the tissues eventually result. The so-called 'tapir nose' is characteristic, although like many classic features of disease it is seldom seen in its typical form: it results from involvement and collapse of the anterior part of the cartilaginous septum, with loss of the columella and the lower parts of the alae.

The leishmanias are usually easily found in the lesions in the earlier stages of the infection (Fig. 4.14). Later, they are fewer: at this stage the diffuse scattering of the infected macrophages throughout the lesion may give way to a strikingly tuberculoid picture. This change in the character of the lesion and the parallel fall in the number of recognizable parasites suggest that a change has taken place in the patient's state of immunity.

New World leishmaniasis, like Old World leishmaniasis, is seen from time to time in practice in countries like Britain where neither occurs naturally.[58] The importance of knowing the patient's geographical history is clear, assuming the doctor to be sufficiently familiar with geographical medicine. It is worth noting again that care is needed

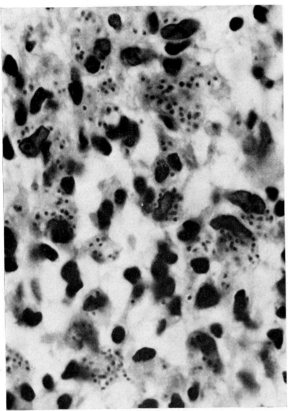

Fig. 4.14.§ *Leishmania brasiliensis* in the cytoplasm of macrophages in an ulcerated granuloma of a nostril and the upper lip. The patient was an Irishman who had travelled widely in Amazonia. He had had a primary cutaneous sore on the inner aspect of one knee about 12 months before the mucocutaneous lesion began to appear. He had been back in Europe for several weeks before the first sign of the latter, which then continued to become slowly more extensive during the further year that passed before its nature was recognized in the biopsy specimen illustrated. When the sections were first examined the leishmanias were taken for histoplasmas. *Haematoxylin–eosin.* × 860.

to avoid mistaking *Histoplasma capsulatum* for a leishmania, or a leishmania for the histoplasma.[59] Both are intracellular parasites of the macrophages, and their similarity of size can cause them to be confused. The leishmanias do not give a positive periodic-acid/Schiff reaction and are not shown by the hexamine–silver (methenamine–silver) method of staining fungi.

Viral Granuloma

A patient who had recently received a cadaver kidney transplant developed fatal herpes simplex infection. The infection manifested itself as a progressive, ulcerating, destructive granuloma of the nose, complicating herpes of the upper lip.[60] This exceptional experience is noteworthy because it may presage similar cases as immunosuppressant measures come to be more frequently used.

Rhinophyma

Rhinophyma is preceded by a rosacea type of dermatitis, with transient episodes of erythema and vasodilatation: indeed, it is now generally believed to be an outcome of rosacea (see Chapter 39). Its development is slow, taking anything from 5 to 20 years. Papules and pustules appear in crops, and repeated recurrence over the years leads to the characteristic picture. Hypertrophy of the tissues of the nose produces lobulate, dull red or purplish masses, ranging from 3 mm to several centimetres in diameter. When the condition is advanced the nose may be greatly enlarged, and the changes may affect other parts of the face that are liable to rosacea, such as the cheeks and forehead.

Histopathology.—The essential microscopical features are hyperkeratosis of the epidermis, and hypertrophy and hyperplasia of the sebaceous glands. The follicles are distended by large accumulations of keratin, and abscesses may develop within them. There is overgrowth of the connective tissue of the affected parts, and dilatation of the blood vessels. Lymphocytes and sometimes plasma cells and macrophages accumulate round the follicles and, particularly, the adjacent blood vessels.

The incidence of rhinophyma is decreasing, perhaps because of earlier and more effective treatment of rosacea.

There is no evidence that excessive consumption of alcohol plays any part in its causation, and this formerly popular theory has been abandoned by most dermatologists. The small metazoan parasite, *Demodex folliculorum*, is often present in large numbers in the follicles—it has no pathogenic significance (see Chapter 39).

The Non-Healing Nasal Granulomas of Unknown Cause[61–63]

Among the considerable variety of granulomatous diseases of the nasal region (see above) there is very important group of progressive necrotizing granulomas that are of unknown causation and that have no tendency to heal spontaneously. The multiplicity of names that have been given to these conditions indicates the unresolved nature of the aetiological problem. While two main and distinct forms of these non-healing granulomas are now widely recognized, Wegener's disease and the so-called Stewart type of necrotizing granuloma, these represent the different ends of a spectrum of related conditions. These two conditions are histologically of quite different pattern, and typical cases of each are readily recognized and cannot be confused with one another: in the intermediate series of cases that do not fall clearly into one category or the other there is represented every shade of histological pattern, linking the two extremes in a continuous series.

Wegener's disease is a giant-celled, tuberculoid, necrotizing granuloma that arises in the upper air passages and eventually involves the lungs, kidneys and small arteries throughout the body. The Stewart type of necrotizing granuloma, in contrast, is a non-tuberculoid, histiocytic and lymphocytic granuloma, frequently confined to the nasal region and without accompanying visceral and vascular changes. Its granulomatous nature is less apparent than that of Wegener's disease, and it has, with good reason, been much oftener taken for a malignant tumour than the latter, although both diseases spread and destroy after the manner of cancers and time and again are liable to be confused with cancer both clinically and pathologically.

Many attempts have been made to clarify the conflicting biological concepts and histological interpretations of these two forms of necrotizing granuloma of the nose. Their study has been hampered by unresolved aetiological and terminological problems, and confusion has been added to by the multiplicity of descriptive names.

Neither of these diseases is as rare as the comparatively small number of published cases might seem to indicate. Both have been recognized as entities only comparatively recently: yet they are already familiar to most pathologists and ear, nose and throat specialists from personal experience. In the past, the Stewart type of necrotizing granuloma was generally mistaken for carcinoma, and most clinicians and pathologists of today can look back on cases of supposed cancers of the face or nose that, in the light of present knowledge, would probably be regarded as examples of this disease. It must be pointed out, however, that some cancers arising in the nose—particularly lymphosarcoma and reticulum cell sarcoma—may exactly reproduce the clinical features of the Stewart granuloma. This may cause serious practical difficulties, especially because it is often hard to distinguish confidently between the latter and these types of sarcoma on histological grounds, particularly in biopsy specimens from early lesions.

Wegener's Disease (Wegener's Granulomatosis)

This condition was originally defined in 1936 and 1939 by Wegener, who described it as a rhinogenic form of polyarteritis.[64] Essentially, it takes the form of a necrotizing giant-celled granuloma that usually presents first in some part of the upper respiratory tract, with the subsequent development of confluent, necrotic lesions in the lungs (see page 371). An arteritis of polyarteritic type affects the pulmonary and systemic vasculature.

The presenting symptoms may relate to the nose, or nasal manifestations may be trivial and overshadowed by purpura, haematuria, abdominal pain and renal failure. Malaise, fever and loss of weight may be out of proportion to other clinical findings, the significance of such local symptoms as 'catarrh' and 'sinusitis' being then readily overlooked. Sooner or later, signs that point to the respiratory system, and particularly to the upper respiratory tract, usually develop. Rarely, however, evidence of nasal or pulmonary involvement is not evident until necropsy. The more obtrusive symptoms of upper respiratory tract disease, such as blood-stained nasal discharge or frank epistaxis, hoarseness, and deafness or earache, are less likely to be neglected in diagnosis.

The earlier intranasal changes take the form of crusted, bleeding granulations on the septum and conchae, with thickening of the mucosa. Later, protuberant granulomas form, especially on the septum, and become ulcerated, with conspicuous destruction of the tissues. In one series of 25 cases the presenting lesion was in the nose in 11 cases, in a maxillary sinus in 6, in the hard palate in 2, in an ear in 3 and in an orbit in 3.[65] As the disease advances, external signs often appear: oedema of the orbits and face, proptosis, antro-alveolar fistula and even collapse of the nasal bridge are among these. Spreading ulcers may develop in the mouth, pharynx and larynx.[66]

Death occurs within six months to a year of the onset of symptoms and is generally the result of renal failure caused by the vascular changes in the kidneys: characteristically, there is a necrotizing glomerulitis as well as renal arteritis. Necrotizing

H

granulomas similar to those in the respiratory tract, but small and discrete, and sometimes mistaken for miliary tubercles, are found in the spleen ('speckled spleen'—see Chapter 9) and other viscera in some cases.

Aetiology.—The disease usually occurs in adults. There is no significant difference in its sex incidence. Little is known of its causation. Allergy to the bacteria that are associated with chronic infections of the nose, sinuses, throat and ears has been suggested, and sensitization to drugs—particularly sulphonamides and antibiotics—has also been named as a possible factor, as in other cases of polyarteritis (see page 144). It is relevant that patients who develop the disease seem to be unusually liable to sensitivity reactions of one sort or another: this is indicated by the high incidence of urticarial drug reactions and of blood transfusion reactions of the 'serum sickness' type.[67] However, the causal importance of an allergic factor has not been proved.

Histopathology.—The presence of multinucleate giant cells, although not pathognomonic, is helpful in the correct interpretation of the significance of the presenting lesion in cases of Wegener's granulomatosis. In all the cases that we have seen, giant cells were found in the biopsy material, although in variable numbers. In some cases they are scattered widely through the tissue, and are numerous enough to be found readily; in others, they are scanty, and tend to be grouped near to blood vessels (Fig. 4.15). Sometimes the giant cells lie so close to the artery that the picture is very similar to that of giant cell arteritis (see page 141), but the two conditions can be distinguished by the fact that in Wegener's granulomatosis the giant cell reaction (Fig. 4.16) is not related to the breakdown of the elastica in the vessel wall as it is in true giant cell arteritis.

The giant cells may resemble those of tuberculosis, but their nuclei are often peculiarly compact, appearing dense, ovoid, and so intensely haematoxyphile that they frequently look black. The nuclei are often clustered in two sickle-shaped groups at opposite poles of the cell. The cytoplasm is generally more compact, more homogeneous and more eosinophile than in the giant cells of other tuberculoid granulomas. Attention to these cytological details may be helpful in diagnosis.[68]

Patches of necrosis are common in the granulomatous tissue. The necrotic material has a typically granular appearance, with conspicuous stippling

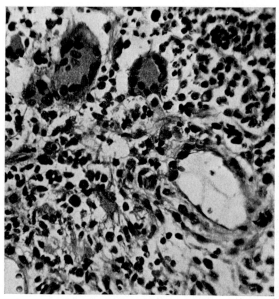

Fig. 4.15. Wegener's disease. Multinucleate giant cells are present. *Haematoxylin–eosin.* × 600.

by haematoxyphile, particulate debris of nuclear origin. The destruction of tissue is not as extensive as in the Stewart type of necrotizing granuloma: in particular, there is less tendency for cartilage and bone to become involved.

The Stewart Type of Non-Healing Necrotizing Granuloma ('Malignant Granuloma')

There are several names still in current use for this condition. The term malignant granuloma was introduced by Woods[69] and has been favoured by most British authors.[70, 71] American authors have given preference to the terms 'lethal midline granuloma of the face', which was introduced by Williams[72] in 1949, and 'midline lethal (or malignant) reticulosis of the face',[72a] while on the continent of Europe the term 'granuloma gangraenescens' is often used.[73] Some writers use the rather unilluminating term, histiocytic granuloma, which might be applied to most granulomas of the nose and other parts of the body. The definitive name for the disease will be decided when its nature is known: pending that time, we have chosen to refer to it as the Stewart type of non-healing necrotizing granuloma of the nose, in recognition of the contribution of J. P. Stewart,[70] of Edinburgh, to our knowledge of the condition.

The disease is almost always preceded by a longstanding, non-specific infection of the nose or nasal sinuses. The initial manifestation of the developing

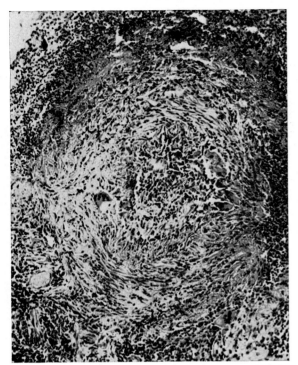

Fig. 4.16. Wegener's disease. Giant-celled arteritis in a nasal biopsy specimen. *Haematoxylin–eosin.* × 230.

granuloma is an indurated swelling of the tissues of some part of the nose: this may be the vestibule, the septum, or, more rarely, one of the conchae. Ulceration of the affected part follows (Fig. 4.17), and epistaxis may be the presenting symptom, often with some obstruction of the airway. In some cases the initial changes are in one of the maxillary sinuses.

The ulcerated mucosa is covered by sticky, black or brownish-yellow crusts. Removal of the crusts reveals what looks—clinically—like a simple granulation tissue. Cartilage and bone are eroded, and as the condition progresses sequestra may form. Ulceration develops on the conchae and septum, and spreads rapidly throughout the nose, often involving the hard palate, which may become perforated. Bacterial infection of the ulcerated tissues leads to inflammatory oedema of the lips, cheeks and eyelids, and subcutaneous abscesses may follow. Extensive erosion and destruction of the nose, cheeks, lips and hard palate soon result, and in some cases the entire roof of the nose and nasopharynx may be visible through the mouth, with exposure of the roof of the maxillary sinus after destruction of the lateral wall of the nose. Ulceration may occur at any stage in one or both

maxillary sinuses, or in other sinuses, or in the oropharynx, spreading to the nasopharynx and hypopharynx.[74] Sometimes, there is deep ulceration of the alveolar processes, with loss of teeth.

Death may result from septic pneumonia following aspiration of infected material, from haemorrhage due to erosion of a large vessel, from meningitis following invasion of the cranial cavity, or from cachexia, to which the difficulty of getting adequate nutrition contributes.[75]

Histopathology.—The essential histological change is a dense accumulation of cells in the affected tissues. The cells are predominantly lymphocytes; there is an admixture—often considerable—of plasma cells and there are also many peculiar, elongated or spindle-shaped, histiocytes, with a round or kidney-shaped nucleus (Fig. 4.18). Necrosis is not limited to the ulcerated surface, but characteristically affects a very considerable part of the cellular tissue, both superficially and in depth.

In a majority of cases the appearances so closely resemble those of some of the malignant diseases of the lymphoreticular system that it seems possible that the picture of the Stewart type of necrotizing granuloma may sometimes be due to a localized, nasal manifestation of a lymphoreticular disease. It is relevant that the Stewart granuloma may respond well to comparatively small doses of X-rays. Interpretation of the nature of this disease is complicated by the fact that typical lymphosarcomas and reticulum cell sarcomas may also arise in the nose or sinuses, and behave in a manner clinically indistinguishable from the Stewart type of granuloma except that sooner or later foci of the tumour develop elsewhere—for example in the

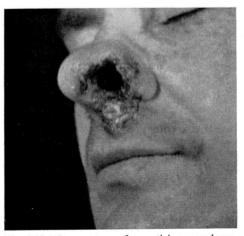

Fig. 4.17.§ Stewart type of necrotizing granuloma.

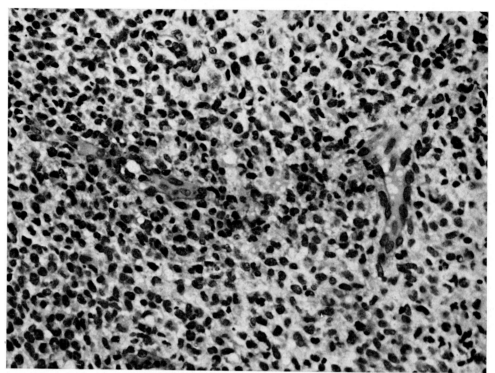

Fig. 4.18.§ Stewart type of necrotizing granuloma. Except that lymphocytes are less conspicuously numerous than in most fields in biopsy material from this condition, this photograph is typical. In particular, there are many of the characteristic pale histiocytes, with rather pale, round or kidney-shaped nucleus, and cytoplasm that seems to merge into the intercellular background. There are several capillary blood vessels in the field. *Haematoxylin–eosin.* × 300.

cervical lymph nodes, mediastinum or skeleton (particularly the cranial bones).

The distinction between tumour-like proliferative diseases and true neoplasms is nowhere less clear than in the lymphoreticular system: the malignant and potentially malignant diseases that arise in that system include conditions of uncertain nature as well as indisputable neoplasms. This is not to say that the Stewart type of granuloma is itself a disease of the lymphoreticular tissues of the nasal region or in any way related to the neoplastic diseases of the lymphoreticular system. It does mean, however, that the greatest care has to be taken to try to distinguish between the true lympho-reticular neoplasms of the nose and the Stewart type of granuloma: this puts the diagnostic responsibility squarely on the histopathologist, for the two entities cannot yet be finally distinguished other than by histological means.

Intermediate Varieties of the Non-Healing Nasal Granulomas of Unknown Cause

It has been indicated above that Wegener's disease and the Stewart type of necrotizing granuloma are at the extremes of a nosological spectrum. Every grade of histological pattern may be found linking these extremes. Lesions that exactly correspond histologically to the granulomas of Wegener's disease may remain strictly localized to the nasal region ('limited Wegener's disease'). Such cases may present both widespread polyarteritic changes characteristic of Wegener's disease and the accompanying renal lesions; or only the latter may be present; or there is no disease at all apart from the nasal lesions themselves. Nearer the Stewart end of the spectrum are those cases that histologically present the features of the latter but in addition are characterized by a scattering of the giant cells typical of Wegener's disease. In other 'Stewart' cases there are not only the occasional giant cells among the lymphocytes and histiocytes but also the giant-celled arteritis in the mucosa that is a frequent feature of Wegener's disease and lacking in fully typical cases of the Stewart granuloma. As a further variant, the lesions of the latter in the nose may be associated with widespread cutaneous, visceral or generalized polyarteritis.[76]

There is a form of Wegener's disease with excep

tionally extensive and deep necrosis of the midline structures of the nose, in this respect resembling the Stewart lesion although histologically fully consistent with the former.[77] Again, there are cases of Wegener's disease with no lesions in the nose but typical changes in the lungs.[78]

The Nature of the Non-Healing Nasal Granulomas of Unknown Cause

At present, the cause and therefore the nature of these conditions remain unknown.[79] We agree with those who regard Wegener's disease, the Stewart type of granuloma and the spectrum of diseases intermediate between them as variants of a single disorder, probably vascular in its basis, and possibly due to a disturbance that is immunologically determined. It is likely that diseases affecting other systems and parts of the body, and similarly associated with angitis, may belong to the same general category.

TUMOURS OF THE NOSE
AND NASAL SINUSES

It cannot be urged too strongly that *all tissues removed from the nose and nasal sinuses should be examined microscopically.* Many nasal neoplasms present as polyps, and on clinical examination may exactly simulate simple polyps. Further, tumours arising in the nasal sinuses and in the nasopharynx also frequently present as polyps. Unless *all* polyps are sectioned, the diagnosis of some cases of nasal cancer will inevitably be unnecessarily delayed.

It is important to note, too, that for the histological examination to be adequate, *all the pieces excised must be sectioned and not merely one or two supposedly representative samples* of the tissue.

Exfoliative cytology occasionally has a part in the recognition of the presence of cancer in the nasal region.[80, 81] Its potential is limited by the frequency of infection, which results in an inflammatory cellular exudate that confuses or totally obscures the cytological evidence of malignant disease.

Topographical Pathology of Nasal Tumours.— Although there is no sharp anatomical division between the nasal cavities and the nasal sinuses, and in spite of a considerable similarity in the types of tumours that arise in the two situations, there are good reasons for paying attention to the distinctions between the tumours of the nasal

cavities and those of the nasal sinuses. First, among the great variety of tumours that occur in the upper respiratory tract there are some that tend to arise more frequently or even exclusively in one or the other of these regions. Second, the relative proportions of benign and malignant tumours differ markedly in the two regions: in our experience, over a period of 21 years, the ratio of benign to malignant tumours in the nasal cavities is about six to one; in the nasal sinuses the ratio has been almost exactly the reverse of these figures. Third, tumours of similar histological type may differ in their behaviour in the two regions: for example, the survival rate in cases of squamous carcinoma of a nasal cavity is almost three times that of squamous carcinoma of equivalent differentiation arising in the sinuses.

However, it must be appreciated that the precise site of origin of a carcinoma in a sinus can seldom be determined, for by the time of diagnosis a large part of the sinus may be involved and the tumour may have extended into adjoining parts. It may, therefore, be impossible to tell whether a carcinoma within the nose has arisen in the nasal cavity or in one of the sinuses.

*Classification.—*Classification of the tumours of the nasal region is often based on their behaviour. We believe that the close relation between certain benign and malignant tumours makes it more convenient and more appropriate to adopt a classification based on tissue of origin.

1. Tumours Arising from Surface Epithelium

Benign Tumours

*Squamous Papilloma.—*The commonest benign tumour of the region is the squamous papilloma. It arises almost exclusively in the vestibule. Usually hyperkeratotic, it is often indistinguishable from the common skin wart (see Chapter 39). In a series of 555 benign tumours of the nasal cavity that we have studied there were 222 squamous papillomas. They occurred over a wide range of age and were commoner in females.

*Keratoacanthoma.—*The skin of the vestibule is occasionally the site of a keratoacanthoma.[82] There were four in our series of 555 benign nasal tumours.

*Transitional Type of Papilloma.—*This is both the most important and the most interesting of the benign tumours of the nasal region. It arises from epithelium of respiratory type but is characterized by squamous differentiation, its structure including a range of epithelial types from columnar to fully keratinized squamous. It was because those tumours that represent intermediate stages of squamous differentiation may mimic papillomas of the urinary tract in their appearances that this group as a whole came to be described as the transitional papillomas or transitional cell papillomas of the nose. They account for about 25 per cent of tumours of the nasal cavities. They occur over a wide age range, with the peak in the fifth and sixth decades; men are affected five times oftener than women. They are usually unilateral but affect the mucosa over a considerable area, often involving the nasal sinuses.

Macroscopically, the transitional type of papilloma is polypoid (Fig. 4.19). Although usually firmer to the touch than simple polyps, and liable to bleed during removal, it may be confused with these.

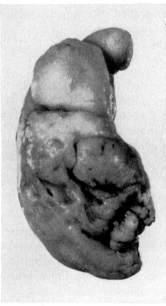

Fig. 4.19. Transitional type of papilloma of the nose. The condition presented with the clinical picture of a unilateral 'nasal polyp'. The specimen had the firm consistency that is one of the characteristics of this neoplasm. *Natural size.*

The microscopical appearances are characteristic. Rapid and extensive proliferation leads to true stratification of the neoplastic epithelium, with or without persistence of ciliate columnar cells at the surface. The degree of squamous differentiation varies: there may be none, with total persistence of columnar cells throughout the growth, or any degree up to a completely squamous epithelial

structure. The increase in the surface area that results from the cellular proliferation is accommodated by infolding of the oedematous stroma (Fig. 4.20): this may give a false microscopical impression of an invasive growth in which cell masses, sometimes with central degeneration, appear to lie deep to the surface—however, the basement membrane

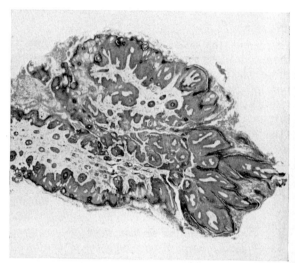

Fig. 4.20. Transitional type of papilloma of the nose. This example included areas of differentiated stratified squamous epithelium. *Haematoxylin–eosin.* ×2·5.

is intact and continuous with that of the adjoining normal surface epithelium. As infolding proceeds, the stroma becomes reduced in amount and the cells that were originally at the surface come to lie at the centre of the deeper masses (Fig. 4.21), where desquamation and sometimes incipient keratinization simulate central necrosis and thus heighten the impression of malignancy. In spite of the variation from columnar to squamous cell type, the arrangement of the cells is generally regular. The nuclei in the basal layer may be hyperchromatic and somewhat variable in appearance, and mitotic figures are not infrequent. Cholesterol granulomas may form in the stroma (Fig. 4.22), particularly when infection has led to breaking down of some of the epithelial masses.

The nature of these tumours is controversial. This is reflected in the use of such descriptive synonyms as 'inverted papilloma', 'papillomatosis' and—by those who regard them as inflammatory—'chronic hypertrophic rhinitis'. A broad histological spectrum can be drawn, ranging from what appears to be strictly local epithelial hyperplasia in an otherwise typical simple nasal polyp to solid growths of unquestionably neoplastic epithelium.[83] It is by

In a series of 170 cases that we studied over periods ranging from 3 to 21 years, the frequency of recurrence was high, and indeed rose to 50 per cent and more in those patients who had been longest under observation:[84] frank carcinoma developed in two cases. Apart from the cases in this series, all of which were instances of benign papillomas at the time of the initial histological examination, there are rare instances in which the original biopsy shows undoubted carcinoma in association with the otherwise typical picture of the transitional type of papilloma. If an observation of this sort is accepted as evidence of malignant change in the papilloma, the frequency of such change in our series is of the order of 5 per cent; if one accepts the stricter criterion of demanding that malignant change first be observed in the course of studying successive biopsy specimens in a given case, following an initially benign picture, the incidence of malignant change is under 2 per cent. In a review of some 300 published cases only three were considered to be acceptable as instances of the development of carcinoma.[85]

The potential malignancy of these tumours will be discussed below in the context of the carcinomas of transitional type. It is possible to state here that in the great majority of cases of the transitional type of papilloma there is no evidence of malignant change, even after there have been multiple

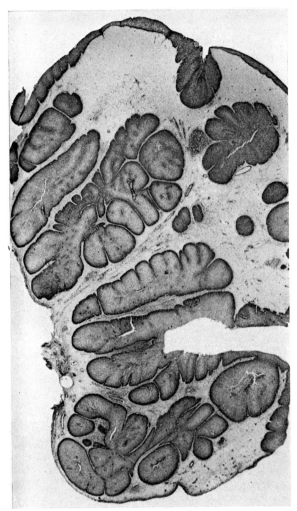

Fig. 4.21. Transitional type of papilloma of the nose. It is easy to see how such a picture may give an initial but incorrect impression of malignant invasion. However, the circumscribed epithelial masses have formed, in continuity with the surface of the tumour, by the process of infolding in the course of their growth. An area where this process is illustrated is seen at the top of the picture, to the right of the centre. *Haematoxylin–eosin.* × 10.

no means sure that this range in the extent and cellularity of the changes should be seen as representing a single process, an epithelial proliferation of one origin and one nature. This must be kept in mind when considering the often raised question of the malignant potential of these changes. Quite apart from the occasionally equivocal histological picture, the fact that some of these lesions recur and that some manifest frank carcinomatous change has led many to regard the transitional type of papilloma as at least premalignant. Such a view calls for very careful evaluation.

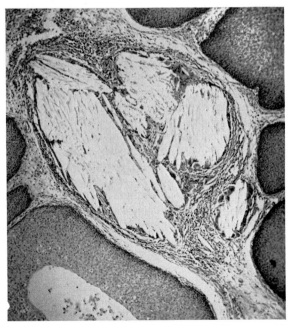

Fig. 4.22. Transitional type of papilloma of the nose, with cholesterol granuloma. *Haematoxylin–eosin.* × 40.

recurrences over a period of many years. However, the difficulty of prognostication in individual cases is real, as a report of metastasis to the regional lymph nodes in a case of microscopically typical transitional papilloma exemplifies.[86]

Carcinoma

Carcinomas—squamous carcinomas, carcinomas of transitional type, anaplastic carcinomas and adeno-carcinomas—account, perhaps surprisingly, for only about 50 per cent of malignant tumours of the nasal cavities. In the nasal sinuses they account for about 80 per cent. The combined incidence in these two situations amounts to substantially less than 1 per cent of all carcinomas in man. The peak age incidence is in the sixth decade; there is no significant sex difference, taking the tumours as a whole. It may be noted, from the point of view of aetiology, that, contrary to what is sometimes said, no correlation has been established between chronic sinusitis and the occurrence of carcinoma.

In the nasal cavity about 75 per cent of carcinomas are squamous and arise anteriorly. Because of their situation these tumours are diagnosed earlier and have a better prognosis than those arising in the nasal sinuses. The carcinomas that arise farther back in the nasal cavities are about equally divided between transitional and anaplastic growths, with only an occasional adenocarcinoma. In the sinuses, in contrast, squamous tumours account for fewer than half the carcinomas, transitional for one in about four, anaplastic for one in about four and adenocarcinomas arising from seromucinous glands for the rest.[84] The site of origin of the tumours of the sinuses may be difficult to determine: two thirds or so appear to arise in the maxillary sinus, especially its antro-ethmoidal angle, and the others are ethmoidal.[87] Carcinoma of a frontal sinus is rare: in our series of 154 carcinomas arising in the sinuses only one was in a frontal sinus.[88] Carcinoma of a sphenoidal sinus is even rarer.

The spread of a carcinoma of the nasal region depends to some extent on its site of origin. Most nasal carcinomas tend to remain localized for a considerable time; in contrast, antral and ethmoidal tumours frequently involve the lateral nasal wall and the nasal cavity at a comparatively early stage. The orbital cavity is much more frequently invaded by carcinomas arising in the antro-ethmoidal angle than by those strictly of ethmoidal origin.[87] Invasion of the anterior and lateral walls of the maxillary antrum by carcinoma arising there

often leads ultimately to involvement of the soft tissues of the cheek, sometimes with ulceration of the skin; the palate may also be invaded. Less frequently, there is extension from the antrum to the sphenoidal or frontal sinuses and the anterior cranial fossa. This may also occur, less rarely, in cases of ethmoidal carcinoma.

In our series, haematogenous spread occurred in 14 per cent of cases. Histologically confirmed lymph node involvement was much less frequent.[87]

Histopathology.—The *squamous carcinomas* of the nasal cavities and sinuses are usually moderately well differentiated, but there is often great variation within a single tumour and it is important to note that the degree of malignancy is determined by the least differentiated parts of any growth (Fig. 4.23).

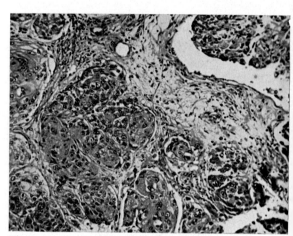

Fig. 4.23. Poorly differentiated, invasive, squamous carcinoma of maxillary antrum. *Haematoxylin–eosin.* × 100.

The *anaplastic carcinomas* may be pleomorphic or of spheroidal cell or spindle cell type; they are liable to be confused with amelanotic malignant melanoma and with myeloma. The 'oat cell' type of anaplastic carcinoma, so frequent in the lower parts of the respiratory tract (see page 396), is rarely—if, indeed, ever—seen in the nasal region.

The *transitional type of carcinoma* is of particular interest, for two reasons. First, because it resembles and may be related to the transitional type of papilloma (see page 217), and, second, because of its distinctive behaviour. The histological resemblance to the papilloma is readily apparent in the better differentiated tumours: the two have all too often been confused. The pattern of surface proliferation is the same, leading to infolding of the neoplastic epithelium: this is delineated by long stretches of basement membrane, which appears to be intact even when the polarity of the cells is disturbed and dedifferentiation marked. The persistence of the basement membrane results in the 'ribbon' or 'garland' appearance that has been considered characteristic (Fig. 4.24).[89, 90] In many areas the appearance is essentially that of an intraepithelial carcinoma: careful search may be necessary to establish the presence of areas of invasion, which are always present. Apart from this, the distinction from the transitional type of papilloma may be facilitated by recognition of disorientation of the epithelial structure, even in areas where the basement membrane is unbroached. Points that may be of further help in assessment are that the transitional type of carcinoma is relatively much less common in the nose than in the sinuses, in contrast to the papilloma, and that the predominant incidence of the benign growth in men is not a feature of the carcinoma.

It is possible that the benign papilloma may become malignant (see above). Most of the evidence, however, indicates that the transitional type of carcinoma is usually frankly malignant from the outset.

It is noteworthy that the tendency for the basement membrane to persist in cases of the transitional type of carcinoma indicates a relative inability of the tumour to grow invasively and so implies a better outlook. The five years survival rate in cases of this type of carcinoma of the nasal cavities (36 per cent) is about twice that of squamous and anaplastic carcinomas arising in these situations.[84]

Malignant Melanoma[91, 92]

It tends to come as a surprise to the general histopathologist to learn that malignant melanoma is second only to squamous carcinoma among the cancers that arise in the nasal region. Of 91 malignant nasal tumours seen in our practice over 21 years, 28 were malignant melanomas. The incidence of malignant melanoma in the nose is highest in the sixth decade. There is no significant sex difference. Most of the tumours arise in the nasal cavities; the small remaining proportion arises in the sinuses.

The pathogenesis, particularly the cytogenesis, of these tumours has recently been clarified by

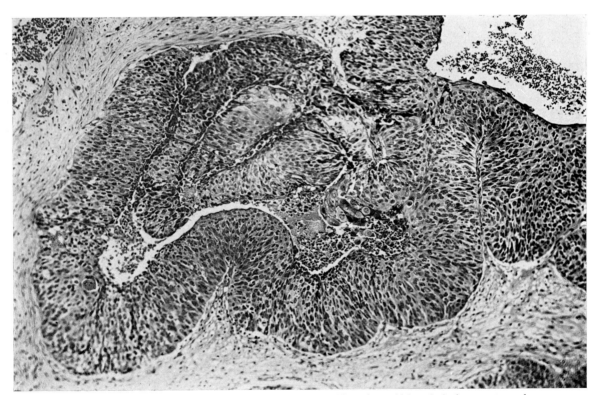

Fig. 4.24. Well-differentiated transitional type of carcinoma of a maxillary sinus. Although the basement membrane appears to be intact in the field photographed, the polarity of the epithelial cells is disturbed. The general pattern, with well marked folding of the epithelial layer, is that often described as the 'ribbon' or 'garland' appearance. *Haematoxylin–eosin.* × 85.

H*

the recognition, with the aid of silver staining methods, that melanin-containing dendritic cells are normally present in the nasal mucosa.[93] For long it had been generally believed that melanin is not found in the normal nasal mucosa except in the olfactory area, the natural brownish colour of which is due to the presence of this pigment in the supporting cells; in contrast, it was recognized that melanocytes are a regular constituent of the squamous epithelium of the nasal vestibules, as may be shown, for instance, by the DOPA-oxidase reaction.[94] It seemed a paradox that melanomas should be exceptionally rare in the vestibules, where melanocytes occur, and arise in the great majority of cases in a part of the mucous membrane where melanocytes were thought to be absent under normal circumstances. The demonstration of melanocytes in the respiratory epithelium of black people, and in nasal glands, and commonly in the superficial and deep stroma of the septum and of the middle and inferior conchae, in both blacks and whites, has indicated that the seeming paradox was based on inaccurate observation of the normal condition:[91] it may be concluded that the melanocytes of the mucosa are the source of the malignant melanomas that arise in these parts. In our experience, melanocytes are relatively seldom seen in the general run of biopsy specimens of the nasal respiratory mucosa: in contrast, they are conspicuously numerous in the respiratory mucosa adjacent to a primary melanoma. The explanation of this observation is obscure. It has been shown that melanogenesis in the oropharyngeal and nasal mucosa may be activated in the presence of a malignant melanoma of the oral cavity.[95]

The relation that exists between malignant melanoma and junctional naevus in the skin (see Chapter 39) has no counterpart in the nose, where the occurence of junctional naevi has not been demonstrated. In contrast, examination of malignant melanomas of the nose often reveals conspicuous changes in the immediately adjoining surface epithelium that may be compared with junctional activity in skin (see Chapter 39) (Fig. 4.25). Such a finding would seem to establish beyond doubt that a given melanoma in the nose is a primary tumour. It is of diagnostic interest to mention that such were the findings in two patients with intranasal melanoma whom we saw, each of whom had previously had a primary malignant melanoma of the skin of a limb. It is relevant here to recall that patients who have had a malignant melanoma are likelier to develop a second primary malignant melanoma than others are to develop a melanoma

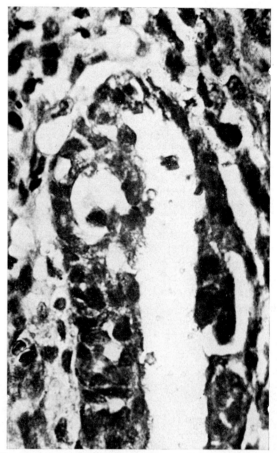

Fig. 4.25. Crypt-like fissure in the epithelial surface of the nasal mucosa. The crypt is lined by pseudostratified columnar ciliate epithelium of respiratory tract type. Two clear areas within this epithelium, enclosing nuclei, are melanocytes: the picture is that of junctional activity. It accompanies a primary malignant melanoma, the cells of which have diffusely infiltrated the subepithelial tissue included in the field. *Haematoxylin–eosin.* × 650.

at all.[96] The finding of junctional activity not only in the vicinity of primary nasal melanomas but also in what are regarded clinically as locally recurrent growths suggests that the latter are, in fact, fresh primary tumours and a manifestation of the multicentricity of the disease.

Macroscopically, malignant melanomas of the nose are usually polypoid. They may be pigmented or unpigmented. Microscopically, they show the pleomorphism characteristic of these tumours wherever they arise (see Chapter 39). The sarcoma-like spindle-celled form is the most frequent. Melanin is usually abundant: when it is scanty or absent the tumour is liable to be mistaken for an anaplastic carcinoma or sarcoma.

The prognosis is bad. Involvement of regional lymph nodes occurs at an early stage and there is often early and widespread dissemination through the blood stream.

2. Tumours Arising from Mucosal Glands

The mucous and seromucous glands of the upper respiratory tract can give rise to any of the range of tumours that characteristically are associated with the salivary glands (see Chapter 11). Such tumours account for about 5 per cent of all neoplasms of the nasal region. There are important differences in the frequency of the various types of tumour in the two situations. Pleomorphic tumours, exactly corresponding in structure and behaviour to the pleomorphic tumours of the salivary glands, are found only occasionally among the tumours of the glands of the nose and sinuses. Even rarer are the mucoepidermoid and acinar cell tumours, which again are in every respect comparable to those of the salivary glands. In contrast, adenomas and adenocarcinomas arising from ducts are relatively frequent in the nasal region.

Adenomas

The adenomas may be of a simple type, often formed of brightly eosinophile epithelium such as is characteristic of the salivary adenolymphomas, but without the lymphoid tissue that characterizes the latter. Alternatively, they may include a large proportion of mucus-secreting cells and, particularly when there is a cystic and papillary structure, the distinction from adenocarcinoma may be difficult. Such tumours may be referred to as *microcystic papillary adenomas* (Fig. 4.26): they are found most frequently in elderly people, and although their proliferative appearances and tendency to recur after excision may seem ominous there is no evidence that they are ever malignant.

Adenocarcinomas

Two distinct histological types of adenocarcinoma arise from the mucosal glands. The more frequent

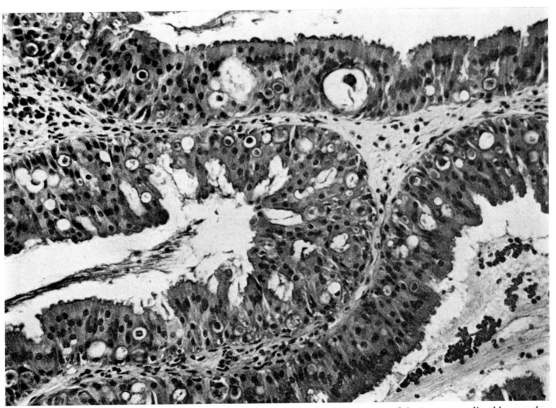

Fig. 4.26. Microcystic papillary adenoma of a maxillary sinus. The gland-like spaces of the tumour are lined by pseudo-stratified ciliate columnar epithelium in which there are numerous rounded mucigenic cells. The latter are sometimes grouped to form superficial crypts in the epithelium. The mucigenic cells have been mistaken for coccidia or other intra-epithelial protozoal parasites (by the editor, for instance). *Haematoxylin–eosin.* × 250.

type is usually found in the nose or ethmoid sinuses. It has a tubular, cystic and papillary structure and is formed of columnar or mucus-secreting cells (Figs 4.27 and 4.28). Sometimes the production of mucus is very abundant. Occasionally, tumours of this type are occupational in origin, developing in those whose work exposes them to the dust of fine woods used in the furniture trade (Fig. 4.27).[97]

The second type of adenocarcinoma, the adenoid cystic carcinoma (cribriform adenocarcinoma, or 'cylindroma') (Figs 4.29 and 4.30), occurs most frequently in the maxillary sinuses. It is sometimes confused with the ameloblastoma (see Chapter 12), particularly in view of its situation: the distinction is important, particularly prognostically, for the cribriform adenocarcinoma, while initially radio-sensitive, has a marked tendency to recur locally and ultimately to metastasize widely.

3. Neurogenic Tumours

Neurofibroma and Neurolemmoma

These tumours may be found in the nasal cavities and in the sinuses, particularly the former. They are rare: there were only seven in a series of 646 tumours of the nasal cavities that we collected. Recurrence has been observed, even many years after initial excision, but frankly malignant behaviour is very rare.

Nasal 'Glioma'[98-101]

The so-called 'glioma' of the nose is a very rare tumour-like lesion that is seen almost exclusively in young children. It presents as a rounded projection beneath the skin at the root of the nose or under the mucosa of the upper part of a nasal

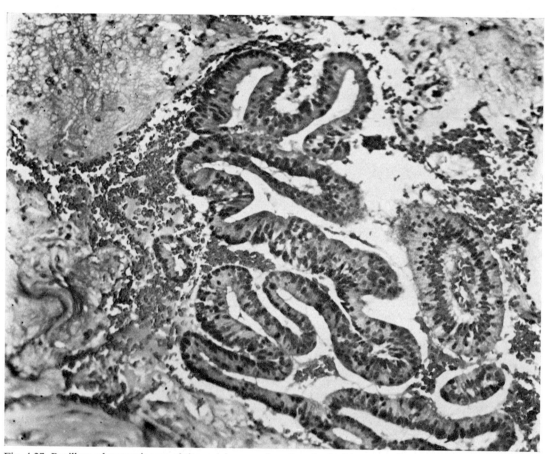

Fig. 4.27. Papillary adenocarcinoma of the nose in a wood-worker. In this biopsy specimen the papilliform epithelium has become separated from its stromal attachment except in relatively small areas, such as the transected papilla to the right in the picture. Much mucus and blood are included in the specimen. In such biopsy material it may be difficult to find recognizable tumour tissue. It is for such reasons that it is essential to section *all* the material obtained by the surgeon. *Haematoxylin–eosin.* × 180.

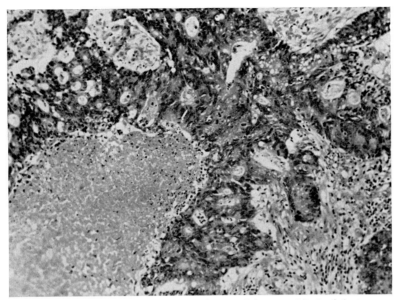

Fig. 4.28. Papillary and tubular adenocarcinoma of the nose. Much of the tumour is necrotic (lower left quadrant) and its papillary structure is scarcely evident in this field. *Haematoxylin–eosin.* × 110.

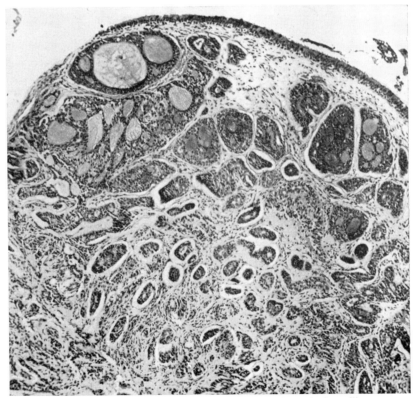

Fig. 4.29. Adenoid cystic carcinoma (cribriform adenocarcinoma) of maxillary antrum. The tumour presented with the clinical picture of a unilateral 'nasal polyp'. *Haematoxylin–eosin.* × 75.

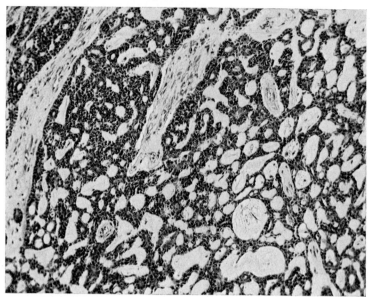

Fig. 4.30. Adenoid cystic carcinoma (cribriform adenocarcinoma) of maxillary antrum, showing characteristic 'cylindromatous' pattern. *Haematoxylin–eosin.* ×110.

cavity. It may be extranasal or intranasal, or both, with or without an intracranial attachment by a stalk traversing a gap in the skull. It is quite benign, and—apart from some enlargement during the first weeks or months of life in a minority of cases—it shows no tendency to grow. There seems little doubt that it is a congenital anomaly, arising in glial tissue that has been sequestered in the nasal region as a developmental fault. Those exceptional examples that are recognized in older children or adults[102] may also be regarded as congenital.

Microscopically, the 'glioma' consists of mature glial tissue (Fig. 4.31). Most of the cells are astrocytes and some of these are multinucleate. The cells are usually sparsely scattered throughout the matrix of glial fibres; in places they may assume a rosette formation. Neurons are not present.

Olfactory Neuroblastoma (Olfactory Neuroepithelial Tumour)

The great rarity of this tumour—the olfactory aesthesioneuroepithelioma of French authors[103]—is indicated by the fact that only one instance was included among 750 consecutive cases of tumour of the nasal cavities in the practice of the Royal National Throat, Nose and Ear Hospital, London, during a period of 24 years. It arises from the neural component of the olfactory epithelium. Its peak incidence is in the second decade, but an

appreciable proportion of the cases occurs among adults, particularly the middle-aged and elderly.[104]

The tumour presents in the upper part of a nasal cavity, often as a haemorrhagic mass with evidence of bone destruction. Microscopically, it is characterized by rounded, compact, cellular foci separated by very vascular stroma. The nucleus of the tumour cells is oval or round and stains deeply, and the growth often has some resemblance to a lymphocytic tumour; in general, however, the cells have more cytoplasm than lymphocytes, although it tends to be so poorly defined that the appearances are those of 'naked' nuclei. The presence of rosettes is diagnostically important: they may be of the type conventionally referred to as 'pseudorosettes', consisting of cuboidal or columnar cells about a central space, thus resembling a glandular structure, or they may be the so-called 'true rosettes', the cells enclosing fibrillary or granular material (Fig. 4.32).

Electron microscopy shows that the cytoplasm of the tumour cells contains small granules, consistent with catecholamine storage.

The olfactory neuroblastoma differs from neuroblastomas of the adrenal glands and sympathetic nervous system in its age incidence and in prognosis. It is said to have a five years survival rate of 50 per cent.[104] Metastasis occurs both by lymphatics, with involvement of regional and more distant lymph nodes, and in the blood. Haematogenous secondary deposits are seen most frequently

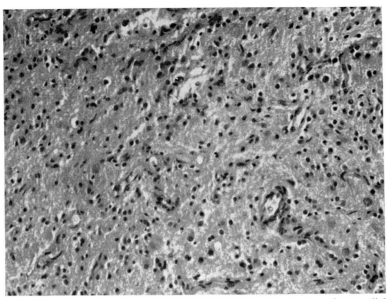

Fig. 4.31. 'Glioma' of the nose. The histological structure is that of neuroglial tissue. *Haematoxylin–eosin.* × 200.

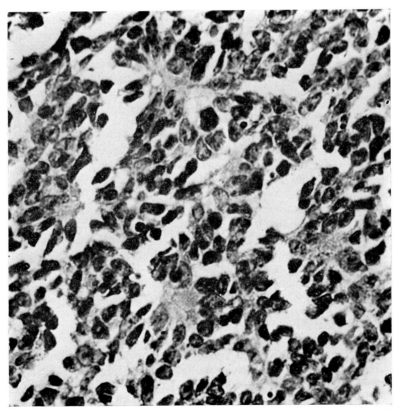

Fig. 4.32. Olfactory neuroblastoma. Several rosette-like formations are included in the field. *Haematoxylin–eosin.* × 800.

in the lungs and liver. Interestingly, they have occasionally been found in the skeleton, leading to a diagnosis of 'Ewing's tumour', as may occur in cases of secondary neuroblastoma of adrenal origin.[102]

Meningioma

The very rare extracranial meningioma may present as a polypoid nasal lesion.[105]

4. Tumours of Vascular Origin

The lesions that may be considered under this heading include some that are not true tumours. As the clinical presentation may be like that of a neoplasm, and as the histological interpretation is sometimes debatable, it is appropriate to consider these various conditions in the present context.

Capillary Haemangioma

Many tumour pathologists regard all benign vascular growths as hamartomatous malformations,[106] a view presupposing their presence in some form at the time of birth. As so many of these lesions occur in young patients this view would seem in general to be acceptable. In the nasal region, however, the angioma has its peak incidence in the fifth and sixth decades, and its history is usually short—less than six months in most of our cases: such a lesion is more easily explained as of recent origin than as a result of activation in middle life of a congenital condition. Confusingly, these nasal angiomas are often referred to as *angiofibromas*, although in structure they resemble haemangiomas of other parts of the body. They must not be mistaken terminologically for juvenile angiofibroma, another benign condition but of totally different origin and presentation (see below).

Macroscopically, the capillary haemangioma is usually a sessile or polypoid swelling, a few millimetres across. In 9 out of 10 instances it is situated on the septum; the tenth is on a concha or on the lateral wall of the nasal cavity. The usual site of the septal angioma is Little's 'bleeding area'—the anteroinferior part of the septum where the main septal branch of the sphenopalatine artery anastomoses with the septal branch of the superior labial artery. In exceptional instances, the angioma becomes a large, tense and very hyperaemic mass that protrudes from the nostril.

Microscopically, well-formed capillaries are arranged in a lobular pattern; the intervening connective tissue is of varying density but often rather oedematous. Some of the vessels may be obliterated by thrombosis: different stages in organization and scarring will then be seen. Iron pigment may be scattered in the tissue, usually sparsely. Very rarely, there is so much pigment, much of it within macrophages, that the unwary may misinterpret the lesion as a malignant melanoma. Inflammatory cells are sparse or absent unless ulceration has occurred.

It is those lesions in which there is a heavy inflammatory infiltrate that acquired the name 'pyogenic granuloma' or 'telangiectatic granuloma', both of them misleading terms (see also Chapters 12 and 39). The term 'haemangiomatous granulation tissue' has been suggested;[107] other authorities regard the lesions as true capillary haemangiomas.[108]

Juvenile Angiofibroma (Juvenile Fibroma)

This is a lesion less common and more serious than the capillary haemangioma. It is unrelated to the latter, although confusion has been caused by the occasional designation of the angioma as angiofibroma (see above). While the juvenile angiofibroma is often said to be a nasopharyngeal growth, it is more appropriately discussed here, for reasons that should become evident.

It is a disease pre-eminently of boys. It is rare before the age of 10 years: most cases present at about the time of puberty. Although significantly commoner in the Far East than elsewhere, and particularly among Chinese, this growth may be found in patients in any part of the world and of any race. Ten cases were recognized at the Royal National Throat, Nose and Ear Hospital in London in a recent period of 21 years. Sometimes the disease is familial.

Contrary to a frequently expressed view, there is no doubt that the disease may occur in girls,[109] but this is exceptionally rare. Indeed, it is important to note that when the clinical picture in a girl or woman seems to be that of juvenile angiofibroma the cause is almost always a fibrosarcoma (see page 232).

Clinical Manifestations.—The first symptoms are nasal obstruction and, less constantly, bleeding. Severe epistaxis is unusual, except as a complication of surgery: bleeding following a biopsy operation has occasionally been uncontrollable and followed by death. As the tumour grows it tends to fill the nasal and postnasal cavities; its bulk may cause those bones of the base of the skull that have not yet completed osseous union to be forced apart. Although the tumour does not invade the bones its mass may lead to extensive local destruction of the cranium through pressure atrophy, and in rare cases this has been complicated by suppurative meningitis. As the space between the orbits gradually widens to accommodate the growing tumour, the characteristic 'frog-face' deformity results: this has been described particularly among Chinese patients and occurs only rarely among those of other races. The disfiguration persists permanently after the angiofibroma has finally become inactive.

Histopathology.—Macroscopically, the lesion appears vascular, oedematous and often haemorrhagic. In most cases its principal attachments are at the margins of the choanae and it extends both forward into the nasal cavities and backward into the postnasal space.[110] It is usually symmetrically disposed; rarely, the condition is confined, or largely so, to one side, and the resultant disfiguration is correspondingly unilateral. Occasionally, it arises in a maxillary sinus.[111, 112] Although the growth may have some attachment in the postnasal region, this is generally trivial in comparison with the involvement of the structures of the nasal wall: it is for this reason that the disease is better considered in the context of the nose than among diseases affecting the nasopharynx primarily. In exceptional cases the growth spreads so far forward within the nasal cavity that it presents at the nostril on one or both sides.

Microscopically, the angiofibroma consists of numerous vascular channels embedded in fibrous tissue (Fig. 4.33). The latter varies in texture from

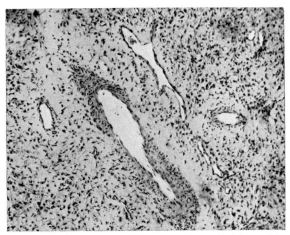
Fig. 4.34. Juvenile angiofibroma, showing a blood vessel in which there is an abrupt transition between stretches with a thick, muscular wall and others with only an endothelial lining. *Haematoxylin–eosin.* × 55.

a compact, hyaline mass to an oedematous granulation tissue; in general it has a laminar pattern, reminiscent of scar tissue, rather than the whorled and fascicular arrangement more characteristic of fibromas. The wall of many of the vessels is no more than a layer of endothelium: the liability to bleeding is readily understood. Some vessels, however, have a muscular wall; this often varies remarkably in the degree of its development, and there are abrupt transitions between stretches where there is a thick, well-defined muscle coat and those with no more than the simple endothelial layer between lumen and fibrous tissue (Fig. 4.34). These vessels probably represent a malformation of the structures concerned in the formation of the nasal erectile tissue (see page 193).[110] Other microscopical features of the lesions are more or less extensive foci of reparative granulation tissue, haemorrhages and scattered clusters of mast cells.

Nature of Juvenile Angiofibroma.—Earlier views of the nature of juvenile angiofibroma of the nose were coloured by preoccupation with the fibrous component, to the exclusion of considering the significance of the peculiar vasculature, and by confusion regarding the anatomical site of its origin.[98, 113] It was thought by some that the disease is a form of dysplasia of specialized vascular and connective tissue of the nasopharyngeal mucoperiosteum, and perhaps related to the various forms of fascial and aponeurotic 'fibromatoses' that are familiar in the plantar and palmar tissues and elsewhere (see Chapter 38).

More recently, the angiofibroma has been seen

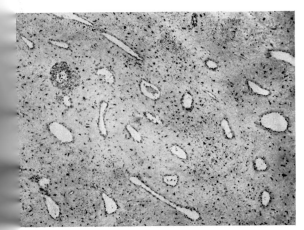
Fig. 4.33. Juvenile angiofibroma, showing numerous thin-walled blood vessels. *Haematoxylin–eosin.* × 65.

as a malformation of vascular tissue.[110, 114, 115] The nasal erectile tissue, because of its complex development and its concentration toward the back of the nasal cavities (see page 193), is the likeliest source.[110] Transmission of the arterial blood pressure directly into the capillaries can result in oedema and bleeding: reparative activity follows, and as this sequence is repeated, proliferative fibrosis becomes more extensive and accounts for the growth of the lesion. The eventual distribution of these changes is ultimately limited by the degree and anatomical extent of the vascular malformation. This also accords with the observed facts that the development of the condition is seen progressively less frequently in successive age groups, and not at all after early adulthood, while existing lesions become progressively less vascular and have run the whole of their self-limiting course before the patient is 25 or so.

The sex incidence of juvenile angiofibroma could be thought an impediment to accepting the malformation theory. The explanation of the remarkable preponderance of boys among patients with the disease remains obscure. The possible relation between the nasal erectile tissue and the erectile tissue of the genital organs (page 193) may have some potential aetiological significance,[107] perhaps in terms of an anomalous hypertrophic response to the physiological hormonal changes associated with puberty.

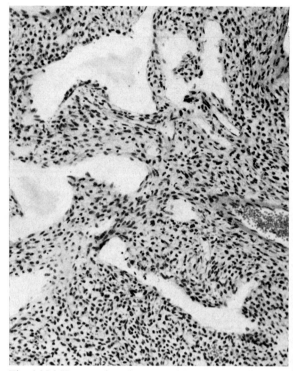

Fig. 4.35.§ Haemangiopericytoma of the nose. See Fig. 4.36 also. *Haematoxylin–eosin.* × 100.

Malignant Vascular Tumours

Angiosarcomas are rare in the nose. They include the haemangiopericytoma and, even rarer, the haemangioendothelioma. The former occurs at any age, but usually in older adults. It presents as a haemorrhagic mass. It has some tendency to recur after treatment, but while unquestionably sarcomatous, its malignant potential is often low. The histological picture varies and may be difficult to interpret: in typical areas, endothelium-lined spaces are separated by relatively solid masses formed of rounded, spindle-shaped or stellate cells (Figs 4.35 and 4.36). The distinction between pericytoma and angioendothelioma may be facilitated by reticulin impregnation, which delineates the basement membrane of the vascular spaces: the cells of the endothelioma are inside the area delimited by the membrane whereas the cells of the pericytoma are outside the membrane. In some cases, however, the findings are equivocal: these are usually the less differentiated tumours and they are correspondingly more malignant in their behaviour.

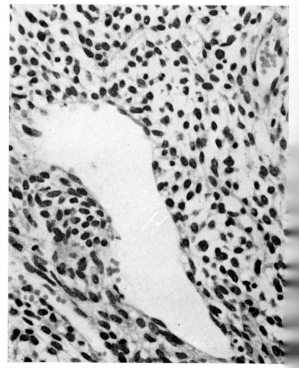

Fig. 4.36.§ Haemangiopericytoma. Same specimen as in Fig. 4.35. *Haematoxylin–eosin.* × 250.

5. Tumours of Lymphoreticular Tissue

Lymphomas

Lymphomas, particularly immunoblastic and histiocytic lymphomas, may arise in the nasal cavities or sinuses. They account for well under 10 per cent of all malignant tumours of the nasal region: this reflects the relative paucity of lymphoreticular tissue in these parts in contrast to its abundance in the nasopharynx and the relatively much greater frequency of lymphomas there (see page 243).

Myeloma (Plasmacytoma)

The upper respiratory tract is the most frequent site of extraosseous myelomas.[116] Although these tumours are not generally considered with the lymphomas, this seems a reasonable place to discuss them in the context of this chapter. The extraosseous myeloma is usually solitary: it arises most frequently in the mucous membrane of the nasal cavity itself; exceptionally, its origin is in the sinuses, usually a maxillary sinus. It must always be regarded as a malignant tumour In a small proportion of cases it is a manifestation of myelomatosis, usually antedating the symptoms of the latter: this means that in every case of nasal myeloma biochemical and radiological investigations must be carried out. It may be emphasized that examination of the urine by concentration methods may disclose the presence of Bence-Jones protein even when there is no apparent abnormality of the plasma protein pattern.[117] Only when the results of these examinations remain negative over several years can the prognosis be regarded as favourable, and even then it has been known for the nasal growth itself to give rise to widespread metastasis, usually to extraskeletal sites, after many years of latency. Similarly, myelomatosis has been known to appear as long as 15 years after the initial diagnosis of an extraosseous nasal myeloma. The prognosis of the latter is therefore always difficult to assess: even in the presence of myelomatosis the course of the disease may be long.

Nasal myelomas tend to obstruct the airway. They become ulcerated and may be the source of troublesome and even dangerous bleeding. They are usually radiosensitive and their early recognition is therefore of practical importance. A diagnostic difficulty lies in the fact that plasma cells may be present in large numbers in many simple nasal polyps (see page 199) and other inflammatory lesions of the upper respiratory tract. In the latter plasma cells may so greatly outnumber other inflammatory cells that the term *plasma cell granuloma* is sometimes applied, although this says nothing of the cause and nature of such lesions and serves no useful purpose beyond the important one of reminding us of the liability to mistake inflammatory conditions for myeloma. Among the specific infections that may be histologically misinterpreted in this way, scleroma deserves more attention than it usually gets (see page 204): we know of two cases of scleroma, acquired in Central Africa and first investigated when the patients returned to Europe, in which the appearances in biopsy specimens were interpreted as myelomatous and not reconsidered until long afterwards, when repeated courses of radiotherapy and cytotoxic drugs had failed to cure the disease (Fig. 4.6).[118]

Some nasal myelomas contain extracellular, eosinophile, crystalloid material that is probably a globulin precipitate. Such material may be present in solitary tumours and does not necessarily indicate that the lesion is a manifestation of myelomatosis. Similarly, amyloid may be deposited in the stroma of solitary extraskeletal myelomas without ominous significance; generalized amyloidosis, in contrast, is not found unless the local tumour is associated with skeletal myelomatosis.

Russell bodies are sometimes found in myelomas but are more characteristic of plasma cell granulomas.

Myeloma cells may be so well differentiated that it is impossible to distinguish them individually from non-neoplastic plasma cells; equally, they may be so atypical that many fields and even many samples of tumour must be examined before their nature is recognized. Most myelomas in the nasal region are quite readily identified correctly. The less differentiated tumours are sometimes confused with lymphosarcoma or anaplastic carcinomas. Electron microscopy demonstrates the presence in the myeloma cell of abundant rough endoplasmic reticulum: this may be invaluable in distinguishing myeloma from anaplastic tumours.[119]

6. Tumours of the Skeletal and Fibrous Connective Tissues

Benign Tumours and Tumour-Like Lesions

Benign Skeletal Growths.—The least rare benign growths of connective tissue in this region are chondromas and osteomas. *Chondromas* are occasionally found in the nasal cavities, usually arising from the septum (cartilaginous tumours in the sinuses are generally sarcomatous, even when slowly growing). *Osteomas* occur most frequently in the frontal sinuses. They may reach a large size, filling the sinus and leading to its considerable distension: they form a sessile or pedunculate mass, often with a coarsely lobulate surface; the overlying mucosa may be intact, although atrophic, or ulcerated if infection has developed. Microscopically, they range from the dense 'ivory' osteoma to the rarer cancellous osteoma, which may be finely or coarsely trabeculate. The structural differences may reflect the degree of osteoblastic activity.

The maxillary sinuses and, less often, the nasal cavities may be involved by disorders of bone that affect the maxilla.[120] The latter include *ossifying fibromas*, *reparative granulomas* (see below), *fibrous dysplasia* (see below) and *solitary bone cysts*. The histological distinction between these conditions is not always straightforward, particularly when only small biopsy specimens are available, and particularly when inflammatory changes have been added in consequence of ulceration and infection (see Chapter 37). The disfiguring appearance that is sometimes described as *leontiasis ossea* may result from the presence of certain of these disorders, including Paget's disease of bone and fibrous dysplasia.

Paget's disease of the bones of the nose is usually a manifestation of general skeletal involvement (see Chapter 37).

Fibrous dysplasia of bone may involve any part of the nasal skeleton.[121] It may occur at any age and is usually of the monostotic type. The histological appearances are described in Chapter 37.

The *giant-celled reparative granuloma* of bone (see Chapter 37) may simulate a neoplasm both clinically and histologically. It is especially liable to be confused with osteoclastoma because the haemorrhagic granulation tissue contains small, irregularly scattered clusters of osteoclasts (Fig. 4.37).[122]

Fibromas.—True fibromas are very rare in the nasal region. They must be distinguished from fibrosarcomas (see below) and neurofibromas (page 224), juvenile angiofibroma (page 228) and the skeletal disorders noted above, as well as various other non-neoplastic conditions, even including atypical manifestations of infections (for instance, leprosy—see Fig. 4.38).

Sarcomas

Sarcomas of the nose and sinuses are much less frequent than carcinomas. The surprisingly high incidence reported by earlier workers probably

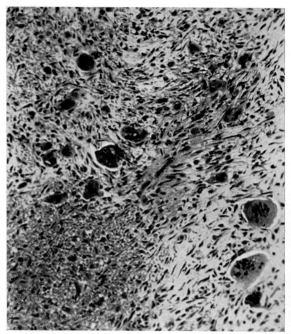

Fig. 4.37. Reparative granuloma of the jaw, with osteoclasts in dense fibrous tissue adjacent to a small haemorrhage. *Haematoxylin–eosin.* × 150.

reflected misinterpretation of anaplastic carcinomas as sarcomatous. The least rare varieties, in descending order of frequency, are fibrosarcoma, chondrosarcoma, lymphosarcoma and reticulum cell sarcoma (see page 231), osteogenic sarcoma and rhabdomyosarcoma.[123, 124] Overall, they account for about 15 per cent of all malignant tumours of the nasal region. They arise in the sinuses more frequently than in the nasal cavities. They occur at any age and are about equally distributed between the sexes.

The *fibrosarcomas* grow comparatively slowly. For this reason patients survive appreciably longer with a fibrosarcoma of the nasal region than with most forms of nasal carcinoma. Confusion with juvenile angiofibroma has to be avoided (see page 228).

Chondrosarcomas vary greatly in behaviour, which in general reflects the apparent degree of malignancy indicated by the histological picture. Many of the more slowly growing chondrosarcomas are distinguishable only with difficulty from the benign cartilaginous tumours of the region.

Osteogenic sarcomas are generally regarded as occurring much less frequently than fibrosarcoma and chondrosarcomas. However, it must be remembered that an unrepresentative biopsy specimen of

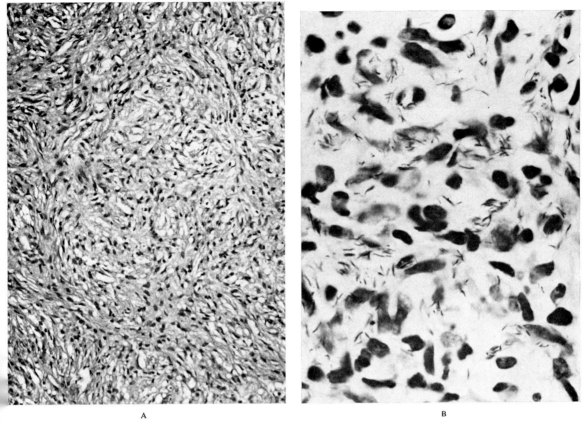

A   B

Fig. 4.38.§ Lepromatous leprosy. The clinical presentation was atypical: the lesion was a small, pale, discrete, hard, solitary nodule in the mucosa of the atrium of the middle meatus. It was thought to be a tumour—possibly a fibroma—and excised *in toto*. The initial histological diagnosis was 'fibromatoid histiocytoma' (Fig. 4.38A), supposedly related to the common dermatofibroma (see Chapter 39). Another microscopist was unconvinced and asked for a Ziehl–Neelsen preparation (Fig. 4.38B), which confirmed his suspicion, showing large numbers of leprosy bacilli to be present. Fig. 4.38A: *haematoxylin–eosin;* ×150. Fig. 4.38B: *Ziehl–Neelsen stain;* ×750.

a pleomorphic osteogenic tumour may include no tissue indicative of its real nature: a small but significant proportion of tumours initially diagnosed as chondrosarcomas turn out to be osteogenic.

Rhabdomyosarcomas are among the rarest nasal tumours. They are notably less rare in the naso-pharynx (see page 243), where most examples involving the nose originate.

7. Secondary Tumours

A too frequent cause of misdiagnosis is failure to consider the possibility that a tumour in the nasal region may be a secondary deposit from a cancer elsewhere in the body. Metastatic tumours in the nose may present as polyp-like lesions, a fact that justifies reiteration of our view that all polyps and polyp-like lesions removed from the nose must be examined, and sufficiently examined, histologically.

In a review of secondary tumours in the nose, throat and ears it was found that more than half occurred in the nose and sinuses.[125] Adeno-carcinoma of renal origin and anaplastic carcinoma of bronchial origin are the primary growths that most frequently metastasize to the nasal region.

REFERENCES

STRUCTURAL AND FUNCTIONAL CONSIDERATIONS

1. Merker, H. J., *Arzneimittel-Forsch.*, 1966, **16**, 509.
2. Rivera y Pomar, J. M., Sanchez, F., *Rev. Fac. Med. Sevilla*, 1969, **1**, 29.
3. Friedmann, I., Bird, E. S., *Laryngoscope (St Louis)*, 1971, **81**, 1852.
4. Fawcett, D. W., Porter, K. R., *J. Morph.*, 1954, **94**, 221.
5. Anderson, R. G. W., *Primate News*, 1971, **9**, 5.
6. Sade, J., Eliezer, N., Silberberg, A., Nevo, A. C., *Amer. Rev. resp. Dis.*, 1970, **102**, 48.
7. Swindle, P. F., *Ann. Otol. (St Louis)*, 1937, **46**, 600.
8. Mackenzie, J. N., *Johns Hopk. Hosp. Bull.*, 1898, **9**, 10.
9. Proetz, A. W., *Essays on the Applied Physiology of the Nose*, 2nd edn. St Louis, 1953.
10. Negus, V. E., *The Comparative Anatomy and Physiology of the Nose and Paranasal Sinuses*. Edinburgh and London, 1958.
11. Krauss, B., Kitamura, H., Latham, R. A., *Atlas of Developmental Anatomy of the Face*. New York and London, 1966.
12. McKenzie, J., *Arch. Dis. Childh.*, 1958, **33**, 477.

INFLAMMATORY CONDITIONS

13. *Report of the Medical Research Council for the Year 1959–1960*, page 18. London, 1961.
14. Tyrrell, D. A. J., Bynoe, M. L., Hitchcock, G., Pereira, H. C., Andrewes, C. H., *Lancet*, 1960, **1**, 235.
15. Tyrrell, D. A. J., Bynoe, M. L., *Brit. med. J.*, 1961, **1**, 393.
16. Cherubino, M., *Boll. Mal. Orecch.*, 1956, **74**, 360.
17. Henriksen, S. D., Gundersen, W. B., *Acta path. microbiol. scand.*, 1959, **47**, 380.
18. Anderson, P. S., Jr, Cowles, P. B., *Nature (Lond.)*, 1958, **181**, 350.
19. Anderson, P. S., Jr, Cowles, P. B., *J. Bact.*, 1958, **76**, 272.
20. Lucas, H. A., *J. Laryng.*, 1952, **66**, 480.
21. Berdal, P., *Acta oto-laryng. (Stockh.)*, 1954, suppl. 115, 7.
22. Donovan, R., Johansson, S. G. O., Bennich, H., Soothill, J. F., *Int. Arch. Allergy*, 1970, **37**, 154.
23. Blackley, C. H., *Experimental Researches on the Causes and Nature of* Catarrhus aestivus. London, 1873.
24. Urbach, E., Gottlieb, P. M., *Allergy*, 2nd edn. New York, 1946.
25. Manson-Bahr, P. H., *J. Laryng.*, 1956, **70**, 175.
26. Hunter, D., *The Diseases of Occupations*, 4th edn, page 457. London, 1969.
27. Hebra, F., *Wien. med. Wschr.*, 1870, **20**, 1.
28. Shaw, H. J., Martin, H., *J. Laryng.*, 1961, **75**, 1011.
29. Symmers, W. St C., *unpublished observations*.
30. Oomen, H. A. P. C., *Docum. Med. geogr. trop. (Amst.)*, 1952, **4**, 124.
31. Mott, F. W., *Proc. roy. Soc. B*, 1905, **76**, 235.
32. Thiéry, J. P., in *Cellular Aspects of Immunity*, edited by G. E. W. Wolstenholme and M. O'Connor, page 59. London, 1960.
33. Friedmann, I., *Sci. Basis Med.*, 1963, 302.

34. Friedmann, I., *Trans. Amer. Acad. Ophthal. Otolaryng.*, 1963, **67**, 261.
35. Shaw, H. J., Martin, H., *J. Laryng.*, 1961, **75**, 1011.
36. Symmers, W. St C., *personal observations*, 1967–1975.
37. Osborn, D. A., *J. Laryng.*, 1963, **77**, 29.
38. Martinson, F. D., *Amer. J. trop. Med. Hyg.*, 1971, **20**, 449.
39. Emmons, C. W., Bridges, C. H., *Mycologia*, 1961, **53**, 307.
40. Bras, G., Gordon, C. C., Emmons, C. W., Prendegast, K. M., Sugar, M., *Amer. J. trop. Med. Hyg.*, 1965, **14**, 141.
41. Martinson, F. D., Clark, B. M., *Amer. J. trop. Med. Hyg.*, 1967, **16**, 40.
42. Andrade, Z. A., Araújo Paula, L., Sherlock, I. A., Cheever, A. W., *Amer. J. trop. Med. Hyg.*, 1967, **16**, 31.
43. Grueber, H. L. E., *J. Christ. med. Ass. India*, 1969, **44**, 20.
44. Symmers, W. St C., *personal observation*, 1969.
45. Symmers, W. St C., *Ann. Soc. belge Méd. trop.*, 1972, **52**, 365.
46. Williams, A. O., *Arch. Path.*, 1969, **87**, 13.
47. Baker, R. D., in *Human Infection with Fungi, Actinomycetes and Algae*, page 832. New York, Heidelberg, Berlin, 1971.
48. Gregory, J. E., Golden, A., Haymaker, W., *Bull. Johns Hopk. Hosp.*, 1943, **73**, 405.
49. Symmers, W. St C., *Proc. roy. Soc. Med.*, 1965, **58**, 341.
50. Sandison, A. T., Gentles, J. C., Davidson, C. M., Branko, M., *Sabouraudia*, 1967, **6**, 57.
51. Milošev, B., Mahgoub, El S., Abdel Aal, O., El Hassan, A. M., *Brit. J. Surg.*, 1969, **56**, 132.
52. Symmers, W. St C., *personal communication*, 1973.
53. Satyanarayana, C., *Acta oto-laryng. (Stockh.)*, 1960, **51**, 348.
54. Karunaratne, W. A. E., *Rhinosporidiosis in Man*. London, 1964.
55. Symmers, W. St C., *Amer. J. clin. Path.*, 1966, **46**, 51 [cases 34–37].
56. Manson-Bahr, P. E. C., Winslow, D. J., in *Pathology of Protozoal and Helminthic Diseases with Clinical Correlation*, edited by R. A. Marcial-Rojas and E. Moreno, chap. 4. Baltimore, 1971.
57. Jaffé, L., *A.M.A. Arch. Otolaryng.*, 1954, **60**, 601.
58. Emslie, E. S., *Brit. med. J.*, 1962, **1**, 299.
59. Woo, Z.-P., Reimann, H. A., *J. Amer. med. Ass.*, 1957, **164**, 1092.
60. Montgomerie, J. Z., Becroft, D. M. O., Croxson, M. C., Doak, P. B., North, J. D. K., *Lancet*, 1969, **2**, 867.
61. Friedmann, I., *J. Laryng.*, 1971, **85**, 631.
62. Moschella, S. L., *Cutis*, 1973, **11**, 650.
63. Harrison, D. F. N., *Brit. med. J.*, 1974, **4**, 205.
64. Wegener, F., *Beitr. path. Anat.*, 1939, **102**, 36.
65. Friedmann, I., *personal observations*.
66. McKinnon, D. M., *J. Laryng.*, 1970, **84**, 1193.
67. Walton, E. W., *Brit. med. J.*, 1958, **2**, 265.
68. Symmers, W. St C., *J. clin. Path.*, 1960, **13**, 1.
69. Woods, R., *Brit. med. J.*, 1921, **2**, 65.
70. Stewart, J. P., *J. Laryng.*, 1933, **48**, 657.

71. Friedmann, I., *J. Laryng.*, 1955, **69**, 331.

72. Williams, H. L., *Ann. Otol. (St Louis)*, 1949, **58**, 1013.

72a. Fechner, R. E., Lamppin, D. W., *Arch. Otolaryng.*, 1972, **95**, 467.

73. Walton, E. W., *J. clin. Path.*, 1960, **13**, 279.

74. Ellis, M., *Ann. Otol. (St Louis)*, 1957, **66**, 1002.

75. McKinnon, D. M., *J. Laryng.*, 1970, **84**, 1193.

76. Appaix, A., Pech, A., Cadoccioni, J. M., *J. franç. Oto-rhino-laryng.*, 1959, **8**, 737.

77. Nieberding, P. H., Schiff, M., Harmeling, J. G., *Arch. Otolaryng.*, 1962, **77**, 512.

78. Liebow, A. A., Carrington, C. R. B., Friedman, P. J., *Hum. Path.*, 1972, **3**, 457.

79. Harrison, D. F. N., *Brit. med. J.*, 1974, **4**, 205.

TUMOURS OF THE NOSE AND NASAL SINUSES

80. Friedmann, I., *J. Laryng.*, 1951, **65**, 1.

81. McGrew, E. A., *Postgrad. med. J.*, 1961, **37**, 456.

82. Venkei, T., Sugar, J., *Derm. Wschr.*, 1958, **138**, 957.

83. Osborn, D. A., *J. Laryng.*, 1956, **70**, 574.

84. Osborn, D. A., *Cancer (Philad.)*, 1970, **25**, 50.

85. Fechner, R. E., Alford, D. O., *Arch. Otolaryng.*, 1968, **88**, 507.

86. Schoub, L., Timme, A. H., Uys, C. J., *S. Afr. med. J.*, 1973, **47**, 1663.

87. Osborn, D. A., Winston, P., *J. Laryng.*, 1961, **75**, 387.

88. Osborn, D. A., Wallace, M., *J. Laryng.*, 1967, **81**, 1021.

89. Ringertz, N., *Acta oto-laryng. (Stockh.)*, 1938, suppl. 27.

90. Lewis, M. G., Martin, J. A. M., *Cancer (Philad.)*, 1967, **20**, 1699.

91. Mason, M., Friedmann, I., *J. Laryng.*, 1955, **69**, 98.

92. Mesara, B. W., Burton, W. D., *Cancer (Philad.)*, 1968, **21**, 217.

93. Zak, F. G., Lawson, W., *Ann. Otol. (St Louis)*, 1974, **83**, 515.

94. Szabo, G., in *Pigment Cell Biology*, edited by M. Gordon, page 99. New York, 1959.

95. Takagi, M., Ishikawa, G., Wataru, M., *Cancer (Philad.)*, 1974, **34**, 358.

96. Allen, A. C., Spitz, S., *Cancer (Philad.)*, 1953, **6**, 1.

97. Acheson, E. D., Hadfield, E., Macbeth, R. G., *Lancet*, 1967, **1**, 311.

98. Ringertz, N., *Acta oto-laryng. (Stockh.)*, 1938, suppl. 27.

99. Bratton, A. B., Robinson, S. H. G., *J. Path. Bact.*, 1946, **58**, 643.

100. Zettergren, L., *Acta path. microbiol. scand.*, 1948, **25**, 672.

101. Cuthbert, N. M., *Med. J. Aust.*, 1950, **1**, 46.

102. Symmers, W. St C., *personal communication*, 1973.

103. Berger, L., Luc, R., *Bull. Ass. franç. Cancer*, 1924, **13**, 410.

104. Lewis, J. S., Hutter, R. V. P., Tollefsen, H. R., Foote, F. W., *Arch. Otolaryng.*, 1965, **81**, 169.

105. Kjeldsberg, C. R., Minckler, J., *Cancer (Philad.)*, 1972, **29**, 153.

106. Willis, R. A., *Pathology of Tumours*, 4th edn, page 718. London, 1967.

107. Zaynoun, S., Juljulian, H. H., Kurban, A. K., *Arch. Derm.*, 1974, **109**, 689.

108. Lever, W. F., *Histopathology of the Skin*, 4th edn, page 646. Philadelphia and London, 1967.

109. Osborn, D. A., Sokolowski, A., *Arch. Otolaryng.*, 1965, **82**, 629.

110. Osborn, D. A., *J. Laryng.*, 1959, **73**, 295.

111. Munson, F. T., *Ann. Otol. (St Louis)*, 1941, **50**, 561.

112. Hora, J. F., Brown, A. K., Jr, *Arch. Otolaryng.*, 1962, **76**, 457.

113. Brunner, H., *Ann. Otol. (St Louis)*, 1942, **51**, 29.

114. Harma, R. A., *Acta oto-laryng. (Stockh.)*, 1959, suppl. 146.

115. Schiff, M., *Laryngoscope (St Louis)*, 1959, **69**, 981.

116. Emslie-Smith, D., Johnstone, J. M., Whyte, I. C., *J. clin. Path.*, 1955, **8**, 104.

117. Martin, N. H., *Brit. J. Hosp. Med.*, 1970, **3**, 662.

118. Symmers, W. St C., *personal communication*, 1973.

119. Friedmann, I., *Proc. roy. Soc. Med.*, 1961, **54**, 1064.

120. Jaffe, H. L., *Ann. roy. Coll. Surg. Engl.*, 1953, **13**, 343.

121. Cooke, S. L., Powers, W. H., *Arch. Otolaryng.*, 1949, **50**, 319.

122. Radcliffe, A., Friedmann, I., *Brit. J. Surg.*, 1957–58, **45**, 50.

123. Lichtenstein, L., Jaffe, H. L., *Amer. J. Path.*, 1943, **19**, 553.

124. Lichtenstein, L., Jaffe, H. L., *Amer. J. Path.*, 1947, **23**, 43.

125. Friedmann, I., Osborn, D. A., *J. Laryng.*, 1965, **79**, 576.

ACKNOWLEDGEMENTS FOR ILLUSTRATIONS

Figs 4.4–6, 8, 13, 14 and 38. Photomicrographs provided by W. St C. Symmers.

Fig. 4.7. Reproduced by permission of the editors from: Symmers, W. St C., *Lancet*, 1953, **2**, 1068; Symmers, W. St C., *Nurs. Mirror*, 1963, **117**, xi (Dec. 13).

Figs 4.9–12. Reproduced by permission of the editor from: Symmers, W. St C., in *Deep Mycoses of the Tropics— Proceedings of the Second International Colloquium on Medical Mycology, Antwerp, 3–5 December 1971*, page 131; Antwerp, 1972 [published simultaneously in: *Ann. Soc. belge Méd. trop.*, 1972, **52**, 365].

Fig. 4.17. Photograph provided by Mr Gavin Young, Western Infirmary, Glasgow.

Figs 4.18, 35, 36. Photography of the authors' specimens by Mr R. S. Barnett, Department of Histopathology, Charing Cross Hospital Medical School, London.

5: *The Nasopharynx*

by I. FRIEDMANN *and* D. A. OSBORN

CONTENTS

5: *The Nasopharynx*

by I. FRIEDMANN *and* D. A. OSBORN

STRUCTURAL AND FUNCTIONAL CONSIDERATIONS

The nasopharynx lies behind the nasal cavities and is the widest part of the pharynx. Anteriorly, it is continuous with these cavities through the posterior nares, or choanae, which are separated by the posterior edge of the nasal septum. The roof of the nasopharynx is formed by the thick layers of mucous membrane and periosteum on the under-surface of the basilar part of the occipital bone. The posterior wall of the cavity is formed by the mucous membrane that overlies the prevertebral muscles and fascia; the anterior arch of the atlas vertebra can be felt a little below the upper limit of the posterior pharyngeal wall. During swallowing, the nasopharynx is closed below by the soft palate: at other times there is free communication with the oropharynx.

The pharyngeal ostia of the auditory tubes (Eustachian tubes) are on the lateral walls of the nasopharynx, behind the inferior conchae; they are vertical clefts, bounded above and behind by the tori. These are expansions of the cartilage of the tubes, and behind them lie deep recesses, the pharyngeal recesses or fossae of Rosenmüller. The mucosa of this part of the nasopharynx contains much lymphoid tissue, sometimes known as the tubal tonsils. They form part of Waldeyer's ring of pharyngeal lymphoid tissue. A much more important part of Waldeyer's ring is the naso-pharyngeal tonsil (Luschka's tonsil)—a single mass of lymphadenoid tissue, or 'adenoids', situated in the area where the roof and posterior wall of the nasopharynx merge into one another.

The surface epithelium of most of the naso-pharynx is of pseudostratified ciliate columnar type, characteristic of the respiratory tract. There are, however, considerable areas that are nor-mally covered by stratified squamous epithelium.[1] Squamous metaplastic changes are common also, particularly in adults, and are probably the con-sequence of chronic inflammation. Keratinization of the squamous areas is always pathological.

The natural pathway taken by the secretions of the mucosal glands of the nose, including Bowman's glands in the olfactory area, is backward to the nasopharynx. The mucous blanket covering the epithelium of the nasal cavities and sinuses is constantly propelled in that direction by the action of the cilia, part of the stream passing above and part below the openings of the Eustachian tubes. This flow of mucus is wholly normal, and is part of the defences of the upper respiratory tract against infection.

ABNORMAL POSTNASAL DISCHARGE

It is only when the quantity, odour and other characteristics of the nasal and postnasal secretions change that it becomes necessary to regard them as possibly abnormal. The most important causes of abnormalities are neoplasms, but chronic rhinitis and sinusitis are very much commoner. A blood-stained, purulent discharge should always be regarded as suggesting the presence of a neoplasm until some other cause has been clearly demon-strated to be alone responsible.

Bleeding into the nasopharynx may result from trauma or disease. Fracture of the base of the skull is the commonest traumatic cause, apart from haemorrhage following adenoidectomy. Among the conditions in which bleeding is noteworthy are acute ulcerative forms of nasopharyngitis, infection complicating the presence of foreign bodies, spon-taneous rupture of dilated superficial blood vessels in patients with arterial hypertension, and haemo-rrhagic states such as may accompany leukaemia and thrombocytopenia.

INFLAMMATORY CONDITIONS

Any of the inflammatory diseases that occur in the nose and nasal sinuses may affect the nasopharynx

238

(see pages 194 to 217 in Chapter 4). Further comment here will be confined to a few points of particular local relevance.

Acute Nasopharyngitis.—The nasopharynx is commonly involved during the course of acute infections of the nose or of the oropharynx—for instance, acute tonsillitis, in which the pathogenic organism is usually *Streptococcus pyogenes*. Rarely, diphtheria may be confined to the nasopharynx, a localization particularly prone to occur in children whose tonsils have been incompletely removed.

In acute nasopharyngitis, hyperaemia and oedema of the mucous membrane are accompanied by increased secretion of mucus. Severer changes, such as ulceration or membrane formation, are sometimes found, their presence depending chiefly on the nature and pathogenicity of the responsible organism.

Chronic Nasopharyngitis.—Chronic inflammation of the nasopharynx occurs in association with certain nasal diseases, among them chronic sinusitis, obstruction of the airways by deviation of the nasal septum, and allergic rhinitis. It may be a troublesome consequence of working in a dusty atmosphere, the nasopharynx bearing the brunt of the irritation caused by the inhaled particles. The presence of residual adenoid tissue after incomplete excision predisposes to persistence of chronic nasopharyngitis. A special form of chronic nasopharyngeal inflammation is the atrophic form; it is usually associated with atrophic rhinitis, and its causes are the same (see page 196).

Tuberculosis of the nasopharynx is rare, but its frequency in cases of chronic respiratory tuberculosis is appreciably greater than has generally been recognized. Two types have been distinguished— the open ulcerative form, and the closed type in which the mucosa is intact and the disease can be demonstrated only by microscopical examination. The lymphoid tissues are those most involved.

Nasopharyngeal Abscesses.—Two varieties of nasopharyngeal abscesses have been described; both are very rare. *Tornwaldt's abscess* is a chronic suppurative lesion in the midline of the adenoid, and is believed to result from infection in the remains of the median recess of the posterior nasopharynx (pharyngeal bursa).

Internal Bezold abscess is the name given to a peculiar complication of acute suppurative otitis media in which pus tracks anteriorly alongside the Eustachian tube, but outside it, until it reaches the pharynx, where a retropharyngeal abscess forms and eventually ruptures into the postnasal space. This lesion acquires its name from the supposed similarity between its pathogenesis and that of the traditional form of Bezold's abscess, in which pus in the mastoid points into the soft tissues of the neck in the digastric fossa (see Chapter 41).

In osteomyelitis of the sphenoid bone, complicating sphenoidal sinusitis, the pus may discharge into the nasopharynx.

Enlargement of the Pharyngeal Tonsil

Although the term '*adenoids*' has been used as a synonym for the pharyngeal tonsil, without implying the presence of any pathological state, it is generally used in clinical practice to denote an abnormal enlargement of this collection of lymphoid tissue. Adenoidal enlargement is common, especially in children from 5 to 10 years old. Its pathogenesis is still obscure. It may be part of a generalized hyperplasia of the lymphoid tissues throughout the body, or a purely local condition developing as a response to repeated infections of the adenoid tissue, possibly by viruses of the adenovirus group. Just as the adenoids are usually involved together with the faucial tonsils in acute inflammatory conditions of the throat, so chronic tonsillitis is likely to be accompanied by chronic inflammatory hyperplasia of the adenoids.

Chronic sinusitis may be both the cause and the consequence of adenoidal hyperplasia. Allergic rhinitis may aggravate the local condition, for the added obstruction of the airways that is caused by the local swelling of the mucosa both increases the difficulty in breathing through the nose and helps to perpetuate the adenoidal enlargement by hindering the free drainage of discharges.

There are wide differences in the severity of the symptoms produced by adenoidal enlargement. It is possible that individual variations in the internal configuration of the nasopharynx may influence the effects of the enlargement on the airway, and help to determine the clinical significance of the condition in different cases.

The typical symptoms are nasal obstruction, which leads to mouth breathing, especially at night, and a characteristic facies, with broadening and flattening of the nasal arch. Enlargement of the upper deep cervical lymph nodes is common. Children with enlarged adenoids suffer in general health; they tend to be nervous and irritable, backward at school, and prone to colds and other infections of the upper respiratory tract. Hearing may be impaired as a result of obstruction of the Eustachian tubes, and this blockage also predisposes to infection of the middle ear.

Histological examination of adenoids removed surgically shows a non-specific hyperplasia of the lymphoid tissues, often with many large, closely packed follicles with prominent germinal centres. It has been from fragments of such tissues that many of the adenoviruses have been cultured. There may be a narrow zone of hyaline fibrous tissue immediately deep to the epithelium, and also between the deep aspect of the adenoids and the tissues underlying them. Fibrosis of the lymphoid tissue itself is seldom conspicuous. Suppuration is much less frequent than in the faucial tonsils. The respiratory type of epithelium that normally covers the adenoids is often replaced by squamous epithelium.

Nasopharyngeal Polyps

Polyps similar to those of the nose may be found in the nasopharynx (see page 198). They usually arise in the maxillary antrum, whence they extend into the nasal cavity and eventually through the choana into the nasopharynx (*choanal polyps*).

NEOPLASMS OF THE NASOPHARYNX

Most of the tumours of the nasopharynx are malignant; probably well under 10 per cent are benign.

Benign Tumours and Tumour-Like Lesions

Among the benign tumours is the *transitional type of papilloma*, which occasionally is confined to the nasopharynx,[2] but more usually arises in the nose and nasal sinuses (see page 217). *Adenomas* of the seromucous glands and *cavernous haemangiomas* also occur.

Juvenile angiofibroma usually extends backward from its choanal origin to occupy the postnasal space: it is described in Chapter 4 (page 228).

Malignant Tumours

The nasopharynx has been described as a 'silent area' of cancer, for the primary malignant tumours that arise there may remain small and symptomless after widespread metastasis has occurred, whether to the regional lymph nodes or through the blood to the lungs or other viscera. Moreover, such tumours may easily be overlooked during clinical examination, and they may be difficult to find at necropsy unless the region is dissected with special care. When the possibility of a small primary nasopharyngeal growth cannot be resolved by ordinary direct examination *post mortem*, it is necessary to remove the whole of this region by the comparatively simple methods described by Gräff[3] and Teoh.[4]

A series of 142 malignant tumours of the nasopharynx that we collected over a period of 23 years included 91 carcinomas, 33 lymphomas, 8 sarcomas, 3 chordomas, 1 myeloma and 1 secondary tumour (a metastatic deposit of a carcinoma of the larynx). Five of the tumours remain unclassified, illustrating the occasional difficulty of histological interpretation that is a feature of cancer of this region.

A special source of diagnostic difficulty is the almost inevitable presence of lymphoid tissue in specimens from the nasopharynx. As well as the problem of the so-called lymphoepithelioma (see below), this association leads to confusion because of the proneness of lymphocytes to become peculiarly altered by artefact, with consequent misinterpretation. Crushing or stretching the tissue during excision of a biopsy specimen may so distort lymphocytes that they come to resemble hyperchromatic tumour fibroblasts or anaplastic carcinoma cells of the small spindle-shaped type that characterizes, for example, the so-called 'oat cell' carcinoma of the lower respiratory tract. Again, delayed or otherwise insufficient fixation may result in confusing artefacts. For this reason, many of us whose work is in this field prefer the use of rapid fixatives such as Zenker's fluid to the more usual formol saline.

Many cancers of the nasopharynx have become ulcerated and infected by the time of biopsy. The secondary changes that result add to the difficulty of interpretation. They are not always avoided by taking material for histological examination from parts of the lesion that are not ulcerated, although such are generally preferable. In these cases it is, of course, important to remember that induration round a tumour may result from circulatory or inflammatory changes: a biopsy might thus be taken from tissue not directly involved by the nearby neoplasm, and an unwary report could then delay the correct diagnosis that might be made immediately by repeating the biopsy operation in another site.

Carcinoma

Anaplastic Carcinoma (Figs 5.1 and 5.2)

More than half the 91 carcinomas in our series (see above) were anaplastic. Such tumours are not always easily distinguished from reticulum cell sarcomas, for the tumour cells and their histological presentation are sometimes closely similar in the two forms of cancer in spite of the very different origins. Moreover, the intimate association with the lymphoreticular tissue of the part tends to mask the identity of the malignant epithelium: the very frequent intermingling of cells of such different provenance and behaviour was the basis of the continuing controversy about the concept of

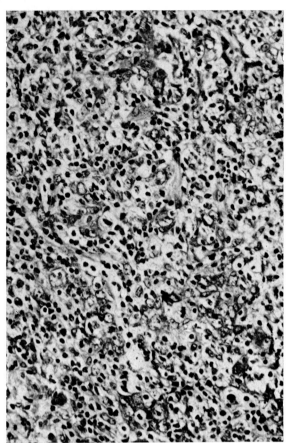

Fig. 5.2.§ Primary anaplastic carcinoma of the nasopharynx. In this field, from the same biopsy specimen as Fig. 5.1, it would be very debatable whether the growth should be regarded as an anaplastic carcinoma or as a poorly differentiated reticulum cell sarcoma. The former diagnosis was correct in this case, and was initially based essentially on the presence elsewhere in the specimen of the more frankly carcinomatous areas such as that illustrated in Fig. 5.1 *Haematoxylin–eosin.* × 215.

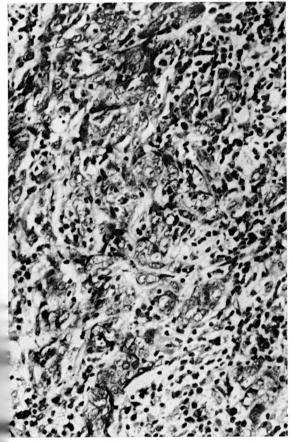

Fig. 5.1.§ Primary anaplastic carcinoma of the nasopharynx. It requires little experience to recognize the distinction in this field between the sheets of large, pale carcinoma cells, with their large and predominantly clear nuclei, and the lymphocytes and plasma cells. The picture is one of those that formerly would have been regarded as characteristic of a 'lymphoepithelioma' (see text). Compare this appearance with that illustrated in Fig. 5.2. *Haematoxylin–eosin.* × 215.

See *Acknowledgement*, page 245.

'*lymphoepithelioma*', which dates from the observations of Regaud[5] in 1912 and of Schmincke[6] in 1921, both of whom regarded the lymphocytes and the epithelial cells as integral components of the neoplastic process. The already existing arguments over the functional relation between lymphoid tissue and its epithelial covering, seen particularly in Waldeyer's ring and in the intestines, provided a background to this concept of the tumours, which attracted more interest and support among clinicians than in the laboratory. Thus, a picture evolved of a highly radiosensitive tumour that metastasized early and extensively to the lymph nodes on both sides of the neck. The predisposition of the Chinese to develop malignant epithelial tumours of this region (see below, *Epidemiology*), and at an age significantly lower than among people of other races, led to a belief that 'lymphoepithelioma' was particularly common in China and occurred there particularly among comparatively young patients.

Today, few pathologists accept that there is such an entity as the lymphoepithelioma. Most consider the tumours that have been so named to be anaplastic carcinomas with a conspicuous contribution of lymphocytes to the histological picture.[4, 7] The presence of the lymphocytes is explicable in two ways. It may merely reflect invasion of the lymphoreticular tissues of the nasopharynx and, of course, of the regional lymph nodes by the carcinoma. Alternatively, it may represent active infiltration of the tumour by lymphocytes, possibly in the nature of an immunological defence, albeit an ineffectual one. The latter explanation accords better with the observation that distant metastatic deposits of these carcinomas, as in the liver, often are also notably infiltrated by lymphocytes, although in some cases this feature is lacking.[8]

Some tumours that have been called 'lymphoepitheliomas' are not carcinomas but examples of reticulum cell sarcoma.

Squamous Carcinoma

About a quarter of the 91 carcinomas in our series were of squamous type, and of this proportion at least half were poorly differentiated. This marked liability of the epithelial tumours of the nasopharynx to be poorly differentiated is a feature of the transitional type of carcinomas also (see below).

Transitional Type of Carcinoma

A somewhat smaller number of the tumours could be classified as of the transitional type (see Chapter 4, page 220). As with the squamous growths, most were poorly differentiated. They are often taken for anaplastic carcinomas; formerly, they were usually diagnosed as lymphoepitheliomas. Careful study, however, shows the tendency to retain the basement membrane that also characterizes their counterparts in the nasal region. They have the same comparatively high survival rate as the latter.[9]

Adenocarcinoma

Adenocarcinomas, arising from mucosal glands, are occasionally found in the nasopharynx. Only four were found among the 91 carcinomas in our series; one was of well-differentiated papillary type, with abundant production of mucus (Fig. 5.3) and the other three were cribriform (Fig. 5.4).

Adenoid Cystic Carcinoma.[10]—The histogenesis of the adenoid cystic carcinoma (cribriform adenocarcinoma, cylindroma) is uncertain: there is evidence that it may be of myoepithelial origin.[11]

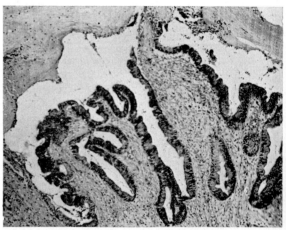

Fig. 5.3. Well-differentiated papillary adenocarcinoma of nasopharyngeal origin. *Haematoxylin–eosin.* × 60.

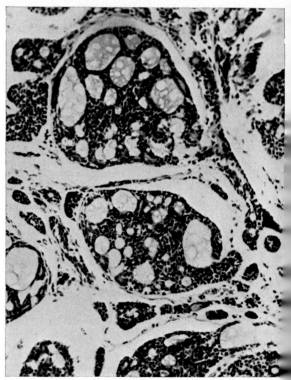

Fig. 5.4. Adenoid cystic carcinoma (cribriform adenocarcinoma) of the nasopharynx. *Haematoxylin–eosin.* × 160.

It occurs at any age but is least rare in young adults. Its prognosis is very poor:[12] although initially radio-sensitive, its recurrence is almost inevitable; this has been explained on the grounds that the tumour has a special propensity for infiltrating alongside and within nerves. Haematogenous metastasis is common, especially to the lungs.

Epidemiology of Nasopharyngeal Carcinoma

Carcinoma of the nasopharynx accounts for less than 1 per cent of all carcinomas among Caucasians: the corresponding figure among the Chinese in the region of Canton exceeds 50 per cent.[13] The incidence of the disease among Chinese people born outside China is considerably less, although higher than among Caucasians. The possibility of a genetic factor cannot be excluded, but environmental factors must also be considered in view of the striking geographical differences in the frequency of these tumours among Chinese of similar ethnic background living in different areas.

Adenovirus infection is commoner among patients with nasopharyngeal carcinoma than in a given population in general. These patients often have high titres of antibodies to the Epstein–Barr virus, which has been associated also with infectious mononucleosis (see Chapter 8) and Burkitt's lymphoma (see Chapter 9).[14]

There is some evidence that there are relatively high levels of oestrogens in the body among people who belong to population groups with a particular liability to nasopharyngeal carcinoma. This, it has been suggested, may be a factor that alters the sensitivity of the nasopharyngeal mucosa to other carcinogenic agents, viral or chemical.[13]

Lymphomas

Any variety of lymphoma may arise in the lympho-reticular tissue of the nasopharynx. Hodgkin's disease in its various histological forms is comparatively infrequent in this region; most nasopharyngeal lymphomas are of the immunoblastic or histiocytic types. The histiocytic lymphomas vary greatly in their differentiation: in general, the more anaplastic they are, the more difficult it becomes to distinguish them confidently from anaplastic carcinomas. Among the better differentiated histiocytic lymphomas, the lack of cohesion of the tumour cells to form continuous groups or sheets of cells is a point that may help to eliminate the possibility of carcinoma. The histological picture of the immunoblastic lymphomas merges into that of the lymphocytic lymphomas: the cells are separate, rounded and often devoid of pleomorphism, and they have relatively sparse cytoplasm—they are, however, larger than the cells of the lymphocytic lymphomas. As the prognosis of the lymphomas is, in general, less bad than that of the anaplastic carcinomas, there is point in trying to distinguish between these two groups in biopsy material. Failure to differentiate correctly between the various histological types of lymphoma is, perhaps, of less practical importance, as there is little evidence that in the long term they differ significantly in their response to the various forms of treatment that are available, although the better differentiated tumours are, in general, less rapidly progressive than the anaplastic ones.

About a third of the lymphomas n our series of 33 cases could be classed as lymphocytic lymphomas. The lymphocytic lymphomas may be very difficult to recognize, particularly when biopsy material is meagre and the tissue has been traumatized or inadequately preserved (see above). Tumour lymphocytes cannot be distinguished from normal lymphocytes: the biopsy diagnosis is not made at cytological level but from the histological picture as a whole, and in an appreciable proportion of cases the working diagnosis must be derived from an assessment of all the facts. Clinical history and findings often prove more crucial than the biopsy appearances, which may well be no more than consistent with a diagnosis of lymphocytic lymphoma rather than indicative of that interpretation. The presence or absence of lymphoid follicles is not necessarily helpful: a lymphoma may invade or arise in tissue rich in well-formed follicles, and follicles may be absent in tissue heavily infiltrated by lymphocytes in the course of a chronic inflammatory reaction.

Widespread lymph node involvement eventually occurs in well over half the cases of lymphoma originating in the nasopharynx. Leukaemia often develops as a terminal event.

Other Sarcomas

Rhabdomyosarcoma

The lateral wall of the nasopharynx is one of the sites of election of this tumour. The patients are usually very young children and the tumour has been known to be congenital. Rapid extension into the nasal cavities and sinuses and into the base of the skull and the orbit is usual, with early death from haemorrhage, infection or widespread dissemination. The tumour is not usually very radio-sensitive. Microscopically, it is bizarrely pleomorphic; the most characteristic feature is the presence of long, strap-like cells with hyperchromatic nucleus and eosinophile cytoplasm: cross-striation may be found in a very small proportion of these cells, and the search for this feature may entail hours of examination of many sections. In some of the tumours there is a conspicuous vascular component formed of atypical and complexly ramifying vessels.

Electron microscopy has proved of much help in the diagnosis of these tumours by facilitating the recognition of myofibrils in the cells.

Fibrosarcoma

Fibrosarcomas are least rare in adolescents and young adults but may be seen at any age. Extensive invasion of the skull may result in death well within a year of the first sign of the growth, or progress may be spread over many years, with or without recurrence after treatment. Often it is difficult to decide whether the histological picture is that of a sarcoma (Fig. 5.5) or of a benign lesion. In some cases there are associated angiomatoid features (Fig. 5.6), but these do not indicate any relation to the juvenile angiofibroma (see Chapter 4, page 228), which is an altogether different and distinct condition, clinically as well as pathologically.

Chondrosarcoma

While chondrosarcomas occur in the nasopharynx, they are less frequent than in other parts of the upper respiratory tract. They grow slowly and have little tendency to metastasize, although local recurrence after excision is not infrequent. Their differ-

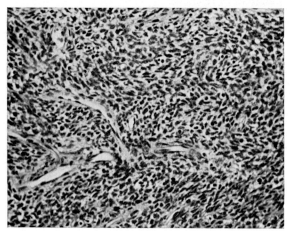

Fig. 5.5. Fibrosarcoma of nasopharynx. *Haematoxylin–eosin.* × 170

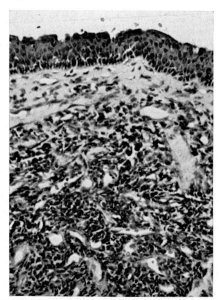

Fig. 5.6. Fibrosarcoma of nasopharynx, invading the mucosa The tumour is notably vascular. *Haematoxylin–eosin.* × 170

entiation from benign chondromas may be difficult (see Chapter 37).

Chordoma

While a chordoma may arise at any site along the line of the notochord, from remnants of which it takes origin, the nasopharynx is one of the two sites most frequently involved clinically, the other being the sacrococcygeal region.[15, 16] Presentation in the nasopharynx is typical of chordoma arising in the base of the skull and is associated with invasion of the cranial cavity also and often of the sphenoidal sinuses and the orbits. Compression of the brain stem and ulceration, infection and secondary haemorrhage are the outcome, the predominant manifestation being determined by the direction in which the tumour mainly extends.

Chordomas are lobulate or globular tumours of whitish, translucent appearance and firm or gelatinous consistence. The cut surface may be loculate or solid, and there may be foci of calcification.

Microscopically, they consist of large cells, occurring singly or in sheets, and separated by amorphous mucoid material (Fig. 5.7). Many of the tumour cells are vacuolate, and when this is particularly developed their cytoplasm has the characteristic bubble-like appearance that led Virchow to coin the name 'physaliphorous cell' (Fig. 5.8).[17] Those chordoma cells that are not vacuolate are often stellate in form. Electron microscopy has confirmed

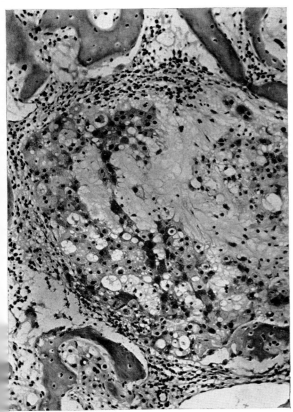

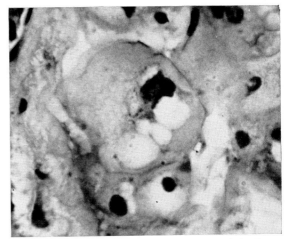

Fig. 5.8. Physaliphorous cell in a nasopharyngeal chordoma. *Haematoxylin–eosin.* × 550.

Myeloma (Plasmacytoma)

A myeloma in the nasopharynx may be solitary or a manifestation of myelomatosis. Its occurrence in either circumstance is very much rarer than in the nose (see page 231). As in the latter situation, electron microscopy may be helpful in the diagnosis of doubtful cases, the very characteristic and plentiful rough endoplasmic reticulum being readily demonstrated in the myeloma cells.[19]

Fig. 5.7. Chordoma invading bone. See Fig. 5.8 also. *Haematoxylin–eosin.* × 145.

that they and the physaliphorous cells are of similar nature.[18]

REFERENCES

1. Ali, M. Y., *personal communication*, 1964.
2. Radcliffe, A., *J. Laryng.*, 1953, **67**, 682.
3. Robb-Smith, A. H. T., *J. tech. Meth.*, 1937, **17**, 66.
4. Teoh, T. B., *J. Path. Bact.*, 1957, **73**, 451.
5. Regaud, C., Crémieu, R., *C. R. Soc. Biol. (Paris)*, 1912, **72**, 523.
6. Schmincke, A., *Beitr. path. Anat.*, 1921, **58**, 161.
7. Willis, R. A., *Pathology of Tumours*, 4th edn, page 300. London, 1967.
8. Symmers, W. St C., *personal communication*, 1974.
9. Osborn, D. A., *Cancer (Philad.)*, 1970, **25**, 50.
10. Conley, J., Dingman, D. L., *Arch. Otolaryng.*, 1974, **100**, 81.
11. Hamperl, H., *Curr. Top. Path.*, 1971, **53**, 161.
12. Harrison, K., *Ann. roy. Coll. Surg. Engl.*, 1956, **18**, 99.
13. Clifford, P., *Int. J. Cancer*, 1970, **5**, 287.
14. De Schryver, A., Friberg, S., Jr, Klein, G., Henle, W., Henle, G., De The, G., Clifford, P., Ho, H. C., *Clin. exp. Immunol.*, 1969, **5**, 443.
15. Harvey, W. F., Dawson, E. K., *Edinb. med. J.*, 1941, **48**, 713.
16. Dahlin, D. C., MacCarty, C. S., *Cancer (Philad.)*, 1952, **5**, 1170.
17. Stewart, M. J., *J. Path. Bact.*, 1922, **25**, 40.
18. Friedmann, I., Harrison, D. F. N., Bird, E. S., *J. clin. Path.*, 1962, **15**, 116.
19. Friedmann, I., *Proc. roy. Soc. Med.*, 1961, **54**, 1064.

ACKNOWLEDGEMENT FOR ILLUSTRATIONS

Figs 5.1, 2. Photomicrographs provided by W. St C. Symmers.

6: *The Larynx*

by I. Friedmann *and* D. A. Osborn

CONTENTS

6: *The Larynx*

by I. Friedmann *and* D. A. Osborn

ANATOMICAL CONSIDERATIONS

For descriptive purposes, the larynx may be divided into three regions—(i) the superior or *supraglottic region*, which includes the epiglottis, the aryepiglottic folds, the arytenoid cartilages and the interarytenoid fold, the vestibular folds (false vocal cords), and the laryngeal sinuses (ventricles); (ii) the middle or *glottic region*, which includes the vocal folds (true vocal cords), and the anterior commissure; and (iii) the inferior or *subglottic region*, which is the part of the larynx that lies below the level of the vocal folds.

The hypopharynx is the part of the pharynx behind the larynx, and it extends, therefore, from the level of the top of the epiglottis to the beginning of the oesophagus at the level of the lower margin of the cricoid cartilage. Its named regions are (i) the *piriform fossae*, which lie one on each side of the lower half of the laryngeal opening, between the aryepiglottic fold medially and the lamina of the thyroid cartilage and thyrohyoid membrane laterally, and (ii) the *postcricoid region*, behind the cricoid cartilage.

Two further topographical terms—intrinsic and extrinsic—are used clinically, particularly in describing the site of primary carcinomas. These tumours are often known as *intrinsic* if they are limited to the vocal folds, and as *extrinsic* if they arise in the subglottic and supraglottic region or in the piriform recesses.

Attention to the anatomical situation of the lesions is important in diseases of the larynx, and particularly in relation to cancer, for therapeutic measures and prognosis depend to an important extent on the part of the larynx that is affected. Thus, the abundance and extent of the anastomosis between the lymphatics of the extrinsic parts of the larynx and those of the adjoining parts of the throat and mouth account for the early and extensive spread of carcinomas arising in this region of the larynx: in contrast, there is relatively little communication between the lymphatics of the intrinsic parts and those of the adjacent structures, and this is one of the factors that account for the very much better prognosis of intrinsic cancers.

Histology of the Normal Larynx

Much of the epithelium covering the supraglottic and subglottic regions of the larynx is pseudostratified columnar ('respiratory') epithelium with interspersed goblet cells, although scattered metaplastic patches of stratified squamous epithelium or of transitional epithelium may also be found. The vocal folds are covered by non-keratinizing stratified squamous epithelium.

The elastic fibres in the lateral part of the conus elasticus (cricovocal membrane) become attenuated as they approach its free border, which forms the edge of the vocal fold (true vocal cord). Although the mucosa is attached firmly to each aspect of the edge of the membrane over which it is stretched, there is a potential space between the lines of attachment: separation of the mucosa in the plane of this potential space is important in the pathogenesis of polyps of the vocal folds (page 253).

Seromucous glands are present in the mucosa of various parts of the larynx. Their distribution is variable, but they are generally most numerous (and best developed) in the laryngeal sinuses, in the region of the ventricular folds and on the epiglottis. They are also numerous in the subglottic region but absent from the vocal folds and their immediate vicinity.

The Lymphatic System of the Larynx

The lymphatic system of the interior of the larynx is poorly developed and is subdivided by the vocal folds into supraglottic and subglottic regions. The vocal fold itself has a sparse lymphatic supply. The supraglottic region is drained through lymphatics running alongside the superior laryngeal vein directly to the deep cervical lymph nodes. The sub glottic region is drained through the anterior laryngeal nodes (along the lower margin of the thyroid cartilage) to the deep cervical lymph nodes.

MALFORMATIONS AND ACQUIRED DEFORMITIES OF THE LARYNX

The cartilaginous skeleton of the larynx may vary in size and shape; individual cartilages may be malformed or even absent. A man may have a small, female-type larynx and a woman may have the large and more spacious male-type larynx.

Laryngeal Web

The so-called laryngeal web is the commonest congenital malformation of the larynx. The web may be a thin and translucent membrane, or more fibrous and thicker: it is spread between the vocal folds near the anterior commissure. There may be adhesions in the supraglottic and subglottic regions.

Stenosis of the Larynx

This may be congenital or acquired. Congenital stenosis may be due to compression of the larynx or to cysts or webs. Acquired stenosis of the larynx is due to scar formation or destruction of cartilaginous parts of the larynx, and may be traumatic in origin (including surgical measures) or, more frequently, due to burns or caustic poisons. Stenosis may also result from syphilis, tuberculosis, scleroma, typhoid, diphtheria, measles and other infections.

Perichondritis accompanying or following irradiation of laryngeal tumours may lead to destruction of the cartilaginous skeleton of the larynx and so give rise to stenosis or severe deformities.

Laryngocele

A laryngocele is an enlargement of the laryngeal ventricle and saccule. It is of congenital origin and regarded as an atavistic structure, homologous with the air sacs of monkeys. Its enlargement is furthered by increased intralaryngeal pressure due to coughing and, perhaps, the playing of wind instruments. It may become infected, the condition of *laryngopyocele* resulting, which, if untreated, may prove fatal.[1]

INFLAMMATORY CONDITIONS

Misuse of the Term 'Laryngitis'

In many textbooks of laryngology various non-inflammatory conditions are included under the term 'laryngitis'. It has, indeed, become a clinical convention to describe as laryngitis any laryngeal disturbance that presents with a history of hoarseness and is not the result of paralysis of the vocal folds or of cancer. The more important conditions that are thus mistakenly described as laryngitis are the various polyps and polypoid lesions of the vocal folds, and keratosis. This carelessness in terminology is doubly regrettable, first, because it discourages an adequate investigation of the patient's condition, and second, because the nomenclature of many of these lesions is already confused by the application—and misapplication— of many synonyms.

Acute Laryngitis

Various infections, both bacterial and viral, may cause acute laryngitis. The bacteria most commonly concerned are beta-haemolytic streptococci, *Haemophilus influenzae* and, possibly, pneumococci. In diphtheria, and exceptionally in typhoid fever, the larynx may be acutely inflamed and ulcerated. The importance of viruses in relation to laryngitis has been much underestimated in the past. In addition to influenza virus, the adenoviruses are now well-recognized causes. Smallpox and chickenpox may cause pustular laryngitis.[2] Exposure to dust or to irritant fumes can be the direct cause of acute laryngitis.

In acute laryngitis, the mucosa is hyperaemic and infiltrated by neutrophils. The epithelium may become necrotic, and the resulting areas of ulceration become covered by fibrinopurulent exudate. In some cases, the necrosis may extend into the underlying tissues. Acute oedema of the glottis is a rare complication, except after exposure to particularly irritant fumes.

Acute Epiglottitis

Acute epiglottitis is a rare but important disease of early childhood.[3, 4] The illness develops with startling rapidity, often within a few hours, and is rapidly fatal. It is caused by *Haemophilus influenzae* type B, and the organism can be recovered from the blood and from the inflamed epiglottis.

The epiglottis is grossly swollen, brawny and red (Fig. 6.1). No obvious ulceration can be seen with the naked eye, and generally no other part of the larynx or of the mouth or pharynx is involved. No lesions are found elsewhere in the body, apart from the non-specific effects of the overwhelming

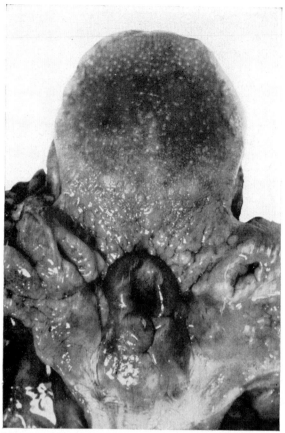

Fig. 6.1. Acute epiglottitis due to infection by *Haemophilus influenzae* type B. The organism was isolated from the throat. The patient, a boy of $3\frac{1}{2}$ years, died within 12 hours of the onset of the illness.

toxaemia, often with septicaemia, that accompanies the infection. Microscopically, there may be superficial ulceration of the epiglottis, but the changes are essentially those of an acute, histologically non-specific inflammation.

Chronic Laryngitis

Non-specific, chronic inflammatory changes are commonly found in the larynx, particularly in smokers, town-dwellers, and those who persistently over-exert their voices. In some cases, atrophic changes are found in the mucosa (atrophic laryngitis). Non-specific inflammatory changes are frequently seen near other chronic laryngeal lesions, such as the various polyps and tumours. Plasma cells may be numerous in the exudate, but ordinarily lymphocytes predominate.

Specific Forms of Chronic Laryngitis

Tuberculous Laryngitis.—Tuberculous infection of the larynx was frequent in cases of advanced pulmonary tuberculosis before drug treatment became effective. Nowadays, tuberculous laryngitis is less common, not simply because of the great fall in the incidence of all forms of tuberculosis, but also because treatment of chronic pulmonary tuberculosis, even when it fails to cure the disease in the lungs, is still likely to lessen the number of viable tubercle bacilli in the sputum and thus to hinder infection becoming established in the mucosa of the upper air passages. Nevertheless, tuberculous laryngitis continues to demand clinical consideration, for it may be confused with carcinoma of the arynx.

During recent years it has been observed that there is a slight, but incontrovertible, increase in the frequency of tuberculosis of the larynx in patients in late middle age admitted with a provisional clinical diagnosis of laryngeal cancer to the Royal National Throat, Nose and Ear Hospital in London. Biopsy in these cases reveals characteristic tuberculous tissue beneath the surface epithelium, which shows no malignant change. There is little or no pulmonary disease associated with the laryngeal condition in these cases, and this may indicate the same trend in the incidence of tuberculosis in this portion of the upper respiratory tract as has been observed in the comparable cases of tuberculosis of the nose and ear seen in the same hospital in middle-aged patients. The disease usually takes the form of multiple, small, superficial ulcers, with a tendency for the interarytenoid fold, the ventricular and vocal folds and the epiglottis to be involved, in that order. Often the underlying cartilage becomes exposed and undergoes necrosis. The infected mucosa may be swollen and reddened, as in any form of acute inflammation, even when histological examination shows only tuberculous granulation tissue (Fig. 6.2). The condition may present clinically as keratosis.

Even before the discovery of drugs effective against tuberculosis, tuberculous laryngitis sometimes healed, but with the formation of much scar tissue and eventual stenosis of the larynx.[5]

Laryngeal Lupus.—In a few cases of lupus vulgaris of the face or nasal cavities and nasopharynx, the infection spreads to the larynx, and particularly to the epiglottis, whence it involves the aryepiglottic folds. Ulceration and consequent fibrosis and stenosis are the main sequelae, different areas

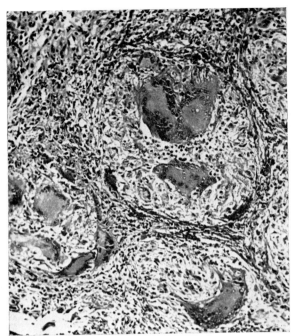

Fig. 6.2. Tuberculous laryngitis. Biopsy of left vocal fold. The patient was a man, aged 62, whose laryngeal infection was at first mistaken clinically for a carcinoma. *Haematoxylin–eosin.* × 140.

showing different stages in the progress of the lesion.

Syphilis of the Larynx.—A primary chancre of the larynx is a rarity. Secondary syphilis causes diffuse erythema, which may be mistaken for diffuse acute non-specific laryngitis. At this stage, mucous patches are as common in the acquired disease in the adult as in congenital syphilis of the newborn.

More important is the gumma of tertiary syphilis, which may appear as a well-defined 'tumour' or as a diffuse infiltration of the larynx that leads sooner or later to the formation of a characteristic punched-out ulcer. Secondary infection results in perichondritis and then necrosis of the adjacent cartilage; subsequently, the formation of abundant scar tissue causes stenosis or other deformities of the upper air passages. The healing of congenital syphilitic lesions may also lead to stricture of the larynx.

Other Chronic Specific Infections.—Some of the deep-seated fungal infections may cause proliferative and ulcerative, granulomatous lesions of the larynx. These occur notably, if rarely, in the North and South American forms of blastomycosis, in histoplasmosis and in rhinosporidiosis. Superficial infections of the laryngeal mucosa by *Candida* may complicate severe thrush in the mouth and throat.

Leprosy (Chapter 39) and *scleroma* (page 204) may involve the larynx.

Cricoarytenoid Arthritis

The cricoarytenoid joint is overtly inflamed in about a quarter of all patients with rheumatoid arthritis. It has been accepted by most observers as the cause of the laryngeal stridor that may develop at a late stage of this disease.[6, 7] During remission, the mucous membrane over the cartilage becomes thickened and movement is limited or the joint becomes fixed.

Rheumatoid arthritis is believed to impair laryngeal function both by involving the cricoarytenoid joint and by direct injury to the nearby muscles. The muscle lesion may be either specific rheumatoid laryngeal polymyositis or neurogenic atrophy (due to compression of the nerves by the inflammatory reaction round the affected joints).[8] It may be difficult to distinguish between cricoarytenoid arthritis and bilateral neurogenic abductor paralysis of the vocal folds as the cause of stridor. Clinical examination seldom, if ever, provides sufficient evidence to enable this distinction to be made, and often only a full microscopical study of the joints, muscles and nerves of the larynx gives the answer.[7]

Rheumatoid nodules have been observed in the larynx. Studies using the method of microlaryngoscopy indicate that they are by no means uncommon.[9, 10]

GOUT AND THE LARYNX

An uncommon cause of hoarseness is the deposition of sodium urate in the vocal folds or in the subglottic region.[11] This occurs only in the presence of longstanding gout. The deposits may form nodules up to several millimetres in diameter. There may be an accompanying giant-celled granulomatous reaction, as in gouty deposits in other parts of the body (see Chapters 38 and 39).

OEDEMA OF THE LARYNX

The larynx may become oedematous in cases of cardiac, renal or other generalized forms of oedema. In such cases, the swelling of the laryngeal tissues seldom causes respiratory embarrassment.

However, if the oedema is due to obstruction to the venous return from the head and neck—as happens, for instance, if there is thrombosis of the superior vena cava—the laryngeal swelling may be acute and extensive, with correspondingly greater risk of impeding respiration.

'Angioneurotic oedema' sometimes involves the soft tissues of the larynx as a manifestation of allergic hypersensitivity to a particular food or drug. Stings of wasps and bees may prove fatal from the same cause. But the commonest and most dangerous causes of laryngeal oedema are diphtheria and streptococcal infection (including Ludwig's angina—Chapter 13), and the acute inflammation that results from exposure to steam or irritant gases.

Fluid can collect in the soft areolar tissues of certain parts of the larynx: its spread in some directions is limited by the firmer adherence of the mucosa to the underlying tissue—in oedema, therefore, the swelling is characteristically seen first over the arytenoid cartilage and in the aryepiglottic folds, spreading thence into the epiglottis and the vestibular folds; it does not, however, extend into the vocal folds or past the pharyngoepiglottic folds. It is mainly the swelling of the posterior ends of the aryepiglottic folds that obstructs the passage of air.

AMYLOID DISEASE OF THE LARYNX

The larynx may be involved in primary and secondary generalized amyloidosis; there is also a form of amyloid disease that is confined to the larynx. The deposition of amyloid in the laryngeal tissues as part of generalized amyloidosis is unlikely to cause any functional disturbance.

Localized Primary Amyloidosis of the Larynx[12]

Amyloid disease limited to the larynx is a rare condition. It may present either as tumour-like deposits, which may be solitary or multiple and reach a centimetre or even more in diameter, or as a diffuse thickening of parts of the mucosa. The surface of the deposits is smooth or nodular and the mucosa remains intact. Either form may eventually obstruct the laryngeal airway, necessitating tracheotomy and surgical excision. Primary amyloidosis of the larynx is rarely followed by generalized amyloidosis.

Aetiology and Pathogenesis.—Primary laryngeal amyloidosis occurs mainly in middle-aged or old

people; its cause is unknown. Sometimes the deposits are related to accumulations of plasma cells in the affected parts of the mucosa, an observation in keeping with other instances of the association between amyloid disease and plasma cells or their neoplastic counterpart, myeloma cells. It is noteworthy that localized amyloidosis is occasionally a complication of the rare, so-called primary extra-skeletal plasma cell myeloma, one of the commonest sites of which, in the upper respiratory tract, is the larynx. In fact, the topographical distribution of localized amyloidosis of the respiratory tract is essentially the same as that complicating extra-skeletal solitary myeloma.[13] However, such myelomas are rare, and it is likely that the deposition of amyloid at these sites is ordinarily associated with the liability of the respiratory tract mucosa to chronic infection that evokes the local accumulation of plasma cells and much local production of antibody globulin. This view is supported by the fact that the secondary type of generalized amyloidosis is apt to be associated with chronic infections characterized by prolonged production of globulin, or with other conditions, such as myelomatosis, in which globulin production is excessive.

Localized amyloidosis may also occur in the nasal sinuses, the nasopharynx, the trachea and the bronchi. The respiratory tract is much the commonest site of localized amyloid disease.

Microscopical Appearances.—In haematoxylin-eosin preparations amyloid appears as a pale pink, homogeneous substance that is indistinguishable from other hyaline materials (Fig. 6.3). However, it has some staining characteristics that help to distinguish it from other abnormal protein deposits. The tentative diagnosis may be suggested by the histological finding of homogeneous deposits, with or without giant cells. This must be confirmed by using additional methods of identification:[12] meta-chromatic staining; strong affinity for Congo red; negative birefringence and dichroism when stained with Congo red; strong secondary fluorescence in ultraviolet light when stained with thioflavin T; and a high degree of resistance to extraction with proteolytic enzymes, such as pepsin.

Homogeneous deposits in the tissues that satisfy these criteria may be regarded as amyloid. These reactions usually establish the sometimes difficult distinction between amyloid and the hyaline material that is found in some laryngeal polyps (see page 254). In some cases there is a well-marked

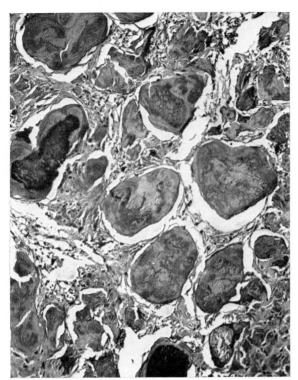

Fig. 6.3. Amyloid deposits that formed a subglottic mass. The patient was a man, aged 51. *Haematoxylin–eosin.* × 100.

foreign-body type of giant cell reaction round the amyloid deposits.

POLYPS OF THE VOCAL FOLDS[14, 15]

The study of polyps of the vocal folds has been complicated unnecessarily by a confusing nomenclature that is largely the outcome of discrepancies between clinical impressions and histological findings. Some clinicians freely describe simple polyps by such pathological terms as myxoma, fibroma and angioma, without microscopical confirmation and merely because of a superficial resemblance between the lesion and these tumours. Again, the term *chorditis tuberosa* is commonly used in some clinics, although the implication of an inflammatory process is not strictly substantiated. The least objectionable clinical terminology is that based on occupation and has the merit of indicating that polyps occur predominantly in those whose work involves much strain on the voice. Such terms are singer's, hawker's, teacher's, preacher's, lawyer's, politician's, heckler's, ranter's and chairman's nodes or nodules.

I*

It must be emphasized, before describing the lesions more fully, that the nature of such polyps can be determined only by microscopical examination, and that this should never be omitted. Failure to take this precaution may allow the occasional early, but identifiable, carcinoma that presents as a polypoid nodule to pass undetected at a stage when the chance of cure is greatest.

Aetiology and Pathogenesis.—Conflicting statements about the incidence of polyps of the vocal folds are to be found in different textbooks of laryngology. Experience at the Royal National Throat, Nose and Ear Hospital in London has been that they are commonest in the fifth decade, and that they occur twice as often in men as in women.[15] But no age is exempt, and—to some extent—the patient's occupation may determine the age at which polyps appear.

The polyps result from mechanical injury to the connective tissue of the vocal folds.[16] This injury is incurred mainly through misuse of the voice, and especially through persistent misuse when there is an incidental laryngitis, or after symptoms of polyp formation have already appeared. Faulty voice production is as important a cause as over-use, and the commonest fault is forcing the voice after most of the available air has been exhaled, in an effort to compensate for the sharp fall in the air flow. This leads to the vocal cords being pressed unduly firmly together at a time when their rapid vibrations are liable to cause injury. Altering the pitch of the voice in order to make it better heard in noisy surroundings, a means commonly adopted to avoid shouting, is another frequent source of 'voice strain', a colloquial expression that aptly describes the effect on the vocal folds. That straining the voice in such ways can bring about immediate changes in the vocal folds has been shown—for instance, by indirect laryngoscopy after conversation for a few minutes in a noisy London underground railway carriage; efforts even by experienced speakers to converse under such conditions may be followed by hyperaemia and increased secretion of mucus, and occasionally by slight swelling of the vocal folds.[17]

The polyps that develop in consequence of vocal stresses are believed to be the result of vascular engorgement, oedema and focal haemorrhage in the subepithelial tissue, all of which lead to distortion of the vocal fold. The distortion is usually localized, and the commonest site for polyps is the medial aspect of the vocal fold at about the junction of the anterior and middle thirds. In many cases the lesion is bilateral, but often the polyps of the two sides differ in size. In some cases, the changes are more extensive, and in extreme instances there is polypoid degeneration of the entire membranous part of the vocal fold—that is, its anterior two-thirds.

Microscopical Appearances.—The internal structure of the polyp seems to depend upon the fate of the initial exudate. Ingrowth of blood vessels from the deep aspect of the upper part of the crico-thyroid membrane may produce a predominantly vascular tissue that can be mistaken for an angioma. By contrast, if proliferation of simple connective tissue predominates, a fibrous nodule simulating a fibroma may be formed (Fig. 6.4). Myxomatoid degeneration in such fibrous tissue has sometimes led to the mistaken diagnosis of myxoma. The resemblance of these varied histological pictures to tumours is not, in fact, especially close, and with care mistakes are unlikely.

Bleeding into the stroma is common, especially in angiomatoid polyps, and occasionally the resulting haematoma may interfere with respiration. Organization of the clot leads to fibrosis, and the

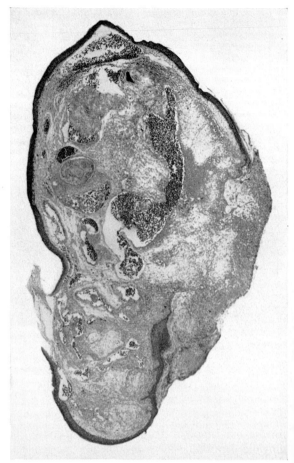

Fig. 6.5. Large polyp of a vocal fold, with extensive hyaliniza-tion and haemorrhage in the stroma. A considerable area of the overlying stratified squamous epithelium is ulcerated. *Haematoxylin–eosin.* × 15.

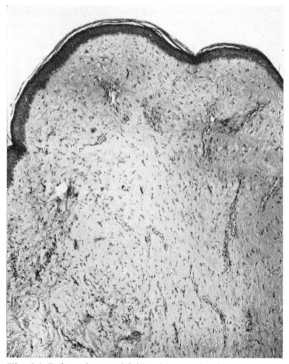

Fig. 6.4. Polyp of a vocal fold, with vascular fibrous stroma covered by keratinizing squamous epithelium. *Haematoxylin–eosin.* × 50.

resulting scar tissue is often heavily pigmented with haemosiderin.

Hyaline change is found in many polyps, either through hyalinization of the collagen or through some alteration in the proteins of the exudate in the interstitial tissue. Hyaline material may even occupy most of the polyp (Fig. 6.5): oftener it forms small, discrete deposits. These may be found in three situations: as rings round blood vessels; within blood vessels, as a result of hyaliniza-tion of thrombi, the affected vessels appearing as plexiform, distended, thin-walled channels, occluded by the hyaline mass; and in the stroma, usually in the form of fine, thread-like deposits. It may be difficult to distinguish between amyloid and hyaline material (Fig. 6.6) without the use of selective stains (see page 252).

It must be stressed again that all polypoid lesion

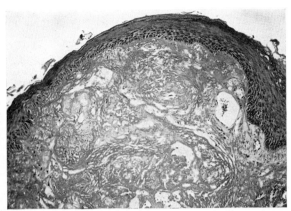

Fig. 6.6. Part of a polyp of a vocal fold, with extensive hyalinization of the stroma. The polyp is covered by hyperplastic stratified squamous epithelium. *Haematoxylin–eosin.* × 40.

of the vocal folds should be examined microscopically, for only by so doing is it possible to determine the diagnosis precisely. Although in most cases the microscopical examination confirms the clinical impression that the polyp is a simple one, such lesions may prove to be amyloid foci, squamous papillomas, keratotic nodules or even early squamous carcinomas.

'*Plasma Cell Polyps*'.—Some laryngeal polyps consist of dense accumulations of plasma cells throughout an oedematous stroma. Small numbers of lymphocytes and macrophages are also present. Although these infiltrates may be no more than an extreme example of the chronic inflammatory reaction often seen in laryngeal polyps, two unusual features suggest that this view is not always correct: first, the presence of small, faintly haematoxyphile, globular clumps of material that histochemically can be identified as precipitates containing ribonucleic acid;[18] and second, though less constant, fine deposits of amyloid. The only practical significance of these peculiar lesions, as far as is yet known, is that the precipitates may be mistaken for fungi or other parasites.

Myelomas (plasmacytomas) may also occur in the form of polypoid lesions (see page 266).

KERATOSIS OF THE LARYNX[19]

The terms keratosis, hyperkeratosis, leucoplakia and pachydermia have been applied to a form of hyperplasia of the laryngeal epithelium. This state has its counterpart in the mucosa of the mouth and pharynx and of the vulva and vagina. In fact, the changes may occur in any mucous membrane with epithelium that normally is of non-keratinized, stratified squamous type. They are the outcome of chronic irritation, which stimulates keratin formation in ordinarily non-keratinized squamous cells. This process is accompanied by hyperplasia of the basal and prickle cell layers. Although much effort has been expended in seeking to define the supposed differences between keratosis, hyperkeratosis, leucoplakia and pachydermia, it now seems apparent that they are merely variants of a single type of reactive change and that little is to be gained by trying to distinguish between them. In this chapter they are considered inclusively under the term keratosis.

Microscopical Appearances.—There is hyperplasia of the prickle cell layer (acanthosis), with or without keratinization; the relative proportions of acanthosis and keratinization vary greatly. The proliferating basal cell layer sends downgrowths into the connective tissues; the basement membrane, however, remains intact and in most cases the arrangement of the cells is orderly. Should the appearance and disposition of the epithelial cells become irregular, it may be difficult to be certain whether the lesion is benign or malignant.

Changes in the underlying tissues are confined to the superficial zone of the lamina propria of the mucosa. They comprise oedema, a variable amount of fibrosis, proliferation of thin-walled capillaries, deposition of haemosiderin, and accumulation of lymphocytes, plasma cells and macrophages.

Microscopical Differential Diagnosis.—The conditions to be considered in the differential diagnosis of keratosis of the larynx are carcinoma *in situ* and well-differentiated squamous carcinoma. Carcinoma *in situ* has to be considered particularly when there is conspicuous variation in the size, shape and intensity of staining of the nuclei, with irregularity in the arrangement of the cells throughout most of the lesion. Malignant change, whether of the in-situ type or frankly invasive, however, may be very localized, and this greatly increases the difficulties of diagnosis.

In practice, it is often harder to distinguish confidently between a well-differentiated squamous carcinoma and keratosis than between keratosis and carcinoma *in situ*. This is because the disorderliness of nuclear arrangement and variations in nuclear shape and size are much more distinct in carcinoma *in situ* (Fig. 6.13). There is, indeed, no well-defined borderline between keratosis and well-differentiated squamous carcinoma that is invasive *ab initio*: the interpretation of an equivocal histological picture is a subjective assessment the correctness of which can only be judged by appropriate follow-up studies.[20, 21] The verrucous type of squamous carcinoma is specially liable to misinterpretation (see page 262).

Biopsy often needs to be repeated, even more than once, because the finding of equivocal appearances requires examination of other parts of the lesion before the presence of carcinoma can be excluded. These difficult cases may cause much anxiety both to the laryngologist and to the microscopist, for their correct treatment and their microscopical interpretation are comparably difficult.

CYSTS OF THE LARYNX

Most laryngeal cysts result from obstruction of the ducts of mucous glands, due either to inflammation nearby or to contraction of scar tissue after healing of a local ulcer. These retention cysts are found on the lingual aspect of the epiglottis or in the aryepiglottic folds, and only exceptionally at other sites, such as the vocal folds.[22] They are smooth-surfaced, tense, translucent structures, ranging from 5 to 15 mm in diameter, and filled with thick, very glairy mucus (Fig. 6.7). They are liable to become infected, and they may occasionally cause death through suffocation.

Rarely, excision of what had seemed to be a simple retention cyst is followed by recurrence of the lesion. This may be merely the result of incomplete removal of the wall of a benign cyst, which then formed again from the remnant. Sometimes, however, such a recurrence proves to be evidence

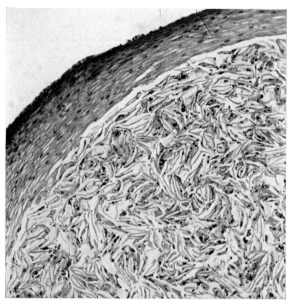

Fig. 6.8. Epidermoid cyst of a vocal fold. The cyst is filled with desquamated squames. *Haematoxylin–eosin.* × 100.

that the original cystic lesion was in fact a neoplasm (see page 265).

Some cysts of the epiglottis appear to arise within the substance of the cartilage as a degenerative change in its matrix.

Epidermoid cysts (Fig. 6.8), dermoid cysts and branchial cysts occur as developmental anomalies.

BENIGN TUMOURS OF THE LARYNX

Before considering the pathology of the benign tumours of the larynx it is important to make the point that more than 80 per cent of laryngeal tumours are malignant. This fact demands a high index of suspicion of cancer when dealing with tumours of this region.

Benign Epithelial Tumours

Papillomas

Papillomas are the commonest of the benign tumours of the larynx. There are two important varieties, juvenile and adult, differing not only in age incidence but also in clinical features and histological structure.

Juvenile Papilloma of the Larynx

The juvenile papilloma occurs in very young patients. Both sexes are equally liable to the

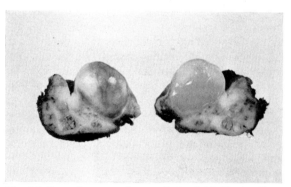

Fig. 6.7. Retention cyst of a ventricular fold. The cyst was removed by laryngofissure.

disease. The lesion is often multiple, tending then to be widely distributed over the mucosal surface of the larynx. The papillomas are soft, pale pink, finely lobulate growths, usually from 2 to 5 mm in diameter. Characteristically, they are mobile, a feature that is diagnostically important, since a tumour that is fixed must arouse suspicion of malignancy. Histologically, a juvenile papilloma has the features of a squamous papilloma, but with a characteristic lack of keratinization. It comprises multiple, small, papillary processes that are formed of stratified squamous epithelium with a relatively meagre core of vascular stroma. There is a notable lack of cellular and nuclear atypia, which is in sharp contrast to the marked tendency for the lesions to recur after removal.

The typical history of these patients is of frequent attendance for local removal of recurring tumours in the early years, the intervals lengthening progressively as puberty approaches. In spite of the high recurrence rate, the microscopical appearances remain constant in the great majority of cases. Malignant change is sometimes observed,[23] especially in cases of long standing with a history of repeated treatment by irradiation or cauterization.

The cause of juvenile papilloma is unknown. Virological and electron-microscopical studies have suggested the presence of a virus in some cases.[24, 25]

Papilloma of the Larynx in Adults

The laryngeal papilloma of adults is unequivocally distinguished from the juvenile type not only by the age of the patient but also by its almost exclusive origin from the vocal folds and by the invariable occurrence of keratinization (Fig. 6.9). It is commoner than the juvenile papilloma. Its relation to laryngeal cancer presents diagnostic difficulties, for primary carcinoma of the larynx may present as a papillomatoid mass without gross evidence of invasion, and the histological distinction between carcinoma and papilloma may be far from easy. Follow-up studies of such histologically debatable tumours suggest that many of them are benign, in spite of cellular and nuclear atypia reminiscent of carcinoma *in situ.*[26]

The adult type of papilloma rarely recurs. Frank malignant change is even rarer; most of the tumours in which it develops are near the anterior commissure.[27] As a generalization it is justifiable to state that the prognosis is better than has usually been suggested;[28] nevertheless, every specimen must

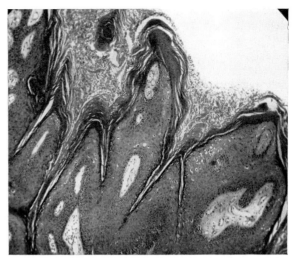

Fig. 6.9. Keratotic squamous papilloma of a vocal fold. *Haematoxylin–eosin.* × 35.

be interpreted on the basis of its own characteristics.

Adenomas

For convenience, the laryngeal adenomas are dealt with in the section on tumours of the seromucous glands (see page 264).

Paraganglioma (Chemodectoma)[29–31]

Paragangliomas are among the rarest of the laryngeal tumours (see also Chapter 41). Eleven cases had been reported by 1970;[29] since then, greater awareness of the occurrence of the tumour has led to its more frequent recognition.[30, 31] It may arise from any of the paraganglia of the larynx: there are two pairs of these bodies, upper and lower, and it is the upper pair—situated just above the anterior end of the vocal fold—that is the usual source of the tumours. In exceptional cases there is more than one tumour.

A paraganglioma is well defined. Although it often protrudes into the airway it seldom becomes ulcerated. Usually it is from 0·5 to 1·0 cm in its longest dimension but it may be several times larger than this. Severe pain is occasionally an accompaniment of the tumour and may be episodic in character. In a case in which the cause of the pain was initially overlooked, because the tumour was very small, the patient was driven to attempt suicide: the tumour, which was detected eventually on dissection of the tissues underlying a small area of relative pallor of the mucosa, was a flattened disc, 2 mm in diameter; its removal completely relieved the patient's symptoms.[32]

The potential secretory activity of the paragangliomas must be remembered when operation is undertaken. Catecholamines are likely to be released during removal of the growth, sometimes in large amounts; the considerable transient rise in blood pressure that results may endanger the patient's life unless it has been foreseen and the appropriate measures are taken to counteract it.

Histologically, paragangliomas consist of cuboidal or columnar cells, corresponding to the chief cells of the normal paraganglion. The tumour cells are arranged in an alveolar pattern (Fig. 6.10) or, often, have a distinctive disposition about vascular spaces, which may be abundant. If the tissue has been fixed by formalin vapour there

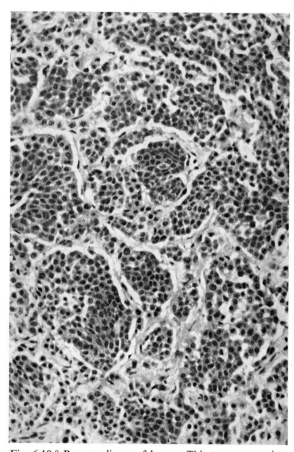

Fig. 6.10.§ Paraganglioma of larynx. This tumour consists of cuboidal cells arranged in an alveolar pattern and surrounded by delicate stroma in which thin-walled blood vessels are numerous, although difficult to make out because of some shrinkage of the tissue during histological preparation. *Haematoxylin–eosin.* × 150.

§ See *Acknowledgement*, page 267.

may be autofluorescence of the cells. Electron microscopy shows what are assumed to be granules of catecholamine in the cytoplasm.[29]

Benign Tumours and Tumour-like Lesions of Connective Tissue

Lipoma

Laryngeal lipomas are very rare. The tumour usually arises in the region of the aryepiglottic folds. If pedunculate, it may fatally obstruct the larynx or pharynx.

Neural Tumours

Neurofibromas and neurolemmomas occur in the larynx both as solitary tumours and as a manifestation of von Recklinghausen's neurofibromatosis.[33] They are uncommon.

Angioma

Angiomas of the larynx are rare. Most of the lesions that have been so diagnosed were probably angiomatoid polyps (see page 254). However, haemangiomas of considerable size are sometimes encountered in children[34, 35] and may cause disastrous bleeding during attempted intubation of the larynx: the widespread involvement of the laryngeal mucosa may lead the anaesthetist to misinterpret the appearances as simple local hyperaemia. As elsewhere in the body, such haemangiomas are hamartomas rather than true tumours.

Chondroma[36]

A chondroma may arise from any of the laryngeal cartilages. The cricoid cartilage is affected oftenest. The tumour grows very slowly; eventually it may interfere with phonation and respiration.

'Granular Cell Myoblastoma'[37]

About 10 per cent of all 'granular cell myoblastomas' arise in the larynx. There were five examples in the collection of over a thousand laryngeal tumours studied in the Institute of Laryngology and Otology in London during a recently ended period of 23 years. The peak incidence of the laryngeal 'myoblastoma' is in the fourth decade; the tumour may be seen at any age from early childhood. The commonest site is the posterior third of a vocal fold.

Histologically, the essential feature is the characteristic cell (Fig. 6.11), which has abundant, coarsely granular, eosinophile cytoplasm. The cytoplasm often contains distinctive, polygonal or rod-shaped, intensely periodic-acid/Schiff-positive bodies—the 'angular bodies of Bangle'.[38] Electron microscopy shows the cells to be packed with rounded, membrane-bound structures, a micrometre or so in diameter; these contain material of greatly varying electron density; the appearances suggest that they are lysosomes.

The histological diagnosis of 'granular cell myoblastoma' may be confused in some cases by the presence of well-marked pseudocarcinomatous hyperplasia of the overlying epithelium (Fig. 6.12). A mistaken diagnosis of squamous carcinoma of the vocal fold often results.

The nature of the laryngeal 'myoblastoma' is as debatable as that of the corresponding tumours arising elsewhere in the body (see Chapter 39). Recurrence is unusual;[39] in one of our cases the disease recurred 13 years after its initial recognition.

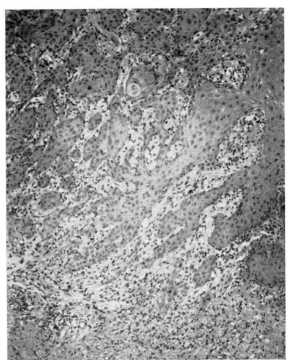

Fig. 6.12. 'Granular cell myoblastoma' of a vocal fold, with pseudocarcinomatous hyperplasia of the overlying squamous epithelium. The pattern of the epithelial proliferation could be mistaken for that of a well-differentiated squamous carcinoma, particularly when—as here—relatively little of the characteristic 'myoblastomatous' tissue is included in the biopsy specimen. *Haematoxylin–eosin.* × 60.

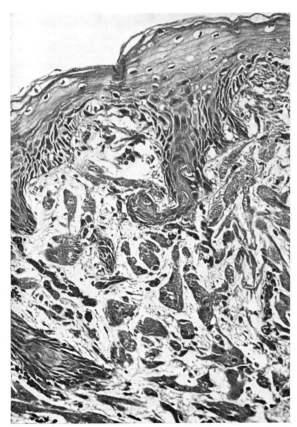

Fig. 6.11. 'Granular cell myoblastoma' of the larynx, showing the characteristic cells. There is some hyperplasia of the overlying epithelium. *Haematoxylin–eosin.* × 175.

MALIGNANT TUMOURS OF THE LARYNX

Squamous Carcinoma

Carcinoma *in situ*
(Intraepithelial Carcinoma)[40, 41]

It follows from the views expressed on pages 255 and 256 that the role of the histopathologist in laryngology is not so much to elaborate upon the more or less distinctive features of the various degrees of keratosis as to recognize the presence of malignant change at as early a stage as possible. While carcinoma *in situ* may be regarded as the earliest recognizable stage of carcinoma, it must be noted that at least some carcinomas are invasive from their outset and do not pass through an in-situ phase. Further, it is not certain that every untreated carcinoma *in situ* becomes an invasive cancer. Undoubtedly, however, the finding of a carcinoma *in situ* demands appropriate treatment, for to ignore the microscopical evidence in the hope that the lesion might not be progressive could prove disastrous for the patient.

Carcinoma *in situ* is commoner in men. Most cases are recognized after middle age, but generally at an age somewhat below that of patients with invasive carcinoma.

Structural Changes

Carcinoma *in situ* may arise in any part of the larynx, intrinsic or extrinsic, but is very much commoner on the true vocal folds, especially their anterior part. Its distribution thus corresponds with that of invasive carcinomas. It is doubtful whether the lesion always starts in areas normally covered by stratified squamous epithelium; when the condition develops in areas ordinarily covered by transitional epithelium or by pseudostratified columnar epithelium of respiratory tract type, it seems likely that metaplasia to squamous epithelium has preceded the neoplastic change.

The initial change in carcinoma *in situ* is believed to take place in the basal layer of the epithelium. As the neoplastic cells gradually extend toward the surface they also spread laterally, in all directions, within the epithelial layers (Fig. 6.13). The cells often migrate into the mucous glands, but there, as in the surface epithelium, they are always confined by the basement membrane. This involvement of the ducts of the glands has to be distinguished from squamous metaplasia of their epithelium, which is by no means uncommon.

Carcinoma *in situ* may be multicentric in origin.

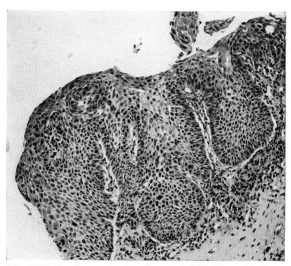

Fig. 6.13. Carcinoma *in situ* of a vocal fold. The epithelium is much thickened, and many of its cells have an unusually darkly stained nucleus or are enlarged. *Haematoxylin–eosin.* × 100.

If specimens are examined thoroughly, appearances typical of the condition are often found in isolated fields of otherwise apparently normal epithelium, or in a number of separate glands or their ducts. Examination of serial sections confirms that these lesions may be completely isolated from one another by areas of apparently healthy epithelium. The extent of the disease may range from small foci of microscopical size, some or all of which may eventually fuse, to involvement of almost the whole mucosa of the larynx.

The changes of carcinoma *in situ* may sometimes be found near an invasive cancer. This must be taken into account when correlating clinical and microscopical findings, especially if the biopsy specimen has included only the edge of a suspect lesion.

A feature of carcinoma *in situ* that adds to the difficulties of microscopical diagnosis is the widely varying degree of anaplasia. Some cells may be very bizarre, and many are giant forms or otherwise atypical. Even where the deviation from cellular normality is slight, and grounds for regarding the condition as malignant are minimal, there is a risk that invasive cancer may develop. It is for this reason that even 'minor' degrees of carcinoma *in situ* may not be disregarded.

Invasive Squamous Carcinoma

Invasive squamous carcinoma of the larynx accounts for 1 to 2 per cent of all cases of human cancer. It occurs at any age after early childhood, the incidence being highest in the seventh decade.

Aetiology and Pathogenesis

Carcinoma of the larynx is often associated with a history of chronic laryngitis, heavy smoking or persistent over-use of the voice. Keratosis may precede the cancer (see page 255). Rarer antecedent conditions include papilloma and lupus vulgaris of the vocal folds. However, in many cases the predisposing conditions are not followed by cancer, and in many cases of cancer there is no history of any recognized predisposing factor.

Hormonal factors have been supposed to have some part in the genesis of laryngeal cancer. Testosterone has been suggested because it is believed to influence the growth of the larynx in males at puberty. The greater incidence of this cancer in men, however, may very well be due to other factors, still unknown.

Topographical Classification

The old-established practice of classifying laryngeal carcinomas as 'intrinsic' or 'extrinsic', according to their situation, is giving way to a system that is more useful in practice, particularly in relation to advances in treatment. Carcinoma of the piriform fossa, formerly classed as an extrinsic growth, is now usually considered as an entity or, along with postcricoid carcinoma (see Chapter 11), as a 'laryngopharyngeal carcinoma'.

Studies of the natural history of laryngeal carcinoma and of the problems—and results—of radiotherapy and surgery have led to international recognition of three main anatomically defined groups of these tumours. The classification that has been evolved relates the tumours to topographical situations that have been designated in accordance with the following anatomical schema:[42]
1. *Supraglottis*: (a) epilarynx (the posterior surface of the suprahyoid part of the glottis, including the tip of the epiglottis, the aryepiglottic folds and the arytenoid region, including the marginal zones); (b) elsewhere than the epilarynx (the infrahyoid level of the epiglottis, the vestibular folds and the ventricles);
2. *Glottis* (the vocal folds and the anterior and posterior commissures);
3. *Subglottis*.

Tumours in the glottis are the most frequent and carry the least unfavourable prognosis. Tumours in the subglottic region are comparatively rare; the prognosis in these cases is very poor. Supraglottic tumours are intermediate in frequency and in outlook.

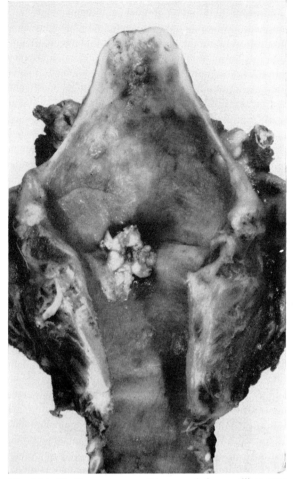

Fig. 6.14. Glottic carcinoma: this example is a papillary type of squamous carcinoma of the anterior end of the left vocal fold.

Macroscopical Appearance

The gross appearances of laryngeal carcinomas may vary considerably. When the vocal folds are involved, as they are in most cases, they may be thickened and indurated by infiltration, destroyed in some degree by ulceration, or obscured by the proliferation of the tumour tissue (Fig. 6.14). Naked-eye examination of laryngectomy specimens of primary carcinoma of a vocal fold may show a degree of subglottic extension (Fig. 6.15); systematic microscopical examination shows such extension to be substantially commoner than has generally been thought.

Excavating ulcers (Fig. 6.16) may cover a large area of the interior of the larynx, with exposure and destruction of cartilage. Bacterial and fungal infections often follow. In contrast to these florid lesions, some laryngeal carcinomas are very small, involving only a segment of a vocal fold at the time of clinical presentation; in such cases the biopsy operation itself may prove to have been in effect a complete excision.

Histology

Most laryngeal carcinomas are squamous and well differentiated, with a varying degree of keratinization. Characteristic 'cell nests' are sometimes formed (Fig. 6.17). A few tumours are anaplastic, presenting either a pleomorphic picture, with bizarre cells and nuclear irregularity, or a predominantly spindle-celled pattern (see below). Like carcinomas of other parts of the body, laryngeal carcinomas may vary in differentiation within the extent of any given tumour.

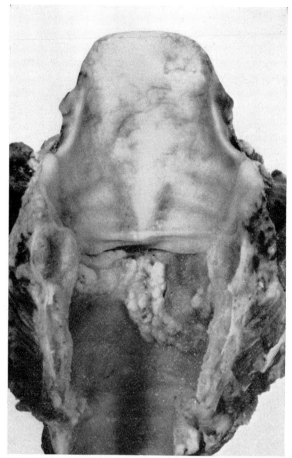

Fig. 6.15. Subglottic carcinoma: this tumour, a squamous carcinoma, arose from the right vocal fold and extended into the anterior commissure.

Areas of intraepithelial carcinoma may be found, sometimes in continuity with the invasive tumour and sometimes separated from it by uninvolved epithelium. These areas are regarded as evidence of the multicentric origin of the disease.

Spindle-Celled Carcinoma ('Laryngeal Pseudo-sarcoma').[43]—The predominantly spindle-celled tumours may closely resemble certain types of sarcoma. They form a controversial group that is sometimes described as pseudosarcomatous.[44] The origin of these 'pseudosarcomas' from surface squamous epithelium is often discernible, and their carcinomatous nature cannot be doubted (Fig. 6.18). The prognosis is poor: 40 per cent of the patients die within two years.[45]

Verrucous Carcinoma.[46–49]—Particular diagnostic difficulties may be caused by the relatively rare verrucous carcinoma of the larynx, which accounts for under 2 per cent of all laryngeal cancers. This tumour, which is seen macroscopically as a warty mass, is characterized microscopically by its uncommonly well differentiated, keratinizing, squamous epithelial structure, which generally lacks recognizable cytological features of malignancy. The epithelium forms broad, club-shaped or finger-like processes that penetrate deeply into the underlying tissue. Anaplastic transformation is occasionally seen.[50] There is a conspicuous inflammatory response in the invaded tissues.

It is notable that the clinician tends to overestimate the malignancy of verrucous carcinoma on examination of the larynx; in contrast, the microscopist tends to misinterpret the lesion, par-

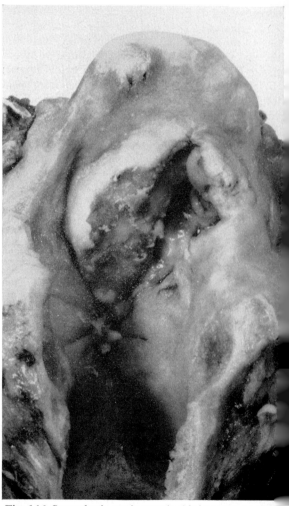

Fig. 6.16. Supraglottic carcinoma: in this instance, a squamous carcinoma of the epiglottis forms a deep, crater-like ulcer at the base of the epiglottis.

ticularly in small biopsy specimens, as an adult type of papilloma (see page 257) or, oftener, as benign keratosis of the vocal fold (see page 255).[51] The possibility of verrucous carcinoma should regularly be considered when the histological picture suggests a diagnosis of keratosis: if the keratotic epithelium is folded into parallel rows or enclosures that contain hyperkeratotic debris, or if there is a broad, pale band of prickle cells just superficial to the basal layer of epithelial cells, the possibility of verrucous carcinoma is strengthened.[51]

Verrucous carcinomas are said to respond poorly to irradiation, which indeed may encourage their recurrence and dissemination.[49]

Spread

Direct extension of laryngeal carcinoma within the mucosa and submucosa is common. The conus elasticus is almost invariably found to be involved in laryngectomy specimens of primary tumours of the vocal folds; the anterior commissure and the

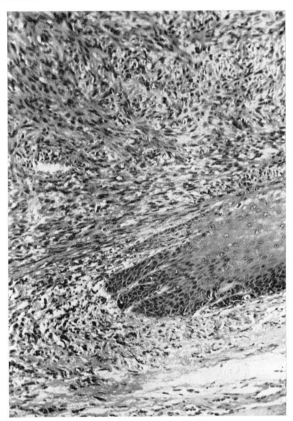

Fig. 6.18. Anaplastic squamous carcinoma of the larynx, composed of spindle-shaped cells (so-called 'pseudo-sarcoma'). *Haematoxylin–eosin.* × 115.

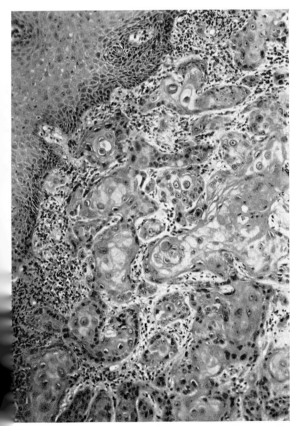

Fig. 6.17. A well-differentiated squamous carcinoma of a vocal fold, with invasion of the lamina propria of the mucosa. *Haematoxylin–eosin.* × 110.

thyroarytenoid muscles are frequently affected. Upward and forward extension, particularly of supraglottic tumours, may involve the post-hyoid space: it is because of the possibility of invasion of this region that the hyoid bone is regularly removed during laryngectomy.

Glottic tumours tend to remain for a long time localized within the larynx. However, tumours involving the anterior commissure may penetrate the cricothyroid ligament, the thyrohyoid membrane or even the thyroid cartilage, to appear in the prelaryngeal region (Fig. 6.19), occasionally reaching the skin of the front of the neck. Systematic examination of operation specimens shows that invasion of cartilage is by no means uncommon: the thyroid cartilage is affected most frequently. Areas of cartilage that have become ossified are most readily invaded. Absence of fixation of the vocal fold does not indicate that invasion of cartilage has not occurred.

Both supraglottic and subglottic tumours metastasize to regional lymph nodes early in their

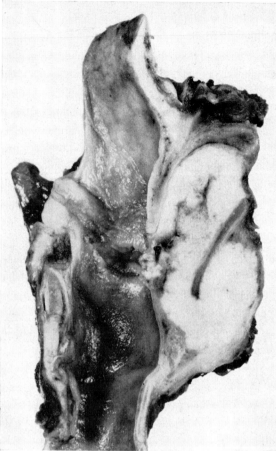

Fig. 6.19. Carcinoma of the larynx. The larynx has been divided sagittally through the midpoint of the right vocal fold, where there was a barely visible ulcer with everted edges. It is seen that the tumour has extended in an exuberant manner from this point anteroinferiorly, through the crico-thyroid ligament, to invest the lamina of the thyroid cartilage, apparently without invading the perichondrium. The tumour has also extended anterosuperiorly, through the thyro-epiglottic ligament and into the pre-epiglottic space. The specimen illustrates the extent to which a superficially small carcinoma may have spread into the more deeply situated structures of the larynx and its vicinity.

course.[52, 53] This is due partly to the abundance of lymphatics in these regions and partly to the higher proportion of such tumours that are less differentiated and more actively growing, and therefore likelier to spread early and widely. Tumours that do not arise from the vocal folds often remain clinically silent until they have reached a relatively advanced stage. It is for these reasons that the prognosis of extraglottic laryngeal carcinomas is so unfavourable.

Recurrence and Metastasis Following Surgical Treatment.[54]—Stomal recurrence and distant metastasis are two of the most important complications that may follow surgical treatment of carcinoma of the larynx. Four factors have been blamed for stomal and peristomal recurrence: at the time of operation the tumour may already have reached the margin of the resection, although not detected; tumour cells may be implanted in the wound during the operation; recurrence may be the result of extension of tumour from metastatic deposits in paratracheal or pretracheal lymph nodes; the apparently recurrent tumour may be in fact a further primary carcinoma. Contamination of the tracheal wound with tumour cells is probably the most usual explanation.

The lungs are the most frequent site of secondary deposits of laryngeal carcinoma. The deposits tend to be small and multiple.[54]

Histological Considerations in Relation to Treatment of Carcinoma of the Larynx[53]

Moderately differentiated and well differentiated tumours respond about equally well to treatment, whether by excision or by irradiation. Poorly differentiated tumours, and anaplastic tumours particularly, respond better to surgery. Attempts to grade histological appearances in biopsy specimens are fraught with difficulty, mainly because the tissue removed is small in amount and therefore may not be truly representative. In practice, modern methods of radiotherapy enable a high proportion of carcinomas of the vocal cords to be treated initially by irradiation; surgery remains the treatment of choice for carcinomas involving other parts of the larynx.

Tumours of the Laryngeal Seromucous Glands
(Including Benign Tumours)

The abundant seromucous glands of the laryngeal mucosa are relatively rarely the source of tumours. The tumours that arise from them are of the types that occur in salivary glands (see Chapter 11); more than half are malignant.

Benign Tumours of Seromucous Glands (Laryngeal Adenomas)

The most frequent benign tumour of seromucous glands is the *simple adenoma*. It usually presents as a swelling no more than a few millimetres across. Rarely, multiple adenomas are found.[55] Microscopically, the adenoma has a simple tubulocystic structure (Fig. 6.20), sometimes with epithelial projections into the lumen of the cysts that justify the name *papillary cystadenoma* (Fig. 6.21). Sometimes the distinction between hyperplasia of the glands and neoplasia is equivocal—what seems to have been a simple retention cyst of one of these glands (see page 256) may turn out to be a tumour, the eventual recurrence of the lesion indicating its real nature.

The adenomas are formed of cuboidal or columnar cells. The cells are sometimes conspicuously eosinophile (the so-called 'oncocytes'): the presence of such cells is believed to indicate that the tumour has arisen from the ducts of the glands rather than from their acini. Similar cells are a feature of some tumours that arise from the ducts of salivary glands (see Chapter 11). Recurrent tumours may assume the appearance of the microcystic type of papillary adenoma that occurs in the nasal mucosa (see page 223): this underlines the close relation between these growths.

Malignant Tumours of Seromucous Glands[56]

A *pleomorphic tumour* corresponding to the pleomorphic ('mixed') type of tumour of salivary

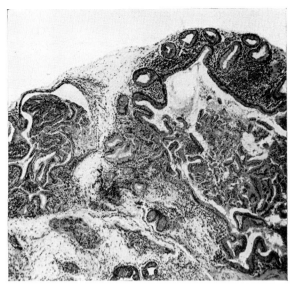

Fig. 6.21. Papillary type of cystadenoma of a ventricular fold. *Haematoxylin–eosin.* × 45.

glands (see Chapter 11) is occasionally found in the larynx.[57] There were no examples in our series of over a thousand laryngeal tumours.

The commonest malignant tumour of the laryngeal glands is the *adenoid cystic carcinoma* (cribriform adenocarcinoma, or cylindroma).

Other Adenocarcinomas

Other types of adenocarcinoma, among which the mucoepidermoid carcinoma may for convenience be included (see Chapter 11), are occasionally found in the larynx.[58] They are all very rare. Taken together, the adenocarcinomas (including those arising from the seromucous glands—see above)[59] account for less than 1 per cent of all cases of cancer of the larynx.[60]

Metastatic adenocarcinoma is an occasional finding in the larynx. It may be mistaken for a primary growth. Renal adenocarcinoma is the most frequent source of such secondary deposits.

Other Malignant Tumours

Sarcomas

Sarcomas account for about 1 to 2 per cent of all malignant neoplasms of the larynx.[61] Most of them are *fibrosarcomas*,[62] and these must be distinguished from the spindle-celled anaplastic carcinomas ('pseudosarcomas') referred to above (page 262). *Chondrosarcomas*[63] are next in frequency; they correspond in structure and behaviour to chondro-

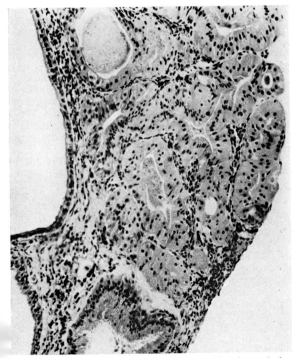

Fig. 6.20. Simple adenoma of the larynx, showing tubules and cyst formation. The tubules are formed of the eosinophile type of cell that is associated with the ducts of the seromucous glands. *Haematoxylin–eosin.* × 150.

sarcomas arising in bone (see Chapter 37), and they pose the same problems in histological interpretation. *Rhabdomyosarcoma*,[61] *liposarcoma* and *angiosarcoma* are among the tumours that have been recorded occasionally.

Lymphomas, particularly lymphocytic lymphomas, have been recognized in the larynx. In most cases the larynx seems to have been involved secondarily, but both lymphocytic lymphomas and Hodgkin's disease may be confined to the interior of the larynx, presenting with appearances clinically indistinguishable from those of carcinomatous ulceration.[64]

Myeloma

The mucosa of the larynx is one of the extramedullary sites of myeloma (plasmacytoma). The tumour may form a polypoid mass that interferes with phonation and obstructs the airway. Ulcera-

tion may lead to serious bleeding. The tumour may be solitary, or—more rarely—there are several myelomas in the larynx, either in the absence of disease elsewhere or associated with extramedullary myeloma of the nose (see page 231). Amyloid may be laid down in these tumours (see page 252).

Scleroma must always be considered in the differential diagnosis of myeloma of the larynx (see page 204).

Myelomatosis.—The larynx is sometimes involved in myelomatosis. This exceptional occurrence is virtually confined to those older patients whose laryngeal cartilage has ossified, the foci of tumour developing within the marrow cavity. In one such case, laryngeal foci of unsuspected myelomatosis resulted in pathological fractures during thyroidectomy, with fatal obstruction of the larynx, which collapsed when the anaesthetist withdrew the laryngeal tube at the close of the operation.[64]

REFERENCES

1. Lindahl, J. W. S., Robertson, M. S., *Lancet*, 1963, **1**, 635.
2. Carstairs, L. S., Emond, R. T. D., *Proc. roy. Soc. Med.*, 1963, **56**, 267.
3. Camps, F. E., *Proc. roy. Soc. Med.*, 1953, **46**, 281.
4. Jones, H. M., Camps, F. E., *Practitioner*, 1957, **178**, 223.
5. Ormerod, F. C., *Tuberculosis of the Upper Respiratory Tracts*. London, 1939.
6. Lofgren, R. H., Montgomery, W. W., *New Engl. J. Med.*, 1962, **267**, 193.
7. Montgomery, W. W., Lofgren, R. H., *Arch. Otolaryng.*, 1963, **77**, 29.
8. Darke, C. S., Wolman, L., Young, A., *Brit. med. J.*, 1958, **1**, 1279.
9. Webb, J., Payne, W. H., *Ann. rheum. Dis.*, 1972, **31**, 122.
10. Abadir, W. F., Forster, P. M., *J. Laryng.*, 1974, **88**, 473.
11. Bonito, L. di, Ferlito, A., *Clin. oto-rino-laring.*, 1971, **22**, 94.
12. McAlpine, J. C., Radcliffe, A., Friedmann, I., *J. Laryng.*, 1963, **77**, 1.
13. Symmers, W. St C., *J. clin. Path.*, 1956, **9**, 187.
14. New, G. B., Erich, J. B., *Arch. Otolaryng.*, 1938, **28**, 841.
15. Epstein, S. S., Winston, P., Friedmann, I., Ormerod, F. C., *J. Laryng.*, 1957, **71**, 673.
16. Chiari, O., *Arch. Laryng. Rhin. (Berl.)*, 1895, **2**, 1.
17. Symmers, W. St C., *unpublished observations*.
18. Symmers, W. St C., *unpublished observations*, 1956.
19. Kleinsasser, O., *Arch. Ohr.-, Nas.-, u. Kehlk.-Heilk.*, 1959, **174**, 290.
20. Miller, A. H., Fisher, H. R., *Laryngoscope (St Louis)*, 1971, **81**, 1475.

21. Bauer, W. C., McGavran, M. H., *J. Amer. med. Ass.* 1972, **221**, 72.
22. Asherson, N., *J. Laryng.*, 1957, **71**, 730.
23. Grimaud, R., Pierson, B., Wiadzalowski, G. J. *J. franç., Oto-rhino-laryng.*, 1961, **10**, 587.
24. Meessen, H., Schultz, K., *Klin. Wschr.*, 1957, **35**, 771.
25. Hollinger, P. H., Johnston, K. C., Conner, G. H., Conner, B. R., Holper, J., *Ann. Otol. (St Louis)*, 1962, **71**, 443.
26. Altmann, F., Basek, M., Stout, A. P., *A.M.A. Arch. Otolaryng.*, 1955, **62**, 478.
27. Webb, W. W., *Laryngoscope (St Louis)*, 1956, **66**, 871.
28. Kleinsasser, O., *Arch. Ohr.-, Nas.-, u. Kehlk.-Heilk.*, 1958, **174**, 44.
29. Vetters, J. M., Toner, P. G., *J. Path.*, 1970, **101**, 259.
30. Lawson, W., Zak, F. G., *Laryngoscope (St Louis)*, 1974, **84**, 98.
31. Helpap, B., Koch, U., *Z. Laryng. Rhinol.*, 1974, **53**, 410.
32. Symmers, W. St C., *personal observation*, 1974.
33. Cummings, C. W., Montgomery, W. W., Balogh, K., Jr, *Ann. Otol. (St Louis)*, 1969, **78**, 76.
34. Baker, D. C., Jr, Pennington, C. L., *Laryngoscope (St Louis)*, 1956, **66**, 696.
35. Cameron, A. H., Cant, W. H. P., MacGregor, M. E., Prior, A. P., *J. Laryng.*, 1960, **74**, 846.
36. Walter, W. L., *Ann. Otol. (St Louis)*, 1959, **68**, 1144.
37. Booth, J. B., Osborn, D. A., *Acta oto-laryng. (Stockh.)*, 1970, **70**, 279.
38. Bangle, R., Jr, *Cancer (Philad.)*, 1952, **5**, 950.
39. Walter, W. L., *Ann. Otol. (St Louis)*, 1960, **69**, 328.
40. Stout, A. P., *Amer. J. Roentgenol.*, 1953, **69**, 1.
41. Kleinsasser, O., Heck, K. H., *Arch. Ohr.-, Nas.-, u. Kehlk.-Heilk.*, 1959, **174**, 210.
42. International Union against Cancer, Committee on

TNM Classification, *The TNM Classification of Malignant Tumours*. Geneva, 1972.

43. Sherwin, R. P., Strong, M. S., Vaughan, C. W., *Cancer (Philad.)*, 1963, **16**, 51.
44. Grigg, J. W., Rachmaninoff, N., Robb, J. M., *Laryngoscope (St Louis)*, 1961, **71**, 555.
45. Hyams, V., *Canad. J. Otolaryng.*, 1975, **4**, 307.
46. Ackerman, L. V., *Surgery*, 1948, **23**, 670.
47. Kraus, F. T., Perez-Mesa, C., *Cancer (Philad.)*, 1966, **19**, 26.
48. Biller, H. F., Ogura, J. H., Bauer, W. C., *Laryngoscope (St Louis)*, 1971, **81**, 1323.
49. Nostrand, A. W. P. van, Olofsson, J., *Cancer (Philad.)*, 1972, **30**, 691.
50. Demian, S. D. E., Bushkin, F. L., Echevarria, R. A., *Cancer (Philad.)*, 1973, **32**, 395.
51. Fisher, H. R., *Canad. J. Otolaryng.*, 1975, **4**, 270.
52. Putney, F. J., *Ann. Otol. (St Louis)*, 1958, **67**, 136.
53. Ormerod, F. C., Shaw, H. J., *J. Laryng.*, 1956, **70**, 433.
54. Batsakis, J. G., *Tumorous Conditions of the Head and Neck*. Baltimore, 1974.
55. Ranger, D., Thackray, A. C., *J. Laryng.*, 1953, **67**, 609.
56. Toomey, J. M., *Laryngoscope (St Louis)*, 1967, **77**, 931.
57. Sabri, A. J., Hajjar, M. A., *Arch. Otolaryng.*, 1967, **85**, 332.
58. Rosenfeld, L., Sessions, D. G., McSwain, B., Graves, H., *Ann. Surg.*, 1966, **163**, 726.
59. Whicker, I. H., Neel, H. B., III, Weiland, L. H., Devine, K. D., *Ann. Otol. (St Louis)*, 1974, **83**, 487.
60. Fechner, R. E., *Canad. J. Otolaryng.*, 1975, **4**, 284.
61. Batsakis, J. G., Fox, J. E., *Surg. Gynec. Obstet.*, 1970, **131**, 989.
62. Norris, C. M., *Ann. Otol. (St Louis)*, 1959, **68**, 487.
63. Huizenga, C. H., Balogh, K. J., *Cancer (Philad.)*, 1970, **26**, 201.
64. Symmers, W. St C., *unpublished observations*, 1966–1974.

ACKNOWLEDGEMENT FOR ILLUSTRATION

Fig. 6.10. Photomicrograph of authors' preparation by Mr R. S. Barnett, Department of Histopathology, Charing Cross Hospital Medical School, London.

7: The Lungs
including the Trachea and Bronchi and the Pleura

by G. Payling Wright *and* B. E. Heard
revised by B. E. Heard

CONTENTS

7: *The Lungs*

including the Trachea and Bronchi
and the Pleura

by G. PAYLING WRIGHT *and* B. E. HEARD
revised by B. E. HEARD

THE LUNGS

THE STRUCTURE OF THE NORMAL LUNG

Anatomical Segments.—Before 1949, the names of the segments of the lungs were not generally agreed. For instance, the apical segment of the upper lobe of the right lung was termed the pectoral, or anterior, or anterolateral segment by different authors. In that year, an international nomenclature was introduced: this is illustrated diagrammatically in Fig. 7.1.[1-4] The branches indicated by the letters on the diagram are named according to the anatomical segments noted in the following paragraph. It is desirable that pathologists use only this terminology in their records.

The following anatomical features are common to both lungs (Fig. 7.1): each *upper lobe* has anterior (C,T), apical (D,U) and posterior (E,V) segments; each *lower lobe* has apical (J,AA), anterior (M,BB), lateral (N,CC) and posterior (O,DD) segments. In the following respects the two lungs differ: (i) the *right main bronchus* (A) continues through a lower part (F) to become the bronchus to the basal segments (L); the *left main bronchus* (P) continues as the lower lobe bronchus (Z); (ii) the *middle lobe of the right lung* is served by a branch (G) of the lower part of the right main bronchus (F), whereas the *lingula of the left lung*, which is the homologue of the right middle lobe, is served by a branch (W) of the upper lobe bronchus (Q); (iii) unlike the left lung, the *lower lobe of the right lung* bears a small extra segment called the medial basal (or cardiac) segment (K); (iv) the two *subdivisions of the right middle lobe* are respectively medial (H) and lateral (I), while the two *subdivisions of the lingula* are superior (X) and inferior (Y).

The inspired air passes through many divisions

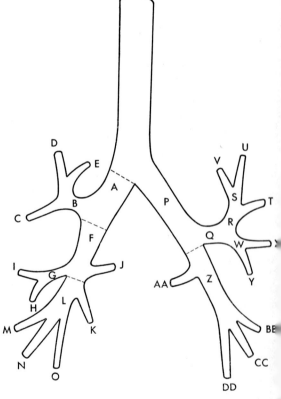

Fig. 7.1. Diagram of the common arrangement of the bronchial tree, based on *The Nomenclature of the Bronchial Tree* (*Thorax*, 1950, **5**, 222). The lettered branches are referred to in the text (this page).

of the bronchi (which possess muscle, cartilage and mucous glands in their walls) and the bronchioles (which have muscle but neither cartilage nor glands) before it reaches the first alveoli the

270

bud from the walls of the respiratory bronchioles. Between the tracheal bifurcation and the smallest bronchi of the right upper lobe about eight divisions are passed.[5] Three or four further divisions of the bronchioles follow, the last element in the sequence being the terminal bronchiole. From this point onward there are three orders of respiratory bronchioles and one order of alveolar ducts; the alveoli bud from the walls of the respiratory bronchioles and alveolar ducts, and it is only in the alveoli that the main gaseous exchange takes place (Fig. 7.2).

Lung substance is divided into secondary lobules, each measuring 1 to 2 cm in diameter and clearly demarcated in some parts of the lung by fibrous septa that are visible both on the cut surface and on the outer surface.[6] Each secondary lobule is formed by a cluster of about five acini. The term acinus is applied to all the respiratory tissue

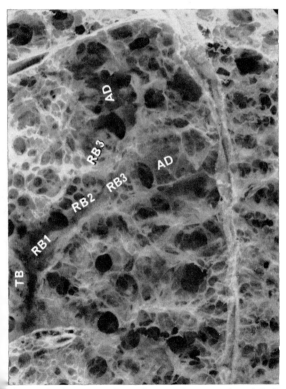

Fig. 7.2.§ The cut surface of part of a secondary lobule, showing some of the branches of an acinus. TB—terminal non-respiratory bronchiole. RB 1, RB 2, RB 3—successive orders of respiratory bronchioles. AD—alveolar duct. The fibrous septa that border the lobule are also seen. There is some loss of alveolar walls, indicating a mild degree of destructive panlobular emphysema (see page 292). *Pressure fixation; barium sulphate impregnation.* × 10.

§ See *Acknowledgements*, page 428.

supplied with air by one terminal bronchiole. Each acinus contains about 2000 alveoli. It is estimated that both lungs together contain about 300 million alveoli, and that the surface area that they present to the respiratory gases is about 100 square metres.[7]

The pulmonary arteries accompany the bronchi and enter the secondary lobules centrally.[8] The pulmonary veins, on the other hand, leave the lobules at their periphery and run in the surrounding septa. The blood entering the lungs by the pulmonary arteries flows mainly through the capillaries in the walls of the alveoli.

The bronchial arteries[9] supply the lungs with oxygenated blood. The right artery is usually single and arises from the third posterior intercostal artery or from the upper left bronchial artery. It joins the posterior surface of the right bronchi and follows and supplies them. The left bronchial arteries are usually two in number and arise from the descending thoracic aorta. The bronchial veins, usually two on each side, open into the azygos vein on the right and the superior intercostal vein or superior hemiazygos vein on the left. Blood from the bronchial and pulmonary arteries mixes to a limited extent, and the bronchial veins do not necessarily drain only blood supplied by the bronchial arteries.

The lungs have abundant lymphatic drainage. The lymph channels close to the surface of the lung open into the subpleural plexus; those deeper in its substance pass to the hilar lymph nodes. The infratracheal group of nodes collects lymph from both lower lobes, while the tracheobronchial nodes on each side of the trachea receive lymph from the remaining lobes on the respective sides. The lymph from the left tracheobronchial group of nodes drains into the thoracic duct, while that from the nodes on the right side passes into the right bronchomediastinal trunk; each of these main channels empties into the subclavian vein of its own side. The lymphatics of the two lungs communicate freely.

Microscopical Structure[10]

Light Microscopy.—The bronchi are lined by a pseudostratified ciliate epithelium that decreases in height distally, becoming single-layered in the bronchioles. Non-ciliate cells may be present at the surface among the ciliate ones, but the latter are present as far as the respiratory bronchioles. Mucus-secreting goblet cells usually lie singly among the ciliate cells; they decrease in number as the bronchioles are approached.

The epithelium lies on a basement membrane over a vasculofibrous layer interrupted by collections of longitudinally-arranged elastic fibres that correspond in position to the longitudinal ridges in the mucous membrane. Smooth muscle fibres run circumferentially or obliquely in the submucosa in the form of a geodesic network;[11] they give rise to transverse ridges. The ducts of the bronchial glands pass toward the bronchial lumen through this network of fibres. Relative to the size of the lumen, the musculature is thickest in the terminal bronchioles. The acini of the compound bronchial glands are part mucous and part serous. Many lymphatics are present in the walls of the bronchi and of all the smaller air passages as far as the alveolar ducts.

The alveolar walls contain an enormous number of blood capillaries arranged in a fine meshwork that enables the ready passage of gases to and from the blood stream. The stroma of the alveolar walls contains reticulin fibres, occasional elastic and collagen fibres, and some histiocytes.

Alveolar Pores.—Small holes, the pores of Kohn,[12] are found in the alveolar walls. They are a normal feature in all animals and in man: their diameter ranges from 2 to 13 μm and there are from one to seven pores in each alveolus. They are absent at birth, and in man develop at the end of the first year of life. For this reason some argue that they are an abnormality and represent the beginnings of emphysema. Others believe that they are normal and provide collateral ventilation to lobules when bronchioles are obstructed by mucus.[13]

Pores can sometimes be seen in paraffin sections of pneumonic lesions when threads of the fibrinous exudate pass through them from one alveolus to another. They are seen better in thick histological sections than in those of usual thickness. They are evident in electron micrographs, which show their edge to be formed by intact alveolar wall.[14] They are best demonstrated with the scanning electron microscope (Fig. 7.3).

Electron Microscopy.[15, 16]—Owing to the speed of autolysis of dead cells it is necessary to place tissues into a 1 to 5 per cent solution of glutaraldehyde within a few minutes of surgical removal if preservation is to be at its best for electron microscopy. Human necropsy material is unsuitable.

Bronchial epithelium can be studied in far greater detail than by light microscopy.[17] For instance, it has been possible to demonstrate about 250 cilia on each ciliate cell, each cilium being about 5 to 8 μm long and 0·25 to 0·30 μm wide. The cilium has a covering three-layered unit membrane that is continuous with the membranes of the cell. Internally there are 11 filaments, two centrally placed and nine arranged in a circle round them. Between the cilia are about 150 filiform villi up to 1 μm long. The mucigen granules of the mucosal goblet cells originate near the Golgi apparatus and enlarge as they pass toward the surface before extrusion. The less common brush cell is recognized by the regular, broad, blunt microvilli on its surface, 0·5 to 1·0 μm long and 150 to 180 μm wide.[18, 19] Occasional argentaffin cells are seen at the basal level of the surface epithelium; they are recognized by their neurosecretory granules.

Bronchiolar epithelium is simpler than bronchial. Its ciliate cells are shorter, and protruding between them are the occasional, distinctive Clara cells:[20] the latter contain peculiar, oval, cytoplasmic bodies that are believed to be mitochondria.

Electron microscopy has settled an old argument by demonstrating quite clearly that there is a continuous epithelial lining to the alveolar walls. Normally, this lining is without interruptions, although in places the cytoplasm of the cells thins to 100 nm and cannot be resolved by the light microscope in tissue preserved with the older fixatives.[21, 22] The electron microscope has also confirmed that there are two kinds of alveolar epithelial cell (pneumonocyte)—the type 1 pneumonocyte, which is flat and rather featureless, with similarities to an endothelial cell, and the type 2 pneumonocyte, which is larger and contains some dense, laminate, osmiophile inclusions that are about 2 μm in diameter (Fig. 7.4). These cells had been observed by light microscopy and termed membranous and granular pneumonocytes (pneumocytes) respectively.[23, 24] Type 2 cells secrete surfactants that coat the interior of the alveoli and, by reducing surface tension, help prevent collapse.[25, 26] The osmiophile bodies in these cells represent surfactants in course of formation. The surfactant material on the surface of the alveolar lining can be visualized by special methods.[27–29] Recent evidence suggests that type 1 cells are derived from type 2 cells by mitotic division.[30] This would explain why type 2 cells often become more numerous in alveoli that are the site of injury and repair.

The epithelial cells lie on a basement membrane. This is separated by the interstitial space from the capillary basement membrane, which abuts on the

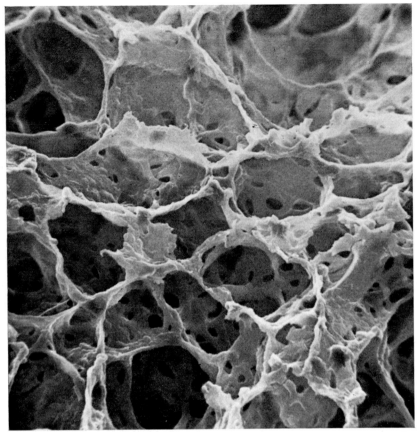

Fig. 7.3. Lung of a normal mouse viewed with the scanning electron microscope. The small holes in the alveolar walls are the pores of Kohn. × 540.

endothelial cells. The capillaries of the alveolar septa are without pores and fenestrae, unlike renal and pancreatic capillaries. Septal cells lie in the interstices, as well as collagen, elastic and reticulin fibres. There is muscle near the mouth of the alveolus. Nerves and nerve endings have been demonstrated in the alveolar wall in mice.[31]

A few free-lying macrophages are generally present within the lumen of the normal alveolus. They have a vital part in clearing dust from the lungs and are of major importance in the pathology of pneumoconiosis. They are larger than lymphocytes and have a round or indented nucleus; dust particles are commonly present in their cytoplasm. Under the electron microscope the cytoplasm is seen to contain many lysosomes: these bear hydrolytic enzymes that are injected into the intracellular vesicles that form round foreign material as it is ingested by the cell.

Lymphatics can be seen by electron microscopy in the pleura and in the connective tissues round arteries, veins and bronchi. They have also been identified very near the alveolar walls (the so-called juxta-alveolar lymphatic capillaries) but not with certainty in the alveolar walls themselves.[32]

Scanning Electron Microscopy.—The scanning electron microscope is proving invaluable in the study of the respiratory tract. It enables the internal surfaces of airways to be observed at higher magnifications than previously. Its use in studying the pores of Kohn has been mentioned above (Fig. 7.3): one method of achieving this is to distend fresh lung with buffered glutaraldehyde and examine small pieces after drying by the critical-point method[33]—the fixative washes away mucus and surfactant that would otherwise obscure the pores.

CONGENITAL MALFORMATIONS

Congenital Bronchopulmonary Anomalies

At the fourth week of development, the trachea becomes separated from the ventral surface of the

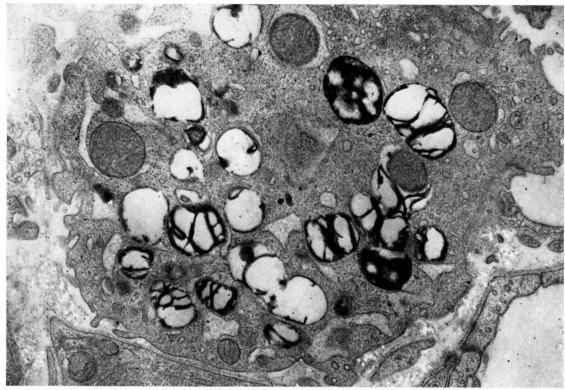

Fig. 7.4. Electron micrograph of normal rat lung showing a type 2 epithelial cell. The intracytoplasmic bodies containing strongly osmiophile material are characteristic of these cells: they represent surfactants in process of formation. × 18 000.

foregut through the formation of the tracheo-oesophageal septum.[34] Two bronchial buds appear at its lower end and grow into each half of the thoracic cavity as the primary bronchi, branching later to form lobar and segmental bronchi. A defect in this branching may subsequently cause profound abnormalities of the anatomy of the lungs. On very rare occasions, only a malformed trachea may be present, or, following the failure of one primary bronchus, there may be agenesis of one lung—an anomaly surprisingly compatible with long life. Some variation in the arrangement of the segmental bronchi is common, and seldom of pathological significance. For example, if the eparterial bronchus on the right side fails to develop, a more peripheral branch of the first ventral main bronchus takes its place. Anomalies in bronchial architecture can be induced experimentally in rats—for example, by subjecting the mother to vitamin A deficiency during pregnancy.[35]

A minor malformation of a segmental bronchus or of structures near it may cause distal air-trapping and the condition known as congenital lobar emphysema (see page 292).

Hypoplasia.—One or both lungs may be hypoplastic, and this condition may accompany other congenital anomalies, such as congenital diaphragmatic hernia.[36] Hypoplasia of the right lung is a feature of the 'scimitar syndrome', so-called because of the radiological appearance produced by an anomalous pulmonary vein along the right cardiac border.[37]

A very rare disorder is total lack of mucous glands in the respiratory tract. This occurs as a part of the condition known as congenital anhidrotic ectodermal dysplasia.[38]

Congenital Cystic Diseases of the Lung

Congenital Cysts of Bronchial Origin.—Developmental errors that involve deficiencies of bronchial or bronchiolar cartilage, elastic tissue and muscle may be responsible for one form of congenital cystic disease of the lungs.[39–41] The number and size of the cysts in this condition vary greatly. A single large cyst that occupies most of one lobe is termed a *pneumatocele*. Oftener, the cysts are smaller and multiple, and so widespread that the lung has a sponge-like appearance (Fig. 7.5). The affected portion of the bronchus dilates into a thin-walled cyst, several millimetres in diameter, and sometimes much larger, that is generally lined by rather flattened, ciliate, mucus-secreting epithelium. As a rule, these cysts contain air and have a smooth lining; occasionally they are filled with opalescent fluid and lack attachment to their bronchus of origin. Those that still communicate with the parent bronchus are liable to become infected and converted into abscesses. Occasionally, a cyst ruptures into a pleural cavity, giving rise to pneumothorax.

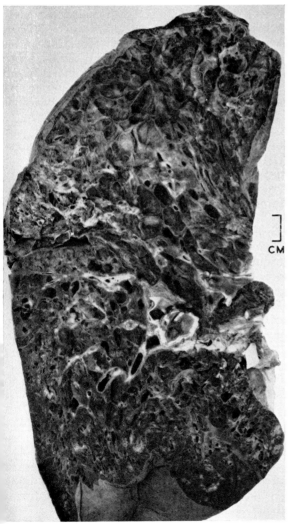

Fig. 7.5.§ Congenital cystic disease of lung. The cystic spaces range from 1 to 10 mm in diameter: they are thin-walled and have a smooth lining, and there is no evidence of infection.

Other Congenital Cysts.—Congenital pulmonary lymphangiectasis is characterized by the presence of lymph cysts and dilated lymphatic channels in the connective tissue beneath the pleura and in the interlobar septa.[42]

Cysts of pleural origin are an occasional congenital anomaly.[43, 44]

The description 'congenital' should not be applied, as sometimes it has been, to acquired varieties of lung cysts, simply because they develop during the course of hereditary metabolic diseases (for instance, Hand–Schüller–Christian disease and xanthomatosis) or of certain diseases of early childhood (for instance, Letterer–Siwe disease).

Congenital cystic adenomatoid malformation is described on page 276.

Accessory Pulmonary Lobes.—An *azygos lobe* is occasionally found on the medial side of the right upper lobe and separated from it by the azygos vein, which has curved too far laterally. Since it is extrapleural, the vein brings down a fold of pleura, termed the mesazygos.

The *cardiac lobe* (medial basal lobe) is sometimes separated from the right lower lobe: this is a condition normally present in certain quadrupeds, such as rabbits. A so-called *tracheal lobe* arises occasionally from the right side of the trachea just above the bifurcation. Very rarely, an accessory lobe arises from the oesophagus.

Sequestration.—The term sequestration refers to the presence of abnormal masses of lung tissue that have no bronchial connexion with the main body of the lung. In *extralobar sequestration* the mass may be at the base of the left lung, or below the diaphragm, near the left kidney. Its arterial supply is from the aorta or the left adrenal artery. In *intralobar sequestration* a bronchopulmonary mass or cyst is included in either of the lower lobes.[45-48] Sometimes the sequestered tissue projects from the lung on a narrow stalk: this form has been referred to as *intermediate sequestration*. In most cases the misplaced tissue is supplied by an accessory branch of the aorta; the wall of this vessel resembles a pulmonary artery histologically.

Sequestration of the lung may present with haemoptysis or repeated chest infection in early life; in contrast, it may be symptomless for many years.

Extralobar sequestration is believed to originate from an accessory pulmonary bud arising from the lower part of a normal bronchial bud or from an oesophageal diverticulum. The origin of intralobar sequestration is still uncertain: the accessory bud may arise from the foregut, the aberrant artery developing independently;[49] alternatively, an aberrant branch of the aorta may be the primary anomaly, causing sequestration by traction. It is also possible that in some cases the condition is not congenital but the outcome of inflammation in early life.

Congenital Cystic Adenomatoid Malformation.— Sequestration of the lung has to be distinguished from this condition, in which part of one lung is cystic.[50, 51] Histologically, the cysts resemble overgrown bronchioles and are lined in places by tall mucigenic epithelial cells. The air spaces in the affected parts communicate with the bronchi, unlike those in sequestration.

Congenital Vascular Anomalies

The pulmonary vascular bed initially appears as a capillary plexus embracing the pulmonary anlage. It arises independently of the primary pulmonary arteries, which are derived from the sixth pair of aortic arches.[52] As they grow caudally the pulmonary arteries normally separate from the dorsal aorta, except for the ductus arteriosus; the bronchial arteries continue throughout life to supply blood to the lungs directly from the aorta.

Defects in the complicated development of the pulmonary arches and plexus result in a wide variety of anomalies.

Stenosis.—This may affect one segment of the vasculature or there may be multiple constrictions. It may affect the main pulmonary arteries or their lobar and segmental branches. It is usually associated with poststenotic dilatation of the affected vessel. There may be accompanying cardiac anomalies (see page 96).

Aplasia.—Aplasia (agenesis) of a pulmonary artery occurs with equal frequency on the right and left. In nearly half the cases an anomalous systemic artery arises from the aorta or one of its branches to supply the lung of the affected side; in the others a collateral circulation develops from the bronchial arteries. *Hypoplasia of a pulmonary artery* can occur. These conditions are recognized more readily now than formerly, owing to improvements in angiocardiography. On the affected side, there may be diminution of lung movement and of breath sounds; recurrent pulmonary infections are common, but the anomaly may be symptomless.[53]

Pulmonary Arteriovenous Fistula.—A pulmonary arteriovenous fistula is a persistent communication between a pulmonary artery and vein, bypassing part of the capillary bed. Such shunts may be single or multiple. They may lead to cyanosis, polycythaemia and clubbing of the fingers. About half the patients with congenital pulmonary arteriovenous shunts suffer from hereditary haemorrhagic telangiectasia (see page 166), a condition characterized by weakness and dilatation of capillaries and an accompanying tendency to capillary bleeding.[54]

Anastomoses Between Bronchial and Pulmonary Arteries.—Studies of normal fetal and neonatal lungs have shown the presence of small anastomoses between bronchial and pulmonary arteries. These anastomotic channels are from 40 to 240 μm in diameter. In normal children they become fewer during the first two years of life, and they are rarely seen later than that.[55, 56] They persist and may enlarge in the presence of some congenital cardiac and pulmonary diseases.

An *anomalous systemic artery* may supply part of a lung,[57] as occurs also in some cases of sequestration. There is usually then some degree of anastomosis with branches of the pulmonary arteries in addition to the common circulation through the capillary bed.

Anomalies of Pulmonary Veins.—There may be abnormalities of the origin, connexions and distribution of the pulmonary veins. Varicosity is an occasional form of venous malformation.

Extrapulmonary Causes of Congenital Anomalies of Pulmonary Vessels.—The pulmonary vasculature may be abnormal at birth as a consequence of an extrapulmonary disorder. For example, hypoplasia of the chambers of the left side of the heart results in less blood passing through the foramen ovale than is normal and correspondingly more passing into the right ventricle and pulmonary arteries. This leads to an abnormal increase in the amount of muscle in the medial coat of the pulmonary arteries before birth.[58] Conversely, pulmonary stenosis may result in a subnormal muscle mass in these vessels. The normal postnatal decrease in the amount of pulmonary artery muscle is not found in infants who are born at high altitudes.[59]

'Plexiform Structures'.—Repeated thrombosis and recanalization of pulmonary arteries results in the development in the former lumen of a spongework

of vascular spaces, the so-called plexiform structures. Such lesions are sometimes congenital and sometimes a result of postnatal thrombosis (see page 283).

(see page 283)

VASCULAR DISTURBANCES

Pulmonary Embolism and Infarction

The sequelae of embolism in the pulmonary arterial tree are often seen at necropsy, especially in elderly and obese people who have been confined to bed with congestive cardiac failure, and in adults of any age who have undergone a major surgical operation.[60] Experiments using radioactive fibrinogen have shown that deep vein thrombosis occurs in at least a third of patients over 40 who are convalescent after operations.[61] In most cases, fortunately, it does not extend above the calf.

Pulmonary embolism also occurs following parturition. This complication of childbirth is much less frequent than formerly because of recognition of the prophylactic value of massage and exercise. Puerperal thromboembolism is seen oftener among women whose lactation has been inhibited by administration of oestrogen than among those who feed their babies at the breast.[62, 63] The part played by oestrogens in promoting thromboembolism has been established also by study of the effects of oral contraceptives. A regimen providing more than 100 μg of oestrogens daily is said to be more dangerous than others.[64] The most consistent changes in the blood have been acceleration of factors VII and X and of platelet aggregation.

Embolism after operations and in the post-partum period usually follows thrombosis in tributaries of the main veins of the legs and thighs, where the vascular stasis that follows immobilization in bed is known to be most pronounced.[65] Less often, the emboli originate in the veins of the arms or pelvis, or in the appendage of the right atrium; they are then smaller and less liable to cause sudden death.

Sometimes the embolus is a massive one, and its lodgement in the pulmonary conus or main pulmonary artery is at once fatal because of virtually complete obstruction of the circulation through the lungs (see below). More frequently, the embolus is smaller, and by coming to rest more distally may lead to infarction in the region supplied by the obstructed artery. In these cases there may be more than one embolic episode, each indicated clinically by an attack of localized pleural pain,

with dyspnoea and haemoptysis: at necropsy, infarcts of different ages are found.[66]

Sudden Fatal Pulmonary Embolism

In the cases in which sudden death follows the release of a large thrombus from the leg veins, the embolus is found at necropsy to be coiled on itself, straddling the bifurcation of the pulmonary trunk (Fig. 7.6). The chambers of the right side of the heart and the venae cavae are distended; the left atrium and ventricle are contracted and empty, and the lungs are pale.

When the embolus is removed from the site of its impaction and uncoiled it is seen to be on average about a centimetre in diameter, corresponding to the calibre of the vessels in which it had formed. Its surface is marked in correspondence with the venous valves; the broken ends of the thrombotic cast of the tributary veins can also be recognized and it may be possible to match these with the thrombus remaining in the veins.

Thrombi that have been carried to the pulmonary arteries as emboli must be distinguished from those that have formed in these vessels. The latter are more firmly attached to the wall of the vessel and are likelier to show a laminate pattern when incised. Both thrombi formed *in situ* and

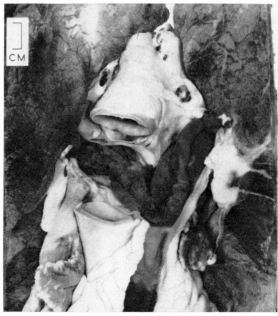

Fig. 7.6.§ Massive pulmonary embolism. The dark V-shaped mass in the centre of the photograph is a coiled-up thrombus from the veins of a leg. It plugged the left and right main pulmonary arteries completely, causing immediate death.

K

thrombotic emboli are firm but friable, and show lines of Zahn, indicative of their development during life: these features distinguish them from clots formed *post mortem*. The latter are shiny, soft and elastic: when pulled carefully from the vessels they also show the characteristic 'horse's tail' appearance of the cast of blood from the smaller branches of the pulmonary arteries. The post-mortem clots may show a transition from red to yellow, corresponding to sedimentation of the cellular constituents in the stagnant blood, leaving a paler zone of serum in the eventual coagulum: this demarcation lacks the multiple layering that characterizes the lines of Zahn in the thrombi.

Often, the thrombus breaks into several fragments at its origin or during its passage through the heart, and these smaller pieces are carried farther into the pulmonary tree. The lodgement of such multiple emboli in the major or smaller branches of the main pulmonary arteries may obstruct the circulation sufficiently to cause acute pulmonary hypertension and death from right ventricular failure.

The sudden impaction of a large embolus in the main pulmonary artery brings the circulation virtually to a halt. The small volume of blood that can percolate past the mass is quite insufficient to fill the left side of the heart and maintain a normal systemic arterial pressure and an adequate circulation through the cerebral and coronary arteries.

Non-Fatal Pulmonary Embolism

The train of events that follows the impaction of a medium-sized embolus in a pulmonary artery depends largely upon the state of the general circulation at the time. Since the bronchi and part of the parenchyma are supplied with oxygenated blood by the bronchial arteries,[67] the closure of a branch of the main pulmonary arteries does not as a rule cause infarction of the whole area supplied by the occluded vessel. The sufficiency of the bronchial circulation for the survival of the lung parenchyma after complete obstruction of the pulmonary arteries has been demonstrated by experiments on animals.[68] In man, it is only when the general circulation is depressed, as in congestive cardiac failure or pneumonia, that the flow of blood through these alternative arterial channels is insufficient: ischaemic necrosis of lung tissue then follows the impaction of a medium-sized embolus.[69] One reason for the greater vulnerability

of infected or passively congested lungs may be that the accumulation of large numbers of neutrophils and macrophages ('heart failure cells') in the alveoli adds to the local requirements for oxygen, rendering the tissues in the area more than usually susceptible to impairment of their circulation.

Pulmonary infarcts of some days' standing can generally be recognized at necropsy by their firmness and haemorrhagic appearance, the prominence that they are given by the elastic retraction of the surrounding, air-containing lung substance, and the thin layer of fibrin that usually covers their pleural surface. When the lung is cut through a recent infarct, the area stands out conspicuously as a deeply plum-coloured, rather sharply demarcated triangle, its base to the pleura and its apex pointing to the hilum of the lung (Fig. 7.7). When large, such areas may have been seen in radiographs taken during life, although seldom in the form of a wedge-shaped or triangular shadow, because the lesion is not usually oriented to the X-rays in a plane that allows this classic outline to be projected.[70]

With care, the impacted embolus can often be found near the apex of the infarct in one of the branches of the pulmonary artery.

Histologically, the infarcted area is seen to be stuffed with blood, which, because of the porous structure of the lung and its constant movement with respiration, may spread beyond the confines of the initially ischaemic area. It is apparent that ischaemic injury to small vessels in the alveolar walls leads to local extravasation of blood, with later spread by pulmonary movements into nearby lobules by way of the air passages.

During the subsequent weeks, the extravasated blood in the infarct gradually disappears through lysis of its cells and digestion of its fibrin. If the infarct is large, and the patient is suffering from congestive cardiac failure, the serum bilirubin may rise and mild jaundice may develop. Large numbers of macrophages collect in the area and contribute to resolution of the lesion; many of these cells stain heavily by Perls's method for iron because of their content of haemosiderin, derived from breakdown of the red blood cells. Such macrophages may still be found at the site of the infarct many months later. If tissue necrosis has taken place the area ultimately undergoes organization, with the formation of a scar that is often recognizable beneath a small, depressed and thickened area of pleura. But usually the circulation through the bronchial arteries in the affected area increases soon after the branch of the pulmonary artery has

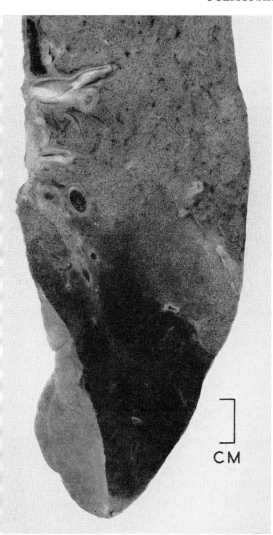

CM

g. 7.7.§ Recent infarct of lung. The dark area in the
notograph is infarcted lung in which the air-spaces have
:come filled with blood. Just above the top of the lesion on
e left can be seen the pulmonary artery supplying the
fected part: the artery is distended with ante-mortem
rombus.

:en blocked, and thus the extent of the destruction
f the parenchyma is reduced.[71]

In most cases, pulmonary emboli are sterile.
ometimes, if the thrombus has originated in
nfected tissue, it may contain bacteria. In these
rcumstances, the resulting infarct may suppurate,
lung abscess developing.

Micro-Embolism of the Lungs

Videspread embolization of the lungs may result
om the presence in the circulating blood of various
kinds of material. The most important of these,
next to thrombus, are fat droplets, small clumps
of tumour cells, gas bubbles, and material present
in amniotic fluid.

Fat Embolism.—Pulmonary fat embolism is a
common finding after serious injury, particularly
fractures of the long bones but in some cases as a
result of bruising or tearing of adipose tissue elsewhere. It may also occur as an accompaniment
of injury that at first may seem of little importance:
injury to the thoracic bones during external cardiac
massage is often sufficient to result in fat embolism.[72]
In cases of injury to bones, fat embolism results
from disintegration of the cells of the fatty marrow,
their contained fat escaping as globules into the
circulation. Sometimes small groups of adipose
cells are forced into the blood, causing *fatty marrow
embolism*, which is histologically recognizable in
the pulmonary capillaries. When haemopoietic
marrow is injured, whether through involvement
in an obvious fracture or merely by contusion or
severe deceleration injury, as in a fall, *haemopoietic
marrow embolism* may occur.

A rare cause of fat embolism is injury to the
liver in cases of severe fatty change in its parenchyma, globules of fat escaping from the cells into
the radicles of the hepatic veins.

In general, it seems that even widespread micro-
embolism of the finer pulmonary vessels, as judged
by the amount of fat disclosed on chemical analysis
of the lungs and by the appearance of the lungs in
frozen sections, has little effect on the pulmonary
circulation, so great is the vascular reserve of these
organs to meet the needs of heavy exercise.[73] When
many emboli reach the lungs, fat droplets may
escape into the alveoli and be recognizable in the
sputum.[74] The importance of fat embolism is that
it assumes a much graver form when some of the
droplets pass through the pulmonary circulation
and lodge in small vessels in the brain (see Chapter
34), where they create minute, but maybe fatal,
foci of necrosis in the vital centres and elsewhere.

Oil Embolism.—Oil embolism has been reported as
a complication of lymphangiography.[75] The radio-
opaque oil passes through the lymphatic system
and enters the blood by the thoracic duct or other
tributaries of the venae cavae; the droplets may
fuse into globules large enough to obstruct pulmonary arterioles. Respiratory difficulties may
follow the circulatory disturbance, especially if the
function of the lungs is already defective because
of some pulmonary disorder; death may result.

Oil droplets sometimes appear in the sputum, as in cases of fat embolism (see above).

These potentially serious complications of lymphangiography can be avoided if the amount of oil injected is kept to a minimum and if patients with pulmonary disability are not subjected to the procedure.[76]

Cotton Embolism.[77]—It has long been recognized that tangles of cotton filaments commonly lodge in the small arteries and arterioles of the pulmonary circulation as a supposedly insignificant hazard of pouring fluids for injection through cotton gauze. The gauze was intended to prevent access of dust to the glass funnel and rubber tubing that, particularly in the years between the world wars, was a commonplace means of administering fluid and solutions of drugs intravenously. Microscopical granulomas, sparse or numerous, were found in the lungs of many patients so treated:[78] the cotton fibres could be identified in the giant cell granulomas by the pattern of their birefringence in polarized light and by their destruction on microincineration. Similar granulomas are seen today, in the vasculature of the lungs and elsewhere,[79] perhaps mainly as a result of contamination of needles when they are stored on or wiped with cotton gauze. Their effects are, it seems, seldom serious.

Talc Embolism ('Drug Addicts' Lung').—Some addicts break tablets of drugs in water and inject the suspension intravenously. One of the substances used as a lubricant or excipient (filler material) in the manufacture of tablets is talc: injected, this may lodge in pulmonary vessels and induce thrombosis and a local foreign body granulomatous reaction.[80] When the injury to the vessels becomes extensive, pulmonary hypertension may result.

Trophoblastic and Decidual Embolism.—Fragments of trophoblastic tissue, often including recognizable chorionic villi, may be found in the lungs in a large proportion of women who die during pregnancy or the puerperium, particularly in cases of eclampsia or when there is a hydatidiform mole.[81] It is believed that normal uterine contractions during pregnancy, and especially those accompanying labour, dislodge the trophoblastic tissue and enable it to enter the blood stream. The emboli appear to be immunologically inert, in spite of their fetal origin.[81] They usually undergo early lysis. Thrombosis is a rare consequence. In very exceptional cases, persistence and even growth of trophoblastic emboli have been noted, with eventual regression and disappearance.[82] Trophoblastic embolism has to be distinguished from metastatic choriocarcinoma.

Decidual tissue has been found in the lungs, both within blood vessels[83] and in the lumen of alveoli.[84] In the former instances the condition is presumably embolic in origin; in the latter, too, embolism is the least unlikely cause, the emboli remaining viable and in the course of their continued growth bursting through the blood vessel wall into the alveolus. If endometriosis occurs in the lungs, as has been claimed (see page 388), decidual change might appear in the stroma of the foci during pregnancy.

Emboli Formed of Other Tissues.—Emboli of fatty marrow and of haemopoietic marrow have been mentioned above. Emboli of brain tissue have been found in the lungs in cases of serious head injury[85] and, in the neonatal period, in association with malformation of the brain[86] or following injury to the fetus *in utero*.[87] Emboli of liver tissue have been recognized in the pulmonary vessels after injury to the liver.[88] Fatal embolism by pancreatic tissue occurred during partial pancreatectomy when an anomalous vena cava was accidentally incised and the tissue forced into it during efforts to stem the bleeding.[89]

Tumour Embolism.—Tumour emboli, especially from cancer of the stomach, are common in the lungs. A few of the cells survive to form metastatic deposits:[90] the rest die very soon and the embolus becomes enclosed by platelet thrombi and finally undergoes organization. The vascular occlusion that follows is sometimes so widespread and leads to such obstruction to the pulmonary circulation that right-sided heart failure may follow.[91]

Air Embolism.—Rarely, at operations on the neck, air enters exposed veins through minor incisions and is drawn toward the lungs by the negative pressure created during inspiration. The fine bubbles into which the air is churned during its passage through the heart are carried into the pulmonary arteries, and sometimes through the lungs into the cerebral circulation. The volume of air needed to produce fatal air embolism if introduced into a systemic vein—even when injected under pressure as in some methods of blood transfusion—may be 100 to 200 ml or more. The cause of death in these cases is acute heart failure associated with frothing of the mixture of air and blood in the chambers of the right side of the heart.

If air is introduced directly into a pulmonary vein, as occasionally happened inadvertently during the production of artificial pneumothorax in the treatment of respiratory tuberculosis, the quantity needed is far less; probably a few millilitres could then prove fatal through obstruction of small vessels in the brainstem or, more rarely, in the heart.

'Caisson Disease' (Decompression Sickness).[92]— Formerly, before the industrial hazard was recognized and guarded against, men working at high atmospheric pressures, such as are used in submarine tunnelling and similar engineering operations, were liable to the formation of nitrogen bubbles in the blood and tissues if decompressed too quickly. Under these circumstances, the condition of caisson disease ('the bends') results from the release of the increased amounts of nitrogen that have gone into solution in the lipids of adipose tissue and of the central nervous system at the higher pressure (see Chapter 34): the released nitrogen forms bubbles unless decompression is sufficiently gradual for the excessive nitrogen to diffuse from the fats into blood and so across the alveolar membrane into the air. While cases of caisson disease still occur—for instance, among divers working from offshore oil rigs—they are much less frequent than previously.

Amniotic Fluid Embolism.—Occasionally, near the natural termination of pregnancy, amniotic fluid with its content of particulate debris—mostly epidermal squames and meconium—may be forced by strong uterine contractions into the maternal circulation at the placental site. These particles may be so numerous that they can lead to generalized, and sometimes fatal, micro-embolism in the small pulmonary arteries of the mother (Fig. 7.8).[93]

Micro-Embolism and Pulmonary Hypertension.— Interest has recently been awakened in micro-embolism of the lungs as a possible cause of certain forms of pulmonary hypertension and cor pulmonale that cannot be explained on other grounds (see page 283).

Experimental Pulmonary Embolism

The functional disturbances that follow occlusive changes in the pulmonary arteries have been much studied experimentally.[94, 95] These experiments have shown that the sequelae depend greatly on the rate of development as well as on the extent

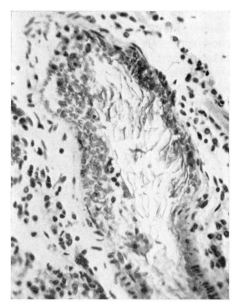

Fig. 7.8.§ Amniotic fluid 'embolism'. A small pulmonary artery is shown; most of its lumen contains short, fine, slightly wavy structures, which are epidermal squames that had been shed into the amniotic fluid from the skin of the fetus. *Haematoxylin–eosin.* × 200.

of the obstruction. A single large embolus that blocks the pulmonary artery of a dog kills the animal at once, with clinical and pathological manifestations like those in man. But if the main branches of the pulmonary artery are obstructed one by one, the dog may survive the occlusion of three-quarters of the pulmonary circulation through adaptive changes in still patent vessels.[96]

When emboli formed from blood that has been allowed to clot are introduced into a systemic vein in rabbits, the size of the emboli and the anatomy of the pulmonary arterial tree both affect their subsequent distribution in the lungs. While large emboli lodge in any of the main arteries, those of medium size—formed from blood that has clotted in capillary tubes—are carried disproportionately often into the vessels of the posterior basal segments.[97] In man, pulmonary infarcts are commoner in the posterior segments of the lower lobes (solitary metastatic tumours in the lungs are also more frequently basal than apical[98]). The explanation lies in the anatomy of the pulmonary arteries: they have a large axial trunk that gives off its branches at an angle and terminates in the posterior basal segment.[97]

Ever since Virchow initiated the experimental study of pulmonary embolism over a century ago, a wide variety of materials has been employed in such investigations. Some of them may erode through the wall of the artery in which impaction has occurred,[99] but the great majority remain within the lumen. In rabbits, autogenous blood clots may undergo organization, and in four to six weeks become converted into fibrous tissue. Some emboli of this kind, however, seem to disappear, and it is presumed that they are destroyed by fibrinolysin.[100] Plaques of intimal thickening in the pulmonary arteries may be derived from such thrombi.[100, 101]

Defaecation occurs immediately after severe pulmonary embolism in rabbits.[100] This has its parallel in man in the urgent call for a bed pan just before sudden death from massive pulmonary embolism. Experimentally, cutting the vagus nerve prevents defaecation in rabbits under these conditions, indicating that a reflex, presumably initiated in the pulmonary vasculature or lungs, is mediated by this nerve.[102] The dyspnoea typical of pulmonary embolism is similarly abolished by vagal section, so that it, too, is probably reflex in origin. The sudden rise in the pulmonary arterial pressure is probably the stimulus that operates these reflexes.

Pulmonary Hypertension

Normally the pressure in the pulmonary artery, even during exercise, seldom exceeds 30/15 mmHg. Studies during cardiac catheterization in a variety of cardiopulmonary diseases have shown that hypertension may develop in the lesser circulation: pressures can rise to four or more times the normal.[103–105] In the great majority of these cases the hypertension is secondary to a recognized lesion in the heart or lungs; in a small minority—the 'primary' cases—no such cause is apparent.

Secondary Pulmonary Hypertension

There are three varieties of secondary pulmonary hypertension: passive, hyperkinetic and obstructive.[106]

Passive Pulmonary Hypertension.—Passive pulmonary hypertension is the commonest, and is associated with an increase of pressure in the pulmonary veins as a result of either mitral stenosis or prolonged left ventricular failure, such as may follow severe systemic hypertension. In mitral stenosis, the medial muscle of the pulmonary veins becomes hypertrophied, especially in the lower lobes.[107] As a result of the rise in pressure in the pulmonary arteries, the larger vessels develop hypertrophy of the medial muscle and coarsening of their elastic fibres. The smaller muscular arteries show similar hypertrophy, and in severe cases this may be followed by necrotizing arteriopathy.[108] The vessels beyond the first division of the segmental arteries are often narrower in the lower lobes than in the upper.[109] Their walls are often thickened and a decrease in their calibre can be demonstrated in angiographs during life. Focal constrictions may be superimposed on the more diffuse narrowing.

Hyperkinetic Pulmonary Hypertension.—In hyperkinetic pulmonary hypertension, the blood enters the pulmonary arteries in greater volume or at a higher pressure than usual. In cases of atrial septal defect, blood passes from the left to the right atrium, and so adds to the quantity of blood entering the pulmonary arteries. When there is a ventricular septal defect, the increase in the volume of blood in the pulmonary circulation is accompanied by a substantial increase in pressure, and the changes in the walls of the pulmonary arteries are consequently severer. The small muscular arteries undergo hypertrophy and induce a state of raised pulmonary resistance through their hypertonicity, although at this stage they are still capable of relaxation and so there is considerable circulatory reserve to meet the needs of exercise.[110] But when severe hypertension persists for long, the lumen of the small muscular arteries becomes narrowed by intimal fibrosis and the vessels are consequently less capable of adaptive dilatation. The hypertension is now irreversible, and the patient is in a perpetual state of high pulmonary resistance and low circulatory reserve. The practical point that emerges is that septal defects should, if possible, be repaired surgically before the muscular arteries in the lungs are permanently narrowed by intimal fibrosis.

Other changes in the small muscular pulmonary arteries in cases of severe, chronic pulmonary hypertension include the development of plexiform, glomus-like formations and of angiomatoid lesions. The plexiform lesion is characterized by proliferation of fibrous tissue that is continuous with the thickened intima of an arterial branch that has lost its medial muscle: endothelial cells proliferate in the fibrous tissue and line a complex of fine spaces that lead from the arterial lumen to the thin-walled, vein-like vessel that takes the place of the distal part of the artery. The vascular channels of the plexiform lesions may communicate with pulmonary venules and with both venules and small arteries of the bronchial wall. There is no evidence that they establish any effective arterio-venous bypass or any significant communication between the pulmonary and bronchial circulations. The plexiform lesions, which occasionally reach a diameter of almost a millimetre, may be organized intravascular thrombi.[109, 110a] The angiomatoid lesion consists of cavernous spaces linking a muscular pulmonary arterial branch and the capillary bed in the vicinity: the artery is typically and severely affected by hypertensive changes; the sinus-like angiomatoid complex is apparently an irregularly dilated vessel with a poorly formed fibromuscular or fibrous wall in which there are often elastic fibres.

Obstructive Pulmonary Hypertension.—Obstructive pulmonary hypertension may result from progressive diminution of the vascular bed in the lungs. In one form, multiple pulmonary emboli or mural thrombi in the pulmonary arteries become organized; if the onset of such a condition can be recognized during life, some mitigation of its progress can be achieved with anticoagulant drugs. Emboli from malignant tumours, especially gastric carcinomas, may similarly lead to obstruction in the pulmonary circulation (see page 409),[111, 112] while in some tropical countries, severe schisto-somal infestation may block the pulmonary arteries.[113–116] These obstructive forms, with the development of right ventricular hypertrophy, can be mimicked experimentally in rabbits by repeated intravenous injections of minute emboli prepared from clotted human fibrin.[117] Pulmonary fibrosis following pneumoconiosis or other chronic inflammatory conditions may reduce the calibre of the pulmonary arteries and cause some degree of obstructive pulmonary hypertension. In areas of bronchiectasis, the bronchial arteries that supply the affected segment may become enlarged, and the passage of blood at systemic arterial pressure through dilated anastomoses into the pulmonary arteries may cause pulmonary hypertension.[118] While a rise in the pressure in the pulmonary circulation commonly follows fibrosis of the lung, the degree of vascular occlusion that develops in this condition is only rarely sufficient in itself to lead to the severer forms of obstructive pulmonary hypertension. It is possible that in some cases of pulmonary hypertension the rise in the pulmonary arterial pressure may be due to increased tonus in the walls of the arterioles in the lungs, induced by hypoxia and other changes in the blood gases that result from impaired respiratory function.[119]

Drug-induced Pulmonary Hypertension.—During the period 1966 to 1968, a tenfold to twentyfold increase in the number of cases of pulmonary hypertension was observed in Switzerland and a similar rise was also noted in Germany and Austria; other countries appeared not to be involved. It was soon appreciated that a large proportion of the patients had been taking the appetite-suppressant drug, Menocil (aminorex, 2-amino-5-phenyl-2-oxazoline fumarate).[120, 121] This drug had been on sale only in these three countries, and the increase in the frequency of pulmonary hypertension closely followed the rise in its sale. It was withdrawn in 1968 and there has been a corresponding fall in the number of cases of pulmonary hypertension. Experiments on dogs have shown that aminorex produces a rise in pressure in the pulmonary circulation.[122] How the drug produces this effect is unknown.

Primary Pulmonary Hypertension

This uncommon condition is found especially in relatively young women. Its aetiology is obscure. The diagnosis can be made only after excluding the various conditions that are known to cause secondary hypertension.

Two apparently distinct forms of pathological change have been recognized in cases of unexplained pulmonary hypertension.[123] The more frequent is characterized by dilatation of arteries and necrotizing arteritis.[124] In the other form the pulmonary veins and venules are affected predominantly and the pulmonary arteries and arterioles only secondarily:[125] this form has been termed *pulmonary veno-occlusive disease.*

Sequelae of Chronic Pulmonary Hypertension

Irrespective of its pathogenesis, long-continued pulmonary hypertension leads to cor pulmonale,* and eventually to cardiac failure. The main pulmonary arterial tree becomes dilated, and atherosclerotic plaques may be found in the large vessels at necropsy. The atheromatous areas may be covered by thrombus that forms *in situ*, gradually adding to the vascular obstruction. Occasionally, such thrombi may form so rapidly and extend so widely that an infarct develops in the lung.

* Chronic cor pulmonale is defined as: 'Hypertrophy of the right ventricle resulting from diseases affecting the function and/or the structure of the lung, except when these pulmonary alterations are the result of diseases that primarily affect the left side of the heart or of congenital heart disease'.[126]

Pulmonary Congestion and Haemosiderosis

Acute congestion of the pulmonary vessels occurs in acute inflammation of the lungs (see page 316) and in acute failure of the left ventricle of the heart.

Chronic congestion is usually the result of an increase in pressure in the pulmonary veins; this may follow failure of the left ventricle from essential hypertension, advanced disease of the aortic valve, myocardial infarction or mitral stenosis. In this last condition, the congestion is often associated with widespread pulmonary haemosiderosis (see below).

At necropsy on patients with chronic pulmonary congestion, the vessels in the lungs are found to be engorged. This may be partly an agonal change, for in mitral stenosis studies on the blood volume of the lesser circulation during life have shown that it is usually scarcely raised above normal, although it may be increased in left-sided cardiac failure.[127, 128] The lungs are often heavy, and aerated fluid can be expressed from the cut surface of the lower lobes. Histologically, the capillaries are distended and their walls are thickened, and the alveolar spaces contain oedema fluid, red cells and many macrophages laden with carbon dust and haemosiderin—the 'heart-failure cells'.[129] Fresh or organizing fibrin is commonly found in the alveoli.

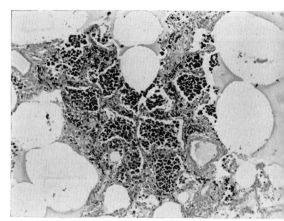

Fig. 7.9.§ Lung in mitral stenosis showing a large collection of iron-laden alveolar macrophages filling about 10 alveoli. They are the consequence of congestion and intra-alveolar haemorrhage. *Haematoxylin–eosin.* ×45.

Haemosiderosis in Pulmonary Congestion

This form of haemosiderosis is a complication of the severe, chronic congestion sometimes met with in mitral stenosis; it also occurs in some cases after several episodes of left ventricular failure.[130] A distinctive mottled or nodular shadowing of the lungs is seen in chest radiographs: this is attributable to the superimposition of aggregates of haemosiderin-laden macrophages. Up to 20 alveoli filled with these cells may be seen near a terminal bronchiole (Fig. 7.9). The elastic fibres of the alveolar walls may be impregnated with iron and subsequently enclosed by giant cells. The condition probably follows numerous small intrapulmonary haemorrhages.

If blood is injected intratracheally in rats it spreads at first diffusely through the alveoli. After 7 to 10 days siderotic macrophages collect in centrilobular masses that closely resemble those seen in congestive pulmonary haemosiderosis in man.[131]

Haemosiderosis in Other Conditions

A rare form of haemosiderosis, of unknown aetiology, is seen mostly in children. The patients suffer from recurring febrile attacks characterized by cyanosis, pallor, dyspnoea and haemoptysis.[132] Jaundice and enlargement of the liver and spleen may follow. Chest radiographs show diffuse speckling throughout the lung fields and mottled shadows that are most marked in the hilar areas. The condition ends fatally after a year or so, and at necropsy the lungs show brown induration. Histologically, the alveoli are filled with red blood cells, haemosiderin-containing macrophages and free haemosiderin granules.

This disease is now recognized with increasing frequency in young adults. It occasionally undergoes complete remission in these patients.[133, 134]

Pulmonary Vascular Lesions and Glomerulitis.— Pulmonary haemorrhage is sometimes associated with glomerulitis (Goodpasture's syndrome—see Chapter 24).[135, 136] Sometimes, pulmonary arteritis is found in association with glomerulonephritis and systemic polyarteritis.[135, 137, 138] Similarly, Wegener's granulomatosis is characterized by pulmonary arteritis and necrotizing glomerulitis.[139] The overlap between these conditions is considerable and their precise differentiation is often impossible; an immunopathogenetic mechanism may be concerned in all of them.[135]

Pulmonary Oedema

Pulmonary oedema is a common clinical manifestation of heart failure and of some renal and other diseases. It may be acute or chronic. It is also a very common post-mortem finding as a terminal event in the course of many forms of illness.

The interstitial space of the normal lungs contains about 200 ml of fluid.[140] Oedema results from the escape of excessive fluid from the small blood vessels into the interstitial space (*interstitial oedema*) and thence into the air spaces (*intra-alveolar oedema*).

Under normal conditions there is a constant, finely balanced circulation of fluid from the arterial side of the pulmonary capillary bed through the interstitial space to return to the blood, either directly on the venous side of the capillary bed or through the pulmonary lymphatic system. Many factors may upset this circulation and lead to oedema. In some circumstances the oedema fluid is like normal interstitial fluid; quite often, however, the permeability of the vessels becomes increased, and blood cells and plasma proteins (including fibrinogen) escape into the tissues.

Types of Pulmonary Oedema

There are two main types of pulmonary oedema, *haemodynamic* and *irritant*. Their most frequent causes are shown in Table 7.1, in which several other important but less common causes of pulmonary oedema are also indicated.

Haemodynamic Oedema.—The pressure in the small blood vessels of the pulmonary circulation normally is under 25 mmHg. When there is left-sided heart failure the pressure rises above that figure and an excessive amount of fluid escapes from the vessels: fluid that cannot be absorbed through the blood vessels and lymphatics accumulates as oedema.[141, 142] Haemodynamic oedema can be produced in the dog by inflating a balloon in the left atrium, causing partial obstruction to the flow of blood returning from the lungs to the heart, and at the same time running saline rapidly into the pulmonary artery:[143] interstitial and intra-alveolar oedema develops; the fluid does not contain fibrinogen and fibrin does not form in it (see below). Haemodynamic oedema can be produced in rats and rabbits by injecting adrenaline intravenously: the explanation appears to be that the pulmonary circulation overfills when the systemic circulation is impeded by the adrenaline-induced vasoconstriction.[144]

When the venous pressure is raised in the isolated perfused dog lung, the pulmonary vascular resistance increases in the dependent part. The circumvascular spaces become distended with oedema

fluid, as in interstitial oedema in man. The increased vascular resistance may be due to collapse of the vessels, an effect made possible by the accompanying loss of the tethering or expanding pull of the pulmonary parenchyma, which normally helps to keep them open.[145]

It remains unclear why the fluid of haemodynamic oedema in the experimental animal should

Table 7.1. *Causes of Pulmonary Oedema*

1. *Haemodynamic Disturbances:* including—
   myocardial infarction
   diseases of the heart valves
   cardiac surgery
   intravenous infusion (including blood)
   shock
   thyrotoxicosis

2. *Irritation:*
   (*a*) Infection and Its Sequelae: including—
   bronchopneumonia
   plague
   anthrax
   rheumatic fever

   (*b*) Inhaled Fumes: including—
   chlorine
   phosgene
   cadmium fumes
   nitrous fumes
   oxygen
   oxyacetylene gas
   smoke

   (*c*) Hypersensitivity: for example, to—
   bee stings
   antiserum
   drugs—such as iodine (in media for angiography), nitrofurantoin and salicylates

   (*d*) Miscellaneous: including—
   eclampsia
   irradiation
   direct action of drugs (for instance, morphia in excess)

3. *Trauma:* for instance—
   injury to the chest (including blast injury)
   thoracic surgery
   head injury
   pleural aspiration
   excessive exertion

4. *Hypoxia:* for instance, at high altitudes (see page 287)

5. *Hypoproteinaemia:* for instance, in renal and hepatic diseases

6. *Lymphatic Obstruction* (most commonly by tumour)

7. *Pulmonary Syndrome of the Newborn* (hyaline membrane disease—see page 288)

be generally fibrin-free, whereas in man it is commonly fibrinous and haemorrhagic. Sometimes the blood urea is raised at the same time in man, and urea (or perhaps other substances that are also present in greater concentration in the blood in uraemia) may damage the capillary endothelium, with the result that fibrinogen and red cells pass through. Other factors, such as hypoxia, may also play a part, for the situation is far more complex in the sick patient than in the otherwise normal experimental animal.

Hypoproteinaemic Oedema. — Lowering of the amount of protein in the plasma is a potential cause of pulmonary oedema, in consequence of the resulting fall in the osmotic pressure, which normally exerts an effect opposite to that of the blood pressure, thus maintaining homoeostasis in the circulation of extravascular fluid. In practice, however, a fall in protein osmotic pressure appears to play little part compared with other factors that are involved in the pathogenesis of pulmonary oedema in man. Sodium retention is far more important. The main evidence for this is that pulmonary oedema subsides when the output of sodium is enhanced by dialysis or by the administration of diuretics. It is believed that an increase in the concentration of sodium ions in the interstitial fluid draws a greater volume of fluid from the blood.

Toxic Oedema.—The term 'toxic oedema', although often inapposite, is currently used in referring to oedema that results when the capillary endothelium is so altered by chemical action as to be abnormally permeable to constituents of the blood. Experimentally, for instance, toxic oedema can be produced in dogs by the intravenous injection of alloxan:[143] the pulmonary artery pressure remains normal. In man, the accidental inhalation of irritant gases used in industrial processes, such as ammonia, sulphur dioxide and fluorine, may cause widespread injury to the parenchyma and to the smaller blood vessels of the lungs.[146] Similar effects are produced when oxides of nitrogen are inhaled in silos of fermenting forage.[147, 148]

Breathing high concentrations of oxygen may cause acute pulmonary oedema (see page 379). A high concentration of urea in the blood is liable to cause pulmonary oedema: it is believed to do so independently of any accompanying haemodynamic changes. Pulmonary oedema accompanying acute infection of the lungs has been attributed to the effects on the capillary endothelium of toxins produced by micro-organisms. Pulmonary oedema occasionally complicates treatment with drugs, particularly hexamethonium[149, 150] and busulphan.[151]

Pathological Findings

At necropsy, an oedematous lung may be as much as twice to three times the normal weight. It feels firm, and fails to collapse when the thorax is opened. Pleural effusion is often also present. When the lung is cut, watery fluid mixed with bubbles of air escapes from the exposed surface. The fluid flows more easily from emphysematous lungs, the deficient alveolar walls retaining it less effectively. The fibrin-containing fluid of 'toxic' oedema does not run from the cut surface as freely as the watery fluid of haemodynamic oedema. The appearances may simulate haemorrhage if red cells have escaped in large numbers into the fluid.

Interstitial oedema is seen to distend the loose connective tissue of the interlobular septa and round bronchi and blood vessels. The subpleural lymphatics may be visibly distended and often the hilar lymph nodes are considerably enlarged by the fluid that accumulates in their sinuses and permeates the rest of their substance.

Light Microscopy.—Non-fibrinous oedema fluid is seen as a homogeneous, eosinophile, proteinaceous material in the interstices of the connective tissue of the septa and round bronchi and vessels, and within dilated lymphatics. Air bubbles are represented by rounded spaces in the proteinaceous contents of the alveoli. At most only scanty threads of fibrin are found. In true fibrinous oedema, in contrast, there is much fibrin in the fluid and there may also be many red blood cells in the air spaces. Iron-containing macrophages may be found in older lesions. Organization of the fibrinous material may occur, leading to fibrosis in the alveoli.[152]

Electron Microscopy.—Electron microscopy has been used in studying the earliest structural changes that relate to the development of pulmonary oedema in experiments on animals. In haemodynamic oedema there is widening of the interstitial spaces in the alveolar walls by fluid, with separation of the collagen fibres; there is no evident damage to the endothelial cells of the capillaries.[143] In contrast, in toxic oedema resulting from intravenous administration of alloxan, the endothelial cells are swollen and disorganized.

Similarly, in the initial stages of the development of pulmonary oedema after intraperitoneal injection of ammonium sulphate, the endothelial cells of the pulmonary capillaries are swollen and stretched over large subendothelial blebs of fluid.[153] Such endothelial changes do not occur in cases of uncomplicated haemodynamic pulmonary oedema. When the endothelial cells are damaged the increase in the permeability of the vessel wall allows fibrinogen to pass, with subsequent formation of fibrin in the oedema fluid.

Radiological Findings

Interstitial oedema is recognizable in radiographs of the chest as horizontal lines, 1 to 3 cm long, at the periphery of the lung fields, towards the base.[154] The lines correspond to the oedematous interlobular septa.[155–157] Another radiological feature is circumvascular and circumbronchial 'cuffing', a shadow that is produced by the interstitial fluid in this situation.[158]

A familiar radiological observation in cases of intra-alveolar oedema is the 'bat's wing' or 'butterfly' shadow that results from the predominant involvement of the hilar region of the lungs. This picture was first described in cases of uraemia: the condition, being thought characteristic of that state, came to be referred to as 'uraemic lung' ('azotaemic lung'). Experience has shown that the same pattern may be seen in cases of pulmonary oedema without uraemia, such as the oedema accompanying left ventricular cardiac failure. Similarly, other patterns of distribution of pulmonary oedema are also commonly observed in cases of uraemia.[152]

DISORDERS OF RESPIRATORY FUNCTION AT HIGH ALTITUDE

Acclimatization to high altitudes entails complex changes in circulatory and respiratory function. The oxygen-carrying capacity of the blood is increased by a rise in the number of circulating erythrocytes (see Chapter 8). There are important changes in the pulmonary circulation. These accompany the increase in respiratory minute volume and pulmonary ventilation. The heart rate and cardiac output are higher. Interestingly, the pressures in the pulmonary circulation are normally higher in those who live at high altitudes than in other people, and may be markedly so. For example,

those acclimatized to living in Morococha, in Peru, at 4540 metres above sea level, have an average resting pulmonary artery pressure of 41/15 mmHg compared with the average of 26/6 mmHg at sea level.[159] There is an increase in the muscle in the wall of the pulmonary arterioles,[160] thickening of the media of the main pulmonary arteries and hypertrophy of the myocardium of the right ventricle in residents at high altitude.

If the change from low to high altitude is made too quickly, or if the individual exerts himself too actively before acclimatization is effective, the physiological response to the rarified environment may fail. Occasionally, longstanding stable acclimatization deteriorates for no clear reason: the result is comparable to that following exposure of unacclimatized people to high-altitude conditions. Two clinicopathological states illustrate these effects, acute high altitude pulmonary oedema and chronic mountain sickness.

Acute High Altitude Pulmonary Oedema

This dangerous condition results from moving quickly to very high altitudes after living at sea level, without stopping at an intermediate elevation to allow the body to adapt to the change. It is as liable to occur in people born at a high altitude who return there after a few weeks spent at sea level as in those who go to the mountains for the first time. The critical altitude differs appreciably among individuals: symptoms are rare below about 2500 metres. Age, sex, physique and physical fitness seem, in general, to have an inconstant role in liability to suffer ill-effects. In the susceptible, oedema of the lungs commonly appears within three days or so of arrival; it is commonly precipitated by exercise. There is increasing dyspnoea, cyanosis and a dry cough, and later the production of copious, frothy, watery sputum, which sometimes becomes blood-stained. Radiography shows a coarsely mottled opacity of the juxtahilar region of the middle and upper zones of the lungs. If the patient is not given oxygen, or returned to sea level, he may die within a week.[161]

It has been suggested that this condition results from constriction of the pulmonary venules caused by oxygen deficiency.[162] The pulmonary artery pressure is three to four times higher than is normal for the altitude. Respiratory alkalosis due to overventilation is manifested by a striking fall in plasma carbonic acid and a rise in plasma pH. After a short delay, the kidneys compensate for these changes by excreting an increased amount of sodium bicarbonate in alkaline urine. The bio-chemical responses are similar to those of physiological acclimatization, but in these circumstances are exaggerated by the immediacy of the demand for correction of the effects of hypoxia; they may fail.

At necropsy, there is generalized vascular engorgement. Microscopically, blood vessels of all sizes are greatly distended and there is 'sludging' of red blood cells and widespread extravasation of blood.[163] The oedema fluid in the pulmonary alveoli is mixed with air and contains some erythrocytes. In a few cases it is fibrinous and there are more neutrophils than is proportionate to the amount of extravasation of blood.

Chronic Mountain Sickness (Monge's Disease)[164]

Chronic mountain sickness is a state of progressive loss of acclimatization to high altitude. The symptoms include dizziness and excessive liability to fatigue. They are accompanied by cyanosis, clubbing of the digits and a fall in oxygen saturation to as little as 70 per cent. The increase in pulmonary ventilation that normally occurs at high altitude fails to be maintained.[165] Recovery quickly follows return to a low altitude.

Brisket Disease of Cattle[166]

Cattle that graze at an altitude over about 2750 metres sometimes develop chronic pulmonary oedema. The condition, which may be fatal, is recognized by swelling of the subcutaneous tissues of the neck, trunk and limbs: this is a manifestation of dependent oedema. The disease owes its name to the notable involvement of the forepart of the trunk (the 'brisket', or breast), but it is essentially the pulmonary oedema that embarrasses the circulation and leads both to the outward manifestations of the condition and to its fatal outcome.

HYALINE MEMBRANE DISEASE

Membranes of hyaline appearance are found in the smaller air passages in the lungs in a variety of conditions and at all ages. The best known and most important form is that found in the neonatal period and known clinically as the *respiratory distress syndrome*' and *pulmonary syndrome of the newborn*'.[167] This condition is commoner in premature babies,[168] after Caesarean section[169] and in the presence of maternal diabetes.[170] A similar condition has been described in newborn foals.[171]

Shortly after birth, the affected infant develops severe dyspnoea and cyanosis that cannot be relieved by oxygen. Mortality is high, the child dying from hypoxia. In some cases X-rays disclose a granular pattern throughout the lung fields; in others there is an almost uniform density of shadow in the lungs, blending with that of the mediastinum.[172] At necropsy, the lungs are dull red, like liver, and tense, engorged and oedematous; they are poorly aerated and sink in water. Histological examination shows widespread atelectasis and, in addition, some over-distended respiratory bronchioles and alveolar ducts lined by an eosinophile, hyaline membrane (Fig. 7.10). This membrane gives a positive reaction with the periodic-acid/Schiff method and contains a trace of fat; it does not give the staining reactions of iron or fibrin.

Electron microscopy has shown the hyaline membrane to consist mainly of an unidentifiable amorphous ground substance in a granular or

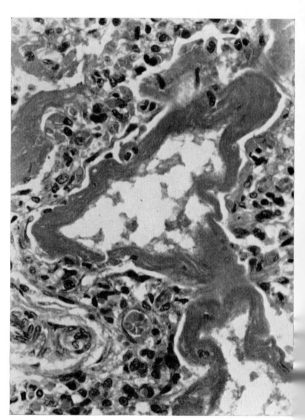

Fig. 7.10.§ Histological appearance of the lung in hyaline membrane disease. The air-space, which may be a partly collapsed alveolar duct, is lined by a thick layer of protein—the hyaline membrane (dark grey in photograph). It communicates in the right lower quadrant with the membrane in an adjacent air-space. *Haematoxylin–eosin.* × 370.

fibrillar matrix, with cell remnants, amniotic squames and osmiophile lamellar bodies.[173] The presence of fibrin is exceptional.

Hyaline membrane disease is related in some way to prematurity and fetal distress *in utero*. The surfactants of normal lung, such as dipalmitoyl-lecithin, which coat the inner aspect of the alveolar lining and lower the surface tension, facilitate pulmonary expansion immediately after birth. These agents are believed to be absent from the parts of the lungs that are collapsed in this disease.[174] It is puzzling that electron microscopy has not shown any consistently present abnormality of the type 2 alveolar cells (see page 272), for the deficiency of their surfactant secretion suggests that such changes might have been expected.

In adults, membranes having this hyaline appearance are seen in the lungs of some fatal cases of influenza. They may also be found following radiotherapy of intrathoracic tumours. Similar membranes sometimes form after inhalation of chemical irritants.

PULMONARY ALVEOLAR PROTEINOSIS

This condition was first described in 1958.[175] It is seen oftener in men than in women. Most of those affected are in the third to fifth decade. The presenting symptom is increasing dyspnoea, with or without pyrexia. Radiography shows feathery or vaguely nodular shadows that spread from the hilar region into the lung fields in a 'bat's wing' pattern. These shadows may clear and the patient recover, or they may continue to enlarge: clinical deterioration is associated with worsening dyspnoea, cyanosis and secondary polycythaemia. The mortality is about 30 per cent.

The lung is firm and contains many consolidated, grey, semitranslucent areas. Histologically, the distal air spaces are filled with a lipid-rich, proteinaceous material that gives a positive periodic-acid/Schiff reaction and sometimes contains crystals and laminate elements of uncertain origin.[176] The presence of this material in the alveoli not only reduces the vital capacity but also impairs gaseous interchange with the blood passing through the lungs and thus accounts for the respiratory disabilities.[177, 178]

The material in the alveoli in pulmonary alveolar proteinosis has to be distinguished from the clustered organisms in pneumocystis pneumonia (see page 361). In most instances its granular appearance is distinctive, contrasting with the foamy appearance of the intra-alveolar colonies of the pneumocystis, but the resemblance may be very close.

Electron microscopy has shown that some cells that are present in the proteinaceous material are granular pneumonocytes; others are macrophages ingesting lipid material, such as surfactants synthetized by the pneumonocytes. The accumulation of surfactants may be due to their inadequate removal or perhaps to overproduction.[179, 180] Serum proteins have also been identified in the alveoli, suggesting that transudation of serum contributes to the formation of the intra-alveolar material.[181]

The cause of the disease is unknown. Similar histological features are seen occasionally in silicosis[182] and tuberculosis.[183] A comparable condition has been observed in association with experimental silicosis in rats, and the possibility of an immunological factor in its pathogenesis has been suggested.[181, 184] However, there is no evidence that the development of alveolar proteinosis in man has been related to exposure to any particular dust. No infective agent has been found that might be a cause of the disease. Terminally, the lungs may become infected with bacteria or fungi. Alveolar proteinosis seems particularly to predispose to infection by *Nocardia asteroides*[185] and, less frequently, *Cryptococcus neoformans*.[186]

DISTURBANCES OF INFLATION

Atelectasis and Pulmonary Collapse

The term *atelectasis* means literally imperfect expansion, and is applied specifically to failure of the lungs to expand fully in the newborn. Once the lungs have been expanded, the development of airlessness, although sometimes referred to as 'secondary atelectasis', is better known as *pulmonary collapse*. Lungs may collapse—at any age—for two reasons: first, as a result of external pressure by air or fluid in the pleural cavity, or as a result of enlargement of a mediastinal structure (for instance, hypertrophy of the heart, an aortic aneurysm or a neoplasm); and second, as a result of bronchial obstruction preventing free entry of air into the lung. Air may be excluded from a lung by obstruction of a main bronchus by a tumour or by viscid mucus. The latter frequently collects during anaesthesia, when respiratory movements are minimal and the cough reflex is suppressed. Bronchial obstruction, especially in children, may result from inhalation of a foreign body.

In time, the air in the alveoli—first the oxygen and later the nitrogen—is removed by the blood that passes through the affected area and the alveoli then progressively collapse. In its collapsed state, the lung appears small and dark red, and has a deeply wrinkled pleural surface. Portions of such lungs sink when dropped into water. Where part of a lobe has recently collapsed, the immediately adjacent, pale pink, aerated secondary lobules are separated from the dark red depressed areas by zig-zag lines that correspond to the interlobular septa. Local foci of collapse are commonly seen at necropsy, particularly in infants. They are found also in adults, predominantly at the base of the lungs, especially when the patient has been in coma for some hours and breathing has been shallow. When collapse has been longstanding, the affected lung and its overlying pleura become fibrotic and reinflation is prevented.

Blood flow through a collapsed lung is reduced, otherwise the degree of saturation of the arterial blood with oxygen would fall markedly.[187] Induction of a pneumothorax in dogs with a volume of air equal to the functional residual capacity of the lung leads to a drop in cardiac output and a rise in pulmonary vascular resistance.[188] Since this resistance is virtually unaffected by vagotomy, it is unlikely to be a mechanical effect of reduced lung volume. Casts of the pulmonary arterial tree in these animals suggest that vascular obstruction may be due to the increased contortion of the small arteries that is probably an accompaniment of vasoconstriction.[189] This contortion does not seem to be due to kinking of the vessels in the collapsed lung.

Atelectasis in the Newborn.—Imperfect expansion of the lungs immediately after birth (*'primary' atelectasis*) is often found in stillborn and very young infants. The opening of the lung to inspired air after birth involves an enormous expansion of the area of the alveolar walls: it is believed that this is facilitated by the surfactants secreted by the alveolar epithelial cells (see page 272). Should these substances be lacking, the strength of the muscles of respiration is insufficient to separate the alveolar walls and thus allow air to enter.

Atelectasis accompanying hyaline membrane disease is considered on page 288.

Pulmonary Collapse in Aircrew

Pulmonary collapse has been seen quite commonly in aircrew of high performance aircraft.[190] Some-times it is related to breathing pure oxygen, which is not only toxic to the lungs but washes the inert nitrogen from the alveoli, and, being more soluble than nitrogen, is more rapidly absorbed into the blood. The addition of nitrogen to the inspired gas reduces the incidence of pulmonary collapse.

Another cause of pulmonary collapse while flying is exposure to positive acceleration. This is in part a consequence of the size of the alveoli in the lower parts of the lungs, which normally are smaller than those elsewhere. When a pilot makes a steep turn or pulls out of a dive, the extra gravitational force on the lungs causes the basal alveoli to collapse: clothing designed to protect the wearer from other effects of high gravitational stress ('anti-G suit') increases the adverse effect on the basal parts of the lungs by raising the diaphragm and reducing lung volume.

The condition causes cough, dyspnoea and pain in the chest. There may be radiological evidence of basal collapse.

Pulmonary Collapse after Surgical Operations

Pulmonary collapse is a frequent X-ray finding after surgery. It presents in two forms—the so-called 'plate' or 'linear' collapse and, less often, collapse of a whole segment or lobe. Accumulation of mucus in the airways is probably an important factor. Attention has been focused also on disturbance of laryngeal reflexes by anaesthetics, allowing pharyngeal secretions to enter the bronchi and obstruct them.[191]

Emphysema

Pulmonary emphysema may be defined as a state of pathologically increased inflation of lung tissue.[192] The proportion of air to tissue rises as a result of greater distension of air spaces, or of loss of parenchyma, or of both these factors. Vesicular and interlobular forms of emphysema are distinguished. Vesicular emphysema is a condition characterized by abnormal enlargement of the air spaces beyond the terminal bronchiole, either from their dilatation or from destruction of their wall.[193] Interlobular emphysema (interstitial emphysema) is the state of inflation of the tissue between the air spaces.[192]

It should be noted that some pathologists prefer to apply the term emphysema only when there is destruction of lung tissue and regard it as inapplicable when overinflation is not accompanied by destruction. Since the word emphysema is derived from a Greek word that means to inflate, and since overinflation and destruction cannot always be precisely distinguished (because the two operate together to varying extents) it does not seem desirable or practicable to consider overinflation as a condition distinct from emphysema.

The classification used in this chapter is set out in Table 7.2.

Table 7.2. *Classification of Emphysema**

Pulmonary Emphysema
   I Interlobular (Interstitial) Emphysema
  II Vesicular Emphysema
      1. Partial Lobular Emphysema
         (*a*) Centrilobular Emphysema
         (*b*) Paraseptal Emphysema
      2. Panlobular Emphysema
      3. Irregular Emphysema

* Heard, B. E., *Pathology of Chronic Bronchitis and Emphysema*. London, 1969.

I. Interlobular Emphysema (Interstitial Emphysema; 'Surgical Emphysema')

Interlobular emphysema may be defined as a state of inflation of the interlobular (interstitial) tissue of the lung.[194] Air in this situation has usually escaped from alveoli that have been ruptured by an excessively high pressure within them, or as a consequence of a very marked fall in the pressure outside them or outside the chest. The alveoli can withstand an interior pressure of 20 to 30 cm of water at birth and of about 150 cm of water in adults.

Interlobular emphysema may be caused by violent artificial respiration, used in the attempt to resuscitate the newborn,[195] or, at any age, as first aid to those apparently drowned or electrocuted. Other causes include intermittent positive-pressure respiration, severe asthma, whooping cough, and exposure to the blast of explosions in air or under water. Sudden decompression in aircraft accidents or after working in a caisson, or in the course of submarine escape training,[196] is also likely to have this outcome: experimental work on the effects of sudden lowering of atmospheric pressure has indicated that the body fluids boil—water vapour may thus be a major constituent of the interlobular bubbles when this type of emphysema results from decompression. Tearing of alveolar walls by fractured ribs or a needle exploring the chest are further causes.

At operation or necropsy interlobular emphysema may be seen as small bubbles of air in the connective tissue immediately beneath the visceral pleura. Large bubbles in this position are termed blebs: they must be distinguished from bullae, which are enlarged air spaces (that is, bullae are a manifestation of vesicular emphysema—see page 293). Air in the interlobular spaces may track along the sheaths round the pulmonary vessels to the hila of the lungs, producing mediastinal emphysema; it may then reach the extrathoracic tissues and present as subcutaneous emphysema. Air embolism may complicate interlobular emphysema.

II. Vesicular Emphysema

Vesicular emphysema may be defined as a condition of the lung characterized by increase beyond the normal in the size of air spaces distal to the terminal bronchioles:[193] it is associated with dilatation or destruction of the wall of the air spaces. The distinction between interlobular and vesicular emphysema was first made by Laënnec in 1819.[197]

Several types of vesicular emphysema may be distinguished by the different ways in which the secondary lobules (see page 271) are affected: these are illustrated diagrammatically in Fig. 7.11. The changes may be localized or widespread.

1 (*a*) Centrilobular Emphysema

This form is characterized by the presence of small rounded foci of emphysema, often pigmented with dust, confined to the centre of secondary lobules (Figs 7.12 to 7.16). If the changes are minimal and little or none of the parenchyma appears to have been destroyed, the term *distensive centrilobular emphysema* may be employed to distinguish it from the severer form, *destructive centrilobular emphysema*.[192]

Distensive Centrilobular Emphysema.—It is common to find a few small distensive lesions in the upper parts of the lungs of town dwellers.[198] The condition that has been called focal emphysema of coal miners is a severe form of distensive centrilobular emphysema:[199] the lesions are, of course, more heavily pigmented with dust than those in other people; distension is believed to predominate over destruction in the pathogenesis of coal miners' emphysema (Fig. 7.67, page 381).

Destructive Centrilobular Emphysema.—The alveolar walls are lost in the lesions of the destructive type of centrilobular emphysema, only some pulmonary vessels surviving to cross the lesions as

VESICULAR EMPHYSEMA

	a. Distensive	b. Destructive
1. Centrilobular emphysema		

	a. Distensive	b. Destructive
2. Panlobular emphysema		

3. Paraseptal emphysema

4. Irregular emphysema   scar →

Fig. 7.11.§ Diagram to illustrate the different patterns of emphysema as they affect the pulmonary lobule, which is represented by the hexagonal figure. In the destructive forms of emphysema, pulmonary vessels remain as strands crossing the spaces. Reproduced by permission of the publishers, Messrs J. & A. Churchill Ltd (Longman Group Ltd), from: Heard, B. E., *Pathology of Chronic Bronchitis and Emphysema;* London, 1969 (Fig. 4.1).

bare strands radiating outward from their parent arteries to supply the alveoli of the periphery of the lobules.[200–202] Centrilobular emphysema tends to affect the upper zone of the lungs more severely than the lower, but any part may be involved. It is quite often accompanied by some degree of panlobular emphysema (see below).

1 (b) Paraseptal Emphysema

This form of emphysema affects air spaces adjacent to septa and thus involves only the periphery of the lobule (Fig. 7.17).[202, 203] It may result from forces pulling on the septa and perhaps also from inflammation. It may occur alone or in association with other forms of emphysema.

2. Panlobular Emphysema

Panlobular emphysema may be defined as a form of vesicular emphysema that involves all the air spaces beyond the terminal bronchiole more or less equally. Panacinar emphysema is an alternative term.[193] Older names include chronic hypertrophic emphysema and diffuse or generalized emphysema. Most classic descriptions of emphysema refer to this variety. Panlobular emphysema is very common, especially in its less severe forms: it was found in 78 per cent of men in a post-mortem study in London.[198]

Distensive Panlobular Emphysema.—This term is applicable when there is dilatation of air spaces without destruction of tissue (Fig. 7.18). The respiratory bronchioles and alveolar ducts throughout the lobule are enlarged to a diameter of a millimetre or more (Fig. 7.18). In histological sections the alveoli appear cup-shaped or saucer-shaped, as a result of stretching.[204] Some pathologists take the view that this condition should be called 'pulmonary overinflation' and not regarded as a form of emphysema (see page 290).[194]

Distensive panlobular emphysema in very young children may take the form of such great distension of a part or the whole of a lung that it presents the radiological picture of a large 'cyst'. This condition is sometimes referred to as *congenital* (or *infantile*) *lobar emphysema.* Its possible causes include a local congenital defect of the bronchial cartilage, compression of the bronchus by an abnormally large or abnormally situated blood vessel, localized bronchial neuromuscular dysfunction, a valve-like fold in the bronchial lining mucosa, and bronchial stenosis.[205] In most cases the mechanism of its production seems to be that air can enter the parts affected during inspiration but cannot escape freely during expiration.

Destructive Panlobular Emphysema.—Destructive panlobular emphysema is seen most frequently in adults. It may involve a remarkable degree of parenchymal destruction as shown in Fig. 7.19.[206] The lungs have a doughy feel, pit on pressure, do not collapse when the chest is opened and overlap the heart because of their great size.[207] They appear very pale because of loss of substance; air-filled bullae, several centimetres across, may be seen at the apices or along the borders.

If the lungs are fixed by distension with aqueous formalin at a pressure of 25 to 30 cm of water for 72 hours and then carefully sliced and the slices impregnated with barium sulphate, the amount of destruction can be appreciated well.[202, 208] When the destruction is moderate in degree (Fig. 7.20) there is loss of some alveolar walls, fenestration

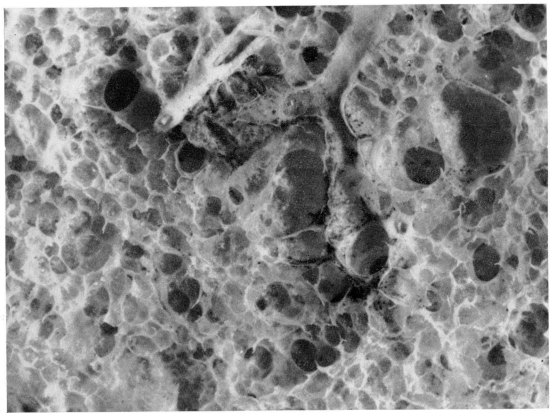

Fig. 7.12.§ Distensive centrilobular emphysema. If the terminal bronchiole at the right of the centre of the field at the top of the picture is traced down to the respiratory bronchiole in the right lower quadrant the latter is seen to dilate to a diameter of 1 mm. There is some dust pigment (black) in the wall of the dilated bronchiole and for a short distance proximally. *Pressure fixation; barium sulphate impregnation.* × 15.

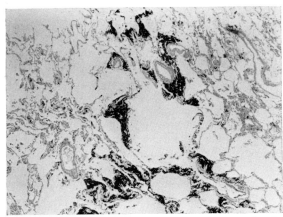

Fig. 7.13.§ Distensive centrilobular emphysema. In the centre of the photograph is a dilated respiratory bronchiole, and in or against the walls of this and of the adjacent air spaces are prominent collections of dust pigment. *Haematoxylin–eosin.* × 30.

of others, and reduction of the capillary bed.[20] Severer changes are characterized by complete loss of most of the wall of the air spaces, bronchiolar as well as alveolar, in the affected parts of the lungs, leaving only a network of blood vessels and some interlobular septa (Fig. 7.19). In places near the pleura the degenerate lung tissue may be distended to form bullae (Figs 7.21 and 7.22).

Examination of histological sections provides less information about the emphysematous state than the study of macroscopical slices. Microscopy confirms that the strands crossing the affected parts are arterioles and venules. These vessels may be patent or they may be obliterated by intimal fibrosis.

The localized areas of panlobular emphysema that are a common incidental finding at necropsy, especially in the anterior parts of the lungs, are probably of little functional significance.

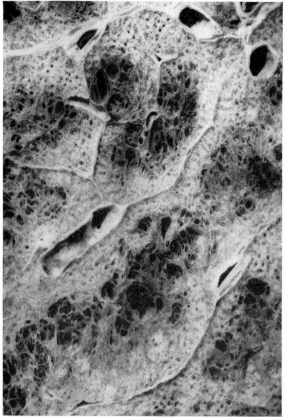

Fig. 7.14.§ Destructive centrilobular emphysema. The affected areas are pigmented with dust. A zone of intact air-spaces (pale) separates the lesions from the septa. *Pressure fixation; barium sulphate impregnation.* × 2.

Mixed Types of Emphysema.—Different types of emphysema, such as centrilobular and panlobular, may be present together (Fig. 7.20). When centrilobular emphysema becomes severe it may be indistinguishable from panlobular; the presence of much pigmentation by dust suggests that the lesions are centrilobular in origin.

3. Irregular Emphysema

This term is useful to describe emphysema that does not affect the lobules uniformly but occurs in small areas near scars, particularly following tuberculosis.

Aetiology and Pathogenesis of Emphysema

The aetiology of emphysema has been the subject of much speculation. Better knowledge of the microanatomical types of the disease is helping toward a better understanding.

Infantile lobar emphysema (page 292) is usually caused by a congenital defect whereby air that enters the lobe during inspiration cannot escape freely during expiration. The same mechanism seems to apply to the development of emphysema beyond a foreign body in a bronchus or an obstructing bronchial tumour.

Panlobular emphysema was also thought to result from local over-distension accompanying bronchial obstruction. Hence it was considered to result from asthma, or to be encouraged by vigorous expiratory efforts such as accompany glass-blowing and the playing of wind instruments: but emphysema proves to be rare in cases of asthma unless there has been much pulmonary infection,[210] and there is no truth in the suggestion about wind instruments.

Extensive destructive panlobular emphysema may be partly a sequel of pulmonary inflammation, but its pathogenesis is still largely unexplained. In some patients with progressively increasing dyspnoea and little or no bronchitis, both lungs may be largely converted into a delicate, fine network of persisting blood vessels with no remaining alveolar walls—this condition is sometimes known as 'vanishing lung'. Since these patients may develop bronchitis only in the later stages of their illness, pulmonary inflammation would seem unlikely to be responsible for the changes in their lungs. Nonetheless, many patients with advanced panlobular emphysema have a long history of chronic bronchitis, with some episodes of bronchopneumonia. Sometimes, dense pleural adhesions overlie localized areas of panlobular emphysema: in such cases the latter are almost certainly attributable to inflammation.

Centrilobular emphysema is thought to be the result of chronic bronchitis (especially bronchiolitis, in which the walls of the respiratory bronchioles are damaged or destroyed).[200, 201, 203] Local air-trapping has been advanced as an explanation of the distribution of the lesions, but it seems unlikely that this could affect only the centre of the lobule.[201] An association has been demonstrated between cigarette smoking and centrilobular emphysema;[211] the possible role of cadmium in this context is noted below. It is also probable that fumes encountered in urban areas and in factories are capable of damaging the delicate pulmonary structure.

In experimental animals, destruction of the wall of the alveoli has been observed after exposure to sulphur dioxide, ozone, oxides of nitrogen and phosgene.[212] In experiments that less closely follow

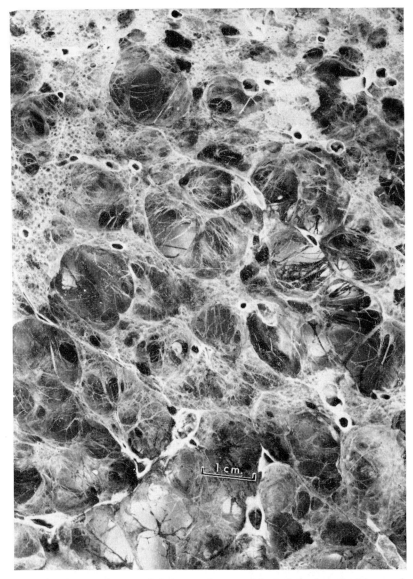

Fig. 7.15.§ Destructive centrilobular emphysema. Most of the lung in this area is emphysematous—very little intact lung is present (mostly in the left upper quadrant). Although whole lobules are destroyed the pattern suggests a primarily centrilobular distribution. *Pressure fixation; barium sulphate impregnation.*

the likely sequence of events associated with inhalation of harmful substances in air, emphysema has been caused by instilling nitric acid into the respiratory tract and also by the introduction of the proteolytic enzyme papain.[213]

Cadmium and Emphysema.—Exposure to cadmium fumes over long periods is a cause of emphysema.[214] This has been confirmed experimentally: introduction of cadmium into the trachea of animals or its

inhalation in the form of an aerosol has caused emphysema.[215] In man, the emphysema that is attributable to inhalation of cadmium affects the upper lobes severely and is mainly of the destructive panlobular type, although the morphological findings, including the presence of dust pigment, suggest that it may commence as centrilobular emphysema.[216, 217] Cigarette smoke is an important source of inhaled cadmium, and recent studies have shown a significant correlation between the

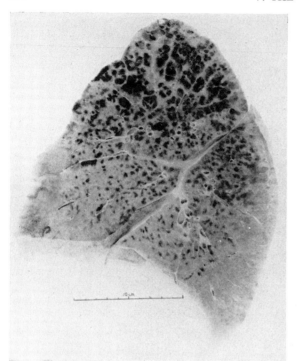

Fig. 7.16.§ Destructive centrilobular emphysema, showing as dark areas in the photograph. The upper part of the lung is most severely affected. *Pressure fixation; barium sulphate impregnation.*

degree of emphysema and the concentration of cadmium in the lungs at necropsy in the case of patients who have not been exposed to cadmium fumes at work.[214] It remains uncertain whether emphysema in smokers is caused by cadmium or by some other material inhaled at the same time.

Deficiency of α_1-Antitrypsin.—Some cases of emphysema, particularly panlobular emphysema, are associated with an inherited deficiency of α_1-antitrypsin, which is normally the chief component of the α_1-globulin of the blood. Deficiency of this substance is inherited through an autosomal recessive gene.[218–220] In homozygotes, the amount of α_1-antitrypsin in the plasma is about 10 per cent of normal; in heterozygotes, various levels have been reported, perhaps in part as a result of the use of different methods by different workers. Emphysema is found in all male homozygotes and in two-thirds of female homozygotes over the age of 40 years.[219, 221, 222] Most of these patients by that age have developed excessive dyspnoea on exertion.

Radiologically, the emphysema affects particularly the lower parts of the lungs. Pathologically, it is of the destructive panlobular type.[219, 223] Its pathogenesis is not certain. The suggestion has

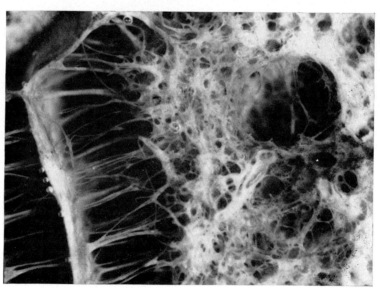

Fig. 7.17.§ Destructive paraseptal emphysema. The thickened septum on the left is separated from the rest of the lobule by a zone of paraseptal emphysema crossed by fibrous strands. There is destructive centrilobular emphysema on the right. Between the two is a band of less damaged, but distorted, lung. *Pressure fixation; barium sulphate impregnation.* × 10.

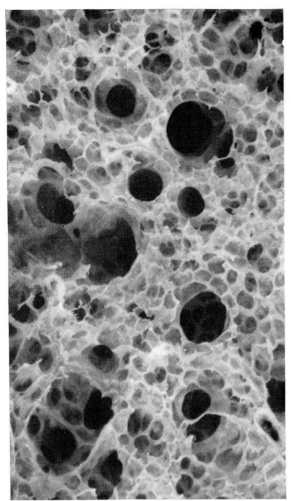

Fig. 7.18.§ Distensive panlobular emphysema. The large spaces are dilated respiratory bronchioles and alveolar ducts. They are recognized by their size—1 mm or more in diameter. There is no destruction of tissue. *Pressure fixation; barium sulphate impregnation.* ×15.

been made that certain proteolytic enzymes, released either from bacteria that have gravitated to the lower lobes or from leucocytes in the blood (the lower lobes have a greater blood flow than the upper), gradually destroy the basal parts of the lungs when there is insufficient α_1-antitrypsin to prevent their action.[224]

Possibly as many as 20 per cent of patients with severe emphysema are deficient in this anti-enzyme. A moderate deficiency of α_1-antitrypsin has been found to be associated with chronic bronchitis and a less striking degree of emphysema than develops when there is a marked deficiency;[225] however, the significance of this finding has not been universally accepted.

Functional Disturbances in Emphysema

Various functional disturbances develop as a result of the structural changes in the lungs in emphysema. They contribute to the dyspnoea, cyanosis and other respiratory disabilities typical of the disease.

Air Flow in the Respiratory Passages.—In emphysema, the rate of flow of air into and, particularly, out of the lungs is reduced. Much of this change seems to be due to increased resistance in the airways, aggravated by loss of the elastic recoil of the lung tissue. The defect is best assessed by measurement of the volume of air expired during the first second of forced respiration. If this volume falls below one litre, the patient is prone to develop ventilatory failure. As a result, many of the accessory muscles of respiration are brought into action, and the oscillations of intrapleural pressure between inspiration and expiration are much increased. This means that the mechanical work involved in breathing is increased, and with it the demand for oxygen.

Lung Capacity.—The obstruction to the flow of air in emphysema leads to an increase in the volume of air in the lungs (total lung capacity, or TLC), often to much beyond that present at full inspiration in a normal person of that sex, age and build. Even more consistently, there is an increase in the resting volume of the lungs, or functional residual capacity (FRC), and in the amount of air left in the lungs at the end of forced expiration, the residual volume (RV). Vital capacity (VC) is diminished, and—more important functionally— so is the 'forced expiratory volume in one second' (FEV$_1$).

Impaired Mixing of Inspired and Alveolar Air.— There is ample evidence that in emphysema a large fraction of the lung substance is poorly ventilated and that the inspired air fails to mix readily with the residual air in the distended air spaces. The extent of the failure to mix can be measured by determining how quickly the concentration of an inert gas, such as helium or nitrogen, when introduced into a closed circuit respirometer, comes into near equilibrium in the reservoir and the lungs.[226, 227] The rate at which nitrogen is removed from the lungs during breathing of pure oxygen is a further valuable index of this function.

Impairment of Gaseous Exchange with the Blood in the Lungs.—In the lungs of patients with chronic

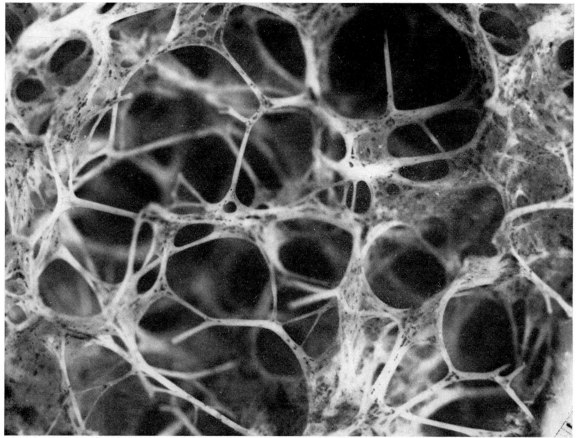

Fig. 7.19.§ Severe destructive panlobular emphysema. Most of the bronchiolar and alveolar walls have been destroyed: the strands that remain are blood vessels. *Pressure fixation; barium sulphate impregnation.* × 20.

bronchitis the normal balance between ventilation and blood flow is disturbed: some portions are overventilated in relation to perfusion and thus act as 'dead space', while others are poorly ventilated and—being well perfused—contribute a 'venous admixture' to the blood that returns to the left atrium from the lungs.[228] Whereas in normal people the average oxygen content of arterial blood is about 96 per cent of saturation, in the presence of severe chronic bronchitis and emphysema it may fall well below 90 per cent. Although there seems to be no greater difficulty in gaseous transfer across alveolar and capillary walls in emphysema, the much reduced surface area available for diffusion necessarily limits the ability of the lungs to promote the uptake of oxygen. As the patient's condition deteriorates, the amount of carbon dioxide in the blood rises; in some patients the sensitivity of the respiratory centre to carbon dioxide declines and respiration is maintained mainly by the stimulus of oxygen lack. It is noteworthy that the rise in

carbon dioxide brought about in these ways leads to the so-called 'carbon dioxide narcosis': consequently, treatment with pure oxygen—by removing the stimulus to the respiratory centre—is often followed by apnoea, which may be fatal.

Emphysema and Chronic Bronchitis

The effects of emphysema are often associated with those of chronic bronchitis: in many cases it is difficult to say which is mainly responsible for the patient's symptoms. Overventilation is often a conspicuous feature in cases of severe destructive panlobular emphysema without serious bronchitis: these patients are seldom cyanotic. In contrast, patients with chronic bronchitis may breathe relatively slowly, although deeply cyanotic. These differences are sometimes helpful in distinguishing the two conditions clinically. However, functional disturbances due to emphysema are mainly responsible for the dyspnoea and cyanosis so common in

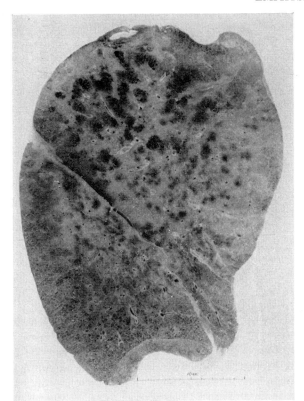

Fig. 7.20.§ Mixture of centrilobular and panlobular emphysema. There is fibrosis and shrinkage of the basal segments and of the lower part of the lingula. The rest of the lung is enlarged and shows panlobular and centrilobular emphysema; it is pigmented by dust. *Pressure fixation; barium sulphate impregnation.*

arteries appear to be reduced in number and calibre, and the background shows an increased translucency of the lungs because of the reduction in the vascular bed.[233] In spite of the diminished vascularity there may be little or no pulmonary hypertension.[234] The concentration of the blood gases may be normal, although the saturation of the arterial blood with oxygen is sometimes reduced.

Some patients with chronic emphysema develop hypertrophy of the right side of the heart, and this may lead to congestive cardiac failure. Pulmonary arteriolar constriction associated with hypoxia and hypercapnia may be the most important factor in causing the rise in pressure in the main pulmonary arteries. In the presence of pulmonary hypertension there may be some dilatation of the pulmonary arterial trunk—a change that can be seen in radiographs—but in only relatively few cases is the extra work so considerable that the right ventricle hypertrophies.[235] It is usually in cases in which deviation in the concentration of oxygen and carbon dioxide in the blood is most marked that gross ventricular hypertrophy is seen: emphysema may be minimal in such cases.

patients with chronic bronchitis. While often present even at rest, they increase distressingly should the patient undertake mild exercise or be exposed to bronchial irritation through inhaling cold or dusty air.[229]

It should be realized, however, that emphysema, while important in this respect, is not the only cause of respiratory distress and failure in such cases. Improved techniques for the display of structural changes in the lungs show that while some patients with chronic obstruction to their airways have severe emphysematous changes, others have little or none.[230–232] In these cases, the cause of the functional disturbances needs further analysis.

Death in cases of severe chronic emphysema is often attributable to purulent bronchitis and bronchopneumonia.

Emphysema and the Heart

n radiographs of the chest in cases of chronic panlobular emphysema, the peripheral pulmonary

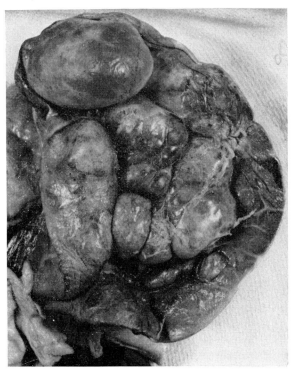

Fig. 7.21.§ Bullae projecting from the diaphragmatic surface of the lung. A slice of this lung is illustrated in Fig. 7.22. *Pressure fixation.* Half size.

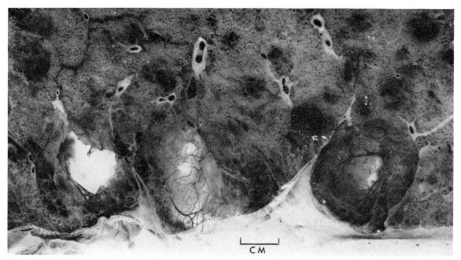

Fig. 7.22.§ Bullae at the base of the lung as seen in a slice. An external view of this specimen is illustrated in Fig. 7.21. In the upper half of the photograph there are scattered dark foci of destructive centrilobular emphysema. Each bulge in the pleura is a bulla, allowing light through the slice. *Pressure fixation; barium sulphate impregnation.*

'Unilateral Lung Translucency'

An increased transradiancy of one lung on X-ray examination may result from a variety of conditions, including obstruction of a major bronchus by a tumour or foreign body, massive emphysematous bullae, and occlusion, obstruction or congenital absence of the pulmonary artery on that side.

A distinctive syndrome is characterized by decreased movements and breath sounds on one side of the chest, a general diminution of pulmonary markings on that side in the radiograph, and absence of obstruction to the larger bronchi.[236, 237] Angiocardiography may show that the pulmonary artery supplying the affected lung is small and that the artery of the opposite side is unusually large.[238] Bronchography may show irregular tapering or dilatation indicative of organic occlusion in the smaller bronchi.

It seems that the condition is usually harmless. Few specimens have been studied in the laboratory: in three cases there was obliteration or distortion of many of the smaller bronchi and bronchioles, hypoplasia of the lung and pulmonary arteries, and emphysema of distensive rather than destructive type.[239]

Patients with unilateral lung translucency often give a history of pneumonia in childhood. It remains uncertain whether pneumonia or congenital hypoplasia of the lung or of its vasculature is the starting point of the condition. Occasionally, only one lobe is affected.

BRONCHIAL ASTHMA

Bronchial asthma, which must be distinguished from the aetiologically quite different cardiac asthma and renal asthma, is a form of dyspnoea in which breathing is rendered difficult by narrowing of the lumen of the bronchi throughout the lungs.[240] The distressing disability becomes particularly apparent during expiration for two reasons: first, because even normally the bronchi undergo some constriction during that phase of respiration; and second, because the thoracic muscles that can be brought into action for expulsion of air from the lungs are less powerful, even with the aid of accessory muscles, than those that act during inspiration.

Bronchial asthma may be *extrinsic* (that is, due to allergy to exogenous substances) or *intrinsic.* Extrinsic asthma is the commoner; it usually begins in childhood whereas intrinsic asthma usually affects older people. Extrinsic asthma is said to be of type 1 when it is a manifestation of type 1 allergy (that is, allergy mediated by IgE and characterized by an immediate hypersensitivity response): this type of allergy is characteristic of atopic individuals (although not confined to them) and type 1 asthma is therefore known also as *extrinsic atopic asthma*. Correspondingly, *extrinsic non-atopic asthma*, which is known also as type asthma and which is characterized by delay in the occurrence of the asthmatic reaction and by fever and leucocytosis, is precipitin-mediated and manifestation of type 3 allergy, which characteristically is found in non-atopic individuals (although not confined to them).[241]

Clinical Features

Clinically, cases of bronchial asthma fall broadly into three main types: those in which the condition is paroxysmal, the attack starting suddenly and lasting a few hours or days; those in which it is chronic, with exacerbation and remission over many years; and the terminal, dreaded, 'status asthmaticus'. In all types of the disease, the dyspnoea, which increases even on minor exertion, is characteristically accompanied by cough, wheezy breathing, some cyanosis, and expectoration.

Paroxysmal asthma is commonest in young children; chronic asthma is more typical of the disease in older people. In the latter, the symptoms are apt to become severer in winter, when the asthmatic disabilities are likely to be complicated by infection of the respiratory tract. It is in general the case that intrinsic asthma tends to worsen with age, in contrast to extrinsic asthma, which becomes less severe as the child grows older and usually ceases during adolescence, particularly in boys (in whom, incidentally, the disease is about twice as common as in girls).

Sputum in Asthma.—The sputum is often viscous, and may contain formed elements, such as Curschmann's spirals and Charcot–Leyden crystals. A Curschmann spiral is a corkscrew-shaped twist of condensed mucus, a fraction of a millimetre to several millimetres long, and usually surrounded by an elongated mass of clear or opalescent mucus that is probably a bronchial cast. Charcot–Leyden crystals have the shape of a pair of long, narrow, six-sided pyramids placed base to base; they are hexagonal when cut across, as is often to be seen in histological preparations. Their nature is uncertain, but they are believed to be derived from eosinophils, which are always present when Charcot–Leyden crystals are found.

Structural Changes

Most of our knowledge of the structural changes in the lungs in bronchial asthma has come from necropsy in cases of status asthmaticus. This has tended to over-emphasize the terminal features and late complications of the condition. When the chest is opened in these cases, the lungs are found to be greatly distended; they fail to retract as normal lungs do when the negative intrapleural pressure is replaced by atmospheric pressure on opening the pleural cavities. Small foci of collapse may sometimes be seen as dark, airless, segmented areas, firm to the touch, and depressed below the level of the surrounding distended lung.[242] While the large bronchi may show reddening of their mucous membrane and contain mucus, the most striking changes are seen in the smaller bronchi.[243] When the cut surface of the lung is exposed, these are seen to be filled with grey plugs of viscous mucus that can be made to protrude from the lumen by compression of the lung. Some degree of bronchiectasis is common. Although the lungs may be fully distended with air at necropsy, very little destructive emphysema is found.[244]

Histologically, the small bronchi and bronchioles are filled with material that is mostly acidophile but partly basiphile. The basiphile portions contain much mucopolysaccharide and give a positive periodic-acid/Schiff reaction. The eosinophile material is presumably in part derived from plasma and in part from secretion of the serous component of the bronchial glands and possibly from the Clara cells of the bronchioles (see page 272); it contains no fibrin. The contents of these bronchi commonly have a concentric or spiral pattern in cross-section, and the included cells are often aggregated in a corresponding distribution (Fig. 7.23). Most of the cells are eosinophils and desquamated epithelium; neutrophils are scanty. In most bronchi the mucous membrane and submucosa are normal; in those occupied by the mucous plugs there may be marked submucosal oedema, with separation and detachment of the superficial columnar epithelium, cells of which can often be found in the sputum,[245] sometimes in the form of aggregates (Vierordt's 'cell balls'[246]). Where desquamation has occurred, regeneration may take place through mitotic division of the basal cells of the epithelium. The basement membrane is only occasionally thickened; deep to it, the small blood vessels are dilated and their endothelium is swollen.

In biopsy specimens of the bronchial mucosa in cases of chronic asthma the serous elements in the glands in the submucosa preponderate over those that form mucus—this is one of the features that distinguish asthma from chronic bronchitis.[247] Superficial, mucus-forming goblet cells are conspicuous in both conditions. The submucosa of the medium and small bronchi and of the proximal bronchioles is infiltrated by eosinophils, lymphocytes and plasma cells; neutrophils are less common.[248]

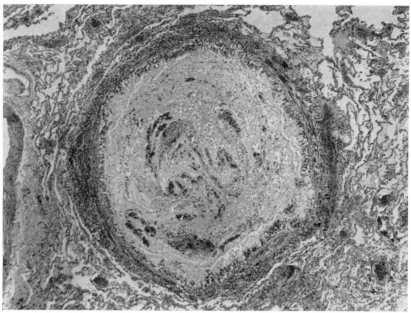

Fig. 7.23.§ Status asthmaticus. The non-respiratory bronchiole occupying the centre of the field is blocked by a mucous plug in which clumps of eosinophils appear as black, granular areas. *Haematoxylin–eosin.* × 40.

Focal Accumulations of Eosinophils in Asthma.— Radiological examination of the chest during an attack of asthma shows the lungs to be over-inflated. Occasionally, scattered shadows are then to be seen: needle or open biopsy shows these to be foci of exudation, with infiltration of the bronchiolar and alveolar walls by eosinophils. These foci are sometimes referred to as a manifestation of 'eosinophil pneumonia', but this is misleading: the foci appear to be transient and may be regarded rather as a feature of the allergic response of the tissues than as a primarily inflammatory condition.

The Bronchial Muscle in Asthma.—An increase in the amount of bronchial muscle is a feature of bronchial asthma.[249] The area of muscle in transverse sections of the bronchi is about three times greater than in control specimens; the number of muscle fibres is also greater, indicating that the increase in the muscle is attributable to hyperplasia rather than to hypertrophy. The cause of the hyperplasia may be extra work imposed by contraction in response to allergens, and perhaps by the lowering of the threshold for a contractile reaction to irritation by fumes or in the course of infection. It is also possible that there is a direct chemical or hormonal stimulus to multiplication of the muscle cells.

Aetiology and Pathogenesis

In the great majority of cases, bronchial asthma has an allergic origin. In very young children, the hypersensitivity is often related to some food, and the proteins of eggs, cow's milk and wheat flour are among those most frequently provocative of an attack. In babies, sensitization to cow's milk may be created by the accidental inhalation of small amounts during the course of artificial feeding.[250] Once allergy has developed, subsequent inhalation of cow's milk can result in severe asthma and even in asphyxial death—one form of the so-called 'cot death'—from the bronchospasm induced.[251] In time, attacks of asthma due to food tend to decrease in severity, and in many children they eventually cease.

More readily understandable is sensitization of the respiratory tract by inhaled particulate allergens; among these, certain pollens, dander from horses, cats, dogs and rabbits, feathers in pillows, and house dust are the most commonly incriminated.

House Dust.—The most important asthma-causing allergen in house dust is a mite, *Dermatophagoides pteronyssinus.*[252, 253] In patients who are sensitive to house dust there is a good correlation of the intensity of the skin reaction to extracts of mites of this species with that to extracts of house dust. Shed human epidermal squames are probably the main food of house mites: for this reason the mites are particularly numerous in dust from bedding, especially mattresses. Damp houses favour the growth of the mites more than dry ones, but very few samples of house dust are completely free of them.

The dermatophagoides occurs throughout the world. There are other genera of house mites that provide the same allergen, or one very like it, but they are numerically less important.

Allergy to Aspergilli as a Cause of Asthma.—In Britain, extrinsic asthma is frequently a manifestation of allergic bronchopulmonary aspergillosis (see page 349).[254, 255] *Aspergillus fumigatus* is the species most commonly concerned, but other species have been responsible for some cases and appear to be relatively more frequent causes in other parts of the world. It is important to note that this condition is not a form of infection by the fungus, since the organism does not invade the tissues (see page 349). Inhalation of fungal elements, presumably conidia (spores), sets up a reaction in the sensitized bronchial tree that is characterized by bronchospasm, accumulation of eosinophils and outpouring of abundant, very viscid mucus. The mucus forms a cast within the affected segment of the bronchial tree, and the cast is colonized by the fungus. Preparation of histological sections of these mucous plugs, expectorated at the end of the acute episode of the illness, permits demonstration of the characteristic hyphae within their substance (silver impregnation methods are often more satisfactory for this purpose[254] than conventional fungal stains, which tend to obscure the hyphae because they also stain the mucopolysaccharides of the mucus so intensely). Immunological tests have largely superseded histological investigation in the diagnosis of this condition,[256] although the latter, properly approached, is a valuable confirmatory measure and in cases with equivocal immunological results may be the only means of recognizing the disease.

Aspergillus antigen causes both immediate and delayed reactions on skin testing, and precipitins are present in the blood.[256] It seems, therefore, that allergic aspergillosis is characterized by both immediate (type 1) and delayed (type 3) hypersensitivity.

Occupational Asthma.—The list of agents that have been recorded as capable of sensitizing the bronchi

is a long one, and noteworthy among them are materials to which prolonged exposure is only likely to occur in particular occupations and industries.[257, 258] Among the commoner of these are the organic dusts inhaled by those working with jute, orris root, or pyrethrum flowers, or engaged in grinding coffee or castor beans. The condition known as 'farmer's lung' is an allergic reaction to moulds in hay (see page 360): it is not accompanied by bronchospasm and therefore is not considered among the asthmatic diseases.

Those who are sensitive to inhaled allergens may develop an attack of asthma within a few minutes of exposure, and the attack may end almost as abruptly. This is well exemplified by the asthma that occurs almost at once in a cat-sensitive person on entering a room with a cat in it, or in a horse-sensitive person on going into a stable. It seems that when the allergenic protein comes into contact with its specific antibody on the surface of cells in the bronchial wall, the combination results in the release of histamine or some agent with a similar pharmacological action (see below). This liberated agent in turn acts promptly on the bronchial muscle to bring about its contraction, on the small blood vessels in the submucosa to cause their dilatation and the extravasation of a fluid and cellular exudate, and on the local glands and goblet cells to cause secretion of mucus. That the agent is released from local structures is well shown by the finding that rings of muscle taken from the bronchus of a horse-sensitive person after surgical lobectomy, and suspended in a saline bath, promptly contract when a small amount of horse serum is added to the fluid.[259]

An asthmatic attack can be provoked experimentally in man and in certain animals by the inhalation of an aerosol that contains the antigen to which the individual is sensitive. In man, the reaction has been studied by bronchoscopy; the mucosa quickly becomes oedematous, mucus is freely secreted and the bronchial lumen narrows.[260] Guinea-pigs can be sensitized to horse dander extract by placing them for several hours in an insufflation chamber into which the extract is introduced as an aerosol. If they are returned to the chamber some weeks later, re-exposure to the aerosol evokes an immediate attack of asthma, which often proves fatal.[261] The structural changes in the lungs are closely similar to those observed in man after an acute paroxysmal asthmatic attack.

Immunopathology of Asthma.—Extrinsic atopic asthma is usually associated with an inborn liability to develop reaginic antibodies to commonplace antigens such as the individual repeatedly meets in everyday life. Symptoms generally begin in childhood, and the disease is often associated with eczema and hay fever. Cutaneous prick tests are usually positive to the antigens responsible, an immediate weal and flare response resulting: the range of allergens that the patient reacts to in this way is often extensive, as is implicit in the atopic state. The reaginic antibody to the asthma-inducing allergen becomes fixed to the cells, particularly the mast cells, and possibly other components of the tissues of the mucous membrane of the bronchial tract: inhalation of the allergen then leads to the antigen–antibody reaction, with consequent release of various bronchoconstrictor substances from the mast cells (see below).

Intrinsic asthma usually affects older people. They are seldom sufferers from hypersensitivity (except in some cases to aspirin and, rarely, other drugs). They do not usually produce reaginic antibodies; skin tests are negative.

Patients with extrinsic atopic asthma can be shown to develop pronounced lymphocyte sensitization only to the antigen that provokes their disease. In contrast, patients with intrinsic asthma show lymphocyte sensitization to a wide range of antigens without specificity to any particular one. Intrinsic asthma appears to be a defect of immunity in general.[262–264]

Studies on isolated lungs of sensitized guinea-pigs have demonstrated that various substances are released when the bronchi are challenged with the antigen. These substances include histamine, 5-hydroxytryptamine, 'slow-reacting substance in anaphylaxis' (SRS-A), prostaglandins of various types, and rabbit aorta-contracting substance (RACS) and its releasing factor (RACS-RF).[265] Their immediate source is principally mast cells, and they cause the bronchial muscle to constrict the airways. As most asthmatic patients react to exercise with some degree of bronchial narrowing, it is believed that mediators may also come from outside the lung, perhaps from the skeletal muscles during exertion.

Emotional stress may act as a triggering factor in asthma. Now that the immunological abnormalities are understood better, the role of stress is thought to be no more than a trigger.

Complications

Longstanding asthma is often followed by other pulmonary lesions.[266] In many patients the disease becomes complicated by infection, and death may occur in an acute episode of the latter. Chronic bronchitis is a frequent development; its complications are often the cause of death (see page 309).[266]

It is commonly estimated that about 3 per cent of all patients with bronchial asthma, irrespective of age and sex, die from the disease. Misuse and abuse of therapeutic measures that, properly applied, are valuable in the control of the disease have contributed to its mortality. For instance, a rise in the number of deaths from asthma in England and Wales from 1175 in 1961 to 1927 in 1965, and a fall then to 1198 in 1971,[267] may have been related to the rise and fall in the sale of certain aerosol bronchodilators, particularly isoprenaline: both refractoriness to the bronchodilatory effect of the drug, when administered in this form, and adverse reactions, particularly those associated with overdosage, appear to have contributed to its dangers.[268] At the peak of this rise in the mortality of the disease bronchial asthma had become responsible for seven times more deaths at ages from 10 to 14 years than previously and was the fourth commonest cause of death among children in this age group.[269]

INFLAMMATION IN THE TRACHEOBRONCHIAL TREE

Acute Tracheobronchitis

Acute inflammation of the trachea and bronchi is common in Britain, especially among young children and the elderly. Its aetiology is far from simple and a number of differing factors, environmental and microbial, may participate in its causation. In the normal person, the defensive mechanisms of the respiratory tract usually destroy or remove any inhaled micro-organisms that may be caught on its mucus-covered surface. But should the combined defences of mucus, ciliate epithelium and the cough reflex be weakened from any cause, such as exposure to cold, irritant dust or vapours, or certain specific diseases, the potentially pathogenic bacteria that are ordinarily resident in the nose and pharynx may succeed temporarily in colonizing the mucosa of the trachea and bronchi. In the pathogenesis of acute tracheobronchitis, therefore these potentiating factors acquire particular significance, for without them the responsible organisms might be unable to establish themselves in these portions of the respiratory tract, which normally are sterile.[270]

Environmental Causes

In industrial cities and large towns the atmosphere is polluted by the products of combustion of coal and oil: from time to time, often provoked by particular meteorological conditions, the concentrations of irritant material in the air may rise to values that initiate an attack of acute tracheobronchitis, especially in elderly people.[271] The notorious 'smogs' in Los Angeles, Liège and London were instances of this kind. While control of air pollution has virtually abolished smog in some areas, such as Greater London, other cities in various countries are not yet free from the dangers of such potentially catastrophic incidents.

In men engaged in certain industries, notably those in which irritant gases or dusts may be inhaled, the mucous membrane of the trachea and bronchi may become acutely inflamed. Occasionally, generally as a result of an accident, noxious gases such as ammonia and sulphur dioxide may be breathed in such concentrations that widespread injury to the respiratory mucosa may follow. In the first world war, the offensive use of chlorine and phosgene as poisonous gases was often followed by destructive lesions throughout the respiratory tract of those exposed.

Acute tracheobronchitis has a marked seasonal incidence (see Table 7.3). In the summer months the mortality is low, but from early in winter it rises steadily to reach a peak in the late winter or early spring. The time of greatest mortality varies considerably from year to year, and depends partly on the severity of the cold and fogs and partly on the prevalence of two epidemic diseases, influenza and measles. For instance, in Britain in 1956, in which February was exceptionally cold, mortality during the first quarter was more than twice that of the same quarter of 1957, which was unusually mild.

Table 7.3. *Mean Annual Deaths from Acute Bronchitis in England and Wales for the Triennium 1956–58*

	Quarters of the year			
	1st	2nd	3rd	4th
Males	748	215	122	435
Females	880	228	102	448

Bacteria and Viruses in Acute Tracheobronchitis

In the aetiology of acute tracheobronchitis, especially in those forms seen typically in infants and young children, great changes have taken place in recent years in the relative importance of bacteria and viruses. Prophylactic immunization against diphtheria and pertussis, and the availability of antibiotics effective against the bacterial causes of secondary pneumonia, particularly pneumococci and *Streptococcus pyogenes*, have together greatly lessened the frequency both of the primary diseases and of their respiratory complications. Similarly, the bacterial complications of measles and influenza can now be effectively treated, although immunization against the primary viral infections is still comparatively unreliable in contrast to that against pertussis and, particularly, diphtheria.

Further advances in the techniques of virus recovery and identification are clarifying the pathogenesis of many forms of hitherto obscure epidemic respiratory infections. For example, investigation of numerous local outbreaks of acute tracheobronchitis is disclosing the frequency with which the many types of adenoviruses and myxoviruses are implicated.[272]

Pertussis (Whooping Cough)

The decline in the incidence of whooping cough in England and Wales since the second world war represents one of the notable contributions of prophylaxis to public health: in 1952, notifications were 116 311, and 10 years later they were 8348—a fourteen-fold reduction. Since then, their level has fluctuated appreciably, perhaps indicating that immunization is, while effective, less so than had been at first thought: the mean annual number of notifications for the years 1963 to 1973 is 17 504, with a fall below 12 945 cases (the figure for 1965) only in 1969 (4995 cases), 1972 (2069 cases) and 1973 (2441 cases).[272a]

In fatal cases of whooping cough, *Bordetella pertussis* can be recovered from the lungs, and microscopical studies have shown that identical organisms can be seen in large numbers in the thick mucopurulent film that covers the mucosa of the trachea and bronchi (Fig 7.24).[273] The mucus may be so viscous that it obstructs the passage of air and so leads to the collapse of the related segments of lung. Although *Bordetella pertussis* itself seems to be capable of establishing an acute inflammatory reaction in the lower respiratory passages, it would appear from bacteriological studies at necropsy that the terminal, fatal bronchopneumonia is caused by *Haemophilus influenzae* or by one of the pyogenic cocci that have been enabled to enter the lungs.[274, 275] In infants, this complication is the chief cause of death in whooping cough, which is

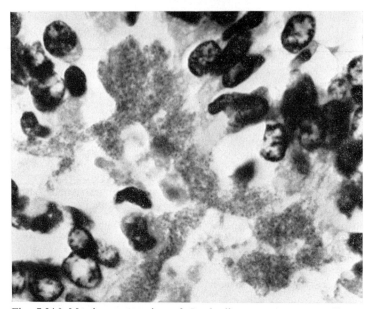

Fig. 7.24.§ Massive aggregation of *Bordetella pertussis* among cilia of bronchial epithelial cells. The individual bacteria can just be made out as coccobacilli forming the bulk of the granular-looking grey mass. From a case of clinically typical, severe whooping cough. *Bordetella pertussis* was isolated in pure culture from the bronchi and bronchopneumonic foci at necropsy. *Haematoxylin–eosin.* × 1150.

still one of the most fatal infectious diseases in the first two years of life; in older children, the collapse of the lung and inflammatory weakening of the walls of the bronchi may lead eventually to bronchiectasis (see page 311).[276]

Diphtheria

In this disease, which a generation ago cost many thousand lives yearly, the bacteria generally infect the pharynx and posterior nares: it is only occasionally that they spread downward and cause acute tracheitis and bronchitis. This pulmonary complication is more frequently associated with infection by the mitis type of *Corynebacterium diphtheriae*. The typical membrane then formed is so insecurely attached to the underlying, readily desquamated, ciliate epithelium that it is readily dislodged and may cause death from asphyxia through impaction in the larynx during a cough.[277] Sometimes, too, the primary injury to the respiratory mucosa by the locally released toxin lays the lungs open to invasion by various other organisms, among them *Haemophilus influenzae* and the pyogenic cocci.

Influenza

This disease, still sometimes known as *grippe*, is epidemic almost annually in winter months in many parts of the world, and at long intervals occurs in pandemic form, as in 1889–92 and 1918–19. In the latter outbreak it is estimated that some twenty to thirty million people died from the disease in little more than a year. The virus responsible was discovered in 1933 by Laidlaw and his colleagues:[278] before then it was widely believed that the disease was caused by *Haemophilus influenzae*, which had been isolated by Pfeiffer from a large proportion of cases in the 1889–92 pandemic. Laidlaw's discovery that the disease could be transmitted to ferrets by intranasal inoculation of filtered washings from the nose of patients, and then passed from the ferrets back to human beings, established its viral nature. Influenza virus (orthomyxovirus) occurs in several variant forms, distinguished by serological methods and identified by the letters A to C; from time to time further strains are added to the types already recognized.

With modern transport, influenza epidemics can spread throughout the world with great rapidity along the major air, sea and land routes, as was well shown in 1957 in the outbreak of Asian influenza.[279, 280] Clinically, the severity of the disease varies much from one epidemic to another and from case to case.[281] In its uncomplicated form, it is usually a mild complaint, with fever, coryza, headache and body aches as its main features, and recovery after a few days. When the viral infection is followed by invasion of the lungs by staphylococci, pneumococci, streptococci or *Haemophilus influenzae*, as is more liable to happen in the winter months, the condition assumes a much graver form, and the case fatality rate may rise alarmingly. Since most of the deaths after influenza are due to secondary bacterial infection, opportunities for studying the pathology of the uncomplicated primary disease are uncommon.[282, 283] It would seem, however, from examination of suitable human cases and of experimentally-infected animals, that the initial injury is inflicted by the virus on the ciliate epithelium of the trachea and bronchi, and that it is because this destruction can be so extensive that the more serious secondary infections follow.

Prophylaxis.—Prophylactic immunization with inactivated influenza virus has, in general, had relatively little success, in part due to the difficulty of keeping the content of the vaccine up to date in relation to the strains of virus prevalent in the community at risk. The development of more effective viral vaccines, and of drugs, particularly adamantan derivatives, is meeting with success.[284]

Measles

In most highly urbanized parts of the world this very infectious viral disease, with its principal clinical features of fever, coryza and rash, is regarded as one of the inevitable diseases of childhood. Its incidence is usually highest in the early spring, when droplet infections are particularly rife. The epidemics in many cities have a remarkably consistent biennial character. This feature of measles was very evident before the second world war: in Britain it was largely lost during the war, probably as a result of evacuation of children from cities to the country: it has since been re-established. The explanation of this biennial epidemic pattern has been the subject of several interesting hypotheses.[285] The one most favoured is that when each outbreak subsides a large proportion of those children who were in contact with an active case have become temporarily immune through a subclinical attack:[286] any resistance thus gained is gradually lost during the two succeeding years. Consequently, together with the influx of two further annual entries into infant schools, a new population of susceptible children is formed and is liable to contract overt disease when the early spring seasonal conditions are again favourable for the spread of the virus. In this way a fresh epidemic wave is developed.

In those parts of the world where measles has been prevalent for centuries the disease is almost invariably mild, and unless complicated by bacterial bronchopneumonia it has a very low mortality. The danger of a complicating secondary respiratory infection has been much reduced by improved hygienic conditions and the introduction of effective antibacterial drugs. In contrast, the mortality from measles may be appallingly high in lands into which the virus is newly introduced.[287] In Polynesia, when the disease was carried there from Australia in 1875, almost the whole population of the Fiji Islands—some 150 000 people—contracted it and a quarter of them succumbed. Similar outbreaks have occurred in recent times: for instance, when the infection was introduced to southern Greenland (in 1951) 4000 people contracted the disease and 80 died.[288]

Measles may also be very severe when it affects patients, both children and adults, who have seriously deficient immunological defences as a result of leukaemia and comparable chronic diseases, or of primary immunological disorders, or of treatment with cytotoxic drugs or immunosuppressants.[289]

Pathology.—The measles virus propagates particularly well in the epithelial cells of the main respiratory passages and leads to the destruction of many of them.[290, 291] In time, when recovery has set in, these losses are made good by regeneration through the multiplication and rearrangement of the surviving basal layer of epithelium, but at the height of the disease the natural defences of the lower respiratory tract are greatly handicapped, and secondary invading bacteria can successfully establish themselves in the lungs.

Giant cell pneumonia as a manifestation of measles is considered on page 323.

Virology.—The viral causation of measles was proved by transmission of the disease to monkeys and to man by intranasal instillation of filtered washings of the secretions from early cases. The virus (a paramyxovirus) can be grown in tissue cultures of monkey kidney cells and produces a striking inclusion body in their cytoplasm.[292] Interestingly, there is a naturally occurring virus in monkeys, the monkey intranuclear inclusion agent (MINIA), that is indistinguishable from human measles virus. This makes monkeys unreliable for research on measles virus except when meticulous precautions can be taken to exclude those carrying MINIA, which, among other problems, may cause serious confusion when present in tissue cultures of monkey kidney cells. Hitherto, only one antigenic type of the measles virus has been identified—a point of importance in relation to prophylaxis and treatment by specific convalescent human serum. Measles virus is antigenically closely related to the viruses of canine distemper and of cattle plague (*Rinderpest*).

Acute Laryngotracheal Bronchitis

This name was given during the first world war to a form of 'non-diphtheritic croup'.[293] The condition, which resembles diphtheria clinically, except that there is no membrane, occurs mainly in the winter months; it is most prevalent during the first year of life and it occurs especially among boys.[294] It is often severe, but seldom fatal; tracheotomy may be needed to relieve the respiratory distress. While in some cases adenoviruses, paramyxoviruses and mycoplasmas have been recovered, in many outbreaks the cause has not been identified.

Acute Viral Bronchiolitis

A number of viruses may cause acute bronchiolitis. An important one is the 'respiratory syncytial virus', a paramyxovirus that was first isolated from an outbreak of coryza in a colony of chimpanzees.[295] Its infectivity for man was shown when one of the investigators of this epizootic contracted the disease. The virus has since been shown to be an important cause of infection of the lower respiratory passages in older children and adults. Specific neutralizing antibodies indicative of an earlier infection[296] can be found in the sera of over 90 per cent of healthy adults in Britain. When tissue cultures of HeLa cells are inoculated with the virus, the cells enlarge, become rounded, and form syncytia that often present a striking microscopical appearance.

Several epidemics of acute bronchiolitis due to this virus have been described among infants in Britain and elsewhere.[297] These outbreaks are often remarkably focal in distribution, affecting only a comparatively small area or community. Secondary bacterial infection may complicate the infection, particularly in babies under about seven months, among whom the mortality is highest and who require intensive antibiotic treatment if the secondary invaders are to be overcome.

Post-Tracheostomy Lesions

The trachea may become narrowed in either of two places after tracheostomy—at the site of the incision, or further down where the balloon causes pressure.[298] Small, shallow ulcers may heal quickly. Deeper ulcers may involve cartilage, which becomes necrotic: healing is then accompanied by stenosis. If the cuff of the balloon is too near the tracheostomy it may act as a fulcrum, causing the tip of the tube to press into the tracheal wall: pressure necrosis and perforation follow, and lead to mediastinitis or erosion of a large blood vessel.

Another cause of obstruction following tracheostomy is the so-called 'granuloma ball', which is a large mass of granulation tissue at the tracheostomy site.[299]

Chronic Bronchitis

The normal human respiratory tract is believed to produce about 100 ml of secretion in 24 hours. This secretion flows up through the glottis into the oesophagus without conscious need to clear the throat or cough: the normal person is thus regarded as having no sputum. Chronic bronchitis has been defined in clinical terms as a persistent or recurrent excess of secretion in the bronchial tree on most days for at least three months in the year, during at least two years.[300] The condition is subdivided into chronic (or recurrent) mucopurulent bronchitis, and chronic obstructive bronchitis accompanying generalized obstruction of the airways.[301] The diagnosis of chronic bronchitis may be made only when other conditions, such as tuberculosis, bronchiectasis and cardiovascular and renal disease, have been excluded by thorough investigation.[302]

Chronic bronchitis affects mainly the middle-aged and elderly. It is commoner in men. Some patients may recall a liability in their earlier years to expectoration for a few days after head colds.[303] Relatives are often similarly affected. The productive cough occurs at first only in the winter months; later it is present all through the year, characteristically with acute exacerbations in winter that usually are precipitated by a viral infection. In some patients breathlessness increases with the years and deterioration in exercise tolerance leads to an inability to continue working, and eventually to complete invalidism and death in respiratory or cardiac failure. The sputum may be purulent continuously; it accumulates in the bronchi during sleep and causes severe obstruction of the airways until it is coughed up in the morning.

Bacteriological examination of the sputum in chronic bronchitis has shown that the most frequent and important pathogenic bacterium is *Haemophilus influenzae*,[304, 305] with *Streptococcus pneumoniae* possibly second in importance but difficult to evaluate because of its frequent presence as a commensal.[305] Purulent sputum usually contains one or both of these organisms in abundance: they tend to disappear after antibacterial therapy and the sputum then becomes mucoid again. The exacerbation of chronic bronchitis by viral infections results from damage to the epithelial lining of the bronchi, with resulting facilitation of bacterial invasion of the mucosa.

While infection by viruses and bacteria is of great importance in the pathology of chronic bronchitis, particularly in relation to the sustained deterioration in the patient's condition as the years pass, other factors contribute significantly to its development and progressive worsening. These factors include cigarette smoking,[306, 307] which is of major importance, air pollution,[308] which accounts for the higher prevalence of the disease in urban communities (in England it reaches its peak in the Merseyside and Manchester conurbations), fumes at work, fog (see below), and a damp, cold climate.[309]

The disease is particularly prevalent in Great Britain (see Table 7.4). About 25 000 deaths are

Table 7.4. *Death Rates per Million from Bronchitis in Certain Countries in 1952**

Country	Males	Females
England and Wales	838	420
Scotland	529	275
Portugal	248	183
Germany	139	86
The Netherlands	127	82
France	55	36
Canada	44	26
Denmark	33	36

* World Health Organization, *Epidem. vital Statist. Rep.*, 953, **6**, 321.

generally believed to be caused by it in England and Wales annually—one in about 25 of all deaths. Of those attributed to its complications—bronchopneumonia, emphysema and cor pulmonale—were

also included, this proportion would be substantially larger. As a cause of sickness and incapacity for work it ranks in terms of 'lost days' with influenza. The social gradient of the disease is steep, for the death rate in the poorest section of the population is some five times that in the most prosperous.

Patients who suffer from chronic bronchitis are particularly susceptible both to acute epidemic respiratory diseases, notably influenza, and to adverse weather conditions.[310–313] The morbidity from the disease rises every winter, and remains high throughout the colder, damper months. The occurrence of fog, especially that form known as 'smog', in which the water vapour becomes heavily contaminated with smoke and sulphurous gases, causes a prompt increase in both morbidity and mortality among older people. The heavy four-day smog in London in 1952 is believed to have precipitated 4000 deaths. Comparable, but smaller, smog epidemics have been recorded in cities in the United States of America and on the European mainland.

Structural Changes[314]

When the lungs of a patient with chronic bronchitis are dissected at necropsy, the exposed bronchi, especially those in the lower lobes, are found to be filled with a mixture of mucus and pus. When the purulent material is washed away from bronchi that have been opened longitudinally, the underlying mucous membrane is seen to be a dusky red. In general, the calibre of the main bronchi remains unchanged; the distal bronchi characteristically become slightly dilated: when they are opened with fine scissors the dilatation is found to reach almost to the pleura (Fig. 7.25).[315] The lung substance is often emphysematous. There may be many small foci of bronchopneumonia in the lower lobes.

The main features of chronic bronchitis become apparent only when the lungs are examined histologically. The glands in the walls of the bronchi are much enlarged, and acini that secrete mucus are much more numerous than the serous variety. The mucigenic acini and their ducts become distended with retained mucus.[316, 317] Indeed, it is possible to correlate the clinical history of chronic bronchitis with the size of the bronchial glands, either by measuring their thickness in transverse sections of selected bronchi[317] or by estimating their cross-sectional area.[318] The epithelium that lines the bronchi may also show signs of increased mucus production, the proportion of goblet cells being increased at the expense of the ciliate ones.

L

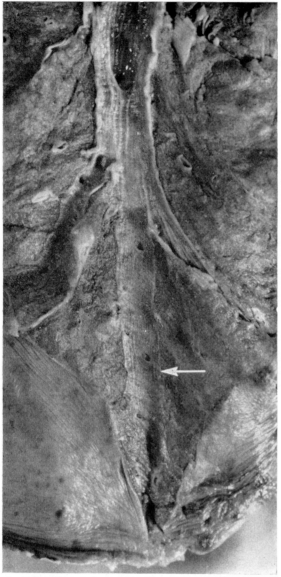

Fig. 7.25.§ Chronic bronchitis. There is a mild dilatation of the distal bronchi (arrow)—a very common finding in this condition. × 1·5.

Patches of the surface epithelium may undergo squamous metaplasia: the accompanying loss of cilia, which ordinarily clear bacteria and dust particles from the lower respiratory tract, predisposes to colonization by micro-organisms.

The submucosa may be infiltrated by moderate numbers of lymphocytes and plasma cells. Its blood vessels are congested. In contrast to bronchiectasis (see below), the musculature and cartilage of the bronchial walls remain intact.

If the inflammation has extended into the smaller bronchi and bronchioles, the exudate in the lumen, which often contains some fibrin, may have undergone organization by cells that have migrated from the submucosal connective tissues through areas denuded of epithelium. In these circumstances, the lumen may become partly or fully closed. This condition is known as *obliterating bronchitis and bronchiolitis*.[319] It may affect many parts of the bronchial tree, leading to irreversible obstruction of the airways.

Although some cases of chronic bronchitis show very little emphysema, recurring exacerbations of pulmonary infection may damage the fine structure of the lungs and give rise to emphysematous and fibrotic changes that cripple the patient further (see pages 297 to 299). Two groups can be distinguished among severely disabled patients. Those in one group tend to be obese and have attacks of respiratory failure with hypercapnia and hypoxia, but are fairly well in the intervals: their lungs may show little emphysema at necropsy. The patients in the second group tend to be sparsely built and to be very dyspnoeic both during and between attacks, although less severely hypercapnic and hypoxic: at necropsy their lungs are severely emphysematous.[320-322]

Bronchiectasis

When a bronchus has been subjected to prolonged inflammation, various elements in its wall, notably the neuromuscular and elastic components that normally modify its calibre during breathing, may become disorganized and, later, lost. The consequent dilatation of the lumen, which usually affects many of the secondary bronchi in a lobe, is known as bronchiectasis. Clinically, advanced bronchiectasis is associated with chronic cough, intermittent fever, much collapse in the corresponding parts of the lung and the expectoration of large amounts—often several hundred millilitres daily—of offensive sputum. This expectoration is particularly copious when the patient rises in the morning and when he changes posture suddenly. In treatment, use may be made of this postural effect to promote the drainage of pus from the affected bronchi.

In its advanced forms, bronchiectasis is a serious suppurative condition, liable to grave complications both in the lungs and elsewhere. Its early recognition is of great importance. Radiological techniques have not only aided the diagnosis of established cases but have also disclosed that minor forms of bronchiectasis are by no mean uncommon as a sequel of acute pneumonia.[323] Cases in the latter category can generally be alleviated by prompt treatment: the pathological changes in the bronchi may then regress.

Much of our present knowledge of the structural changes in the lungs during the earlier stages of the disease has come from examination of lobes removed surgically. This has shown that the likelihood that the lesions may prove amenable to treatment depends largely on the severity of the injury to the elastica and to the neuromuscular elements in the bronchial wall.

Aetiology

Bronchiectasis is not an aetiological entity: it may be the outcome of any of various conditions in which dilatation of the bronchi is the common factor. It may develop at any age; the causes differ in young and older patients. In infants, it may be associated with disorders of mucus secretion, which manifest themselves most conspicuously in fibrocystic disease of the pancreas (see Chapter 23).[324] In older children and young adults, among whom bronchiectasis is common, it generally begins as a sequel to diffuse bronchitis accompanying incompletely resolved pneumonia.[325] Bronchiectasis is often secondary to some specific infection such as primary pneumococcal bronchopneumonia, influenza, whooping cough and measles. It is often associated with persistent infection of the maxillary and other nasal sinuses, but the nature of its relation to sinusitis is not clear. Occasionally, in children, bronchiectasis follows compression of a bronchus by an enlarged tuberculous lymph node; with the great decline in the incidence of tuberculosis, especially among young people, this cause is now uncommon.[326] Sometimes bronchiectasis follows the inhalation of a foreign body which, especially if irregularly shaped or rough of surface, or irritant, is liable to become firmly impacted in a bronchus of the lower lobe, especially on the right side. In adults, bronchiectasis is often found as a complication of partial obstruction of a large bronchus, such as may be caused by an adenoma or carcinoma arising in its wall.

Bacteriology

In the earlier stages of bronchiectasis, *Haemophilus influenzae* is much the commonest bacterium to be recovered from the sputum.[327] Later, a wide variety of different organisms becomes established in the infected air passages. The common commensals of the nasopharynx are typically present. Sometimes, especially when the sputum has become fetid, various spirochaetes (including *Borrelia vincentii*) and *Fusobacterium fusiforme* are found in the mucopus. It is through the activities of these organisms, which are almost always secondary or tertiary contaminants, that the smell of the sputum is so often offensive.

Structural Changes

Bronchiectasis generally affects the secondary bronchi of one (or sometimes both) of the lower lobes. Involvement may be diffuse or segmental.[328, 329] As a result of local pleurisy, the affected lobe is usually adherent to the chest wall. On cutting the lung, the bronchi are conspicuous as widely dilated tubes; their mucosa, after removal of the covering mucopus, is bright red, rather roughened and moist. Generally, the dilatation is more or less uniform throughout the affected parts of the bronchial tree (Fig. 7.26); sometimes, local widening produces a fusiform or saccular appearance (Fig. 7.27). Extensive bronchial distension and the accompanying collapse and fibrosis of the intervening parenchyma may give the lobe a polycystic appearance. Very often parts of the lobe to which air can still gain access are emphysematous.

A striking feature during lobectomy is the enlargement and inflammation of the hilar lymph nodes.

Histology.—On microscopical examination, the bronchial wall is seen to be chronically inflamed. In the early stages, ciliate epithelium may persist, but in time the lining cells lose their cilia and large areas undergo squamous metaplasia. The submucosa is swollen and extensively infiltrated by neutrophils, lymphocytes, plasma cells and macrophages. As the condition deteriorates, the various specialized elements in the bronchial wall —elastic tissue, muscle, glands and cartilage—are lost. Ultimately, the air passages may consist of a tube of granulation tissue lined irregularly with epithelial cells, many of which are squamous, and filled with stagnant pus. The inflammation involves the arteries, many of which become partly obstructed by endarteritis. In most cases, too, the inflammation spreads into the surrounding lung substance, and the resulting interstitial pneumonia is a further complication.

Follicular Bronchiectasis.—This common variety of bronchiectasis has a characteristic histological

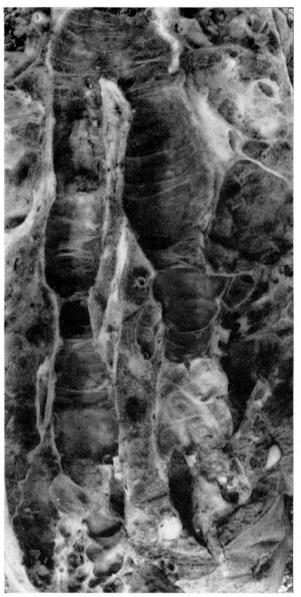

Fig. 7.26.§ Cylindrical bronchiectasis. The bronchi are dilated throughout their length, but more in some stretches than in others. Bulging occurs especially between the transverse muscular folds. *Pressure fixation; barium sulphate impregnation.* × 1·7.

appearance. The amount of lymphoid tissue in the affected bronchi becomes greatly increased; the mucous membrane is consequently much thickened and projects into the lumen, which becomes distorted and partially obstructed (Fig. 7.28). Follicular bronchiectasis may involve many of the bronchi: generally it begins in the smaller ones and extends to the larger.[330]

Pathogenesis

Much discussion has centred on the cause of the dilatation of the bronchi in bronchiectasis—whether it results from the pressure exerted by the copious exudate and secretions inside the lumen, or whether it is brought about through retraction of the surrounding collapsed and fibrotic lung substance.[331, 332] Both views agree in attributing major importance to the structural weakening of the walls of the bronchi, first through paralysis of the neuromuscular elements and later through their destruction. The bronchi are normally held open by traction by the surrounding lung. It would seem reasonable to expect them to dilate when their walls have been damaged by inflammation. Nevertheless, bronchiectasis is often found associated with collapse of the related lung and, in that event, there would be no traction to explain the dilatation. It is probable that the rise in intrabronchial pressure that results from the replacement of air by the much heavier column of purulent secretion is of greater importance, especially in the lower lobes. Not only is the internal pressure raised, but since this is now applied to a greater surface area of wall, the total stretching force that tends to dilate the bronchi is more than proportionately increased.

Complications

Bronchiectasis is essentially a suppurative condition of the lungs, and may be followed by the development of a lung abscess or of a pleural empyema. The latter is the less common of these complications, because adhesions often form early and obliterate the pleural cavity. Pyaemia is an occasional complication; the formation of a metastatic abscess in the brain is a more frequent danger.

The disorganization of the lung structure may become so severe that the pulmonary circulation is embarrassed and cor pulmonale develops.

The prolonged suppuration may lead in time to the development of generalized amyloidosis.

Lung Abscess

A lung abscess is a localized suppurative lesion that forms in the substance of the lung. Once formed, lung abscesses have many features in common, irrespective of their causation, which can vary widely. They may originate in the lung or be secondary to a focus of infection elsewhere. An abscess may develop as a complication of pneumonia (usually staphylococcal pneumonia, but

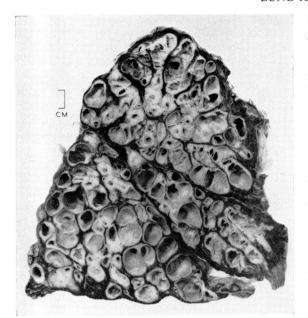

Fig. 7.27.§ Saccular bronchiectasis. In all segments of the lung there are saccules, about 1 cm in diameter, with thick fibrous walls, sometimes showing the remains of the mucosal folds of the bronchi from which they were derived.

may be found. Some of these, such as *Streptococcus pyogenes* and pneumococci, are primary pathogens that may normally be present in the nasopharynx and throat. Others, among them spirochaetes and fusiform bacilli, ordinarily are oral saphrophytes but may thrive in the contents of the abscess: the fetid nature of the pus, so distinctive of many lung abscesses, is attributable to the proteolytic action of these organisms on the exudate. Abscesses are commoner in the right lung than the left, possibly because of the more direct course of the right main bronchus, and in the upper lobes rather than the lower. They may be single or multiple. They are generally more or less spherical (Fig. 7.29), and their contents render them dense enough to be visible in radiographs. On opening the thorax, there may be localized pleurisy over the affected portion of the lung, and, on cutting into the abscess, pus—often fetid—escapes. The wall

sometimes pneumonia caused by the pneumococcus or by Friedländer's bacillus).

Oftener, lung abscess is the result of inhalation of infected material. The patient who is unconscious —for instance, in diabetic or uraemic coma, or under general anaesthesia, or following a head injury, alcohol or narcotic drugs—may inhale infected matter, even into the finest ramifications of the bronchial tree. The inhaled substances include food, vomitus, extracted teeth, parts of guillotined tonsils, blood clot and many others. The posture of the patient at the time largely determines the distribution of the resulting lesions in the lungs—gravity is the major deciding factor.[333]

Septic embolism is another, and now the least common, cause of lung abscess. The marked fall in the frequency of lesions of this origin is a result of the introduction of antibiotics. Formerly, multiple pyaemic abscesses were common in the lungs, especially as a complication of such staphylococcal infections as acute osteomyelitis and carbuncle.

With so diversified a pathogenesis, it is scarcely surprising that many kinds of micro-organisms can be recovered from lung abscesses. Sometimes, as in abscesses complicating a primary pneumonia or due to pyaemia, only a single species of organism is present in the pus, but in those following inhalation of foreign material many different species

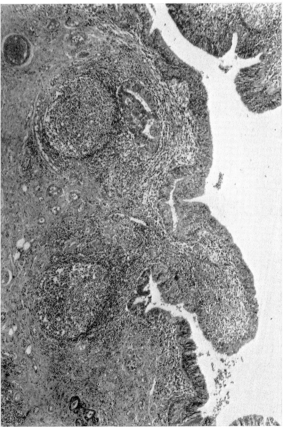

Fig. 7.28.§ Histological appearance of wall of a dilated bronchus in follicular bronchiectasis. Two lymphoid follicles are seen (right), each with a large germinal centre; there are many lymphocytes between these and the respiratory epithelium. *Haematoxylin–eosin.* × 45.

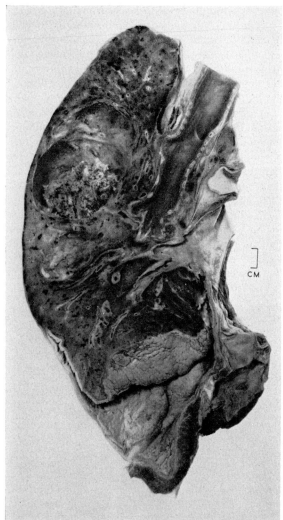

CM

Fig. 7.29.§ Lung abscesses. In the lower half of the right upper lobe is an abscess containing shaggy, broken-down lung substance. There is a smaller abscess in the lower lobe. The rest of the lung is consolidated, and there is compression by a basal empyema.

of the abscess is formed of compressed lung substance and has the structure of a pyogenic membrane, with varying degrees of fibrosis externally.

The subsequent fate of pulmonary abscesses depends much on their size and situation. Often they rupture into a bronchus and their contents may then be partly or wholly expectorated. If the infection is overcome in such cases, a shrinking cavity is formed and becomes lined by epithelium from the nearby bronchi.[334] An abscess near the surface of a lung may rupture into the pleural cavity and give rise to an empyema. The empyema may be interlobar in situation.

There may be extensive fibrosis of the lung tissue round chronic abscesses. The affected lobe may become much deformed by scarring. Adhesions may bind the lung to the chest wall and prevent infection of the pleural cavity.

It is by no means rare for a lung abscess to be complicated by pyaemia. Localized metastatic abscesses may develop: they occur most frequently in the brain, as is also the case in bronchiectasis (see Chapter 34).

Gangrene of the Lung

Gangrene occurs when saprophytic organisms multiply in an abscess or infarct, or round a foreign body or tumour. The necrotic lung is greenish in colour and foul-smelling.

ACUTE INFECTIONS OF THE LUNGS

Acute infection of the lung parenchyma is very common at all ages, and is one of the most frequent causes of death. The provocative agent may be one or more of a wide variety of micro-organisms, including bacteria, viruses and fungi. With such a diversity of causative organisms, it is not surprising that the resulting pneumonic lesions present a variety of structural patterns. It is still possible to classify the different forms of pneumonia on the classic basis of the lobar, lobular, bronchial or interstitial distribution of the lesions. Since much is now known of the pathogenesis of pneumonia, an aetiological classification has obvious advantages, and will be followed as far as possible in the present section. Certain features of some of these infections have been considered earlier in the section on acute tracheobronchitis (see page 304).

Acute Bacterial Pneumonia

Acute inflammatory lesions of the lungs can be caused by infection with many kinds of bacteria. Of outstanding importance is the pneumococcus (*Streptococcus pneumoniae*), which is responsible for almost all cases of lobar pneumonia and for a large proportion of cases of primary bronchopneumonia in infants and old people. Other varieties of bacteria that may produce pneumonia, almost always in its bronchopneumonic form, include *Staphylococcus aureus, Streptococcus pyogenes*, Friedländer's bacillus, *Haemophilus influenzae* (Pfeiffer's bacillus) and *Pseudomonas aeruginosa*. Their relative frequency varies from time to time and place to place, and one or more of them may be present—often with the pneumo-coccus—as a mixed pulmonary infection

Pneumococcal Infections

Epidemiological Considerations

Some 80 types of pneumococcus can be distin-guished by the serological differences between their capsular polysaccharides. Although most healthy people of all ages harbour one or more types of pneumococcus in the throat, intermittently or continuously, these are relatively seldom the types that are responsible for pneumonia. For instance, types 1, 2 and 3 are recovered with particular frequency from patients with lobar pneumonia and type 4 from infants with primary bronchopneumonia. It seems, therefore, that al-though any type of pneumococcus may be found from time to time in sputum from normal people, some types and strains are more pathogenic for man than others.

The widespread distribution of all types of pneumococcus in the throat of healthy people is relevant to the pathogenesis of pneumococcal infection of the lungs. The development of acute pneumonia must be regarded as attributable to circumstances that sharply lower resistance to a potentially pathogenic strain of pneumococcus that has been carried in the nose or throat, perhaps over a long period. Pneumococcal pneumonia is, essentially, an endogenous infection, due to failure of the natural defences of the respiratory tract to prevent the spread of a potentially pathogenic strain of pneumococcus from the nasopharynx to the lungs, where it causes acute inflammation.

Although most cases of acute pneumonia occur sporadically, minor epidemics sometimes occur as a result of the spread of newly introduced patho-genic strains in a community, such as a school or military camp, where personal contacts are especially close. Under these circumstances, a rise in the carrier rate for the responsible type generally precedes the outbreak.[335, 336]

In temperate climates, pneumococcal infections of the lungs, especially in infants and in the elderly, are much commoner in the cold seasons;[337] in England and Wales, for example, deaths from lobar pneumonia are three or four times com-moner in winter than in summer. Low external temperature probably has the greatest bearing on the seasonal occurrence of pneumonia—partly directly, by impairing the natural defences of the respiratory tract through chilling of its mucosa by cold air, and partly indirectly, by aggravating the overcrowding that occurs in inclement weather. Further, the carrier rate for pneumococci in the general population tends to rise considerably during the winter and thus to increase dispersal of the more pathogenic strains by droplet.

The identification of the serological type of the pneumococcus responsible for each case of pneu-monia was of great importance in the days when effective treatment depended on the prompt ad-ministration of the appropriate type-specific anti-serum. The introduction of sulphonamides and, later, of antibiotics, the antibacterial action of which is not dependent on the type of the pneumo-coccus responsible, made serum therapy obsolete.

In the pathogenesis of acute pneumococcal infec-tion of the lungs it is evident that predisposing causes acquire particular significance.[338] The ad-verse effect of cold weather on resistance has been mentioned. Other contributory conditions are sudden chilling, as by immersion in water, trauma to the chest, alcoholism, depressant drugs and various debilitating metabolic diseases. Pneumonia is a common and often fatal complication of any condition, such as coma, that depresses the cough reflex and so sets aside this important defence of the respiratory tract.

The Forms of Pneumococcal Pneumonia

The lung lesions in pneumococcal infection may assume one of two principal forms. In the first, *lobar pneumonia*, the inflammation is virtually con-fined to the affected lobe (or lobes), the rest of the lungs remaining uninvolved. In the second, *broncho-pneumonia*, the lesions are centred on the smaller bronchi and may be dispersed throughout the lungs, although they tend to be more widespread and more advanced in the lower lobes. These two forms of pneumonia differ widely in their clinical features.

Lobar Pneumonia

Clinical Features

In most cases the onset of lobar pneumonia is abrupt. The patient feels ill, complains of a sharp pain in the side of the chest that is made worse by deep breathing, coughs up 'rusty' sputum, and quickly develops a fever of 103° to 104°F (40°C). The respiration rate rises fast, and sometimes at the height of the disease reaches 50 or more a minute; the ratio of pulse to respiration may fall from its usual 4 : 1 to 2 : 1. Cyanosis usually appears as the disease advances. A leucocytosis of

15 000 to 20 000 cells/μl, mainly neutrophils, is often an early feature. In a proportion of cases, pneumococci can be cultured from the blood during the height of the fever.

Structural Changes in the Lungs[339]

Before the introduction of effective treatment, the morphological changes in the lungs often presented a classic sequence of changes which, following Laënnec's original description, were known as the stages of engorgement, red hepatization, grey hepatization and resolution. It should be realized that these terms apply to typical appearances, and that each stage shades into the next. In recent years, improved treatment has curtailed and modified the clinical course of lobar pneumonia, and partly for this reason and partly because of the fall in mortality from the disease, these morbid anatomical appearances are seen much less often than formerly.

In lobar pneumonia, as the name implies, it is usual for the typical changes to be confined to one lobe, although not infrequently two or even three lobes may be involved simultaneously or after brief intervals. In such cases, two or three days may separate the onset of involvement of the different lobes. The lower lobes are most commonly affected; there is no significant difference in the frequency of involvement of the two lungs.

Engorgement.—The stage of engorgement generally lasts for less than 24 hours. It is exceptional for patients to die so early in the disease: when such cases are seen at necropsy, the affected lobe is more or less uniformly involved and appears disproportionately large in comparison with the other lobes, which collapse in the usual way when the pleural sacs are opened at necropsy. The pneumonic lobe is heavy and congested with blood. When cut, a blood-stained, frothy fluid oozes freely from the surface.

Histological examination shows the features typical of acute inflammation: the capillaries in the alveolar walls are much dilated, and the air spaces are filled with pale eosinophile fluid in which there are a few red cells and neutrophils. In sections stained by Gram's method, the paired, lanceolate pneumococci can often be seen, mainly free, in the alveolar fluid. At this stage, little fibrin has formed, and the affected lobe has not yet acquired the firm consistence typical of hepatization.

Red Hepatization.—The feature that led Laënnec to popularize Morgagni's term 'hepatization' is the consistence of the affected lobe, which recalls that of the liver. The cut surface of the lung is much drier than in bronchopneumonia. The development of hepatization is accompanied by sero-fibrinous pleurisy, small, rough tags of fibrin covering much of the visceral pleura of the affected lobe.

The change in the gross features of the affected lobe are readily explained by reference to the histological changes that have taken place during the preceding few hours. The copious fluid exudate, which at the time of its formation contained abundant fibrinogen, has clotted in the alveolar spaces: in sections stained for fibrin, innumerable interlacing strands occupy each space and often can be seen connecting with others in neighbouring alveoli through the pores of Kohn. At the same time, more and more neutrophils migrate from the congested capillaries into the fibrin meshwork. Usually, at this stage, the pneumococci are numerous; neutrophils have ingested many of them.

Grey Hepatization.—After two to three days, the affected lobe gradually loses its red colour and assumes the grey appearance that it retains for the next few days (Fig. 7.30). This change in colour, which starts at the hilum and spreads toward the periphery, is brought about by the pressure of the exudate in the air spaces on the capillaries and by the migration of very large numbers of leucocytes, at first mainly neutrophils but later macrophages, into the fibrin in the alveoli. The almost complete obliteration of the vasculature of the affected lobe can be demonstrated in radiographs of the lungs after their injection at necropsy with radio-opaque material. A temporary virtual cessation of blood flow through the unventilated lobe lessens the liability to systemic hypoxia that might otherwise develop. Toward the end of the stage of grey hepatization, pneumococci are less numerous in the lung and appear in degenerate forms, differing much in size, and often no longer Gram-positive in their staining.

Resolution.—Before the days of chemotherapy, resolution generally began on about the eighth or ninth day of the illness. Quite frequently, the fever fell by crisis, sweating was profuse, respiration became deeper and less rapid, and the patient's condition showed much improvement. This stage often followed quickly upon the appearance of specific antibodies against the pneumococcus responsible.

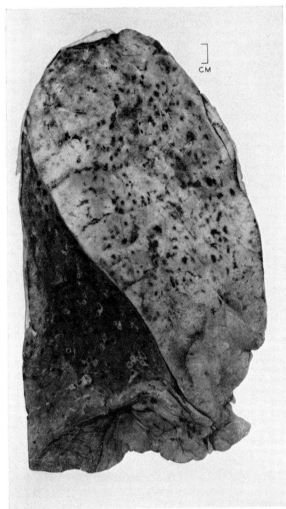

Fig. 7.30.§ Grey hepatization stage of lobar pneumonia. The upper lobe of this left lung has retained its size after death because of the presence of inflammatory exudate in the air-spaces. In contrast, the unaffected lower lobe has collapsed a little on being exposed to atmospheric pressure by opening of the thorax at necropsy. The pallor of the upper lobe is due to the relative bloodlessness of the tissue and the accumulation of fibrinous exudate and leucocytes in the alveoli. The dark areas are small foci of dust-pigmented distensive centrilobular emphysema, an incidental finding common among urban populations.

Structurally, resolution proceeds in a patchy yet progressive manner by liquefaction of the previously solid, fibrinous constituent of the exudate in the air spaces. Soon the affected lobe becomes more crepitant as the air spaces re-open. It is presumed that a fibrinolytic enzyme is liberated, probably from the neutrophils, and digests the intra-alveolar coagulum. The now fluid contents of the air spaces are removed, partly by expectora-

tion but mainly through the lymphatics: this accounts for the soft, moist and swollen appearance of the hilar lymph nodes.

Functional Disturbances in Lobar Pneumonia

Almost all patients suffering from lobar pneumonia show some reduction in the concentration of oxygen in their arterial blood, and in some cases this may give rise to cyanosis.[340] The pathogenesis of the cyanosis has been much discussed, and it seems doubtful whether it can be attributed to any single factor. In some instances it may result from passage of the blood through the airless lung in the stage of grey hepatization and its consequent return to the left side of the heart in unchanged venous state. This explanation cannot account for cyanosis in all cases of this disease, for there is evidence that the circulation in consolidated lobes is reduced —when such a lung is perfused at necropsy with radio-opaque material, X-ray examination shows that little of the medium has entered the affected portions.[341] It seems likelier that impaired oxygenation in the lungs is brought about by the much raised respiratory rate. An important result of the rapid, shallow breathing is that the volume of tidal air is much reduced, and that such ventilation as occurs takes place mainly in the bronchial dead space and only to a limited extent in the finer air spaces where gaseous exchange normally occurs.

The rapid respiration rate so typical of lobar pneumonia seems to be due to heightened sensitivity of the sensory receptors of the Hering–Breuer reflex, perhaps through their exposure to products of the organisms. In dogs, in which this situation is reproduced in experimental pneumonia, section of the vagus nerves restores the rate to normal.[342]

The gravity of severe hypoxia in lobar pneumonia, and in other diseases in which cyanosis is severe, is well pointed by Haldane's remark that 'anoxaemia not only stops the machine but wrecks the machinery'.

By the end of the stage of resolution, completion of which is shown by chest radiographs to require several weeks, the lung ordinarily has recovered its normal structure.

Evolution of the Lobar Distribution

In spite of much experimental work on animals, in which the condition can be reproduced, the mode of evolution of the lobar pneumonic process still has many obscure features. The fact that during the earlier stages of consolidation the lesions near the hilum appear to be more advanced than those toward the periphery suggests that the infective agent spreads centrifugally through the lung substance. It may be that the early formation of a fibrinous clot in the pulmonary lymphatics at the root of the lung impedes the escape of the heavily infected exudate through these channels, and that as a result of gravity and pulmonary movements this fluid is encouraged to flow through the air spaces and the pores of Kohn into the more peripheral parts of the lobe. In this way, the pneumococci become dispersed rapidly through the whole substance of the affected lobe.

Complications[343]

Lobar pneumonia may be complicated by dissemination of the pneumococci throughout the lungs and to other organs.

In some patients, acute pneumococcal bronchitis and foci of bronchopneumonia may be present in lobes other than that mainly involved. These accessory lesions, if severe, may exacerbate the disease by further impairing the respiratory exchange in the lungs.

Although, in patients who recover, the area of lobar consolidation usually resolves completely and again becomes air-containing, several complications may interfere with the completeness of recovery. The initially serofibrinous pleurisy may develop into empyema and be complicated by suppurative pericarditis. Part of the affected tissue may break down, especially in cases of infection by pneumococci of serotype 3, and a lung abscess may form. Resolution may be delayed through incomplete digestion of the fibrin in the exudate within the alveoli, and organization, followed by fibrosis or 'carnification', may develop: this may lead to bronchiectasis, which may affect the whole or part of the lobe (Fig. 7.31).

In many cases of lobar pneumonia there is a bacteriaemia or even septicaemia at the height of the infection. Acute endocarditis may then develop, and this is sometimes followed by the formation of an abscess in the brain after lodgement of an infected embolus. Pneumococcal meningitis, peritonitis and arthritis are rarer manifestations of the dissemination of the organisms by the blood.

Bronchopneumonia

Bronchopneumonia, or lobular pneumonia, is characterized by widespread, patchy areas of

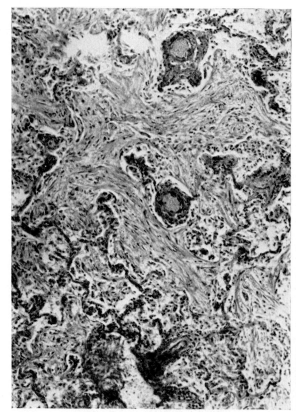

Fig. 7.31.§ Organized lobar pneumonia (carnification of the lung). Pale, cellular fibrous tissue fills all the air-spaces, but their walls can still be seen. *Haematoxylin–eosin.* × 100.

inflammation in which the centre of the pulmonary lobules is particularly affected. The disease may be primary, or secondary to another infective condition of the respiratory tract, such as influenza, measles, pertussis and mycoplasma infection. Bronchopneumonia may also follow inhalation of irritant gases and aspiration of food or vomit.

Primary bronchopneumonia is generally caused by a pneumococcus, which may be of any serotype. It occurs most frequently in infants, debilitated young children and elderly people, and in such patients often proves fatal. It begins as a widely dispersed bronchitis and bronchiolitis (Fig. 7.32); focal areas of pneumonia then develop in the centre of the lobules. The foci are generally larger and more numerous in the lower lobes. Once the organisms are established in the small bronchioles, they spread, partly along the inner airways toward the periphery and partly by penetrating the inflamed bronchiolar wall. When they reach the alveoli, they excite active inflammation, with copious exudation of fluid and immigration of neutrophils

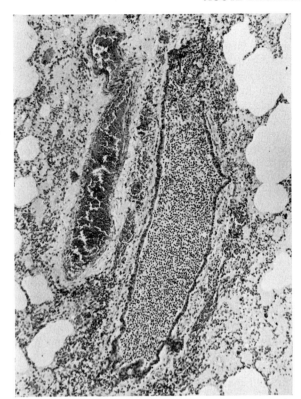

Fig. 7.32.§ Acute suppurative bronchiolitis. Although there is hyperaemia and some oedema of the tissue round the bronchiole there is no pneumonic consolidation of the alveoli (compare with Fig. 7.33). *Haematoxylin–eosin.* × 55.

(Fig. 7.33). The air spaces nearest to the bronchiole show the most advanced degree of inflammation; those at a greater distance may be filled merely with fluid exudate.

The bronchopneumonic areas may be several millimetres across. In the freshly cut lung they are commonly seen as pale, solid, centrilobular foci, often somewhat raised above the surface of the surrounding lung substance (Fig. 7.34). These consolidated areas can be felt as well as seen. Small beads of yellow mucopus can often be expressed from the bronchioles on the cut surface. The lung is much wetter than in lobar pneumonia. In severe cases, the patches of consolidation may enlarge and even become confluent: when this happens the affected area seldom presents the uniformity of texture and colour that is characteristic of lobar pneumonia, in which all parts of the lobe are involved almost simultaneously.

When recovery from bronchopneumonia takes place, the bronchioles again become patent, the exudate liquefies and is expectorated or absorbed, and respiratory function is restored. It is probable that recurring attacks of bronchopneumonia in patients with chronic bronchitis contribute to the development of permanent lung damage in the form of bronchiolar obliteration, emphysema and fibrosis.

Bronchopneumonia may have serious effects on respiratory function. The filling of many air spaces with exudate excludes air from much of the lungs and may lead to serious peripheral hypoxia.

Postoperative Bronchopneumonia

Surgical operations, particularly those on the abdomen, are liable to be followed by bronchopneumonia.[344] The pathogenesis of this complication is complex. In patients anaesthetized with ether or other irritant vapours, the ciliary epithelial defensive mechanism of the bronchial tree may be impaired. Also, the unconscious patient may inhale infected material from the mouth or nose, and the

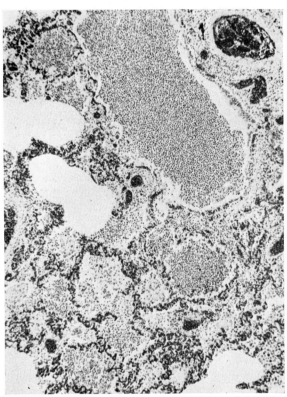

Fig. 7.33.§ Acute suppurative bronchiolitis and bronchopneumonia. The infection has spread from the bronchial tree into the parenchyma of the lung: the leucocytic exudate, in addition to distending the bronchiole (top), has begun to appear in the alveoli also. The interalveolar capillaries and the larger blood vessels are engorged. *Haematoxylin–eosin.* × 50.

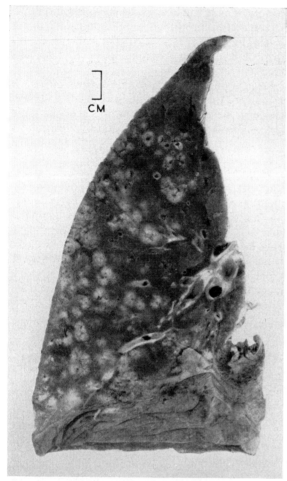

Fig. 7.34.§ Suppurative bronchopneumonia. There are numerous pale foci of inflammation throughout this lower lobe. Compare with lobar pneumonia, Fig. 7.30.

temporary depression of the cough reflex may allow micro-organisms to establish themselves in the lungs. Once the effect of the anaesthesia has worn off, the pain associated with movement, particularly of the abdominal wall, may restrict the normal aeration of the lower parts of the lungs. Finally, some general depression in resistance to infection commonly results from the haemorrhage and shock that may accompany any major surgical operation.

Staphylococcal Pneumonia

Staphylococcal pneumonia has been known for many years as a serious disease with a high case fatality rate.[345] It has been recognized as a common complication of influenza, the organisms often being derived from staphylococcal lesions of the patient's own skin.[346] In the epidemic of Asian influenza in Britain in 1957, staphylococcal pneumonia—often due to antibiotic-resistant strains of the coccus, and fulminating in progress—was the commonest complication of the viral infection.[347] In children, staphylococcal pneumonia may follow measles or whooping cough. In infants a primary staphylococcal bronchopneumonia is known, with a case fatality rate as high as 80 per cent in the pre-antibiotic era and still in the region of 40 per cent.[348] Staphylococcal pneumonia sometimes follows bacteriaemia or septicaemia—for instance, in the course of acute osteomyelitis: oftener, such septicaemia results in solitary or multiple lung abscesses.

In recent years, interest in staphylococcal pneumonia has revived, because, although the mortality from most forms of pneumonia has been reduced by modern drugs, many strains of staphylococcus that are now widely distributed in the population are resistant to the generally used antibiotics.[349] Such strains are common in hospitals, carried in the nose by staff and patients, and fatalities from staphylococcal infection, often with pneumonia, occur among surgical patients who otherwise should have recovered from their operation.

At necropsy, the bronchi are acutely inflamed and the lungs contain many pale centrilobular foci of suppuration, which in the more advanced cases may have enlarged and coalesced to form abscesses a centimetre or more in diameter. Adjacent air spaces contain inflammatory exudate. A superficial abscess may rupture into the pleura and cause empyema, which is a common complication of staphylococcal pneumonia. If the patient survives, there may be permanent damage in the form of pulmonary fibrosis and bronchiectasis.

Klebsiella Pneumonia

Several serotypes of *Klebsiella* are among the less frequent bacterial causes of pneumonia. *Klebsiella pneumoniae* (Friedländer's bacillus) is the species usually responsible. Both typical lobar pneumonia and suppurative bronchopneumonia may result. These infections are comparatively rare in temperate and cold climates: they are notably less so in subtropical and tropical regions. Their mortality is much higher than that of the pneumococcal pneumonias. The abundant mucoid material that the klebsiellae secrete gives the pneumonic lesions a distinctively slimy appearance and feel. This material, like the capsular material of *Cryptococcus neoformans* (see page 353), is mucicarminophile:[350]

this characteristic is often helpful in identifying the infection in histological sections.

Pneumonic Plague

In man, infection with *Yersinia pestis* takes two main forms: *bubonic plague*, in which the bacillus is transmitted from rat to man by infected rat fleas, and *pneumonic plague*, in which the organism is usually spread from man to man by infected sputum droplets, although it can also arise as a complication of the bubonic form. Bubonic plague is prevalent in India and some other tropical countries; pneumonic plague sometimes breaks out in epidemic form in more northerly latitudes, where the climate is colder and less humid.[351] In the past, before the era of effective antibiotics, both forms had a high case fatality rate: indeed, the plague bacillus has been the cause of some of the most widespread and devastating epidemics in human history.

In the pneumonic form the lungs show many areas of bronchopneumonia, which sometimes are confluent; the course of the disease is generally too short for massive consolidation to develop.[352] The pulmonary lesions are often haemorrhagic; they are usually accompanied by serofibrinous pleurisy and great enlargement of the hilar lymph nodes. On histological section, the alveolar capillaries are engorged and the air spaces are full of fluid exudate containing few leucocytes but many bacilli.

Anthrax Pneumonia[353]

Anthrax occurs in many species of domestic animals, especially herbivores. The causative organism, *Bacillus anthracis*, occasionally passes to man. As in plague, human anthrax takes two main forms depending on the portal of entry of the organism—the misnamed 'malignant pustule' that follows its inoculation through the skin (Chapter 39), and the pneumonic form, often termed wool-sorters' disease or 'inhalation anthrax', in which infection of the lungs follows inhalation of anthrax spores. The formerly high case fatality rate in anthrax has diminished greatly in recent years through the use of antibiotics.

Wool-sorters' disease, formerly seen in Bradford and other Yorkshire textile towns, was acquired by inhalation of dust from imported wool and hair, which was often heavily contaminated with the very resistant spores of the organism. Today, effective measures are directed to the destruction of these spores by exposure of the wool to antiseptics before

it is handled by the workers, and as a result the mortality from all forms of anthrax in Britain is now very small.[353]

At necropsy, the bronchi are often acutely inflamed and lined by a membrane. The lungs present widespread, often confluent, areas of haemorrhagic bronchopneumonia. The haemorrhagic inflammatory oedema that constitutes the exudate in the alveoli contains large numbers of the characteristic, large, Gram-positive bacilli.[354] The organisms are readily seen in haematoxylin–eosin preparations (see Figs 39.167A and 39.167B). The later stages of anthrax pneumonia are invariably accompanied by haemorrhagic lesions in the hilar lymph nodes and mediastinum. Septicaemia develops and is often so severe that the organisms are recognizable in films of the circulating blood. The spleen is large, dark and soft. Haemorrhagic lesions may be found in the meninges.

Anthrax can be produced experimentally by causing animals to inhale the spores. However, death is then the result of septicaemia, and there is little or no evidence of infection in the lungs.[355]

Pneumonia in Pseudomonas Septicaemia

Some patients with malignant tumours or leukaemia, especially if under treatment with glucocorticoids and antibiotics, develop septicaemic infection by *Pseudomonas aeruginosa*. The duration of life after the first positive blood culture is about four days.[356] Pneumonia is one of the principal manifestations of the infection; meningitis, arthritis and jaundice may also develop. There may be striking skin lesions, including vesicles and bullae, and sharply demarcated foci of cellulitis that enlarge rapidly and become haemorrhagic and necrotic.

At necropsy, the Gram-negative bacilli are visible in large numbers in the vessel walls, causing an acute necrotizing angitis associated with thrombosis and haemorrhage.[357] In the lungs, this produces infarct-like, haemorrhagic, consolidated areas. Histologically, areas of necrosis are present in which traces of the pre-existing structure remain. The necrotic foci are surrounded by a narrow inflammatory zone containing neutrophils and much granular debris.[358]

Cross-infection by *Pseudomonas aeruginosa* is an important cause of death in hospital. Pneumonia is occasionally a manifestation of this hazard.

Leptospiral Pneumonia

Some patients with acute leptospirosis, particularly infection acquired in tropical or subtropical lands, develop haemoptysis in association with patchy consolidation of the lungs.[359] The lesions are foci of haemorrhagic pneumonia or, in some cases, of simple haemorrhage. In the former instances there is a haemorrhagic fibrinous exudate that contains a few neutrophils and occasional macrophages: the exudate is most conspicuous within the alveoli but is seen also in the interalveolar septa, which are correspondingly thickened.[360] In cases of simple haemorrhage into the tissue of the lung the bleeding is associated with the profound thrombocytopenia that is an occasional accompaniment of leptospirosis. Both types of pulmonary change may be seen in cases of infection by leptospires of various serogroups; they are severest in cases of infection by *Leptospira icterohaemorrhagiae*, but have been a conspicuous feature in a small proportion of cases of canicola fever (infection by *Leptospira canicola*, acquired from dogs) in Europe and of infection by *Leptospira bataviae* in parts of southeastern Asia.[360] The leptospires can be demonstrated in the lesions by Levaditi's method of impregnation with silver.

The pulmonary involvement is part of a general infection and seldom predominates in the clinical presentation (see Chapter 21). Provided the disease is recognized, and treated early and efficiently, the case fatality rate is very low.

Viral, Chlamydial, Mycoplasmic and Rickettsial Pneumonia

(a) Pneumonia Caused by Viruses

Many varieties of virus are among the known causes of pneumonia. They include the orthomyxoviruses (influenza virus), paramyxoviruses (for instance, parainfluenza viruses, measles virus and respiratory syncytial virus), adenoviruses, rhinoviruses and coronaviruses. Undoubtedly there are others that remain to be identified.[361] Occasionally, herpes viruses (for instance, the virus of herpes simplex and varicella virus) and poxviruses (variola virus) may infect the lungs.

Most cases of viral pneumonia end in recovery. In fatal cases the pathological changes in the lungs depend to some extent on the type of virus responsible and, of course, on the effects of secondary bacterial infection, which is a very frequent development in these circumstances. From the occasional post-mortem studies that have been undertaken in uncomplicated cases of viral pneumonia it is apparent that the inflammatory reaction in the lung is mainly histiocytic and interstitial. Neutrophils are numerous only when there is a complicating bacterial infection. Cytoplasmic inclusions may be recognizable in the cells of the alveoli and bronchioles under the light microscope, and viral particles may be found on electron microscopy. Similarly, most of the cells in the sputum in cases of viral pneumonia are histiocytes, except when there is bacterial infection also.

The virus responsible for pneumonia can often be isolated from sputum and from nasopharyngeal washings by cell culture and other methods. Confirmatory evidence of infection by particular viruses is provided by the demonstration of a rising titre of specific antibodies in the patient's serum.

Influenzal Pneumonia

Pneumonia caused by the influenza virus alone is very rare, at least in a form severe enough to be recognized. Although pneumonia is the usual cause of death in epidemics of influenza, it is a secondary bacterial pneumonia that is responsible in the great majority of such cases (see page 318). The pathological changes in influenzal viral pneumonia have been distinguished from those associated with secondary bacterial invasion of the lungs only comparatively recently:[362-364] before the discovery of the influenza virus in 1933[365] no distinction was made between the effects of bacterial and other factors,[366] and the changes that are now known to be due to the viral infection were inevitably confused with those of complicating infections, mainly caused by bacteria.

The macroscopical appearances in influenzal viral pneumonia vary with the severity of the disease. The lower lobes are often affected more than the rest of the lungs. They are bulky, hyperaemic and often of a characteristic plum colour. Blood-stained, frothy fluid oozes freely from the cut surface. Areas of haemorrhage are present and may be extensive. The mucosa of the bronchial tree is hyperaemic and oedematous; ulceration is generally the result of bacterial infection, but some authorities have considered superficial necrosis to be an occasional direct effect of the virus.

The cytopathic effect of influenza virus is seen microscopically in the characteristic degenerative changes in the epithelial cells of the bronchial and bronchiolar mucosa. These changes involve the ciliate and goblet cells of the surface epithelium and often the cells lining the bronchial glands: swelling of the cells, vacuolation of their cytoplasm and degeneration of the nucleus proceed to cell loss, exposing the basement membrane, which is usually notably swollen. There is oedema of the deeper tissues, with hyperaemia and a moderate to marked accumulation of lymphocytes; neutrophils are present but account for only a small proportion of the cellular infiltrate. These changes extend into the interlobular septa. In the alveoli there is conspicuous swelling of the lining cells, which proliferate and in places may virtually fill the lumen. The changes reach their peak on about the third to the fifth day of the disease and then regress. During the stage of recovery regeneration of the epithelium of the bronchial tree may produce a picture of squamous metaplasia (Askanazy's *metaplasierender Katarrh*)[367]: this soon gives place to normal ciliate pseudostratified respiratory tract epithelium. During the phase of recovery the proliferation of alveolar lining cells may continue, and has even produced appearances somewhat resembling a neoplastic state:[366] this condition, which often also involves the terminal bronchioles, eventually subsides completely.

Fulminating Influenzal Viral Pneumonia.[368]—This very rare condition seems to occur only in the course of major epidemics of influenza and is characterized by the exceptional rapidity of the course of the illness, death resulting within a day or two, or even within hours, of the clinical onset of illness. The alveoli contain a fibrin-rich oedema fluid, often frankly haemorrhagic, and macrophages may be numerous in the exudate and particularly in the alveolar walls and interstitial tissue round the bronchioles and in the interlobular septa. Hyaline membranes are often found in the alveoli. Focal necrosis of alveolar walls and thrombosis of capillaries are conspicuous features in the parts most severely affected.

This form of influenzal pneumonia is often associated with changes in other parts of the body that indicate the occurrence of influenzal viraemia. Among these are haemorrhagic encephalomyelitis, apparently an acute infective condition and distinct from postinfluenzal encephalomyelopathy (see Chapter 34).

Measles Pneumonia

Little is known of the occurrence of measles pneumonia other than as a rare fatal complication of measles that is most frequent in children aged from six months to about two years and in those whose resistance is low because of certain other diseases, particularly leukaemia.[369] That pneumonic foci may also develop in the course of severe clinical attacks of measles in other patients is shown by the demonstration in some such cases of patchy opacities in the lungs on X-ray examination: in almost all these cases the condition resolves rapidly. It is unknown if the pathological changes are similar to those in fatal measles pneumonia.

Death from measles pneumonia occurs typically about two weeks after the appearance of the rash. At necropsy, the lungs are heavy and of rubbery consistency; and their cut surface is pale pink. Extensive vascular thrombosis has been a feature of some cases. Close examination may show that the small bronchi are cuffed by a greyish zone that, when recognizable, is a pointer to the diagnosis.

Histologically, there are degenerative changes in the epithelium of the bronchi and bronchioles, often accompanied by hyperplasia, particularly in the latter. As in influenzal pneumonia (see above), squamous metaplasia may occur. The hyperplasia increases the layering of the cells in the surface epithelium; mitotic figures may be numerous. In addition, a characteristic feature of the epithelial reaction is the formation of multinucleate giant cells, such as occur in various other viral infections.[370] In measles pneumonia such cells are seen both in the bronchial and bronchiolar mucosa and in the alveolar ducts and alveoli (Fig. 7.35). Some, at

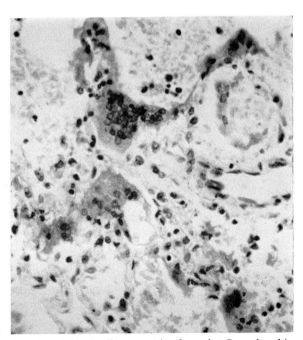

Fig. 7.35.§ Giant cell pneumonia of measles. Several multinucleate giant cells are seen to form part of the lining of the alveoli. The alveoli contain some proteinaceous exudate. There are a few lymphocytes and neutrophils in the interstitial tissue. *Haematoxylin–eosin.* × 250.

least, are formed by fusion of the cytoplasm of several adjoining epithelial cells,[371] with clumping of nuclei and the formation of phloxinophile intracytoplasmic inclusions. These inclusions, which occur in the hyperplastic bronchiolar epithelium also, are thought to be aggregates of measles virus.[372] Electron microscopy has provided support for the view that the giant cells, particularly those in the alveoli, are formed by fusion of epithelial cells.[373] It has also shown that their nuclei contain inclusions that are characterized by the fine filaments of nucleocapsid protein that distinguish measles virus from other paramyxoviruses.[374]

It is important to note that the giant cells in the lungs in cases of measles pneumonia are quite different from the Warthin–Finkeldey giant cells that are found in the lymphoid tissue throughout the body in this infection, mainly in the immediately pre-exanthematous state (see Chapter 9).

There is a heavy accumulation of macrophages, lymphocytes and plasma cells in the alveolar walls. This cellular infiltrate extends into the connective tissue surrounding the bronchioles and small bronchi, accounting for the pale cuff that is seen round them on naked eye examination. Neutrophils are not numerous unless there is a secondary bacterial infection. The appearances are closely comparable to those found in the lungs of dogs that have died of distemper (Carré's disease), which is also caused by a paramyxovirus.[375]

'Giant Cell Pneumonia'.—The form of pneumonia that by convention is known as giant cell pneumonia (Hecht's pneumonia)[376] is histologically of the type described here as measles pneumonia. It is thought to be due to measles virus, which has been isolated from the affected tissue in a number of cases.[377–379] It has occasionally developed in the course of other specific infections, including scarlatina, pertussis and influenza: even in these cases, according to current opinion, it is probably attributable to coincident infection with measles virus. Although clinical evidence of measles may be lacking, and there is no history of a rash, this may be explicable on the basis of an evanescent exanthematous stage, followed by persistence of the virus as a result of deficient antibody formation.[369] Ordinarily, measles virus can be isolated only during the first three days after the appearance of the skin rash: in cases of measles pneumonia it is still recoverable one to two weeks after the rash developed, and in cases of giant cell pneumonia with no history of a rash the infection may well have been present for a similar or longer period.

Smallpox and the Lungs

Acute tracheobronchitis is a feature of severe smallpox and may be associated with specific ulcerative foci in the mucosa. Pneumonia in these cases is ordinarily due to secondary bacterial infection, but histological examination may show interstitial lesions of viral type, although without specific features.

A condition that has been described as *'smallpox handlers' lung'* has been observed on numerous occasions among nursing and medical staff attending patients with smallpox.[380, 381] It is characterized by high fever and prostration: radiological examination shows widespread mottling of the lungs with shadows up to several millimetres across. Typically, there are no catarrhal symptoms. Recovery appears to be the rule. These patients are well immunized by previous vaccination against smallpox and they do not develop a rash. It has been suggested that their acute pneumonia is in fact an allergic reaction to smallpox virus inhaled in the dust of scales desquamated by the patients whom they have been looking after.[381] The nature of the pathological changes in the lungs is unknown.

Cytomegalovirus Infection of the Lungs

Disease caused by cytomegalovirus (salivary virus) is seen most frequently in newborn children infected before birth by virus carried by their mother.[382] The disease may present as an acute fatal infection with jaundice and a form of leucoerythroblastic anaemia. It is rare in adults,[383] but may occur as a late complication in some systemic diseases, especially those of the haemopoietic system and diabetes.[384] It is sometimes a complication of treatment with corticosteroids. The pneumonia may be unilateral or bilateral, and generally involves the lower lobes; advanced lesions may appear as reddish purple, nodular areas.

Histologically, some of the alveolar epithelial cells are enlarged and contain characteristic nuclear inclusions, up to 10 μm in diameter, which are surrounded by a clear zone inside the nuclear membrane (Fig. 7.36). Intracytoplasmic inclusions up to 2 μm in diameter, are often present also; they may give a strong periodic-acid/Schiff reaction.

In some cases there is cellular infiltration of the alveolar walls, particularly by plasma cells: it has been suggested that the latter are present only when there is an associated infection by *Pneumocystis carinii* (see page 360).[384, 385] Similarly, intraalveolar exudate containing neutrophils and fibrin is probably due to an accompanying bacterial

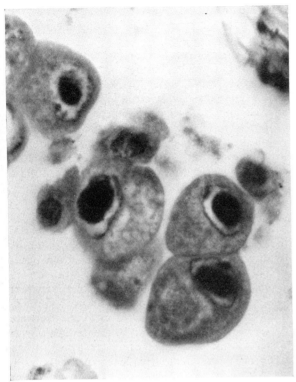

Fig. 7.36.§ Pulmonary infection by cytomegalovirus (salivary virus). The nucleus in several of the alveolar cells in this photograph contains a large, darkly stained inclusion body that is separated from the chromatin adjoining the nuclear membrane by a characteristic, unstained halo (the so-called 'owl eye' appearance). The cytoplasm of the infected cells is also much increased in extent and contains numerous small inclusions. *Haematoxylin–eosin.* × 1300.

infection. There is no good evidence that cytomegalovirus is itself a cause of pneumonia in the strict sense of the term.

(b) Pneumonia Caused by Chlamydiae (Bedsoniae)

Only occasional cases of psittacosis had been described in Britain and on the continent of Europe before the 1920s: the disease then suddenly became much commoner. Many of the cases were severe and the case fatality rate was very high. This epidemic was associated with the importation of a large number of infected parrots from South America, where psittacosis is enzootic: the patients were found to have been in close contact with these birds, either as domestic pets or through working in or visiting pet shops where they were on sale. The importation of parrots into the United Kingdom was stopped in 1930. Temporary

rescindment of the prohibition order in 1951 was followed by further cases, necessitating its reintroduction.

The causative agent of psittacosis was recognized by Bedson and his colleagues in 1930[386] and is sometimes known as *Bedsonia*, although the accepted rules of nomenclature properly give priority to the genus name *Chlamydia*, which had been validly published before *Bedsonia* and is applicable to all members of the psittacosis-lymphogranuloma-trachoma group of organisms (see Chapters 9 and 40).[387] These basiphile agents are no longer regarded as viruses but are commonly thought to be small intracellular bacteria.[388] Similar organisms are found in many species of wild and domesticated birds in various parts of the world: at least some of these are pathogenic for man. For this reason the name of this group of diseases has been changed from psittacosis (parrot disease) to the more generally applicable *ornithosis*.[389]

Infected birds, which may show no signs of disease, excrete the organisms in droppings that, drying at the bottom of their cage, form a highly infective dust. It is usually through the inhalation of such dust while attending to the birds that man becomes infected, and, as is to be expected from the portal of entry of the organism, the disease takes the form of a pneumonia. It is important to bear in mind that the infectivity of ornithosis is high: numerous instances have been recorded of nurses and relatives contracting the disease while caring for patients. The disease has been acquired also through exposure to the organism in the laboratory and in the performance of necropsies.

Pathology.—Macroscopically, the lungs are bulky and patchily consolidated. The consolidated areas, which are usually haemorrhagic, are more numerous in the lower lobes than elsewhere. Where they abut on the pleura there is local fibrinous pleurisy, and petechiae may be conspicuous under the exudate.

Microscopically, the changes are quite distinct from those of viral pneumonia, for exudate within the alveoli is much more marked than interstitial changes. The latter include engorgement and often thrombosis of the capillaries with some lymphocytic accumulation and sometimes a few neutrophils. The thrombosis may cause ischaemia and this can result in foci of alveolar necrosis. Blood, fibrin, macrophages and desquamated alveolar cells are found within the alveoli, which may have a conspicuous lining of swollen epithelial cells showing vacuolation and other degenerative changes. The chlamydiae are just visible with the light microscope, ranging from about 0·25 to rather less than 0·5 μm in diameter: they are to be seen in the cytoplasm of a variable proportion of the alveolar lining cells, and may most easily be found in preparations stained by the prolonged Giemsa method.

The epithelium of the bronchi and bronchioles shows degenerative changes and desquamation.

Diagnosis.—As there is a bloodstream infection during the first few days of clinical illness, which usually starts within one to two weeks of exposure, the presence of the organism may be demonstrated both by transmitting infection to mice by intra-peritoneal inoculation with blood and by cultivation on the chorioallantoic membrane of eggs or in cultures of HeLa cells. The presence of complement-fixing antibodies, particularly when a rising titre is demonstrated, is helpful both in diagnosis of ornithosis during the disease and as a retrospective index. Cross-reactions with other organisms of the psittacosis-lymphogranuloma-trachoma group occur but should not be confusing in practice. A considerable proportion of patients with ornithosis may give a positive skin reaction to Frei (lymphogranuloma inguinale) antigen.[390]

(c) Infection by *Mycoplasma pneumoniae*

During the decade before the second world war, cases of a mild form of pneumonia were reported that clinically were unlike those attributable to bacterial infection. None of the bacteria known to be associated with pneumonic lesions could be recovered from the sputum, and as long as the condition was uncomplicated by secondary bacterial infection the leucocyte count in the blood showed little tendency to rise. Cases occurred sporadically, but oftener appeared in small community epidemics in schools, colleges and camps, although even under these conditions, which are usually conducive to the spread of respiratory infections, the disease was not highly contagious. It became known as primary atypical pneumonia.

The chief clinical features are fever, malaise and cough. On X-ray examination, irregular and ill-defined areas of opacity due to consolidation can be seen in the lungs, usually in the hilar region and sometimes bilaterally. It is characteristic of the disease that the radiological changes are very much more extensive than the comparatively mild clinical manifestations indicate. The case fatality rate is low—of the order of one in a thousand patients—and the pulmonary opacities that are

conspicuous during the 10 days or so that the illness lasts gradually resolve during the ensuing days of convalescence.[391]

There have been few opportunities for post-mortem study of the lesions in primary atypical pneumonia. In a series of 90 cases, however, necropsy disclosed widespread inflammation in the affected lung parenchyma, sometimes progressing to ulceration of the bronchioles, with much muco-pus in their lumen, and surrounding areas of interstitial pneumonia.[392] Neutrophils were less numerous, both in the bronchioles and in the alveoli, than in the bacterial forms of pneumonia.

The aetiology of primary atypical pneumonia has attracted much interest. The first advance came with the isolation of an organism from a number of these cases that became widely known, after its discoverer, as the 'Eaton agent'.[393] That this agent is specifically concerned with the clinical disease is indicated by the rise in specific antibodies that occurs during the course of the illness. The infection, mainly in subclinical form, has become widely prevalent, as is shown by the frequency with which specific antibodies can be detected in the serum of healthy people in the general population.[394]

On account of the ability of filtrates of sputum from cases of primary atypical pneumonia to cause the disease in a large proportion of young volunteers when given by intranasal instillation, and of the transmissibility of the infection to experimental animals, the Eaton agent was at first regarded as a virus. Later studies, in which specific fluorescent antibodies were found to react with coccobacillary bodies visible in the lungs of infected chicks, indicated instead that the pathogen belongs to the group of 'pleuropneumonia-like' organisms (PPLO) —the mycoplasmas—which can pass through a coarse bacterial filter.[395] The organism is now known as *Mycoplasma pneumoniae*: it is one of the considerable number of mycoplasmas that have been recognized in man, animals, plants and soil. For a time, *Mycoplasma pneumoniae* was regarded as the L form of *Streptococcus MG*, a non-haemolytic streptococcus that is agglutinated by the serum of some 10 per cent of patients with mycoplasmic pneumonia and that was isolated originally from a case of the latter at necropsy: comparative studies of the nucleic acids of the two organisms have shown that they are in fact unrelated. The explanation of the presence of agglutinins against *Strep ococcus MG* is unclear. Antibodies to *Mycoplasma pneumoniae* itself form in most infected patients. In addition, in about half the cases the patient's serum agglutinates Group O red blood cells at a temperature between 0° and 5°C to a titre of at least 1 : 30 (cold haemagglutination test).

Pathology.[396]—There is nothing pathognomonic about the macroscopical and microscopical changes in the lungs. Macroscopically, oedema and areas of haemorrhage may be conspicuous. Histologically, oedema fluid, red blood cells and macrophages are found in many groups of alveoli; an occasional alveolus may contain a hyaline membrane. Lymphocytic infiltration is seen in the wall of alveolar ducts and of alveoli in the affected parts.

Although the pneumonic foci have sometimes been said to undergo complete resolution, there is evidence that the more heavily involved parts may become fibrotic. Pleural adhesions are a not uncommon sequel.

(d) Infection by *Coxiella burnetii*

Q fever ('query fever') was so named because of its 'questionable' nature prior to the isolation of the causative organism. It was first recognized in Queensland, Australia, in 1937.[397] It is now known to have virtually a global distribution, and to be essentially an infection of cattle, sheep and goats that occasionally occurs in man. Among cattle, the disease is sometimes transmitted by ticks, but possibly more frequently by the inhalation of contaminated dust from the floor of milking sheds. In man, it is almost always acquired through drinking milk that has been insufficiently pasteurized, or through close contact with cattle, as in dairy farms, abattoirs and hide factories.

The disease is of sudden onset, with general malaise, severe frontal or retro-orbital headache, high fever and muscle pain; most of the symptoms and signs subside after about a week. Pneumonia develops in only a very small proportion of those infected. Radiographs at the height of the disease disclose numerous, relatively small, but widely distributed, patches of consolidation that are due to interstitial pneumonia. The radiological picture, like the clinical condition, has much in common with that of mycoplasma pneumonia (see above).

Q fever is caused by *Coxiella burnetii*, a rickettsial organism that is resistant to drying and that may survive exposure to a temperature of 60°C; the latter characteristic is important in relation to the pasteurization of milk. In human cases, the organism can generally be recovered during the height of the disease by inoculation of the patient's blood or sputum into guinea-pigs. The organisms

can be seen with the light microscope in Giemsa-stained histological sections: they usually measure about 0.25 by 0.45 μm; bacillary forms occur and measure up to 1.5 μm in length. They form microcolonies in infected cells, such as alveolar epithelium, and this facilitates their recognition.

Specific complement-fixing antibodies develop quickly and persist long after recovery. Epidemiological surveys have shown that many more people possess circulating antibodies against *Coxiella burnetii* than have had Q fever clinically: subclinical attacks must be far from uncommon.

The case fatality rate in Q fever is very low, and few necropsies on uncomplicated cases have been recorded.[398] The lungs show nodular or confluent areas of grey consolidation. The fibrinocellular exudate contains lymphocytes, plasma cells and macrophages.

CHRONIC INFECTIONS OF THE LUNGS

Mycobacterioses

Terminology of the Diseases and of the Organisms That Cause Them

Rationalization of the nomenclature of the mycobacteria has led to the replacement of some familiar designations by simpler variants that, once the changes have become established usage, will facilitate accurate identification of the mycobacterioses and of their causative organisms. Thus, the name *Mycobacterium tuberculosis* should now refer exclusively to what hitherto has been known as '*Mycobacterium tuberculosis*, human type' or 'the human type of tubercle bacillus'. What has so long been referred to as 'the bovine type of tubercle bacillus', or '*Mycobacterium tuberculosis*, bovine type', is now to be known simply as *Mycobacterium bovis*: similarly, '*Mycobacterium tuberculosis*, avian type' is now *Mycobacterium avium*.

In consequence of these changes, the name tuberculosis is now applicable only to disease caused by *Mycobacterium tuberculosis*, using the latter term solely in the new, restricted sense that corresponds to what formerly was described as the human type of tubercle bacillus.[399] Disease in man caused by *Mycobacterium bovis* should be described as 'infection with *Mycobacterium bovis*', rather than 'bovine tuberculosis'. Similarly, '*Mycobacterium avium* infection' should be so specified and not described as tuberculosis. Whether such restrictions are likely to be observed, or valuable, remains to be seen.

The great majority of cases of pulmonary mycobacteriosis in man may be termed tuberculosis, being caused by *Mycobacterium tuberculosis*. In a small proportion the organism responsible is *Mycobacterium avium*, mainly in outdoor workers in rural areas: such cases should be described as 'pulmonary infection with *Mycobacterium avium*'. Similarly, the 3 per cent or so of cases of pulmonary mycobacteriosis in Britain that are caused by *Mycobacterium kansasii* and the smaller proportion caused by *Mycobacterium bovis*, should be specified as infection with the organism responsible and not referred to as cases of tuberculosis.

Atypical Mycobacteria

The designations 'atypical' and—sometimes inappropriate—'anonymous' have been applied to some mycobacteria associated with disease in man that are not classifiable as either *Mycobacterium tuberculosis* or *Mycobacterium bovis*. They are all strongly acid-fast but not all are alcohol-fast. Some resemble *Mycobacterium tuberculosis* very closely, particularly when the latter has been modified by antituberculosis drugs. Many of them have been known for a very long time, although it is only comparatively recently that their importance as occasional pathogens has been recognized. Some are common in the environment and may contaminate specimens or culture media. Others are of still unknown origin. A few are pathogens of lower animals. Microbiologists have developed a wide range of biochemical and serological tests, bacteriophage typing and lipid analysis that make it possible to subdivide the large and growing number of atypical mycobacteria—pathogenic and non-pathogenic—into useful groupings, among which those species that are pathogenic to man may be readily identified.

Runyon's classification is widely used:[400, 401] Group I comprises the photochromogens, which form colourless colonies in the dark that become yellow or orange on exposure to light for two days or so; Group II, the scotochromogens, produce orange colonies in the dark as well as in light; Group III, the non-chromogens, remain colourless; and Group IV, the rapid growers, produce colonies within about three days.

Group I includes an important pathogen, *Mycobacterium kansasii*, which most frequently is a secondary invader of pre-existing pulmonary lesions, particularly in middle-aged men living in industrial areas where bronchitis is specially prevalent because of atmospheric pollution. Women are rarely infected by this organism. It is the commonest of the pathogenic atypical mycobacteria in Europe, including Britain, and it is also seen frequently in parts of the United States of America, especially the south-east of the country. Its source is not known. *Mycobacterium balnei* (*Mycobacterium marinum*), the cause of swimming-pool granuloma (see Chapter 39) and a natural pathogen in fish and amphibia, also belongs to Group I. It is widespread in temperate climates, particularly in Europe and North America.

Group II includes *Mycobacterium scrofulaceum*, an increasingly frequent cause of lymphadenitis, especially of the neck in children (see Chapter 9), but there are no serious pathogens in the group and none that has been identified as a cause of disease in the lungs.

Group III includes *Mycobacterium intracellulare* (the so-called Battey bacillus) and the closely related *Mycobacterium avium*, both capable of causing progressive pulmonary disease and death in man, and both relatively insusceptible to anti-tuberculosis drugs. *Mycobacterium intracellulare* is widespread in many parts of the world with a warm climate; it has been recognized with greatest frequency in Western Australia and in the southern and south-eastern parts of the United States of America. Its source appears to be soil. *Mycobacterium avium* is of worldwide distribution: infection is seen oftenest in rural areas, particularly, perhaps, where there is close contact with domestic fowl—in Western Europe it is thought to be least rare in parts of the west of Ireland. *Mycobacterium xenopi*, originally isolated from the South African clawed toad (*Xenopus laevis*), is another member of Group III that may cause progressive pulmonary disease: it is less resistant to drugs than the other pathogens of the group. In Britain it is found mainly in the south. Seabirds have been suggested as its source[402] for, like *Mycobacterium avium*, it is a thermophile organism, growing at 45°C; most of the patients from whom it has been isolated have been resident in coastal or estuarine regions. *Mycobacterium ulcerans*, the cause of Buruli ulcer and similar chronic tropical mycobacterial ulcers of the skin (see Chapter 39), belongs to Group III.

The only human pathogen recognized in Group IV is *Mycobacterium fortuitum*, a cause of disease in cold-blooded animals and occasionally of progressive pulmonary infection in man and in the domestic cat. Oftener, in man, it is found as a commensal or saprophyte in the lungs of patients with chronic pulmonary disease, such as pneumoconiosis. It is also a cause of superficial cutaneous infection, particularly abscesses, which sometimes are a complication of injections, including those self-administered by drug addicts.[403] Unlike *Mycobacterium ulcerans* and *Mycobacterium balnei*, which cause exclusively cutaneous and subcutaneous infection, *Mycobacterium fortuitum* may spread to the regional lymph nodes from the initial lesion in the skin. Sometimes it causes multiple abscesses and ulcers in the skin along the course of the subcutaneous lymphatics between the initial lesion and the lymph nodes, the picture then simulating the lymphangitic form of sporotrichosis and certain other infections that spread in this manner (see Chapter 39).[403] *Mycobacterium smegmatis* (the smegma bacillus) and *Mycobacterium phlei* (the timothy grass bacillus), which are among the best known saprophytic mycobacteria, also belong to Group IV.

Significance of Atypical Mycobacteria in Sputum.— The atypical mycobacteria may be common in the environment and so, as noted above, may contaminate specimens. The occasional isolation of such a strain is by no means uncommon in laboratory practice, and assessment of the significance of such isolates can be difficult. If an atypical mycobacterium is found repeatedly in a patient's sputum, particularly when *Mycobacterium tuberculosis* is absent, its possible role as a pathogen must not be dismissed until full investigation justifies this. The possibility that the atypical strain is present as an 'opportunistic' invader of tissue already diseased, or as a manifestation of lowering of the patient's resistance in consequence of such predisposing conditions as cancer (including leukaemia), diabetes mellitus and malnutrition, has to be kept in mind. Tuberculosis itself may predispose to secondary infection by atypical mycobacteria.

The infectivity of patients with disease caused by atypical mycobacteria is very low. It is exceptionally rare for more than one case to occur in a household.

Drug-Resistant Tubercle Bacilli.[404]—If tuberculosis is properly treated, drug-resistance should not develop. Drug-resistance in the earlier days of the modern antituberculosis drugs seemed to threaten that a situation comparable to that relating to *Staphylococcus aureus* might arise, with even more serious therapeutic consequences. Fortunately, control of the situation was achieved by using more than one drug at a time. Organisms that prove to be resistant to any one of the major drugs used in treating tuberculosis can generally be suc-

cessfully countered with a combination of others. Resistance to all available drugs is very rare, if, indeed, it occurs at all.

The causes of acquired drug-resistance include taking the drugs irregularly, or for too short a time. If two drugs are prescribed and the strain of organism responsible for the patient's infection is already resistant to one of them, resistance to the other may be encouraged to develop. This underlines the practical importance of regularly investigating the drug sensitivity of the strain of mycobacterium responsible for infection: in-vitro resistance to one or more of the drugs under consideration demands the use of *two* effective drugs that the strain is demonstrably sensitive to.

Studies in North America have shown that up to 10 per cent of cases of tuberculosis in children are caused by organisms resistant to one or more of the standard ('first line') drugs—isoniazid, streptomycin and sodium aminosalicylate.[405] In these cases, the reserve ('second line') drugs must be given, as appropriate—ethionamide, thiacetazone and rifampicin are among several possible choices. However, the proportion of cases of drug-resistant tuberculosis is decreasing year by year: generally speaking, therefore, it is always wise to look for an atypical mycobacterium when a patient's infection fails to respond to treatment.

(a) Tuberculosis[406]

Epidemiology of Pulmonary Tuberculosis

In spite of great advances in hygiene and therapeutics, tuberculosis still remains throughout the world as one of the most important of all specific communicable diseases.[407] It has been estimated that there are between 10 million and 12 million people in the world with the disease in an infectious stage, and that between them they infect 50 million to a 100 million contacts every year.[408] The epidemiological situation can be evaluated from the mortality rates in different countries. In most developed countries both the incidence of the infection and its mortality have fallen spectacularly in recent times: the decline in the deaths from all forms of tuberculosis and from respiratory and meningeal tuberculosis from 1949 to 1973 in England and Wales can be seen in Table 7.5. In many less developed countries, especially in those in which industrialization is proceeding actively, the position is much less encouraging and demands unremitting attention on the part of the public health authorities if its spread is to be controlled. Thus, in 1968, when the mortality rate was below

5 per 100 000 of the population in—among other countries—Australia, Denmark, England and Wales, the Netherlands, Norway, Scotland, Sweden and the United States of America, it was 31·2 per 100 000 in Chile and 35·4 per 100 000 in Hong Kong, and probably higher still in some developing countries where adequate records are not available. Such observations confirm that the disease is still epidemic in parts of the world in which neither infection nor environmental factors have yet produced a state of resistance in the community sufficient to stem the progress of the disease.

Table 7.5. *Tuberculosis: Deaths at All Ages for the Period 1949 to 1973 (England and Wales)**

Year	All forms		Respiratory		Meningeal	
	Males	Females	Males	Females	Males	Females
1949	11 918	7 879	10 655	6 816	558	533
1951	8 826	4 980	7 903	4 128	440	442
1953	5 964	2 938	5 447	2 466	177	168
1955	4 533	1 959	4 172	1 665	67	65
1957	3 414	1 370	3 150	1 099	47	63
1959	2 810	1 044	2 620	854	50	37
1961	2 372	922	1 946	647	37	32
1963	2 158	764	1 756	498	39	37
1965	1 614	638	1 303	432	19	29
1967	1 444	622	1 165	415	26	28
1969	1 325	515	841	251	21	19
1971	1 014	425	672	253	15	18
1973	964	388	580	221	22	8

* *The Registrar General's Statistical Reviews of England and Wales for the Years 1949 to 1973;* London, 1950–75.

In England and Wales, most mycobacterial infection is now caused by *Mycobacterium tuberculosis*, and the infection is predominantly acquired through inhalation of this organism into the lungs. Formerly, mycobacteriosis of other parts, particularly the cervical lymph nodes, the bones and joints, and the genito-urinary system, was much commoner than it is today. Intensive efforts to eradicate mycobacteriosis from cattle[409] and to introduce pasteurization of milk on a national scale brought about the virtual disappearance of these forms of disease in man, leaving respiratory tuberculosis, in spite of its diminishing incidence, as outstandingly the most important manifestation of the infection.

The fall in the incidence of fatal tuberculosis in the United Kingdom since mortality records were first kept over a century ago must be attributed to a wide variety of factors that began to operate first among the prosperous classes and that have since extended to all strata of society. During almost the whole of this period an amelioration in social conditions—among which housing has been both the most important and the most easily assessed in numerical terms—had been taking place in an almost uninterrupted, if unspectacular, manner, and it is to these unspecific factors that for many years the progressive fall in mortality was essentially due.[410] The recognition, too, that artisans in certain trades, notably printing and bootmaking, had an exceptionally high incidence of respiratory tuberculosis led to the introduction of more stringent measures of hygiene in these and similar industries. Occupational causes were almost certainly responsible for the fact that, for three decades after 1900, the incidence of tuberculosis among young women failed to fall in parallel with that in other groups of the population: at about that time a large influx of girls into factory industries made great changes in the pattern of their occupations and in consequence led to their greater exposure to people with active tuberculosis.

The peak of the epidemic of tuberculosis in England and Wales was in 1860, when there were 50 000 deaths from this cause among a population that numbered only 20 million at that time. The number of deaths from tuberculosis has fallen in almost every year since then, and most strikingly since the end of the second world war (see Table 7.5). In 1951, when the population was 43 758 000, there were 12 031 deaths in England and Wales from tuberculosis of the respiratory system;[411] in 1973, when the population was 49 248 900, the number of deaths from this cause had fallen to 801.[412] The remarkable decline in mortality from tuberculosis since 1945 must in large measure be ascribed to the introduction of effective anti-tuberculosis drugs, among which isoniazid has been probably the most effective. By bringing about a great fall in the number—often even the complete disappearance—of bacilli in the sputum in cases of active respiratory tuberculosis, these drugs have much reduced the hazard of infection that was formerly incurred by those who inadvertently or by obligatory associations were brought into contact, at work or at home, with an open case of the disease.

In spite of the transformation of the epidemiological situation, there is still a serious tuberculosis problem in Britain. There were 11 180 new notifications of the disease in England and Wales in 1973. In general, immigrants to Britain, as to various other industrial countries, coming from many parts of the world, have a substantially higher incidence of tuberculosis than the indigenous population of the host country. In one English town the number of new cases of the disease rose more than threefold in the period from 1960 to 1970.

Droplet Infection.—In the past, there was much speculation about the possible routes of infection in tuberculosis. Today, there is little doubt that when the lesions are present in the lungs, the infection has taken place as a result of inhalation of tubercle bacilli. That the respiratory tract should be the chief portal of entry is scarcely surprising in view of the great preponderance of the pulmonary form of chronic tuberculosis in man and of the enormous numbers of tubercle bacilli that are eliminated daily in the sputum of most untreated active cases. Children and young adults, when in close contact with such patients, especially in urban surroundings where the population density is high, are liable to inhale the bacilli and so acquire the infection in their lungs. Although the smaller droplets of expectorated sputum, which may remain for many minutes suspended in the air after a cough, are probably the chief vehicle for the transmission of tubercle bacilli, it should be realized that the organisms are resistant to desiccation, and that in consequence dried 'droplet nuclei', or the dust that they ultimately contaminate, may long remain as potential carriers of the infection.

Recognition of Pulmonary Tuberculosis

It is estimated that today, in England and Wales, about 20 per cent of cases of active tuberculosis of the lungs go unrecognized until necropsy.[413] This is particularly true of the elderly, whose resistance to the infection is lowered as an accompaniment of ageing: dormant lesions become active, and spreading disease—even miliary tuberculosis—follows, often with little in the way of clinical manifestations to indicate the seriousness of the danger (see page 344). Similarly, at any age, patients whose resistance is lowered by such serious and debilitating conditions as leukaemia and Hodgkin's disease, or poorly controlled diabetes mellitus, are prone to reactivation of dormant tuberculosis and vulnerable to exogenous reinfection: often the presence of the infection is overlooked, even when it is the immediate cause of death, until disclosed in the post-mortem room.

Many cases of active tuberculosis must go unrecognized, now that the proportion of deaths in hospital that is followed by necropsy is falling markedly in so many medical centres. The danger that persists after the patient's death is that his infection has been passed to his family or associates without awareness of the need for treatment.

The Structural Changes in Tuberculosis of the Lungs

For many years it has been recognized that although the morbid anatomical changes that develop in tuberculous lungs assume a variety of forms, the great majority of cases fall into one or other of two distinctive types. The first type was formerly found mainly in children, and was believed to be associated with infection occurring at an early age: for this reason it became known as the 'childhood type' of respiratory tuberculosis. Further experience has shown, however, that it is not so much the youth of these patients as the fact that they are infected for the first time that accounts for the distinctive structural features of their lesions. In consequence, this form of tuberculosis is now known as the 'primary type', and as the incidence of the disease in the general population has declined and the age of first infection has correspondingly risen, it is now met with increasingly in adults. The second morphological form—previously known as the 'adult type' of the disease—occurs in those patients who have some degree of allergy, and probably also of immunity, as a result of an earlier attack of tuberculosis: this type of disease is now generally termed 'post-primary tuberculosis'. Post-primary tuberculosis is usually due to a fresh infection; sometimes, however, there is pathological evidence that reactivation of a calcified primary lesion is its source.[414]

Primary Tuberculous Infection

The very early stages of a tuberculous lesion in the human lung have seldom been seen,[415] and our ideas on its pathogenesis have been derived almost wholly from study of the development of comparable lesions in experimental animals.[416] When a group of guinea-pigs is placed in an insufflation chamber into which a suspension of tubercle bacilli is introduced in a fine spray, the organisms are inhaled, and those that are not trapped in the upper respiratory tract are carried into the parenchyma of the lungs. If representative animals are killed serially, preferably at daily intervals, during the first two weeks, and subsequently less often, the progress of the pulmonary lesions can be followed in detail.

The presence of tubercle bacilli in an alveolus excites little immediate reaction, and for the first day or two the only response may be a small amount of exudate and a few neutrophils round the organisms. Within the next few days, macrophages collect in increasing numbers, and ingest most or all of the bacilli, some of which are in dead neutrophils. Gradually, the macrophages, with living bacilli in their cytoplasm, aggregate to form microscopical nodules that deform the alveolar architecture of the surrounding lung. After about two weeks, the cytoplasm of some of the more centrally placed macrophages fuses, so forming small, but typical, multinucleate cells of the Langhans type that are such a characteristic feature of the host reaction in tuberculosis. By the third week, the lesion has usually grown sufficiently to be visible to the naked eye as a small, grey tubercle. As these tubercles enlarge, their centre becomes yellowish: microscopical examination at this stage shows that they have undergone necrosis. This evolution from an incipient, mild inflammatory character to the stage of caseous necrosis is typical of tuberculosis in all the mammalian species that have been studied, and is almost certainly representative of the condition in man.

The elastic tissue of the lung persists for a long time in old tuberculous lesions. When stained appropriately, its distribution and pattern give information about the position of blood vessels and of alveolar walls that cannot be recognized clearly, if at all, in haematoxylin–eosin preparations.[417]

In the comparatively small number of cases in man in which there is opportunity to examine the lungs while the lesion of primary tuberculosis is still active, the latter—often known as the 'Ghon focus'[417a]—is generally visible as a pale yellow, caseous nodule, a few millimetres to a centimetre or two in diameter. Characteristically, it is situated in the peripheral part of the lung, underlying a localized area of chronic inflammation and thickening of the pleura (Fig. 7.37).[418] Usually, only one such focus is present, but if the lungs are searched carefully, preferably with the help of post-mortem radiography, it will be found that there is more than one focus in a small proportion of cases. It is a point of importance in the distinction between primary and post-primary tuberculosis of the lungs that in the latter the lesions are almost invariably in the subapical region of an upper lobe, whereas in the former they may be found in any of the five lobes, their frequency in the various lobes being closely parallel to the order of the relative size of these parts.

There is little doubt from studies on primary tuberculosis in man—and insufflation experiments on animals—that within a few days of their deposition in subpleural alveoli some of the bacilli are carried centripetally in the lymphatics to establish infection in hilar lymph nodes (Parrot's law).[418a] Thereafter, the granulomatous changes in the lung and lymph nodes, and the smaller foci that may have formed along the course of the intrapulmonary lymphatics, all develop at about the same rate. The caseating lesions in the lymph nodes tends to be larger than the primary focus in the lung. This combination of a peripheral Ghon focus with corresponding foci of caseation in the regional

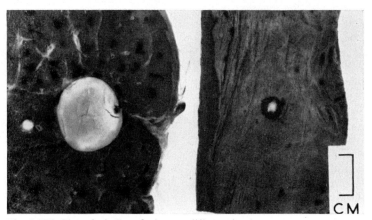

Fig. 7.37.§ Ghon foci. Two foci, very different in size, are seen on the cut surface of the left-hand specimen; the pleura over the larger focus has been pulled inward, being continuous with the fine fibrous capsule that has formed round the caseous mass. In the right-hand specimen (from another patient), a small Ghon focus is seen through the visceral pleura; the black ring round it is due to the presence of carbon pigment trapped in the surrounding scar tissue.

lymph nodes is sometimes known as the primary complex of Ranke (Figs 7.38 and 7.39). The complex is the typical result of a primary tuberculous infection of the lungs.

In a small proportion of cases of primary pulmonary tuberculosis the infection spreads to the pleura, either directly from the primary focus itself or by extension along the lymphatics: the result is often the formation of a pleural effusion (see page 412). Sometimes this is the presenting manifestation of the disease, and it may be the only clinical evidence; in other instances, pleural involvement develops as a complication of a primary focus that has already been recognized.

Further Changes in the Primary Complex

The primary complex may undergo a series of reparative changes, or it may continue to enlarge and in so doing implicate further structures and thus promote dissemination of the infection. The relative frequency and the pathological features of

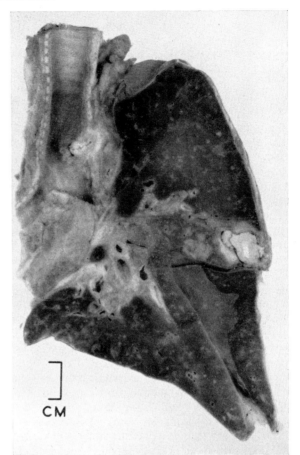

Fig. 7.39.§ Primary complex of tuberculosis. A large caseating Ghon focus, massive enlargement of the infected mediastinal lymph nodes and extensive tuberculous bronchopneumonia are seen. A caseating lymph node to the right of the lower end of the trachea has become adherent to the latter, and the tuberculous process has extended through the tracheal wall to form a sinus, thus contributing to the development of the bronchopneumonia. See also Fig. 7.38.

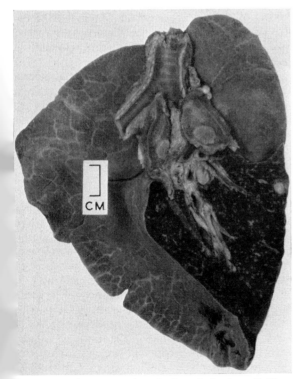

Fig. 7.38.§ Primary complex of tuberculosis. A small Ghon focus in the lower lobe of the lung is accompanied by extensive caseating tuberculous lymphadenitis. The infection has spread from one of the lymph nodes into a branch of a pulmonary artery, resulting in miliary haematogenous tuberculosis of the lower lobe (compare with Fig. 7.39).

healing and progressive primary complexes are considered below.

Reparative Changes.—The slow enlargement of the caseating primary complex is accompanied by development of a fibrous capsule. The fibroblasts that take part in this encapsulating fibrosis are mainly derived from the zone of granulation tissue that forms round the caseous mass in the interstitial tissue of the lung parenchyma. Becoming mobilized in the vicinity of the focus, these cells come to lie more or less circumferentially round it; as the weeks pass they produce first reticulin and later collagen fibres. Thus, in time, the more or less spherical mass of caseous matter becomes enclosed by fibrous tissue that impedes further centrifugal dispersal of the bacilli should any still remain alive.

Later, further changes generally take place in these fibrocaseous masses, though the tempo of the reparative process is much diminished. The most significant of these changes is the deposition of calcium salts. At first calcium carbonate and phosphate are laid down diffusely through the caseous material; sometimes, under the microscope, the focal deposition is seen to occur in more or less concentric rings, not unlike the Liesegang rings created by precipitation in a colloid gel. The rapidity with which calcification takes place depends largely on the amount of calcium that is available, and this in turn depends greatly on the amount of this element in the diet and its absorption from the intestines. Much of our knowledge on this question was gained from follow-up studies in which patients who had recovered from primary tuberculosis were submitted to radiological examination of the chest at monthly or bimonthly intervals. In one such investigation, undertaken in the north-east of London, calcification was recognized early during the second year after the primary infection; half the patients first showed a radiographic opacity after an interval of between 12 and 16 months.[419] This agrees well with a similar study in Baltimore.[420] Probably both studies tended to underestimate the rapidity with which primary foci undergo calcification, for it is only when these lesions exceed a certain minimal size that the deposit of calcium is large enough and dense enough to be recognizable by radiography.

After a long interval, usually several years, such calcified foci may undergo ossification.[421] This begins at the boundary between the calcified mass and its fibrous envelope. The calcified material is slowly transformed through the complementary activities of osteoclasts and osteoblasts: lamellae of bone are formed within the capsule and eventually take the place of much or all of the originally amorphous, calcified mass. Fatty and sometimes haemopoietic marrow may form within the bone. This transformation may affect the fate of the focus, for if bacilli have survived in the caseous material, in spite of conditions there that are adverse to them,[422] they may be carried by phagocytes through the attenuated capsule covering areas where the superficial lamellae of bone have been disrupted by osteoclastic activity.[423]

It has been shown by serial radiography that calcified foci in the lungs, and sometimes calcified

hilar lymph nodes, occasionally undergo resorption, leaving no trace of their presence. This phenomenon is probably commoner than has been appreciated in the past.[424]

Progressive Changes.—In a small proportion of cases of primary tuberculous infection of the lungs the reparative changes fail to stem the progress of the disease. As the infected tissues undergo caseation, the bacilli tend to die in the central areas but to survive and multiply in the surviving zone of granulation tissue that borders the lesion. As a result of this extension, a caseous mass, several centimetres in diameter, may form, either in the lung itself or in the now much enlarged and generally matted regional lymph nodes. Any necrotic mass in the lungs is liable to secondary infection by other bacteria that reach them through the respiratory tract. Enzymes of these newly introduced organisms, or from other sources, such as leucocytes, cause the usually firm caseous matter to soften and even liquefy. The gradual loss of this now viscous and semifluid material through the regional bronchi leads to the creation of a cavity, often of a size little less than that of the parent caseous mass, and surrounded by a ragged lining of partly necrotic tuberculous granulation tissue.

If the necrotic focus breaks through the pleura, the result is pleural effusion, pneumothorax, tuberculous empyema or pyopneumothorax. In the last two the matter in the pleural sac is caseous and not purulent, in spite of the traditional terminology, unless there is a secondary infection by pyogenic organisms (see page 414).

When the infected, semifluid, caseous material enters the main respiratory passages, much of it is expectorated. Many of the bacilli that it contains are expectorated with it; others are dispersed to other parts of the lungs by the deep inspiration that usually follows coughing. Such a widespread and often sudden dispersion of large numbers of organisms within the bronchial tree may lead to an acute, diffuse tuberculous bronchopneumonia in one or both lungs, and this is often fatal. With recovery, a fibrous scar in the bronchial wall may mark the site of the former perforation: even many years later this may become the origin of obstructive changes, leading to bronchiectasis. A rare sequela comparable in pathogenesis to the traction diverticula of the oesophagus (see Chapter 14), is the formation of a bronchial diverticulum: this may become the site of septic infection, complicating stagnation of secretion; squamous metaplasia of its lining has been observed, with the development of carcinomatous change.[425]

Very rarely, when a caseating lymph node erupts into the bronchi, so much matter escapes suddenly that the patient, usually a child, is quickly asphyxiated.

Caseous hilar nodes may compress a bronchus. Partial obstruction may lead to trapping of air and the development of distensive panlobular emphysema (see page 292). Relief from obstruction may be obtainable only by surgical evacuation of the caseous contents of the node or nodes responsible. Massive enlargement of paratracheal nodes, particularly those of the right side, may result in compression of the trachea, causing stridor and sometimes cyanosis.[426]

'Epituberculosis'.—The condition that has been known as 'epituberculosis'[427] is a frequent finding when the lungs are examined radiologically in the course of primary pulmonary tuberculosis. The radiographic picture is of a segmental opacity. It was commonly assumed that this represents segmental collapse of the lung, but such an explanation is now recognized to be unusual. Examination of surgical specimens shows the affected part to be pale, particularly its cut surface. Microscopically, the alveoli contain protein-rich fluid in which histiocytes accumulate and form tubercles, without caseation. The interlobular septa are thickened and oedematous in the earlier stages; later, they are infiltrated by lymphocytes and histiocytes, without tubercle formation, and eventually become fibrotic. The findings thus reflect various combinations of local inflammatory response to the bacilli, hypersensitivity, spread of the infection, and—in some cases—bronchial obstruction.[426] The end result depends on the severity and duration of the active episode and on the earliness and effectiveness of treatment: there may be resolution, 'honeycombing' of the affected parenchyma (see page 369), emphysema, collapse, fibrosis and bronchiectasis.

Haematogenous Dissemination.—In the course of their destructive enlargement, caseating tuberculous foci may involve and finally break through the walls of blood vessels (Fig. 7.38). This is particularly prone to complicate the hilar lymph node component of the primary complex, for these caseous masses are not only larger than those in the lungs but they develop in proximity to the large veins in the mediastinum. It has been recorded that the aorta may be eroded, with consequent rupture and rapidly fatal bleeding. The wall of the affected vessel becomes replaced by tuberculous granulation tissue (the so-called Weigert tubercle[428]); in time, caseation develops, the lesion ulcerates through the intima and tubercle bacilli escape into the passing blood. It is not always possible in cases of miliary tuberculosis to demonstrate such vascular lesions; it seems likely that the organisms may also reach the blood by way of the lymphatics.[429]

A tuberculous bacillaemia may involve the entry into the circulation of few or many bacilli. When few, they are generally destroyed by the cells of the reticuloendothelial system; occasional organisms may escape this fate and—after lodgement in a kidney, bone or joint, the central nervous system, an adrenal or some other organ—set up an isolated focus of tuberculosis that may become chronic and progressive. On the other hand, when many bacilli enter the circulation more or less simultaneously, and a massive haematogenous dissemination ensues, generalized miliary tuberculosis develops. In this condition, as in all forms of bacteriaemia, the organisms are removed from the circulating blood by the cells of the reticuloendothelial system in the liver, spleen, bone marrow and elsewhere. Although—to judge from experimental tuberculous bacillaemias—most of the circulating bacilli are promptly destroyed by phagocytosis, enough survive ingestion to set up innumerable small metastatic foci of infection.[430] Generalized miliary tuberculosis is usually fatal unless treated quickly and appropriately. Even with modern treatment, the case fatality rate is high, particularly if the infection has involved the central nervous system and given rise to tuberculous meningitis (see Chapter 34).

At necropsy in cases of miliary tuberculosis, enormous numbers of small, grey tubercles, a millimetre or less in diameter (the size of a millet seed*), are found, most notably in the liver, spleen, bone marrow, lungs and meninges, and more sparsely in other organs. The preponderant distribution and typically uniform dispersal of tubercles in the parts named may be ascribed to the particularly large number of reticuloendothelial cells in the walls of the capillaries or blood sinusoids of these tissues: these cells engulf bacteria passing in the blood stream. The proportional distribution of the tubercles is mainly determined by the situation of the vessel invaded: if it is a systemic vein in the mediastinum, or the main thoracic duct, the bacilli are first carried to the lungs, where

* The Latin word for millet, *milium*, gives the disease its descriptive designation.

many are filtered out in the pulmonary capillaries; if it is a tributary of the pulmonary veins, they are carried to other organs in the systemic arterial circulation.

On histological examination, miliary tubercles have a characteristic structure. A Langhans-type multinucleate giant cell commonly forms the centre and is enclosed by a zone of epithelioid macrophages and an outer shell of lymphocytes (Fig. 7.40). If the patient survives for a month or more, the tubercles will be larger and their centre is yellowish because of early caseation. Microscopically, these rather more advanced lesions consist of small groups of satellite tubercles that have a general resemblance to the original one and surround the central caseous area that has taken its place.

Today, when many of those patients who develop generalized haematogenous dissemination of the infection are successfully treated, the progressive changes in the tubercles in the lungs can sometimes

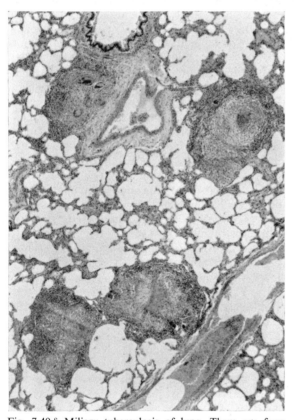

Fig. 7.40.§ Miliary tuberculosis of lung. There are four collections of tuberculous follicles: giant cells are present among the epithelioid cells, and there is an outer mantle of lymphocytes. The intervening lung is unaffected. *Haematoxylin–eosin.* ×40.

be followed in serial radiographs and the findings compared with those in histological preparations of the lungs of patients who died at the corresponding stage. Gradually, during the weeks following the institution of treatment, when the clinical manifestations of the disease come to an end, the finely dispersed opacities can be seen to regress until their presence is no longer detectable. At this stage, microscopical examination of the tubercle shows merely a minute scar composed almost wholly of hyaline collagen with no trace of the former distinctive cellular structure. Should a cure follow at a more advanced stage of the disease, after caseation has occurred, the caseous material becomes calcified: this results in a fine mottling of the lung fields that may be seen on X-ray examination for years after.[431]

Miliary Tuberculosis in the Elderly.—The occurrence of miliary tuberculosis in elderly people is now widely recognized. It is thought to result from activation of old tuberculous foci, primary or post-primary, as a consequence of waning of the immunological defences. In about half the cases the disease takes a 'cryptic' form, characterized by insidious onset and progression, and often lacking any evidence of miliary mottling in the chest radiograph.[432] The diagnosis is usually not made until necropsy.[433, 444] Both cryptic and overt miliary tuberculosis in the elderly may be accompanied by changes in the blood, including pancytopenia and leukaemoid reactions: these may be the first manifestation of the illness, and their significance in such cases is sometimes overlooked. Very occasionally, the blood disorder is primary, and predisposes to disseminated tuberculosis by interfering with resistance.

The so-called non-reactive tuberculosis which occurs with particular frequency in the elderly, must also be considered in this context. It is described on page 344.

Sequels of Primary Tuberculous Infection

The true frequency of tuberculous infection in the general population is very much higher than overt clinical manifestations suggest. This inference is based on two main sources of evidence: first, identification of healed tuberculous lesions in necropsy studies on long series of consecutive cases of patients dying from all causes in large general hospitals; and second, immunological surveys on large samples of the population employing the tuberculin skin test as an indicator of previous infection.

Necropsy Studies.—The realization that primary tuberculosis is followed by recovery in the great majority of those infected was the most important outcome of a pioneer study by Naegeli at the end of the nineteenth century in the post-mortem room of the General Hospital in Zurich.[435] Employing acceptable anatomical criteria for the identification of healed and active tuberculous lesions, he reached two very significant conclusions: first, that practically all the adults who had died in that hospital from diseases of all kinds had, at some site in their body, recognizable tuberculous foci that, in the great majority, had healed; and second, that in only a minority of these patients could death be attributed to tuberculosis. Forty years later, a similar study was made at the same Zurich hospital, and again the traces of a previous infection were detected in the bodies of from 80 to 90 per cent of all adult patients.[436]

The interest and surprise aroused by Naegeli's work stimulated numerous similar studies elsewhere in Europe and in the United States of America: his general conclusions were fully confirmed. It is now recognized that signs of past tuberculous infection, notably calcified mediastinal and mesenteric lymph nodes, are common in any population studies, and particularly so in industrialized urban communities. But although in elderly people the frequency of evidence of such healed infections has changed little during the past half-century, in children and young adults it has shown a decline that reflects the diminished incidence of clinical tuberculosis in occidental countries. These trends will probably continue, and in future a much larger fraction of the population than formerly will reach adult life without a primary infection and—as a corollary—also without the valuable, if partial, immunity that results from an infection that has been overcome.

Tuberculin Surveys.—The tuberculin skin test becomes positive within a few weeks of the infection being acquired and remains so in the great majority. Confidence in the reliability and specificity of the test is based mainly upon evidence from two sources. The first comes from surveys made on cattle just before slaughter: the result of the test correlated very closely with the presence or absence of tuberculous lesions in the carcase. The second is derived from tests on clinically tuberculous and clinically non-tuberculous children under five years of age: 94 per cent of the former, and only 12 per cent of the latter, were positive.[437]

Tuberculin surveys have given incontestable support to the general conclusion drawn from necropsy studies that the infection has been and still is widespread in urban populations. In one of the most carefully conducted tuberculin surveys in London between the two world wars the percentage of positive reactors was found to rise progressively from well below 10 in children under two years to 90 in adults.[437] Yet despite the great frequency of infection and the large number of deaths from the disease, the case fatality rate—the only numerical indicator of the probable outcome of an infection—is comparatively low. This is exemplified by the figures set out in Table 7.6, in which the percentage of positive reactors in three age groups and the death rate from tuberculosis in the same groups are given in parallel columns. From this table it can be seen that even 45 years ago only one out of several thousand children who became infected actually died from the disease: a fatal outcome is even less frequent today.

The most recent study on the prevalence of tuberculous infection in the United Kingdom was undertaken in 1949, and in all the places studied

Table 7.6. *Comparison by Age of Positive Tuberculin Reactors in a Sample London Population with Deaths from Tuberculosis for England and Wales in 1931*

Age group (years)	Positive reactors (per cent)	Deaths from tuberculosis (per cent)
0–5	12	0·076
6–10	30	0·026
11–20	61	0·060

the incidence of the disease had clearly fallen considerably during the preceding few decades.[438] But in spite of this decline—which is the continuing experience in most countries in Western Europe and North America—the conclusion is still valid that most people become infected with tuberculosis early in life and overcome the infection, the primary complex regressing and healing. All that eventually remains of the primary complex in these people is a small calcified or ossified mass in a lung or regional lymph node—the latter may be disclosed by chance at necropsy when the knife grates on a small craggy mass in the mediastinum or mesentery.

The Immunity that Results from Tuberculous Infection

The frequency with which a primary tuberculous infection is overcome, usually without the patient being aware of its presence, roused interest in the possibility that in tuberculosis, as in many other infectious diseases, recovery from an attack leaves a heightened resistance to infection in the event of subsequent exposure to the same organism. Further, as some degree of immunity results from a natural infection, the question was raised whether similar protection could be conferred by some controllable prophylactic procedure. An affirmative answer has been given to both questions.

Immunity from Naturally-Acquired Infection.—The first study that disclosed convincingly that a primary infection conferred some protection was made by Heimbeck in Oslo.[439] In essentials, his conclusions were based on follow-up records of positive and negative tuberculin reactors among probationer nurses entering the municipal hospital in that city. Through a comparative study of the findings on enrolment and their subsequent medical history while nursing, it became apparent that, although all were equally exposed to the same general hospital environment and its hazards, the incidence of overt tuberculosis was significantly less in those girls who were positive reactors at the time of their entry.

Heimbeck's conclusions have since been scrutinized and confirmed in many studies elsewhere. The most extensive of these—the Prophit Fund Tuberculosis Survey—was carried out on nearly 10 000 young people, mainly nurses and medical students, in London over the period from 1934 to 1944.[440] The results of this investigation are summarized in Table 7.7, which shows that there

Table 7.7. *Incidence of Clinical Tuberculosis among Positive and Negative Reactors to Tuberculin in the Prophit Survey in London, 1934 to 1944*

Tuberculin reaction at outset	Number of people examined	Cases of tuberculosis recorded	Incidence per cent
Positive	7130	95	1·33
Negative	1745	69	3·95

* Royal College of Physicians, *The Prophit Tuberculosis Survey*, 1948.

was about three times as high an incidence of clinical tuberculosis among young adults who were negative reactors at the start of the study as among similarly exposed positive reactors in London. This is almost the same as the average ratio derived from nearly 30 comparable surveys elsewhere in Europe and in America. It establishes the conclusion that although a primary infection

does not confer absolute immunity it does give a valuable degree of protection against developing the disease in a clinical form after subsequent exposure.

Specific Prophylactic Immunization.—It is possible to refer here only very briefly to the countless efforts made since the time of Robert Koch to confer immunity to tuberculosis through prophylactic inoculation. For many years these attempts were mainly by veterinary surgeons, in the hope of freeing cattle from the disease: the most significant conclusion from their work was that, unlike what had been found for many other infectious diseases, killed organisms were relatively impotent as immunizing agents.[441] Protection, in fact, could be conferred only through an infection that had been overcome. In consequence of this conclusion, the search for an effective prophylactic agent became a search for strains of the bacillus that were of such low natural virulence, or that had been so attenuated by appropriate methods of culture, that they could be inoculated safely while still alive. Such strains, it was hoped, would produce only a self-limiting infection. Of those that have been found, the organism now widely known, after those who developed it, as bacillus Calmette–Guérin (BCG) has established itself as the agent of choice, and is now widely employed in anti-tuberculosis schemes in many parts of the world.

The effectiveness of BCG has been demonstrated on many occasions: two may be briefly mentioned here.

The first was a long and careful study, made year by year, of the comparative morbidity and mortality from tuberculosis in two large groups of young American Indians in Alaska. At the start of the investigation, in 1935–38, one group was given BCG and the other served as a control.[442] At the end of 20 years, when the study was completed, the mortality records of the two groups were as shown in Table 7.8. To exclude the possibility that one group was inherently less healthy than the other, the number of deaths from diseases other than tuberculosis was included: the rates for these were almost the same in each group.

The second study was made in a Danish school for girls with nearly 400 pupils between 12 and 18 years of age. Because of a case of tuberculosis in the school, more than a third of the girls had been inoculated voluntarily with BCG. A year later, one of the mistresses developed open tuberculosis: this remained for a time unrecognized and led to an outbreak of the disease among the pupils whom

Table 7.8. *Comparative Mortalities from Tuberculosis and Other Diseases in a BCG-Inoculated Group and in a Control Group in Alaska**

	BCG group	Control group
Numbers in group	1547	1448
Deaths: from tuberculosis	13	68
from other causes	91	82
Mortality per 1000: tuberculosis	8·4	47·0
other causes	58·7	56·7

* Aronson, J. D., Aronson, C. F., Taylor, H. C., *A.M.A. Arch. intern. Med.*, 1958, **101**, 881.

she taught.[443] In the subsequent investigation the girls could be divided into three groups: those originally Mantoux-positive through some prior infection; those originally Mantoux-negative and not given BCG; and those originally Mantoux-negative but inoculated with BCG well before the outbreak began. The follow-up study revealed the comparative morbidity in the three groups (Table 7.9). The beneficial result of the previous BCG inoculation is highly significant by statistical test.

Table 7.9. *Comparative Morbidity from Tuberculosis of Girls in a Danish School in Relation to Mantoux Reaction and Inoculation with BCG**

Mantoux state	Number of girls	Number of cases	Per cent affected
Girls originally positive	130	4	3·1
Girls originally negative	105	11	10·5
Girls originally negative but given BCG	133	2	1·5

* Hyge, T. U., *Acta tuberc. scand.*, 1949, **23**, 153.

Lymphocyte Transformation in the Presence of Mycobacterial Antigens.—Skin tests with mycobacterial antigens specifically distinguish hypersensitivity to particular species of these organisms. It has been found that dermal reactivity correlates specifically with the in-vitro transformation of lymphocytes from the peripheral blood into lymphoblasts when the cells are cultivated for five or six days in the presence of the mycobacterial antigen to which the patient is sensitive.[444] Thus the circulating lymphocytes of individuals with known degrees of skin reactivity to purified protein derivative of *Mycobacterium tuberculosis*, *Mycobacterium intracellulare* or other species of mycobacterium can be shown to undergo in-vitro transformation

in corresponding measure in the presence of the same antigen (see Chapter 9).

Passive Transfer of Sensitivity to Mycobacterial Antigens.—There is some evidence that sensitivity to tuberculin and to the corresponding antigens of other mycobacteria may be transferable from a blood donor to a recipient whose skin test to the corresponding antigen was negative before the transfusion.

Sensitization and Immunity in Relation to Post-Primary Tuberculosis.—The pathological characteristics of pulmonary tuberculosis in patients who have had a previous infection by *Mycobacterium tuberculosis* (see below) are different in some important respects from those of a first infection with the tubercle bacillus. Sensitization and increased immunity are regarded as related and complementary causes of these differences: both may result either from a natural primary infection of the lungs or other organs by *Mycobacterium tuberculosis* itself (or *Mycobacterium bovis*, or possibly certain other potentially pathogenic mycobacteria) or from an artificial infection with BCG (or other mycobacteria that from time to time have had a vogue as prophylactic agents—for instance, *Mycobacterium muris*, the vole bacillus[445]).

Post-Primary Tuberculosis

Epidemiological Considerations

There has been a notable lack of agreement among epidemiologists in the past about the origin of post-primary tuberculosis, and difference of opinion still exists as to how often it is endogenous (that is, the result of reactivation of a primary lesion) and how often it is exogenous (that is, reinfection tuberculosis—tuberculosis due to a fresh infection from outside the patient's body). Evidence of endogenous reactivation can sometimes be demonstrated: for example, a post-primary lesion may be continuous with an old calcified primary lesion.[446] Such a finding is rare, and most pathologists regard exogenous reinfection as very much commoner, although this is difficult to prove. In exceptional instances, *Mycobacterium bovis* has been isolated from the primary lesion and *Mycobacterium tuberculosis* from the post-primary. Similar evidence has lately been provided, more frequently, by the recognition of typical post-primary pulmonary tuberculosis, caused by *Mycobacterium tuberculosis*, in a small proportion of individuals whose primary infection was not naturally acquired but the result of inoculation with BCG.

Two pieces of evidence, the first epidemiological and the second experimental, support the belief that the lesions of post-primary tuberculosis in the lungs are the result of exogenous reinfection. Since tuberculosis is so prevalent that by adult life most people have been affected, it is scarcely credible that they would pass the rest of their lives, generally in a wider and more exposed environment, without experiencing further infection. The experimental evidence follows from the anatomical fact that post-primary lesions in the lungs are almost invariably in the subapical region of an upper lobe or in the apex of a lower lobe. If radio-opaque oil is introduced into the upper respiratory tract and its downward passage followed radiologically, it can be seen that when a person is in the horizontal position, on the back or side, the fluid gravitates into those parts of the lungs in which post-primary lesions characteristically first appear.[447] Since these sites are particularly accessible to material reaching them from the bronchial tree, it would seem likely that post-primary tuberculous lesions in the lungs result from infection by this route rather than through the blood stream.

The view that post-primary tuberculous lesions develop at the site of foci of infection resulting from haematogenous dissemination of the bacilli during the primary stage was particularly favoured by some epidemiologists and pathologists of the German school. Essentially, they considered that the organisms survive in a dormant state for many years, both in the lesions of the primary complex and at sites of metastatic infection (the so-called Simon foci) resulting from carriage in the blood. It was considered that such foci, often symmetrically situated near the apex of each lung, might long remain potential centres for recrudescence of the infection, even when clinically the disease appears to have been arrested. According to this view, the development of active pulmonary tuberculosis in young adults is attributable to activation of the latent infection at the vulnerable sites in the subapical region of one or both lungs, perhaps as a result of a breakdown of resistance associated with such stresses as accompany life under industrial conditions. Few authorities adhere now to this thesis.

The Lesions in the Lungs

In contrast with what obtains in primary tuberculosis of the lungs, in which the Ghon focus may develop in any lobe, the early lesions in the post-primary disease are almost invariably found near the apex of one of the upper lobes. Formerly, it was supposed that the post-primary infection develops in the lung immediately deep to the pleura at the apex of the upper lobes, where small pigmented scars are commonly found in elderly people.[448] With the greater application of radiology to the detection of the early stages of progressive pulmonary tuberculosis, interest became directed to the subapical portions of the upper lobes, for it is in these regions that the radiological opacities known as Assmann foci appear early in the course of post-primary tuberculous infiltration.[449] The true significance of these foci became apparent when a comparison was made between radiographs taken at successive stages of the disease and the eventual necropsy findings, for after death the most advanced lesions were found at the sites at which the earliest signs of infiltration had been shown by X-rays.

Usually the early opacities disappear with adequate treatment, so that little is known of the histological structure of these transient infiltrates. Necropsy indicates that in more advanced cases such lesions are probably confluent areas of exudative inflammation, with fluid and many macrophages in the alveoli. In time, some of these pneumonic areas undergo caseation, and it is through the liquefaction of this dead tissue and its expulsion through the regional bronchi that the cavities so typical of the advanced lesions originate.

Once the liquefying contents of a cavity begin to escape into the bronchial tree, the bacilli become widely dispersed to other parts of both lungs, partly by gravity and partly by coughing. This diffuse bronchogenic infection gives rise to innumerable small areas of caseous pneumonia, mostly in the lower lobes. Occasionally, when the bacilli have been disseminated quickly and in large numbers, a rapidly developing tuberculous pneumonia involves almost the whole lower lobe: because of its translucency and viscous consistence this is known as 'gelatinous pneumonia'. Microscopical examination shows tubercle bacilli and macrophages in very large numbers in the consolidated areas. Occasionally, such regions undergo caseation. They may become so confluent as to involve a whole lobe (Fig. 7.41).

At necropsy, the lungs of a patient with longstanding, progressive, post-primary tuberculosis have a characteristic appearance. Large cavities may replace much of an upper lobe, and one or more

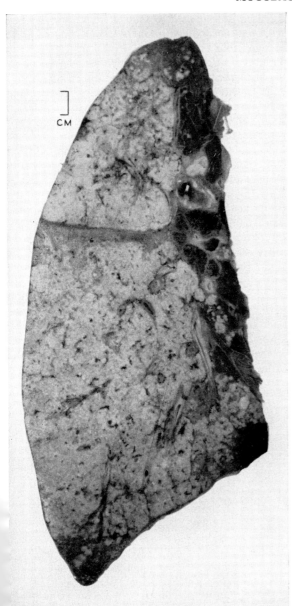

collected, so that the pale caseous areas stand out prominently against the blackened background of fibrotic lung. In this form of tuberculosis, the hilar lymph nodes are much less obviously involved than in the primary form of the disease, but, on histological examination, tuberculous foci—often with small areas of caseation—can generally be seen in them.

Since the time of Laënnec, the cavities in pulmonary tuberculosis have been recognized as originating from the liquefaction of the caseous material. They may be several centimetres in

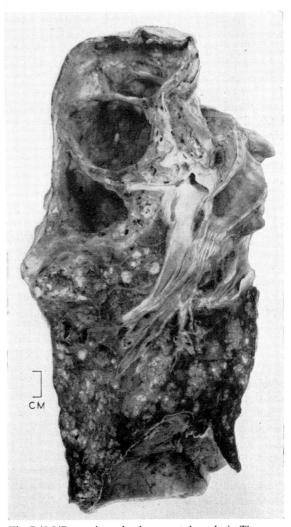

Fig. 7.41.§ Tuberculous bronchopneumonia. Almost the whole of the lung shows pale, confluent areas of caseation.

smaller, but otherwise similar, cavities may be present in the apical part of the lower lobe (Fig. 7.42). Usually the disease is bilateral, with similar, but often less advanced, changes in the opposite lung. The lower lobes are typically mottled with pale yellow, caseous areas, often in small clusters, and the nearby lung substance is in part emphysematous and in part fibrotic. In these latter areas, large amounts of sooty pigment have usually

Fig. 7.42.§ 'Post-primary' pulmonary tuberculosis. The upper lobe is almost completely replaced by a large, chronic, tuberculous cavity. The cords that cross it are the remains of blood vessels. The lower lobe shows many foci of tuberculous bronchopneumonia, the palest areas being areas of caseation.

M

diameter, with walls formed by tuberculous granulation tissue in which the fibrotic remains of the larger bronchi and of branches of the pulmonary arteries form coarse, irregular bands (Fig. 7.42). The loss of so much parenchyma naturally impairs the respiratory functions of the lungs. That the involvement of the blood vessels is not more frequently accompanied by haemoptysis is accounted for by the fact that the destructive process usually advances slowly, so that obliterative endarteritis leads to the closure of the lumen of the pulmonary and bronchial arteries before their walls have been penetrated. Sometimes caseation advances too quickly for the artery to become completely blocked, and an aneurysm may form where the muscular and elastic coats are destroyed on the side nearer the cavity. It is through the rupture of such aneurysms (Rasmussen's aneurysms) that sudden and sometimes fatal haemorrhages occur.[450] In view of the extensive destruction of lung substance and of its blood vessels in most cases of cavitating tuberculosis, it is surprising how relatively uncommon this serious complication is.

Histological examination of the wall of a cavity usually discloses several zones, each grading into the next. The yellowish-grey lining is formed largely of granulation tissue that has undergone caseation but not yet liquefied. Innumerable acid-fast bacilli can generally be seen in this zone: their multiplication there and subsequent escape into the cavity largely accounts for the high infectivity of the sputum expectorated by patients with advanced phthisis. Just deep to this is a zone of living granulation tissue containing a profusion of macrophages and lymphocytes and occasional multinucleate giant cells. If the cavity has been infected secondarily by other organisms, as often happens, this zone may also contain many neutrophils. Still deeper in the wall are traces of residual parenchyma, often with alveoli obliterated by compression and fibrosis. The cavities enlarge by extension of the tuberculous granulation tissue into the surrounding lung substance as the lining progressively caseates, liquefies and is expectorated. Eventually the process of cavitation may reach the pleura, but perforation into the sac hardly ever takes place, for the chronic pleurisy that accompanies the changes within the lungs results in the formation of firm adhesions between the visceral and parietal layers, with obliteration of the pleural sac.

Although the formation of a cavity is a serious development in the progress of a post-primary tuberculous infection of the lung, it does not represent an irreversible stage in the course of the disease. As long as it is small, a cavity may heal by scarring. Ultimately, such a lesion may only be recognizable as an area of fibrosis that stands out from the surrounding parenchyma because of its black pigmentation and the radiating pale strands of fibrous tissue that pucker the neighbouring lung substance (Fig. 7.43). When the cavities are larger than 1 to 2 cm in diameter, particularly when their walls are thick and densely fibrotic, they may persist indefinitely once the tuberculous infection has been overcome. In some such cases the cavity gradually shrinks and may eventually disappear, being represented by a pigmented fibrotic mass. In others, the cavity acquires an epithelial lining: the latter may be of modified respiratory type, formed essentially of columnar cells, with or without a proportion of mucus-secreting cells, or it may be squamous. A squamous lining may take the form of a simple epithelium or include more or less widespread areas of stratification; sometimes keratinization develops, and the lumen of the cavity may become filled by compressed desquamated cells, the appearances being then reminiscent of an epidermoid cyst. If the cavity is not able to drain freely into the bronchial tree, secretion may accumulate in it and

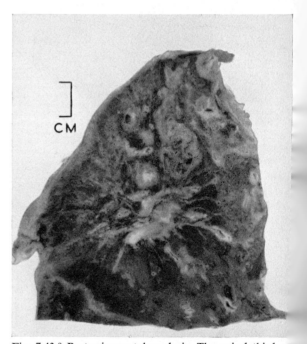

CM

Fig. 7.43.§ Post-primary tuberculosis. The apical third of the right lung contains a tuberculous cavity that has collapsed and partly healed (lowest pale area). It is surrounded by dust-pigmented scar tissue. There is further scarring higher up. Secondary suppurative bronchiectasis is present, with pus in the lumen of some of the affected bronchi.

predispose to secondary bacterial infection, sometimes with the formation of a lung abscess. Fungal colonization may lead to the formation of an aspergilloma or other variety of intracavitary ball colony (see below). The development of cancer in the region of a tuberculous scar is referred to on page 395.

When a cavity has been draining for many months, the surface epithelium of the bronchi through which the infected materials escape undergoes squamous metaplasia. The columnar cells first lose their cilia and later become transformed into squamous epithelium; squamous carcinoma occasionally arises from such areas of metaplasia—more usually, of course, it is cigarette smoking and chronic bronchitis that are associated with metaplasia and cancerous change (see page 395).

Chronic tuberculosis of the lungs is usually accompanied by pleurisy. Although this begins in the neighbourhood of the most active lesions, in time it may extend to involve the whole surface of the lung (Fig. 7.44). The condition advances slowly, generally without the formation of much exudate; by the time of necropsy the pleural lesions have usually undergone fibrosis. The damaged lung becomes firmly attached to the chest wall—indeed the fibrosis may be so firm and extensive that the lung can be removed from the body only by dissection outside the parietal pleura. Occasionally, the entire lung may be enclosed by a dense white layer of hyaline connective tissue, several millimetres thick.

Complications of Chronic Post-Primary Respiratory Tuberculosis

The proliferation of tubercle bacilli that takes place in the caseating lining of cavities in the lungs is often so great that it leads to heavy infection of the exudate and secretions, most of which are expelled by coughing, sometimes aided by the adoption of a posture that promotes gravitational drainage. These organisms form a potent reservoir for infection of the upper respiratory tract and of the alimentary canal.

Upper Respiratory Tract.—In advanced cases of chronic respiratory tuberculosis small ulcers, each a few millimetres in diameter, often develop in the tracheal mucosa. The destruction of tissue is generally slight, and the ulceration amounts to little more than loss of epithelium; occasionally, it may extend more deeply and expose one or more rings of tracheal cartilage. Oftener, the infection involves the larynx (page 250), tubercles forming

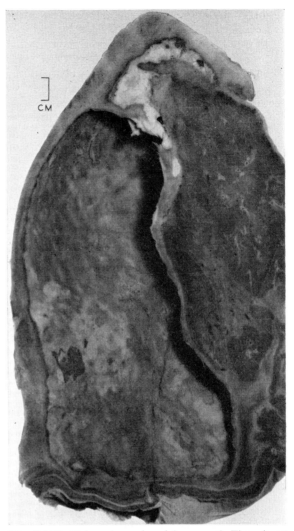

Fig. 7.44.§ Tuberculous pleural 'empyema'. There is an extensive area of caseation between the thickened visceral and parietal layers of the pleura over the apex of the lung; elsewhere, the two layers were separated by fluid exudate that filled the large space between them. Compressed lung is seen on the right.

and ulcers later appearing, particularly on the glottis and the aryepiglottic folds; the subsequent injury to the vocal cords leads both to hoarseness and to frequent stimulation of the cough reflex. Although the damage is generally superficial, it may involve the cartilages.

Alimentary Canal.—The passage through the mouth of sputum teeming with tubercle bacilli may lead to infection of the oral mucous membrane. Most commonly, the lesions appear as ulcers on the margin of the tongue (Chapter 11): these are probably initiated by some minor damage to the mucosa such as results from abrasion by a nearby carious tooth, the resulting breach in the epithelial surface giving access to the organisms. Once these ulcers form, they may penetrate deeply into the muscle. Sometimes, the organisms gain entry to the tonsils and there produce typical changes.

Unless trained not to do so, many patients with respiratory tuberculosis swallow much of their sputum and thus maintain a constant infection of the alimentary canal. Since tubercle bacilli are relatively resistant to acid in the concentrations found in gastric juice, they escape destruction in the stomach and enter the small intestine. The most typical lesions occur in the lowest 2 m of the ileum (Chapter 16); these are chronic, circumferentially oriented ulcers that begin in, and finally destroy, Peyer's patches (Fig. 16.21). Tuberculous ulcers in the ileum differ in several respects from those of typhoid fever (Chapter 16): (i) they are more chronic; (ii) very characteristically they soon extend beyond the limits of Peyer's patches and spread round the bowel wall, following the course of the lymphatics; (iii) small, white tubercles are often visible in the adjacent peritoneal serosa; and (iv) perforation into the peritoneal cavity is rare, the slower rate of penetration of the bowel wall allowing time for the development of adhesions to adjacent loops of intestine and to the omentum or the abdominal wall.

Although intestinal tuberculosis usually involves mainly the lower portion of the ileum, similar invasion and ulceration of the mucosa may occur in the caecum and ascending colon (Chapter 17), and occasionally in the appendix. In almost every case of longstanding pulmonary tuberculosis, typical tubercles can be found in the submucosa of these parts of the intestinal tract.

Anal fistulas may become infected with tubercle bacilli and the infection may spread into the ischio-rectal spaces (Chapter 18). These manifestations may appear early in the course of the disease, and cases have been described in which the first hint of the lung infection was provided by the histological recognition of tuberculous granulation tissue in biopsy specimens removed from an anal fistula. In making this diagnosis, however, the microscopist should be careful not to mistake for tuberculosis the giant-celled tuberculoid reaction to foreign bodies of faecal origin that not infrequently occurs in anal fistulas and fissures.

Secondary Amyloidosis.—Amyloidosis eventually develops in many cases of slowly progressive pulmonary tuberculosis. Although many organs become infiltrated with the amyloid material, renal involvement is the commonest serious manifestation (Chapter 24).

Aspergilloma as a Complication of Tuberculous Cavitation of the Lungs.—When an open cavity (that is, one communicating with the bronchial tree) persists in a lung after healing of the tuberculous infection that caused it, it may become colonized by a fungus, a characteristic intracavitary fungal ball colony resulting. In the great majority of such cases the fungus is a species of aspergillus, and most frequently *Aspergillus fumigatus*—the lesion is a so-called aspergilloma (see page 350). In a survey of 544 patients with persistent pulmonary cavities following tuberculosis, an aspergilloma was demonstrable in 11 per cent: within three to four years after the first survey the proportion had risen to 17 per cent of the 417 survivors examined.[451]

Non-Reactive Tuberculosis

There is a form of generalized haematogenous tuberculosis that differs from miliary tuberculosis (see page 335) in the absence of giant cell granuloma formation.[452–456] This condition may present with chronic fever, sometimes accompanied by anaemia of uncertain cause. Clinical examination shows enlargement of the spleen and sometimes of the liver. There may be fine miliary mottling in radiographs of the lungs, but this is not always conspicuous. The diagnosis may not be made until necropsy, when disseminated miliary tuberculous lesions are found to be widespread. The lesions are appreciably softer than those of classic miliary tuberculosis: histologically, they are foci of virtually structureless necrotic matter, sharply defined from the surrounding tissue, which shows little or no abnormality. Appropriate staining reveals great numbers of tubercle bacilli in the lesions.

This form of generalized tuberculosis is considered to result from a major deficiency in the body's cellular defences. In about a quarter of the cases it develops as a complication of chronic disease of the lymphoreticular system, particularly Hodgkin's disease and leukaemia. In a few cases it has apparently followed treatment with drugs, particularly corticosteroids when given in large doses over long periods, immunosuppressants such as azathioprine and mercaptopurine, and other drugs used in the chemotherapy of cancer. Often however, no predisposing cause is found.

If the diagnosis of non-reactive tuberculosis is suspected during life, tubercle bacilli should be looked for in films of bone marrow. Biopsy may be helpful, any suggestion of a tuberculous reaction being potentially an important diagnostic guide. When *any* biopsy section includes unexplained areas of necrosis, particularly when there is little in the way of a related cellular reaction, it is imperative to look for tubercle bacilli.

It is to be remembered that the tissues in this form of tuberculosis are highly infective. Several cases of tuberculous infection in laboratory staff, including those working in mortuaries, have been traced to this source.[457]

(b) Pulmonary Infection with *Mycobacterium kansasii*

Most of the patients with pulmonary infection by *Mycobacterium kansasii* are middle-aged men living in towns where pollution of the air by industry is a cause of chronic disease of the respiratory tract, particularly bronchitis. The mycobacteriosis is, in fact, usually secondary to other bronchopulmonary disease. Its effects resemble those of tuberculosis. Cough, haemoptysis and loss of weight and strength are among its presenting symptoms. The X-ray findings also are similar to those of post-primary tuberculosis: in some cases there is a radiological clue to the nature of the infection in the presence of homogeneous shadows, each about 1 cm in diameter, grouped round a transradiant area, sometimes with a few radially oriented linear shadows at the periphery of the lesion.[458] Skin tests with purified protein derivative of *Mycobacterium kansasii* may be positive; often they are negative.

Histology.—Only one feature distinguishes the microscopical picture of *Mycobacterium kansasii* infection from that of tuberculosis—the size of the organisms. When stained by a Ziehl–Neelsen method, *Mycobacterium kansasii* is larger than *Mycobacterium tuberculosis*: individual bacilli are up to 20 μm long, rather thicker than tubercle bacilli, coarsely beaded, and often somewhat S-shaped; sometimes they are grouped in curled and intertwined cords.[459]

(c) Pulmonary Infection with *Mycobacterium avium*

Mycobacterium avium is in general a rare cause of disease in man. It is commonly said that the first case in Britain was reported in 1946:[460] however,

cases had certainly been identified in Ireland in the first two decades of this century.[461] In keeping with the fact that its natural source is a disease in birds, the infection in man is usually seen in patients living in rural areas. However, it has repeatedly been observed as a complication of pneumoconiosis, both in coal miners and in patients whose dust disease was acquired in other industries: in some such cases there has been strong circumstantial evidence that the infection was derived from birds kept by the patients as pets or for sporting purposes, or as a supplement to diet or income.

Infection of the lungs by *Mycobacterium avium* may be distinguished from tuberculosis only by identification of the organism. Fatal haematogenous dissemination has been recorded but is very rare.[462]

Syphilis

Syphilitic lesions have never been particularly frequent in the lungs, and probably congenital pulmonary syphilis ('pneumonia alba') has always been the commonest manifestation. All forms are now rare.

Congenital Pulmonary Syphilis.[463]—The pallor and firmness of the lungs, which are larger than normal, account for the old name, pneumonia alba. The condition is usually seen in stillborn syphilitic babies or those who die within a few hours of birth: in the latter, the aerated lobules stand out above the indurated parts. Microscopically, there is widespread thickening of the alveolar walls by reticulin fibres and proliferating fibroblasts, accompanied by an accumulation of plasma cells with some lymphocytes. In places there are microscopical foci of necrosis, maybe with histiocytic proliferation round them, as well as some accumulation of neutrophils: these lesions occasionally merge to form gummatous foci that may be macroscopically evident. Usually there is a conspicuous lining of cubical epithelial cells in the alveoli of the affected parts, and many alveoli may be filled with such cells that have been shed into the lumen. Silver impregnation methods show the presence of great numbers of treponemes in the tissues.

It has to be noted that somewhat similar macroscopical and microscopical changes may result from viral infections in the neonatal period. Also, pneumocystis pneumonia may be mistaken for syphilitic pneumonia in those less common cases in which the interstitial accumulation of plasma cells is accompanied by notably less than the usual degree of colonization of the alveolar lumen by the parasites (see page 361).

Acquired Pulmonary Syphilis.—Gummas, which may be solitary or multiple, and small or large, and interstitial fibrosis are the manifestations of acquired syphilis in the lungs. The gummas, which may also occur in the trachea and bronchi as ulcerative lesions, with a tendency to destroy the cartilage of the wall, have the structure that is common to these lesions wherever they occur in the body. As elsewhere, they tend ultimately to produce dense scars that contract and produce deep cicatricial fissures in the surface of the lungs, an appearance comparable to that of hepar lobatum (see Chapter 21).[464]

It is of the utmost importance to remember that other types of infection, particularly mycobacterioses and mycoses, must be considered and excluded before a diagnosis of gumma can be entertained, even when the patient's serological tests indicate the presence of syphilis. Moreover, primary and secondary tumours are commoner causes of discrete shadows in chest radiographs than gummas, even in patients with syphilis: the correct diagnosis may not be possible without recourse to open biopsy. The necrotic pulmonary lesions of Wegener's granulomatosis (page 371) and even pulmonary infarcts are among other conditions to be considered in the differential diagnosis.

Fungal Diseases[465]

Infections of the lungs that are caused by fungi have attracted growing interest since the second world war. This is due in part to increasing awareness of their occurrence and importance in regions where environmental conditions support the saprophytic phase of such pathogens as *Histoplasma capsulatum, Coccidioides immitis, Blastomyces dermatitidis* and *Paracoccidioides brasiliensis*, which are able to cause disease in previously healthy people. The same period has seen the recognition of infection of the lungs and other parts by fungi that are enabled to invade the tissues only because of lowering of the patient's resistance by some other disease or through side effects of treatment. Some of the fungi that cause these so-called opportunistic infections are seldom, if ever, responsible for illness in unpredisposed individuals—this is particularly so of phycomycetes; others, if they are pathogenic in healthy people at all, cause disease (for instance, asthma from sensitization to aspergilli) of a type very different from the progressive,

destructive, disseminated infection that they set up in those whose resistance has been reduced.

The ease and frequency of international travel make many hitherto 'exotic' diseases the immediate practical concern of doctors who have no personal experience in their recognition and management. The fact that fungi that are frequently the cause of disease in other parts of the world are not indigenous where the doctor is in practice is no longer an excuse for not considering the possibility that his patient may have acquired infection while living in another land or through exposure to contaminated imported materials. Neither histoplasmosis nor coccidioidomycosis, for instance, occurs naturally in the west of Europe, yet every year in countries such as Britain patients are seen whose symptoms are due to these diseases: the cardinal importance of the patient's geographical history, and of the doctor's knowledge of geographical medicine, is self-evident.

(a) Infections Caused by *Actinomyces israelii* and *Nocardia asteroides*

Three of the five families of Actinomycetales include genera of which some species are pathogenic to man—Mycobacteriaceae (genus *Mycobacterium*), Actinomycetaceae (genera *Actinomyces* and *Nocardia*) and Streptomycetaceae (genus *Streptomyces*). Although the Actinomycetales are classed as bacteria, and the infections caused by species of their most important pathogen-including genus, *Mycobacterium*, are invariably considered among bacterial infections, it is established practice in Britain to consider the diseases caused by Actinomycetaceae and Streptomycetaceae along with diseases caused by fungi, under the general heading of mycoses. It will be difficult to change this convention, particularly in consideration of such entrenched nosological nomenclature as actinomycosis and streptomycosis, which by virtue of the ending '-mycosis'—its etymology is usually misinterpreted—are unlikely to be displaced from their customary association with the true mycoses, in spite of such other well-understood terminological paradoxes and pitfalls as mycosis fungoides (essentially a lymphomatous condition of the skin —see Chapter 39) and mycotic aneurysm (the result of embolism by material that is infected, usually with bacteria—see page 147).

The Pathogenic Actinomycetaceae.—The Actinomycetaceae that cause disease in man are *Actinomyces israelii, Actinomyces eriksonii* and *Actino-*

myces naeslundii, which cause actinomycosis, *Arachnia propionica* (*Actinomyces propionicus*), which causes a disease indistinguishable from actinomycosis, *Nocardia asteroides*, which causes the disease that is described simply as nocardiosis, and *Nocardia brasiliensis* and *Nocardia caviae*, which cause mycetomas. *Nocardia brasiliensis*, like the pathogenic species of *Streptomyces*, is an important and frequent cause of mycetoma.* Mycetomas caused by *Nocardia brasiliensis* are seen oftenest in West Africa and in Mexico, Central America and the northern parts of South America. Like the streptomycetes that cause mycetomas, *Nocardia brasiliensis* and *Nocardia caviae* do not cause disease in the lungs, except—rarely—as a result of haematogenous dissemination from a mycetoma of a limb or elsewhere or through direct invasion by a mycetoma originating in the chest wall.

Actinomycosis

Actinomyces israelii, by far the most important and most frequent pathogenic species of actinomyces, is a common commensal or saprophyte in the human mouth and in the contents of the large intestine. It is probable that most infections by this organism are endogenous. About 60 per cent of cases of actinomycosis present with lesions in the region of the mouth, face or neck, the portal of entry being dental or tonsillar. *Actinomyces israelii* is one of the actinomycetes that is found in dental tartar and in the debris in tonsillar crypts. About 25 per cent of cases of actinomycosis involve the ileocaecal region, with or without appendicitis

* Mycetoma is the name given to a type of fungal granuloma that is characterized by the formation of multiple sinuses and that usually is the outcome of penetration of the soft tissues by a thorn, or the like, contaminated by the causative organism. The lesion is most frequent on the extremities ('Madura foot' is the type example—see Chapter 39). Many varieties of fungus cause mycetomas (species of *Madurella* and *Cephalosporium*, *Allescheria boydii*, *Phialophora gougerotii* and others): most of them seldom, if ever, cause other disease.

The term mycetoma has frequently been applied to the intracavitary fungal balls, such as aspergillomas, that occur as a complication of certain diseases of the lungs (see page 350). This is regrettable and should be discouraged. A mycetoma in the sense of a granuloma with sinus formation is a lesion caused by invasion of the tissues by the organism concerned, with the consequent development of a chronic inflammatory reaction. In contrast, an intracavitary fungal ball is essentially outside the tissues, in that characteristically it lies free in the lumen of the colonized cavity and does not, except in most unusual circumstances, lead to extension of the infection into the wall of the cavity itself.

(see Chapter 19) or extension through the portal veins to the liver (see Chapter 21). In the remaining 15 per cent of cases the infection is in the lungs. It is presumed that pulmonary actinomycosis is the outcome of aspiration of infected matter from the tonsillar crypts or mouth, apart from the very small proportion of cases in which the disease has extended from known foci of infection in the abdomen.

Actinomyces israelii is an anaerobic, Gram-positive organism, formed of branching filaments from 0·5 to 1·0 μm wide. The filaments readily break into bacillus-like fragments. They are not acid-fast. Like those of nocardiae (see below), the fragments of the actinomyces may be mistaken for contaminant corynebacteria.

It is only comparatively recently that other species have been distinguished from *Actinomyces israelii* as causes of actinomycosis (with the exception, of course, of *Actinomyces bovis*, the cause of actinomycosis in cattle and long recognized as an exceptionally rare cause of the disease in man). Among these species is *Actinomyces eriksonii*, which has been most frequently isolated from pulmonary lesions.[466] *Actinomyces naeslundii* is another: it was originally regarded as an oral saprophyte, and is now known to be an occasional cause of disease that presents the features of actinomycosis;[467] it has not been recognized as a cause of pulmonary infection. *Arachnia propionica*, an organism closely related to *Actinomyces israelii*, also causes disease indistinguishable from actinomycosis:[468] its source is unknown.

Pulmonary actinomycosis is accompanied by fever and expectoration of mucopurulent sputum. Contrary to a common belief, 'sulphur granules'—the yellow colonial granules of the organisms—are not often to be found in the sputum. The diagnosis depends on recognition of the fine, Gram-positive, sometimes branching filaments in films, and isolation of the organism. It has to be remembered that the organism may be present in sputum only in short bacillary forms that are liable to be misinterpreted. The chest radiograph may show shadows of various sizes scattered through both lungs, particularly in the middle and lower zones.[469] Alternatively, there may be a large pneumonic area, affecting almost all of one or, less often, both lungs, sometimes associated with an empyema: this type of the disease may be accompanied by periosteal new bone formation on the inner aspects of several contiguous ribs.

Characteristically, the affected lung tissue is more or less widely riddled with chronic abscesses that range in diameter from a few millimetres to a couple of centimetres or so. These lesions may communicate with one another, drain into the bronchial tree or extend to the pleural surface and open into the pleural sac. 'Sulphur granules' (see above) are often to be found in the exudate *in situ* in the abscesses and sinuses, even when they are absent from the sputum (Fig. 7.45). Fibrosis is a feature, both surrounding the suppurative foci and more widely through the lungs, particularly involving the septa. The infection may extend into the spine and ribs, whether or not there is an actinomycotic empyema: the latter may be loculate or may involve the entire pleural sac; in many cases obliteration of the sac, locally or throughout its extent, while preventing empyema formation does not present a barrier to the infection as it spreads outward to involve not only the thoracic skeleton but also the soft tissues and skin of the chest wall, often with the establishment of

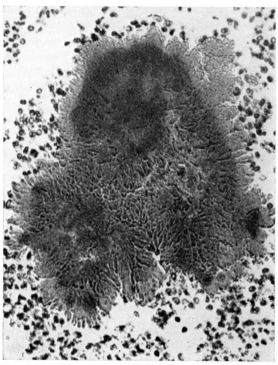

Fig. 7.45.§ Colony of *Actinomyces israelii* in lung. The marginal zone of pale, club-like protrusions is well seen; the 'clubs' consist mainly of fibrin and other substances precipitated from the inflammatory exudate and forming a covering over the fine filaments growing outward from the surface of the colony. The colony illustrated measured about 0·25 mm across; rather larger colonies, 1 mm or so in diameter, are visible to the naked eye as the so-called 'sulphur granules' in exudate from actinomycotic lesions. *Haematoxylin–eosin.* × 320.

draining sinuses. Actinomycosis, including pulmonary actinomycosis, is occasionally complicated by amyloidosis.[470]

Nocardiosis

Nocardia asteroides is not known to occur in the normal flora of the human body. Pathogenic strains can be isolated from soil, and infection is thought to be exogenous. It is an aerobic, Gram-positive organism, formed of filaments from 0·5 to 1·0 μm wide. The filaments may break into fragments during preparation of films of infected exudate. They are commonly acid-fast, but only seldom as strongly so as tubercle bacilli; the acid-fastness is often removed in the course of histological processing. In contrast to *Actinomyces israelii*, and to *Nocardia brasiliensis* and *Nocardia caviae*, *Nocardia asteroides* appears to have no tendency to form colonial granules in infected tissues.

Infection by *Nocardia asteroides* may develop in a previously healthy person, but in most cases there are predisposing factors. These factors include diseases, such as leukaemia, that interfere with resistance, and therapeutic agents, particularly corticosteroids, but in some cases other immunosuppressant and cytotoxic drugs. There is considerable evidence that pulmonary alveolar proteinosis specifically predisposes to infection by this organism, which has been the cause of fatal pneumonic and septicaemic complications (see page 289). The overall incidence of infection by *Nocardia asteroides* appears to be rising, probably in the main because of the increasing use of the drugs that particularly predispose to its occurrence.

In general, the picture of nocardiosis is that of suppuration, with the development of multiple abscesses. The lesions have a notable tendency to confluence. Pulmonary nocardiosis may affect one or both lungs very widely, with extensive consolidation round the suppurative foci: the exudate in the alveoli of these pneumonic foci initially contains much fibrinogen, and a fibrin coagulum forms, often with relatively little leucocytic infiltration until the suppurative process extends from the central abscess. The organisms are present in the exudate, and may be very numerous. Their number is often only inadequately disclosed by a casual glance at Gram preparations, for a considerable proportion of the filaments may have failed to stain; Ziehl–Neelsen preparations, and—often better—modifications designed to show lepra bacilli and other relatively weakly acid-fast organisms, are in general more useful than others, but it must be remembered that the acid-fastness may be lost in processing the tissues for sectioning.

Nocardia asteroides has a particular affinity for the central nervous system, nocardial brain abscess and nocardial meningitis being frequent complications of pulmonary infection (see Chapter 34).

(b) Infections Caused by True Fungi

Aspergillosis

Several species of aspergillus have been identified as causes of infection in man: *Aspergillus fumigatus* is by far the most frequent, particularly in cases of pulmonary disease and of septicaemia (*Aspergillus flavus* as a cause of granulomatous nasal sinusitis and its complications is noted on page 210). Aspergilli, including *Aspergillus fumigatus*, are common saprophytes in decaying organic matter: under certain conditions—for instance, in vegetable compost—their spores may be so numerous that they can be seen as a dense dust cloud raised when piles of such material are disturbed. Although exposure to aspergillus spores is a commonplace experience, the fungus is not a frequent pathogen. Only if the individual is allergic to the spores or if his resistance to invasion of the tissues by the germinating fungus is lowered by other conditions is he likely to suffer ill effects: these, when they occur, may be very serious, endangering life.

In histological preparations of infected tissue, or of expectorated mucous casts of the bronchi in cases of allergic aspergillosis, the fungus has a characteristic appearance and can be generically identified by its morphology (Fig. 7.46). Its hyphae are septate and from 3 to 6 μm in diameter: their fine wall commonly encloses protoplasm that stains to some degree with haematoxylin or eosin. Typically, they branch dichotomously, usually at from 35° to 45°, the branches then tending to orient themselves in a parallel mode. The conidiophores that are so striking a feature of aspergilli when growing as saprophytes are seen in infected tissues only where the mould is exposed to air: they are never found within the solid structure of colonized organs and tissues, but may occasionally be seen on the lining of a bronchus when the mould is present as a saprophyte, growing on stagnant secretion. Aspergillus hyphae are usually visible in haematoxylin–eosin preparations, and sometimes are so intensely haematoxyphile that they are immediately evident under the lowest powers of the microscope: although the periodic-acid/Schiff stain and the Gridley stain for fungi facilitate their recognition the Grocott–Gomori hexamine (meth-

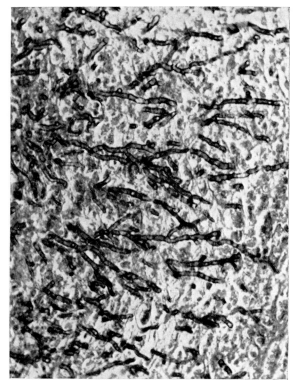

Fig. 7.46.§ Hyphae of an aspergillus invading a pulmonary infarct. The dichotomous branching and transverse septation of the hyphae are characteristic. *Haematoxylin–eosin.* × 380.

enamine) silver nitrate method is very much more reliable.

The occurrence of oxalate crystals in tissue infected by aspergilli is noted below (page 351).

Disease of the bronchi and lungs caused by aspergilli may be considered under the headings of allergic aspergillosis, aspergilloma and aspergillus pneumonia. Aspergillus saprophytosis and septicaemic aspergillosis also require separate attention.

Allergic Bronchopulmonary Aspergillosis.[471–473]— Allergy to aspergilli as a cause of asthma has been discussed on page 303. It is important to reiterate that this condition is not known to be accompanied by invasion of the tissues by the fungus: it appears to be exclusively an allergic response to inhaled aspergillus spores; although the spores may germinate, and the resulting hyphae therefore be found in the expectorated mucous plugs, this is essentially a saprophytic process. The transitory, focal shadows that are commonly seen in chest radiographs during the asthmatic episode are usually due to segmental collapse following obstruction of the bronchus by mucus; occasionally

M*

they are pneumonic.[474] Some of the pneumonic foci are caused by infection: the organisms responsible are bacteria, not fungi, and the infection is a complication of collapse. Oftener, the pneumonic foci are characterized by an intra-alveolar and interstitial exudate formed mostly of eosinophils, apparently as part of the allergic response and not associated with any form of infection. When the mucous plug is expectorated, once its surface begins to liquefy, the collapsed lung tissue becomes re-aerated and any pneumonic process, sterile or bacterial, rapidly subsides. As noted on page 303, serological tests are now the main means of confirming the clinical diagnosis of allergic aspergillosis.

Aspergilloma.[475]—The development of an aspergilloma, or intracavitary aspergillus ball colony, is a particular manifestation of aspergillus saprophytosis, in that the fungus grows in the lumen of a cavity in the lung without invading the tissues, drawing its nutriment from such exudate as may be present. The ball usually forms in an existing cavity, particularly an old tuberculous cavity (see page 350) but sometimes in a cavity associated with such conditions as sarcoidosis, bronchiectasis or a chronic lung abscess, or in a congenital cyst or an emphysematous bulla. In rarer cases the fungus, having saprophytically colonized an infarct that abuts on the bronchial tree, may itself excavate the dead tissue by enzymatic activity, a ball colony eventually developing. Misuse of the term mycetoma as a synonym of aspergilloma is mentioned in the footnote on page 347. While almost all intracavitary fungal ball colonies are formed by *Aspergillus fumigatus*, other species of aspergillus have been identified in some cases and, exceptionally, other fungi have sometimes been responsible. In the latter circumstances the condition might be referred to by a name indicative of the fungus concerned—allescherioma (infection by *Allescheria boydii*[476, 477]), penicillioma (infection by *Penicillium* species[478]) and, perhaps, candidoma or monilioma (infection supposedly by *Candida* species[479]).

An aspergilloma may grow rapidly: a colony 3 cm in diameter was observed radiologically to have formed in nine weeks.[480] Usually, there is no evidence on which to base an estimate of the age of the lesion when it is discovered: in many cases the presence of an aspergilloma has been demonstrated in radiographs over a period of several years, sometimes with little or no detectable change in its appearance, sometimes with appreciable phases of shrinkage and enlargement. Although usually single, aspergillomas may be present in

cavities in both lungs, and in exceptional cases there have been several such lesions. Hitherto, the observation that an aspergilloma rarely develops in association with cancer of the lung has been explained by the relatively rapid course of the latter: however, aspergilloma formation has been observed both in the bronchiectatic lung distal to an obstructing carcinoma[481] and within the cavity resulting from necrosis at the centre of a peripheral squamous carcinoma.[480]

The radiological appearances of an aspergilloma are often characteristic, the fungal ball appearing as a sharply demarcated radio-opaque spheroid that rests on the wall of the dependent part of the cavity and is separated from it elsewhere by a crescent of air. In cases of longstanding the colony may fill the cavity completely.

The colony appears macroscopically as a grey or reddish brown, rarely green-tinged, mass, sometimes firm or rubbery in consistency but often friable. Old colonies may have a gritty feel, from deposition of calcium salts, and exceptionally there may be so much calcification that the ball becomes stony and has been classified among the so-called 'pneumonoliths'.[482]

Microscopically, an aspergilloma consists of a dense mass of hyphae, cemented with hyaline eosinophile material of uncertain origin. Much of the fungal matter is dead, only the hyphae at the surface being well preserved. Occasionally, crystals of calcium oxalate are present, particularly near the surface (see opposite). The lining of the cavity that contains an aspergilloma varies and often is, of course, determined by the nature of the condition that has given rise to it. The wall of an old tuberculous cavity may consist of dense, hyaline fibrous tissue, sometimes devoid of an epithelial covering; in other cases there may be a lining zone of granulation tissue, which usually is without specific features of tuberculosis or other former disease.

Haemoptysis is a common feature of aspergilloma. Usually it causes, at most, some secondary anaemia, but in some cases it has been massive and death has resulted. It often accompanies the development of further excavation of the lung tissue round the colonized lesion: endarteritis obliterans may fail to prevent erosion of a large vessel.

It is exceptional for the fungus to invade the tissues, although aspergillus pneumonia has been observed.[483] Such a change from saprophytosis to invasive growth seems likelier to occur when the patient's resistance is lowered, particularly by immunosuppressant and cytotoxic therapy and les often by administration of corticosteroids.[484] Ordinarily, such chronic inflammatory changes as are seen in the lining of the cavity are attributable either to mechanical irritation by the fungal ball, which often is able to move within the cavity in accordance with the position that the patient adopts, or—occasionally—to secondary bacterial infection.

Most patients with an aspergilloma have precipitins in the serum against the aspergillus.[451] Unless they have developed an associated allergic state, with asthma, the skin test with extracts of the fungus is negative.

Aspergillus Pneumonia. — Excluding saprophytic colonization of pulmonary infarcts (Fig. 7.46) and instances of invasion of living lung tissue round an aspergilloma-containing cavity (see above)—each a relatively very rare occurrence— pneumonia caused by an aspergillus is so exceptional as to be one of the most infrequent of all manifestations of pulmonary mycosis. In most instances of aspergillus pneumonia the patient's resistance has been undermined by corticosteroids or immunosuppressant drugs: aspergillosis in most patients under treatment with these drugs takes the form of a fulminating septicaemia, but in a small proportion a spreading pneumonia develops instead. The resulting lesions are characterized by the outpouring of fibrinous exudate into the alveoli, often with many neutrophils, thrombosis of the capillaries and necrosis of the tissue, which is heavily infected by the fungus. In the early lesions each alveolus may contain a small, star-like cluster of radiating hyphae that clearly have developed from germination of one or more spores; later, the hyphae penetrate the alveolar wall and extend widely into the tissues. In many cases invasion of the larger blood vessels leads quickly to generalization of the infection throughout the body.

Aspergillus Saprophytosis.—It has been mentioned already that the development of an aspergilloma is a special variety of saprophytosis. A frequent and potentially much more serious variety is characterized by growth of the fungus in stagnant secretion in the bronchi in cases of chronic bronchitis and, less often, bronchiectasis. The fungus may be quite harmless in such cases: but if the patient's resistance to its invasion of the tissues is lowered by the effects of corticosteroids or immunosuppressants, given in the treatment of other diseases, the aspergillus may grow through the basement membrane of the bronchial mucosa, reach the blood vessels and set up a fatal septicaemia.[485]

Septicaemic Aspergillosis.—This form of aspergillosis is commonly first recognized at necropsy, and often not until the tissues are examined with the microscope. It is usually attributable to the breakdown of the body's defences in the course of diseases like leukaemia or to treatment with drugs that interfere with resistance. The precise nature of the deficiency that results is unknown. It is possible that there is a plasma factor that under normal conditions inhibits the invasiveness of such organisms.[486]

In many cases the portal of invasion of the blood stream by the fungus is not apparent. In others it is a recognizable local infection such as those already noted (aspergilloma, aspergillus pneumonia or—least rarely—bronchial saprophytosis). There may be a rapidly overwhelming septicaemia, with little to show in the way of focal lesions, or there may be many large foci of necrosis, most frequently in the brain, heart and kidneys. The lesions are often so heavily colonized by the aspergillus that, very soon after exposure to the air at necropsy, conidiophore development occurs and gives a green colour to the necrotic tissue and even an obvious growth of the pigmented mould on the surface. Microscopical examination often shows that the hyphae of the invading fungus are surrounded, in advance of their progress through the tissues, by a spreading zone of necrosis: this is in all probability a result of diffusion through the infected part of toxins produced by the aspergillus.[487] Occasionally, the lesions are suppurative. Infection by other fungi may be present at the same time (see page 363).

Aspergillosis Causing Oxalosis.—Crystals of calcium oxalate have been identified in tissues infected by species of aspergillus, perhaps *Aspergillus niger* particularly, and in aspergillomas.[488] In some cases it has been suggested that local tissue injury and even acute oxalosis and renal failure have resulted from the production of oxalic acid by the fungus.

Candidosis (Moniliasis)[489]

Candida albicans is a yeast-like fungus that is often present in the normal upper respiratory tract and may spread into the lower respiratory tract. It is found as a secondary invader in cases of chronic bronchitis, bronchiectasis and bronchial carcinoma. The commonest form of candidosis is oral thrush, but the organism can attack any mucous or moist cutaneous surface. The fungus is often present in the sputum as an accompaniment of other pulmonary diseases, among them tuberculosis. Its significance in such circumstances is uncertain, but probably it is then no more than a saprophyte. The pulmonary findings have varied according to the primary disease, and the diagnosis of candidosis depends on finding the organism histologically in the cellular exudate in a bronchus or abscess. Very rarely pneumonia can be caused by the candida itself.[489] It is also possible that it may penetrate the bronchi and invade tissue affected with bacterial pneumonia, preventing resolution.[490, 491]

Candida septicaemia is usually a complication of diseases or therapeutic measures that lower resistance.[492]

Phycomycosis[493, 494]

The name phycomycosis is given to any infection caused by a fungus that, by convention, is regarded as a member of the class Phycomycetes. Some of the phycomycoses are primary infections, occurring without predisposing disease: these are subcutaneous phycomycosis (see Chapter 39) and entomophthorosis (primary orificial mucosal phycomycosis—see page 208). Very rarely, dissemination of these primary phycomycoses results in visceral infection: thus, in a case of haematogenous dissemination complicating subcutaneous phycomycosis the causative organism, *Basidiobolus meristophorus*, was isolated from characteristic granulomas in the lungs and other organs,[495] and in a case of longstanding infection of the nose and nasal sinuses by *Entomophthora coronata* death resulted from *Pseudomonas aeruginosa* pneumonia complicating extensive entomophthorosis of the lungs, presumably the outcome of inhalation of infected matter.[494]

The great majority of cases of pulmonary phycomycosis may be attributed to lowering of resistance to invasion of the tissues by moulds of the species *Absidia*, *Mucor* and *Rhizopus*, which ordinarily are saprophytes on decaying organic matter. It is probable that none of these moulds is able to set up progressive infection in patients who are otherwise in good health. The name mucormycosis is sometimes used as a general synonym of phycomycosis complicating other diseases, but it is better restricted to the relatively few cases that are shown by identification of the fungus to be caused by a species of *Mucor*. The predisposing conditions include leukaemia, pancytopenia and myelomatosis, and poorly controlled diabetes mellitus and other

metabolic disturbances that are characterized by persistent, severe acidosis. Certain therapeutic measures also predispose to these infections, particularly administration of immunosuppressant and cytotoxic drugs, antilymphocyte serum and corticosteroids; cannulation of blood vessels, when long continued, is an occasional factor, being a potential portal of infection. Burns, too, have repeatedly become not merely a site of superficial infection but the source of haematogenous dissemination. The predisposing factors to some extent determine the site of predominant infection. For instance, the syndrome of naso-orbitomeningocerebral phycomycosis occurs usually as a complication of diabetes mellitus or renal failure (see Chapter 34): these are comparatively seldom responsible for the development of pulmonary or primarily septicaemic phycomycosis, which in most cases occur as complications of severe blood disease or of the resistance-lowering side effects of drugs. Similarly, severe malnutrition predisposes to phycomycosis of the stomach or intestine (see Chapter 15).

The phycomycetes that cause pulmonary infection are recognizable as such in histological sections by their characteristic morphology (Fig. 7.47), but this does not allow of identification of genus or species. The hyphae are characteristically variable in width, ranging from 3 to 20 μm; because of their irregular appearance and the sometimes striking effects of shrinkage during histological processing they have been likened to lengths of crushed ribbon. They tend to branch perpendicularly, and septation of the hyphae is absent or at most very infrequent (lack of septation, indeed, is often described as a diagnostic feature of the phycomycetes). It must be noted that a false impression of septum formation may be given by folds that result from shrinkage. Although often to be seen in haematoxylin–eosin preparations, particularly when carefully sought, the phycomycetes are best shown by special methods: the hexamine silver stain is often useful, but better results may be obtained by silver impregnation methods, as used in the demonstration of reticulin fibres. As in the case of aspergilli (see page 349), such morphologically specific structures as sporangiophores develop only when the mould is growing in air (see Fig. 4.11, page 209): they are seldom, if ever, seen in pulmonary lesions in the fresh state, but they may form if a specimen is left exposed before being placed in fixative solution.

Pulmonary Phycomycosis.—Macroscopically, phycomycotic lesions in the lungs vary greatly in size and

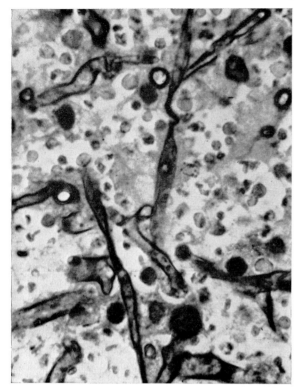

Fig. 7.47.§ Hyphae of a species of *Mucor* in necrotic lung tissue in a case of mucormycosis, one of the varieties of phycomycosis. The hyphae show the folding and irregularity of outline—likened to crushed lengths of ribbon—that are characteristic of the phycomycetes. A further characteristic feature is the infrequency or lack of transverse septa—the septum-like appearance seen in some places is merely due to folding. The rounded structures that look like yeasts or spores are hyphae cut across their long axis. *Grocott–Gomori hexamine (methenamine) silver.* × 600.

number. Multiple lesions are usually the result of haematogenous dissemination, as may occur in cases of naso-orbitocerebral phycomycosis, whereas lesions that are single or few may be the result of direct infection of the lungs by way of the airways. The lesions are firm, hyperaemic or haemorrhagic, and often necrotic. If they extend to the pleura, fibrinous exudate is found over them and there are often petechial or larger foci of bleeding. Microscopically, the most significant finding is fungal invasion of blood vessels of all sizes, with thrombosis and colonization of the thrombus by the fungus, and infarction. It is clear that many strains of these fungi are thrombogenic, and staining the lesions with phosphotungstic acid haematoxylin or by other appropriate methods clearly demonstrates the formation of fine radiating threads of fibrin on the surface of the hyphae within the blood vessels.

The hyphae may be present in great number, not only in the thrombi but throughout the resulting infarcts. The latter soon liquefy, and—if the patient survives—secondary bacterial infection sets in.

As with other fungal infections occurring as a consequence of predisposing illnesses and drug-induced failure of resistance, phycomycosis is very often accompanied by one or more other similar infections, even of the same part. Frequent associations are of phycomycosis with aspergillosis or candidosis, but bacterial, viral and protozoal infections may also be present (see page 362).

Cryptococcosis[496]

Cryptococcosis, a disease of worldwide distribution, is caused by the yeast-like fungus, *Cryptococcus neoformans.* The organism was formerly known as *Torula histolytica,* and the disease as torulosis. Because it was first recognized in Europe, and is caused by a fungus the cells of which reproduce by budding, cryptococcosis was also sometimes known as European blastomycosis (in contrast to the so-called American blastomycoses—see page 359). Although perhaps most familiar as a complication of chronic diseases of the lymphoreticular system, particularly Hodgkin's disease and sarcoidosis (see Chapter 9), in which the infection typically presents as a progressive meningoencephalitis, cryptococcosis is now well known to appear in some cases as a primary disease, without predisposing conditions, affecting the lungs.[497] There may be grounds for believing that infection of the lungs is much commoner than is at present recognized, and that there may be a primary lesion of cryptococcosis, comparable to the initial lesion of histoplasmosis and coccidioidomycosis (see below) and to the Ghon focus of tuberculosis.

Cryptococcus neoformans is a spheroidal or ovoid organism. Its size varies considerably, the cell body measuring from 3 to 20 μm in diameter, although in many instances within the range of 6 to 9 μm. The organism has a mucoid capsule (Fig. 7.48) that stains with mucicarmine, a reaction that is not given by any other pathogenic yeast-like fungus (see also the section on klebsiella pneumonia—page 320). The capsule is sometimes poorly developed, particularly when the organism is proliferating rapidly, but even in these cases some fungal cells can be found that show this characteristic feature unmistakably. Cryptococci are seen well in haematoxylin–eosin preparations and, of course, in those stained by the special methods for fungi.

The fungus occurs as a saprophyte in soil. The

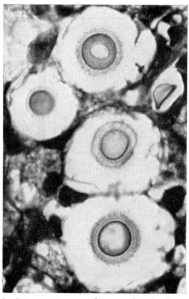

Fig. 7.48.§ *Cryptococcus neoformans* in the lung, showing the characteristic clear halo round each fungal cell. Much of the mucinous material of the cryptococcal capsule has shrunk back in the course of processing the tissue, forming the corona-like covering of the cell bodies. *Haematoxylin–eosin.* × 750.

dried droppings of birds, particularly pigeons and starlings, provide a good culture medium: pathogenic cryptococci can be isolated from buildings that these birds roost on. It is clear that exposure to cryptococci must occur very frequently: equally, the great majority of people must have a high immunity, for cryptococcosis is a rarity in any population.

Pulmonary cryptococcosis takes several forms, ranging from the incidental finding of healing solitary lesions to widespread pneumonia. Isolated, discrete, encapsulate, subpleural granulomas are occasionally seen at necropsy:[498] these are healed or healing lesions, and the implication of their presence is that they are a manifestation of a primary and non-progressive infection. Less rarely, X-ray examination of the chest, in the course of a health check in a patient without symptoms, unexpectedly discloses one or more focal 'coin' lesions in the lungs, up to several centimetres in diameter. These prove to be firm, whitish and rather sharply defined foci of cryptococcal infection; they are encapsulate only when healing. Their cut surface may be dry or gelatinous: the latter is the case when there is less inflammatory reaction to the organisms, which, packed closely in great numbers, account for the mucoid appearance and consistency

of such lesions. Cavity formation is rare, but may occur when the focus is centred on a bronchus: an aspergilloma (see page 350) was found in one such cryptococcal lesion.[499] Confluence and continuing enlargement of these foci may produce a picture of gelatinous pneumonia involving the greater part of one or more lobes: the multicentric origin of this type of lesion can generally be appreciated by the irregular outline of the consolidated parts and the presence of relatively normal lung tissue between the constituent foci where these have not completely merged. In cases of generalized haematogenous dissemination of cryptococcosis the lungs may be studded with miliary or larger foci: close inspection of these discloses their gelatinous nature; they tend to be sharper in outline than miliary tubercles or pyaemic abscesses, the latter being simulated because the gelatinous collection of cryptococci at the centre of the lesion may be washed out during examination of the tissue, leaving a minute cavity.

Microscopically, the lesions may be composed largely of the cryptococci themselves, with little cellular reaction: the alveoli and interstitial tissue contain the closely packed organisms, their cell bodies separated by the variable extent of their mucoid capsule. In other cases there may be a tuberculoid reaction, the fungal cells being found within the cytoplasm of multinucleate giant cells and mononuclear macrophages as well as free in the tissue spaces. In lesions of long standing, lymphocytes and plasma cells may be present in large numbers, and fibrosis may be a feature, although not often conspicuous. Occasionally, neutrophils accumulate in considerable numbers, particularly in miliary haematogenous lesions; in the absence of bacterial infection frank suppuration is not found. Caseation is a rare development, and has to be distinguished from the somewhat similar appearance that may result when large numbers of cryptococci have died and disintegrated into an amorphous, finely granular, eosinophile mass.

The cryptococci may be found in the sputum in cases of pulmonary involvement. They may be seen on microscopical examination of wet films, particularly when the sputum has been mixed with India ink or nigrosin to display the capsule. In dry films the fungal cells disintegrate or become smudged and usually cannot be recognized, although sometimes staining with mucicarmine is conclusive (and may be invaluable when, for whatever reason, more suitable specimens are no longer available).[499] Cultures are generally the preferred means of confirming the diagnosis, but some strains of the cryptococcus do not grow well and several attempts may have to be made before the organism is isolated. It is notable that the cryptococcus is only exceptionally, if ever, found in sputum in the absence of infection, in spite of its near ubiquity in our environment.

It is important to remember that any patient with active cryptococcosis is at risk of developing infection of the central nervous system (see Chapter 34) because of the peculiar affinity of the organism for the brain and meninges and the frequency of its dissemination in the blood.

Histoplasmosis[500]

There are two species of histoplasma that are pathogenic in man, *Histoplasma capsulatum* and *Histoplasma duboisii*. The latter is found exclusively in tropical Africa: the disease that it causes (see Chapter 39) differs significantly from that caused by *Histoplasma capsulatum*, an organism that is geographically far more widespread. In general, when the word histoplasmosis is used without elaboration it refers to disease caused by *Histoplasma capsulatum*. The histoplasmas are diphasic fungi—that is, they are ovoid, yeast-like organisms in cultures at 37°C and in infected tissues (parasitic phase), and they grow in myceliate form, producing characteristic tuberculate macroconidia, in cultures at laboratory temperature (about 18°C) and in their free-living state (saprophytic phase).

Histoplasmosis results from inhalation of dust that contains the infective spores of the histoplasma. This determines the geographical distribution of the disease: in regions where the fungus cannot survive to complete its saprophytic phase in soil or other organic debris, histoplasmosis does not occur naturally—infection does not ordinarily take place from person to person, the tissue form of the fungus being in general unable to convey the disease. In those parts of the world where the soil or the climate is unsuitable for the saprophytic phase of *Histoplasma capsulatum*, the disease is found only among those who have acquired the infection in lands where the fungus is present in the environment, or, much more rarely, as a result of exposure to imported materials contaminated by the infective spores[501] or to laboratory cultures of the saprophytic phase, which develops when the tissue form is grown at laboratory temperature.

Histoplasmosis is endemic in many parts of North America, especially in the basin of the Ohio and Mississippi river valleys, where the prevalence of the infection is indicated by the fact that as many as 90 per cent of the population give a positive reaction to the histoplasmin skin test.[502] The histoplasmin test has the same significance in relation to histoplasmosis as the tuberculin test in relation to infection by *Mycobacterium tuberculosis*.[503] The disease is endemic also in many parts of Central and South America, Africa (where infection by *Histoplasma capsulatum* is endemic over an area far greater than that in which infection by the 'African histoplasma', *Histoplasma duboisii*, occurs) and Asia. Although it is endemic in, for instance, Indonesia, histoplasmosis has not been recognized as an indigenous infection in Australia. Its occurrence in Europe, other than as a result of accidental exposure to the fungus, is exceptionally rare. Histoplasmin surveys in Europe have not disclosed endemic foci of infection, and the organism has been isolated from soil only in parts of Italy. The apparently almost general absence of the fungus from the European environment accounts for the infrequency with which the disease is known to doctors educated and practising in Europe.

Pulmonary Histoplasmosis.—The pulmonary lesions of histoplasmosis may be considered under the headings of primary focus, histoplasmoma, cavitary histoplasmosis and histoplasmosis with multiple primary foci (so-called 'epidemic' histoplasmosis).[500]

The *primary focus* of histoplasmosis resembles that of tuberculosis.[504, 505] It may be solitary or there may be two or more, sometimes many, primary lesions, the number depending on the heaviness of the exposure to the infecting spores. It may occur in any part of the lungs. Generally, and especially when solitary, it is larger than the corresponding lesion of primary tuberculosis. Early calcification is common, and is preceded by caseation and the formation of a fibrous capsule: caseation develops within a few weeks of infection and its appearance is believed to coincide with the development of skin reactivity to histoplasmin. Haematogenous spread of the infection occurs during the primary stage of the disease, with the appearance of foci of infection in any part of the body, but particularly in the spleen and liver. These disseminate foci heal and calcify at the same time as the primary lesion or lesions in the lungs. As in tuberculosis, there is spread of the infection to the hilar lymph nodes, which undergo comparable changes. It is a characteristic of calcified lesions of histoplasmosis that they have a massively chalky appearance and often show a peculiar stippled pattern in radiographs, particularly lesions in lymph nodes. Occasionally, the calcified foci in the lungs have a target-like radiographic shadow because of concentric zones of greater and lesser trans-radiancy.

The typical response to the infecting organisms is proliferation of macrophages. The fungal cells are present in large numbers in their cytoplasm (Fig. 7.49); they are readily seen in haematoxylin–eosin preparations, but only if recently viable. They measure from 2 to 3 μm by 3 to 4 μm and may contain a distinct nucleus. Histoplasmas that have been dead for some time may escape detection in such preparations, although sometimes birefringence, induced by histological processing, may make a proportion of them visible in polarized light. Fortunately, the hexamine–silver stain, provided it is correctly applied, commonly demonstrates histoplasmas very clearly, even when they have long been dead.

Most people who acquire histoplasmosis have no more than a subclinical infection. It has been estimated that clinical manifestations occur in only about 1 per cent of cases and that few of these patients develop serious illness.

The name *histoplasmoma* is given to any circum-

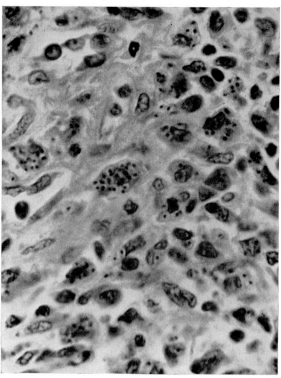

Fig. 7.49.§ *Histoplasma capsulatum* in a pulmonary granuloma. Many of the histiocytes in the field are heavily parasitized by the fungus. *Periodic-acid/Schiff; haemalum.* × 600.

scribed, persistent focus in a lung. The lesion is an outcome of a primary focus. It occurs typically just under the pleura, and is roughly spherical and from 1 to 4 cm, sometimes more, in diameter. Both in radiographs and when examined with the naked eye it has a characteristically concentric pattern of closely set laminae, which may contain appreciable amounts of calcium salts, although by no means invariably. This laminar structure is so characteristic of chronic caseous granulomas of fungal origin that it should guide the diagnostician to consider which fungus is responsible: in many parts of the United States of America it is the histoplasma that most frequently produces such lesions, but in some areas the possibility of a coccidioidal granuloma must be considered, and in other parts of the world a cryptococcal granuloma is the likeliest or indeed the only possibility. Indeed, the concentric pattern in the radiograph is so familiar in some centres that it is regarded as proof of the non-neoplastic nature of 'coin shadows': this is not necessarily justified, for it has been known for carcinoma to arise in the fibrotic capsular zone round such a longstanding mycotic lesion—such a specimen has recently come from a patient in Britain who had acquired a histoplasmic infection in North America many years earlier.[506] In general, histoplasmomas are altogether benign in outlook, and may be left *in situ* with little chance that the infection will be activated and progress; they may become more heavily calcified as the years pass. If resected, they usually prove to be sterile on culture. The causative organism may then be demonstrated most reliably by the hexamine–silver stain, even though it is no longer viable.

Cavitary histoplasmosis may closely or precisely reproduce the clinical and radiological picture of tuberculosis.[507] Moreover, if such patients are exposed to a substantial risk of infection by *Mycobacterium tuberculosis*, as may occur if they are nursed in company with tuberculous patients, tuberculosis may be superimposed on the histoplasmic lesions, with detriment to the chances of successfully treating either infection. In general, cavitary histoplasmosis is seen most frequently in older patients, particularly men, and is attributed to a local breakdown in immunity at the site of dormant subapical histoplasmic granulomas. In some cases it is possible that the condition is due to reinfection, thus adding to the similarities between this manifestation of the fungal infection and tuberculosis.[508] Like the cavities of chronic pulmonary tuberculosis, the lesion of cavitary histoplasmosis may become the site of an aspergilloma. Tuberculoid granulomatous tissue in the lining and vicinity of the cavities contains typical intracellular histoplasmas.

The condition that has been described as *'epidemic' pulmonary histoplasmosis* is a form of severe acute histoplasmosis occurring as a result of a particularly heavy inhalational infection in the unprotected individual. The epithet 'epidemic' has been applied because such cases are commonly seen in several patients simultaneously, all of them exposed on the same occasion to a massive contamination of the air by infective spores. This is an unfortunate name, for such cases may occur singly when individuals are so unfortunate as to stir up large numbers of spores when working in a contaminated environment. These outbreaks have occurred when infected dust is disturbed in the course of cleaning or demolishing buildings, ranging from hen houses to city halls, that have harboured the birds that over years have left the droppings that so perfectly favour the growth of the saprophytic phase of *Histoplasma capsulatum*. Similarly, spelaeologists and others who enter caves where bat and bird droppings have encouraged the histoplasma to proliferate may suffer comparable group outbreaks of acute histoplasmic pneumonia.[509] The multiple foci of histoplasmosis that form in the lungs of these patients have the same structure and run the same course as the solitary primary foci described above. In some cases the infection is so heavy, and the resulting changes in the lungs are so widespread, that death occurs. Those who have not previously had a histoplasmic infection tend to suffer the severest illness in these outbreaks, but even those already known to have had a primary infection may develop fatal pneumonic lesions on re-exposure under such conditions.

Progressive Disseminated Histoplasmosis.—Mention has been made above of haematogenous dissemination of the infection during its primary stage. In most such cases the widespread lesions heal without ill effects. There is another form of disseminated histoplasmosis in which the disease progresses and eventually kills the patient. In some cases of this sort the patient's resistance is lowered by the presence of a lymphoma or leukaemia;[510] in others there are no obvious predisposing factors. Fatal disseminated histoplasmosis is commonly accompanied by the development of painful ulcers at mucocutaneous junction zones or within the orifices of the body or in the pharynx and larynx. Enlargement of the liver and spleen results from the heavy parasitization of the reticuloendothelial cells in these organs. Pneumonic lesions and the development of a few, or many, thin-walled cavities in the lungs may be a feature. Leucoerythroblastic anaemia and other haematological results of heavy parasitization of the bone marrow may develop. Fatal adrenal cortical insufficiency is another important manifestation (see Chapter 30).

Several instances of this type of disseminated histoplasmosis have been seen in Europe, particularly among returned expatriates who had spent some part of their lives in southern or south-eastern Asia.[511]

Diagnosis of Pulmonary Histoplasmosis.—The histoplasma can rarely be demonstrated in sputum, even by culture. Biopsy may be necessary: when it is undertaken the opportunity to set up cultures must not be lost, but good histological material, appropriately stained, is often sufficient to prove the diagnosis. Complement fixation and precipitin tests may also be helpful.

African Histoplasmosis[512]

Histoplasma duboisii, an organism larger than *Histoplasma capsulatum*, has been recognized as a cause of disease throughout much of Africa between the Sahara and the Zambesi. Its distribution overlaps that of *Histoplasma capsulatum*, which, however, is much more widespread on the continent. The source of the infection and the portal of entry of the fungus remain debatable. There is growing evidence that the organism has a saprophytic phase, probably in soil, and that it may enter the body either through the lungs or, in certain cases, by inoculation into the skin. Pulmonary disease as one of its manifestations has attracted less attention than cutaneous and skeletal involvement, but the possibility is under consideration that in many cases the lesions in the skin, like those in bones, are the result of dissemination in the blood from inapparent pulmonary foci.

A feature typical of African histoplasmosis is that the fungal cells provoke a foreign body giant cell reaction, not a simple histiocytosis with or without tuberculoid metamorphosis, as occurs in cases of infection by *Histoplasma capsulatum* (see Figs 39.187A and 39.187B). The organism is ovoid, has a distinct cell wall and some internal structure, and measures from 5 to 12 μm in its longer dimension. It stains well with all the fungal stains, but is unlikely to be overlooked by the careful microscopist in haematoxylin–eosin preparations.

Coccidioidomycosis[513, 514]

This disease occurs especially in the San Joaquin Valley in California but also in the neighbouring states of the United States of America and in some other parts of the Americas. It is caused by the fungus *Coccidioides immitis* (Fig. 7.50). The saprophytic, free-living form of this organism requires special environmental conditions of soil and climate for its survival: these determine its very limited geographical distribution. Indeed, apart from accidental laboratory infections[515] and infection through exposure to contaminated material imported from endemic areas,[516] coccidioidomycosis has only once been found in a patient whose infection may have been acquired naturally outside the Americas (perhaps in Australia).[517]

The initial coccidioidal infection may be symptomless. Oftener, it causes an influenza-like fever, which characteristically may be accompanied by erythema nodosum—hence the popular names in the San Joaquin Valley of 'valley fever' and 'the bumps'. In most cases there is spontaneous recovery from the primary infection. When the disease is severer, which is likelier to be the case in patients of African or Asian origin, it may mimic tuberculosis in any of its manifestations. In such severe infections generalization through the blood is a frequent and particularly grave complication. Meningitis is another common complication (see Chapter 34).

Patients whose resistance is lowered by other

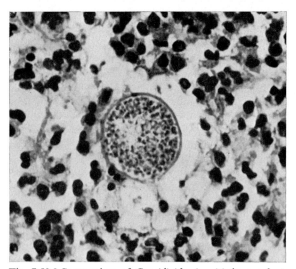

Fig. 7.50.§ Sporangium of *Coccidioides immitis* in purulent exudate in lung (coccidioidal pneumonia). When the sporangium ruptures the innumerable spores that it contains are liberated into the tissues, perpetuating and aggravating the infection. *Haematoxylin–eosin.* × 600.

diseases may develop generalized haematogenous coccidioidomycosis as a consequence of activation of a dormant pulmonary focus. At necropsy, the lungs may show anything from focal consolidation to necrotic, haemorrhagic areas or extensive, necrotic, excavating granulomatous nodules.[513] Histologically, there may be a suppurative exudate in the alveoli, or necrotic haemorrhagic and fibrinous lesions, or a tuberculoid granulomatous reaction.[518] The type of reaction is largely determined by the maturity of the developing fungal cells (see below).

Coccidioides immitis is a dimorphic fungus. Saprophytically, it grows as a mould that produces highly infective arthrospores: these, inhaled in dust, establish the disease. As a parasite, the organism is found almost exclusively in the form of spherules: hyphae develop occasionally in the wall of coccidioidal cavities in the lungs, where there is access of air, but even there it is exceptional to find them and spherules are usually present alone. The coccidioides is one of the most dangerous of all organisms in terms of risk of accidental infection of laboratory personnel and others exposed to its presence. Laboratories dealing with coccidioidal cultures must operate with stringent precautions, including the exclusion of staff not known to have acquired some natural immunity through previous infection. The coccidioidin skin reaction is an invaluable screening test.

Once in the lungs, the arthrospores develop into the parasitic form. The mature parasitic form is the sporangium. This ranges from 30 to 60 μm and sometimes more in diameter (Fig. 7.50). It contains a variable number of sporangiospores ('endospores'), ranging from scores to hundreds. The maturing sporangium is usually accompanied by a histiocytic reaction, with the formation of many multinucleate giant cells: the parasite may be enclosed by the latter or lie free in the tissues. When fully mature, the sporangium attracts neutrophils, which collect to form microabscesses at the centre of the histiocytic granulomatous foci. When the sporangium ruptures, the freshly released sporangiospores, which range from 5 to 10 μm in diameter, at first are free in the purulent exudate but soon are engulfed by mononucleate or multinucleate macrophages. They grow, and eventually become transformed into sporangia, thus repeating the cycle and leading to extension of the infection. The freed sporangiospores are commonly referred to as spherules and the sporangium itself as the endosporulating spherule. The fungal cells are usually well seen in haematoxylin–eosin preparations, except in the early stages when only a few, newly released, small sporangiospores are present: these may be so inconspicuous as to escape detection. The hexamine–silver and other stains for fungi demonstrate all forms of the organism very clearly.

Infection with *Blastomyces dermatitidis* ('North American' Blastomycosis)[519, 520]

It is now recognized that infection with *Blastomyces dermatitidis* occurs very widely throughout Africa and that the geographical designation 'North American', originally intended to distinguish this disease from 'European blastomycosis' (cryptococcosis) and South American blastomycosis (paracoccidioidomycosis), is inappropriate.[521] In exceptional cases, the disease has been acquired in other parts of the world as a result of exposure to contaminated material imported from regions where the fungus occurs naturally.[522] Like the histoplasmas (see above), *Blastomyces dermatitidis* is a diphasic fungus, with a myceliate saprophytic phase in cultures at laboratory temperature and a yeast phase in tissues and in cultures at 37°C. Its natural habitat is soil; infection is believed to occur by inhalation. Grossly, the pulmonary lesions reproduce all the features that may be seen in histoplasmosis. Microscopically, the lesions are characterized by the frequency of a suppurative reaction. The organisms are rounded and usually within the range of 7 to 15 μm in diameter, although some cells may be as much as 30 μm across. They have a thick wall, which may give them a double-contoured appearance. Budding cells can generally be found without difficulty: it is a special feature of *Blastomyces dermatitidis* that it reproduces in tissues by the formation of a single bud that protrudes from the surface of the parent cell, enlarging even until it has reached as much as half the diameter of the latter, or more, before the two separate (Fig. 7.51). Although neutrophils are conspicuous in the reaction to the fungi, tuberculoid granulomas also form: a characteristic feature is the so-called 'suppurating pseudotubercle', in which a central microabscess is enclosed within a complex of epithelioid histiocytes and multinucleate giant cells. The fungal cells may lie free in the purulent exudate or be enclosed in the cytoplasm of the macrophages.

Like histoplasmosis and coccidioidomycosis, infection with *Blastomyces dermatitidis* may become disseminated by the blood stream, foci of the disease appearing in any part of the body. The skin is commonly involved, with the formation of

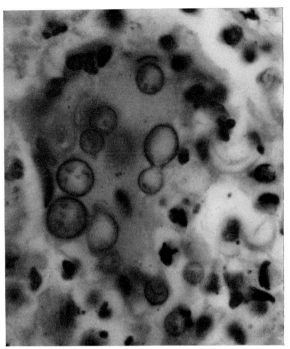

Fig. 7.51.§ *Blastomyces dermatitidis*, the causative organism of 'North American' blastomycosis, in a tuberculoid granuloma in the lung. The fungal cells have a distinct wall, and most of them contain several aggregates of nuclear material. One cell shows a large bud, which characteristically is solitary. *Periodic-acid/Schiff; haemalum.* × 1000.

weeping, verrucose lesions that may become very extensive: these lesions are readily distinguished from the comparatively rare primary granuloma that results from direct inoculation of the organism into the skin. Skeletal involvement is commoner than in other deep mycoses, and infection of vertebral bodies with subsequent collapse has been notably frequent (see Chapter 37).

'South American' Blastomycosis (Paracoccidioidomycosis)[523, 524]

Infection with *Paracoccidioides brasiliensis* occurs most frequently in South America, particularly in parts of Brazil and in Venezuela and Colombia, but also in Central America and Mexico. It has not been proved to occur in any other part of the world. The organism is a diphasic fungus. Its tissue form is characterized by the development of multiple buds over the surface of the parent cell (see Fig. 39.189). The tissue reaction is similar to that in cases of infection with *Blastomyces dermatitidis* (see above). The portal of entry of the infection is now believed to be the lungs:[525, 526] the pulmonary changes reproduce the various pictures seen in such other mycoses as coccidioidomycosis and histoplasmosis (see above).

Rare Pulmonary Mycoses

An intracavitary colony of a penicillium (penicillioma) is mentioned on page 350. Acceptable cases of pulmonary penicilliosis of other types have been reported but are remarkably rare and ordinarily occur as a result of lowering of the body's resistance by other diseases or their treatment.[527] The same is true of most cases of pulmonary geotrichosis (infection by the common saprophytic mould, *Geotrichum candidum*).[528] Sporotrichosis (caused by *Sporothrix schenckii*—see Chapter 39),[529] chromomycosis (caused by species of *Phialophora*—see Chapter 39—or *Cladosporium*—see Chapter 34)[530] and rhinosporidiosis (caused by *Rhinosporidium seeberi*)[531] are very occasionally found as infections of the lungs: in almost all cases such infection has spread, by the airways or in the blood, from a site elsewhere in the body.

Adiaspiromycosis, which is caused by a remarkable fungus, *Emmonsia crescens*, has been seen exceptionally in man.[532, 533] Ordinarily an infection of wild rodents, it is characterized by the formation of multiple tuberculoid granulomas round the cells of the organism. The latter are remarkable for the great size that they may reach—as much as 600 μm in diameter. The fungal cell is usually solitary and has a thick yellowish wall, up to about 8 μm in thickness, surrounding a central mass of amorphous cytoplasm in which there is a single nucleus.

Extrinsic Allergic Alveolitis[534]
(Farmers' Lung)

Although farmers' lung and comparable conditions are not infections but manifestations of allergic sensitization to fungi, it is convenient to consider them here, following the account of the infections that are caused by fungi.

If hay is collected when damp, as often happens after a wet summer, various moulds grow on it during storage. Subsequent handling in late winter may raise a fine dust which, if inhaled, can produce the acute respiratory disease known as farmers' lung.[535] The attack usually begins a few hours after exposure, with fever and a rigor, followed by cough, dyspnoea and, often, expectoration of blood-stained sputum.[536] Mild attacks clear up in two to three weeks, and about half the patients show transient pulmonary opacities on X-ray examination. Further attacks may be severer and more protracted, and recovery may never be complete.

Biopsy specimens taken during resolution show granulomatous lesion in the lungs, with giant cells like those seen in sarcoidosis, and thickening of the alveolar walls; no fungal elements are found.[537, 538] The occurrence of clefts in the cytoplasm of the giant cells is a useful, but not specific, diagnostic aid.[539] In contrast to sarcoidosis, the hilar lymph nodes are unaffected. In fresh cases, the lesions may resolve, but in fatal cases the lungs may show honeycombing, with dense fibrosis.

Similar conditions, also associated with mouldy crops, are *bagassosis*, due to dusts from mouldy sugar cane (bagasse), *maple bark disease* in North America and *paprika splitters' disease* in Hungary. None of these conditions is a manifestation of infection—all are considered to be allergic, resulting from sensitization by inhaled fungal allergens (see page 387).

It has been found that precipitins against extracts of mouldy hay known to produce symptoms of farmers' lung, and against extracts of some micro-organisms recoverable from such hay, are present in the serum of these patients.[539] The fungus *Micropolyspora faeni* is the richest source of the specific farmers' lung hay antigen (FLH antigen) yet found; pure cultures of this organism can form the antigen on artificial media without the presence of hay. Both the spores and the mycelium are rich in FLH antigen, and extracts of the cultures provoke farmers' lung reactions when inhaled by patients with the disease. *Thermoactinomyces vulgaris*, and possibly other thermophile actinomycetes, which multiply rapidly in hay that has become heated by fermentation, may also be involved. Immunoelectrophoresis of extracts of mouldy hay gives a pattern of precipitin arcs with serum from cases of farmers' lung (Fig. 7.52). Inhalation tests with mouldy hay and extracts of mouldy hay produced characteristic reactions in 12 out of 15 patients with farmers' lung but none in 20 control individuals.[540]

The term extrinsic allergic alveolitis is now commonly applied to farmers' lung and similar conditions.[534] It is of help in making the distinction between these conditions and diffuse fibrosing alveolitis, in which there is no demonstrable external cause and no granulomatous reaction (see page 366).

Pneumocystis Pneumonia[541]

Pneumonia due to *Pneumocystis carinii* occurs mostly among premature infants and debilitated babies during the first three months of life. The

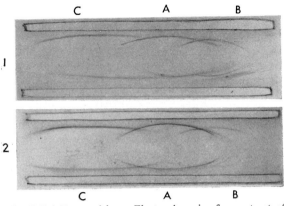

Fig. 7.52.§ Farmers' lung. Electrophoresis of an extract of mouldy hay (1) and an extract of *Micropolyspora faeni* (2). The upper trough in each test contains serum from one patient and the lower trough serum from another. Both were suffering from farmers' lung: there are typical arcs of precipitin reaction in regions C, A and B.

case fatality rate is about 50 per cent.[542] The disease is important also as a serious infection in adults whose immune responses have been impaired by illness or drugs (see below). Both in infants and in adults it has been recognized in many lands and is probably worldwide in occurrence. The causative organism was first described in 1909, in a guinea-pig, by Chagas, who believed it to be a stage in the development of a trypanosome.[543] Although the clinical and pathological features of the human disease were first clearly defined in 1938,[544] the presence of the organism in the alveoli and its pathogenic significance were not recognized until 1952.[545, 546] There is still uncertainty whether the pneumocystis should be classed as a protozoon or as a fungus.[547, 548] Whatever its nature, it is found in a very wide range of animals, inhabiting the lungs without giving rise to any apparent lesion.[549] It has never been cultured.

Pneumocystis pneumonia in babies is ushered in by coryza-like symptoms and soon progresses to respiratory distress. Fatal asphyxia is likely to result after one to six days. Radiographs of the lungs show small, cloudy shadows on both sides, which begin in the hilum and, in severe cases, extend through the whole lung field. At necropsy, the affected parts of the lungs are firm and pale grey, and sink in water. Histologically, the contents of the respiratory bronchioles and alveolar ducts have a finely foamy appearance and stain pink in haematoxylin–eosin preparations. This material consists of aggregated parasites (Figs 7.53 and 7.54); later, with the advent of macrophages, the organisms are ingested and their partially digested remains appear as mucopolysaccharide globules mingled with granules of chromatin. The pneumocystis stains with variable intensity in toluidine blue, Weigert–Gram and periodic-acid/Schiff preparations; it is most conveniently and reliably demonstrated by the Grocott–Gomori hexamine (methenamine) silver method.

Characteristically, the alveolar walls are much thickened and infiltrated by lymphocytes and plasma cells; the capillaries are dilated or compressed, and their endothelium may be unusually prominent. These changes are sufficiently marked to warrant the descriptive term, *interstitial plasma cell pneumonia*, by which the disease is sometimes known. If the resistance of the child is particularly low, as in cases of primary deficiency of immunoglobulin formation, there may be little or no cellular response. Although the organisms are usually confined to the alveolar lumen, they may occasionally be found in the alveolar wall.

Pneumocystis pneumonia is exceptionally rare in the absence of predisposing conditions. In infants, the most important factors that lead to its development are prematurity and congenital hypogammaglobulinaemia;[550] in older children malnutrition (for instance, during famine) and diseases like leukaemia are important. The commonest predisposing conditions in adults are leukaemia and other diseases that specifically lower resistance to infection, and also the administration of corticosteroids and immunosuppressant and cytotoxic drugs.[551]

An unexplained feature of pneumocystis infection is its frequent association with generalized infection by cytomegalovirus (see page 324). This

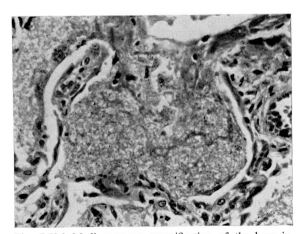

Fig. 7.53.§ Medium-power magnification of the lung in pneumocystis pneumonia, showing an alveolus filled with organisms. See also Fig. 7.54. *Haematoxylin–eosin*. × 100.

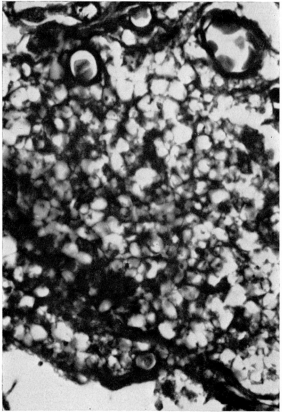

Fig. 7.54.§ High magnification of a collection of *Pneumocystis carinii* in an alveolus. The individual organisms are seen as clear, rounded bodies of various sizes; some of them contain a small granule of chromatin. *Masson's trichrome stain.* × 1000.

has been reported both in cases of neonatal infection and in adults.[552]

Infection of organs and tissues other than the lungs has been recognized only very rarely. Typical colonies of the pneumocystis have been seen in mediastinal lymph nodes in association with pneumocystis pneumonia.[552a, 552b] They have also been seen in the stroma of an ulcerated rectal polyp in an otherwise healthy woman.[552b]

Protozoal Diseases

Pulmonary Amoebiasis[553]

Entamoeba histolytica may spread in the blood from the lesions in the large bowel (Chapter 17), giving rise to metastatic foci of infection. These are most frequently in the liver, lungs and brain, in that order. Although the lesions in these organs are conventionally described as abscesses, they are not accompanied by suppuration unless there is secondary bacterial infection.

If there is amoebic ulceration in the lower part of the rectum, amoebae may reach the rectal venous plexus and, bypassing the liver, make their way directly in the systemic circulation to the lungs. Much oftener, amoebic pulmonary 'abscesses'—which are commonest in the right lung—are secondary to those in the liver: the amoebae pass through the diaphragm to infect the lung. Whether the pleural cavity becomes infected in the course of this extension of the disease from liver to lung depends on whether adhesions that bind the apposed pleural surfaces are sufficient to protect the cavity from invasion (see Chapter 21).

An amoebic 'abscess' in the lung, like that in the liver, is essentially a focus of localized destruction of the parenchyma—an amoebic pneumonia—in which a large part of the lung may be converted into a cavity filled with reddish-brown, viscous fluid. There is little inflammatory reaction in the surrounding tissues; in sections, amoebae may be seen in the zone bordering on the cavity. Often the area of destruction extends to involve one of the bronchi, and much of the characteristic fluid, often blood-stained, may then be expectorated. Should this happen, the condition may be complicated by bacterial infection of the cavity. Such lesions are a grave complication of amoebiasis, and their mortality is high.

'OPPORTUNISTIC INFECTIONS'[554]

It has been recognized since at least Hippocratic times that pneumonia may end the life of the debilitated patient. In recent years the concept has developed that micro-organisms are able to take advantage of a patient's lowered resistance to invade the lungs or other parts of the body, and indeed that organisms that ordinarily are not pathogenic or that cause at most only limited infection may in such circumstances cause widespread, progressive, fatal disease:[555] the organisms have been described as 'opportunists'[556] and the term 'opportunistic infection' has been applied to the diseases that they thus cause. These terms are unfortunate choices, judged at philosophical level,[557] but now so widely current as to serve usefully to designate such organisms and the infections that they cause when other disease or its treatment interferes with resistance.

Many varieties of organisms may cause 'opportunistic' infections, including bacteria, fungi, viruses and protozoa. Even metazoa—for instance, larvae of *Strongyloides stercoralis* (see Chapter 16)—may behave in a comparable manner under equivalent circumstances. The diseases that predispose to microbial 'opportunism' range from diabetes to cancer. The same hazard results from treatment by irradiation, and with corticosteroids, immunosuppressants and cytotoxic drugs, anti-lymphocyte serum, and—in some circumstances—antibiotics and other antimicrobial agents.

Examples of 'opportunistic' infection of the lungs include nocardiosis (page 348), certain forms of aspergillosis (page 351), candidosis (page 352) and phycomycosis (page 352), some cases of crypto-coccosis (page 353), various rarer mycoses (page 360), pneumocystis infection (page 361) and cyto-megalovirus infection (page 324). It is pertinent that the conditions that predispose to infection by organisms that seldom, if ever, cause disease in healthy people may also precipitate activation of dormant or latent infection by acknowledged primary pathogens: for instance, dormant pul-monary mycobacterioses, histoplasmosis (page 357), coccidioidomycosis (page 358) and infection by *Blastomyces dermatitidis* (page 359) and *Para-coccidioides brasiliensis* (page 359) may thus become active, not only causing spreading disease in the lungs but infecting the blood stream and so becom-ing disseminated throughout the body.

It is important to recognize that in most cases of 'opportunistic' infection two or more different organisms are involved and not a single species. In an exceptional case of longstanding Hodgkin's disease with haemolytic anaemia and terminal acute leukaemia, necropsy showed generalized haemato-genous candidosis, aspergillosis, phycomycosis and cryptococcosis, generalized cytomegalovirus infec-tion, pneumocystis pneumonia and staphylococcal pneumonia and pyaemia:[558] earlier in his illness the patient had been successfully treated for acute non-reactive tuberculosis with tuberculous septi-caemia. The potential multiplicity of 'opportunistic' infections in any case has important therapeutic implications. There are equally important diag-nostic implications in the fact that most 'oppor-tunistic' infections are recognized first at necropsy, and, frequently, not until the tissues are examined microscopically.

METAZOAN INFESTATION

Schistosomiasis[559]

Pulmonary schistosomiasis (bilharziasis) may be due to any of the three most important species of human blood fluke, *Schistosoma haematobium*, *Schistosoma mansoni* and *Schistosoma japonicum* (see Chapter 21). Although involvement of the lung is relatively infrequent as a cause of clinical disease in comparison with the major locations of schistosomal infestation, it is recognized wherever schistosomiasis is endemic; its frequency is least where schistosomiasis is due to *Schistosoma japonicum*. Specific changes are found in the lungs in a third of cases of schistosomiasis in Egypt but contribute to death in only 2 per cent of these patients.[560]

Pulmonary infestation may originate in two ways: ova may be carried to the lungs in the blood, having bypassed the portal venous circulation or, indeed, having been produced by flukes inhabiting plexuses that drain into the inferior vena cava; alterna-tively, if adult parasites are present within the pulmonary vasculature itself,[561] ova are produced locally. The ova, which measure from 70 to 170 μm in length by from 50 to 70 μm in breadth, according to the species, are bound by their dimensions to lodge in blood vessels of corresponding calibre: local thrombosis and organization result, with the formation of a characteristic tuberculoid granuloma round the egg itself. Necrotizing angitis often develops in the obstructed arterioles, and eosino-phils may be conspicuously numerous in the vicinity of such lesions. Although the ova may be much distorted during histological processing of the tissues, they are readily seen and recognized, particularly when they were viable at the time when the specimen was obtained. Dead ova often become heavily calcified; they may long retain identifiable traces of the contained embryo. The presence of the eggs is generally the clue to the diagnosis, but in some cases pulmonary arterial lesions, including thrombosis and arteritis, develop where there are no ova demonstrable:[562] these changes may be caused by substances liberated by the parasites, either as a direct effect or through allergic sensi-tization.

When adult flukes reach the lungs they appear to cause no reaction while alive. When they die, thrombosis and arteritis result, and there is com-monly an accompanying focal consolidation of the adjacent parenchyma, giving rise to nodules up to 1 cm and more in diameter that show as small 'coin' shadows in radiographs.

Cor pulmonale may complicate pulmonary schistosomiasis.[562, 563] It may result either from widespread pulmonary endarteritis or from circu-latory obstruction caused by the large number of sclerotic schistosomal granulomas in the lungs. Hyperplasia of the muscle coat of the pulmonary arteries accompanies the rise in pulmonary blood pressure; aneurysmal dilatation of the pulmonary trunk has been observed in cases of long standing.[564]

As in other cases of pulmonary hypertension,[565] peculiar angiomatoid or plexiform appearances may result from recanalization of the obstructed vessels in pulmonary schistosomiasis (see page 283). Disturbance of the pulmonary circulation is notably infrequent in cases of infestation by *Schistosoma japonicum*.

Occasionally, ova reach the respiratory bronchioles and cause a local tuberculoid bronchiolitis.

Schistosomal Granuloma.[566]—Occasionally a tumour-like mass forms in the lungs, sometimes abutting on and obstructing a bronchus: this proves to be a confluent growth of granulomatous tissue and scarring round great numbers of schistosome ova. In one such lesion, removed by pneumonectomy under the impression that it was a primary bronchial carcinoma, the identifiable remains of two pairs of adult schistosomes were present in still patent veins near the centre of the mass:[567] there were hardly any ova or granulomas elsewhere in the lung.

Paragonimiasis[568, 569]

Infestation by lung flukes is endemic in the Far East, and to a lesser extent in Central Africa and South America. In its early stages the disease is characterized by epigastric pain and discomfort; later, when it has become chronic, there is persistent cough and recurrent haemoptysis. In some cases the presence of the parasite is borne well; in others it leads to anorexia and debility. As long as the flukes remain in the lungs the disease is rarely fatal, but should they reach the brain, as happens in a minority of cases, the prognosis is grave.

The fluke responsible is usually *Paragonimus westermani*, which in its adult form is about 1 cm in length. In the lung substance the flukes provoke the formation of small cystic granulomas that eventually enlarge and break into the bronchial lumen. The ova that thus escape from the granuloma pass up the respiratory tract, are swallowed, and eventually are excreted in the stools. The life cycle of the fluke is a complex one: after several weeks in water or moist earth, the ovum hatches into a miracidium, a free-swimming form that eventually enters and parasitizes water snails of the genus *Melania*. After its larval life in the snail, the fluke emerges as a cercaria, which in turn parasitizes small fresh-water crabs and crayfish. It is through the consumption of these crustaceans, raw or insufficiently cooked, that man becomes infested. On reaching the duodenum of the human host, the parasite penetrates its wall and thence passes by way of the peritoneal cavity and diaphragm to the pleura. It attains maturity about five weeks after reaching the lung and so completes its life cycle.

Hydatid Disease (Larval Echinococcosis)

This disease has long been endemic in sheep-raising countries, notably Australia and New Zealand, and in parts of South Africa and South America. Control measures are steadily lessening its incidence. In the United Kingdom it is seen in sheep-raising areas, including Wales. The dog is the usual host of the mature tapeworm, *Echinococcus granulosus*, and sheep and man are the commonest hosts of its larval stage. The ova in the faeces of the dog reach man in contaminated food or water, and after hatching in the small intestine, penetrate its wall and enter the portal circulation. Most of the larvae are retained in the liver, but some negotiate the hepatic barrier and reach the systemic venous circulation and the lungs. Cysts formed by this helminth thus tend to occur most frequently in the liver and the lungs (see Chapters 21 and 34 also).

Pulmonary hydatid cysts are usually solitary (Fig. 7.55) and may form in any lobe. As the cyst enlarges, it may rupture into a bronchus, and the sudden escape of a large amount of its fluid contents may give rise to a grave, even fatal, anaphylaxis-like reaction if the patient has become allergic to the larval material.[570] The presence of allergic sensitization may be demonstrated by the Casoni reaction—an immediate erythematous response that follows the intradermal inoculation of a small volume of sterile cyst fluid.[571]

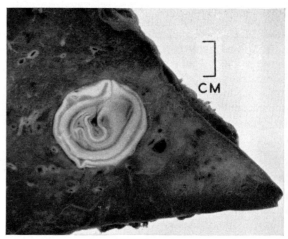

Fig. 7.55.§ Hydatid cyst of lung. The way in which corrugations in the white outermost wall are continuous with the inner folds indicates regression and collapse of the cyst.

Hydatid cysts in the lungs are usually bacteriologically sterile. If they become infected suppuration is likely to develop.[572]

Ascariasis (Pulmonary 'Larva Migrans')[573]

Although essentially an intestinal parasite, *Ascaris lumbricoides* has a complex life cycle, during one phase of which it passes through the lungs. The infestation is acquired by ingesting food or water contaminated with ova passed in the faeces of an earlier host. The ova hatch in the small intestine, where the larvae quickly penetrate the mucosa and are carried either to the liver in the portal blood stream or in lymph to the systemic veins and so to the lungs. Experimental studies on animals indicate that the largest number of larvae reach the lungs about five or six days after ingestion of the eggs: this corresponds with the clinical picture in naturally occurring infestation in man—fever, cough and difficulty in breathing, with general malaise, begin within a week and worsen over a period of some days. During this time there may be radiological evidence of widespread infiltrates, somewhat like miliary tubercles, at least in cases of heavy infestation.[574] Eosinophils and Charcot–Leyden crystals are often conspicuous in the sputum, although the larvae themselves are rarely seen. The illness is usually over within three weeks. In exceptional cases respiratory distress becomes so severe that the patient may die.[575] The subsidence of pulmonary symptoms coincides with the progressive migration of the surviving larvae to the bronchial tree, whence, by coughing, they are carried upward to the pharynx, and, after being swallowed, reach the intestine, where they grow into mature worms.

Except in the rare fatal cases, or when the parasites are present by chance in lungs examined as a result of other disease, microscopical studies of the pulmonary lesions have been infrequent. The larvae may be found in capillaries. Even those that were alive when the specimen was obtained may be accompanied by eosinophils and neutrophils that escape into the interstitial tissue of the alveolar walls and elsewhere. When the larva dies, an intense reaction may develop, with dense local accumulation of eosinophils ('eosinophil microabscess'), often with many macrophages and neutrophils, and the formation of fibrinoid material. Identifiable remnants of larvae may be seen, sometimes in multinucleate giant cells. There may be local haemorrhage. These changes may amount to appreciable foci of alveolar consolidation (focal eosinophil pneumonia).

Now that lung biopsy is more commonly practised, it is particularly important to remember that cases of larval pulmonary ascariasis are likely to be seen, occasionally, even in communities that do not have a high rate of ascaris infestation.[576] The larvae of *Ascaris lumbricoides*, the ascarid parasite of man, must be distinguished from those of other ascarids, such as species of *Toxocara*, that also may be found in the course of biopsy practice. Morphological differentiation of these larvae in histological preparations is commonly beyond the ability even of professional parasitologists; investigation by means of specific immunofluorescent staining may be decisive in such cases. The larvae of the toxocarae have a greater tendency than those of *Ascaris lumbricoides* to die in the lungs when they infest man: they then cause the development of a tuberculoid granulomatous focus that eventually leads to fibrous encapsulation of the remains of the parasite (see Chapter 40 also).[577]

If the infestation is a heavy one, the patient may develop a specific allergy to ascaris, which manifests itself with asthma and eosinophilia; the syndrome resembles that described by Löffler (see below).[578] Skin tests with ascaris antigens usually give rise to an immediate response in any infested person.[579]

PULMONARY EOSINOPHILIA

The term 'pulmonary eosinophilia' was introduced in 1952 to describe pulmonary infiltration associated with eosinophilia in the blood:[580] it is not applied, however, to tropical eosinophilia (see below) or to the conditions that are covered by the term extrinsic allergic alveolitis (pulmonary infiltration characterized histologically by granuloma formation and serologically by the presence of circulating specific precipitins, as in farmers' lung—see page 360).[581] Löffler's syndrome[582] of fleeting pulmonary infiltrates and eosinophilia in the blood* is a classic form of pulmonary eosinophilia, usually in association with infestation by metazoa, including several varieties of microfilariae and larva migrans (see ascariasis, above). Indeed, metazoan infestation is probably the commonest cause of pulmonary eosinophilia in communities in which such parasites

* The name 'Löffler's syndrome' is sometimes also used in referring to the condition of fibroblastic endocarditis with eosinophilia that he also described (Löffler, W., *Schweiz. med. Wschr.*, 1936, **66**, 817). This rare form of endocardiopathy, of unknown aetiology, is sometimes accompanied by 'eosinophil pneumonia' (Brink, A. J., Weber, H. W., *Amer. J. Med.*, 1963, **34**, 52).

are particularly prevalent. In contrast, in Britain, pulmonary eosinophilia is most commonly an accompaniment of asthma and, next in frequency, allergic aspergillosis (see pages 301 and 349). Patients with intrinsic asthma (see page 301) may develop pulmonary infiltrates, with accompanying episodes of high fever and in the absence of sensitivity to fungi: the cause is not known. Systemic polyarteritis has developed in a few of these cases.[583]

Pulmonary eosinophilia, without asthma, may be caused by a number of drugs, most notably the urinary antiseptic nitrofurantoin (see page 378), but occasionally sulphonamides and aspirin, among others.

In a final group no cause has been recognized: such cases are categorized as cryptogenic pulmonary eosinophilia. Some of the patients in this group develop systemic polyarteritis.[584]

Tropical Eosinophilia

The names tropical eosinophilia and tropical pulmonary 'eosinophilosis' have been given to a condition that is found mostly among those who live along the coast of India. It is characterized by very marked eosinophilia in the blood and pulmonary symptoms.[585, 586] The clinical signs are fever, loss of weight, dyspnoea and asthmatic attacks; radiographs of the chest show nodular shadows in the lungs.

The condition is benign and little is known of the changes in the lungs. Such reports as have been published describe irregularly scattered whitish nodules, 3 to 5 mm in diameter, distributed at intervals of 1 to 3 cm throughout the lungs. Histologically,[587, 588] the nodules are composed of a group of 20 to 30 alveoli filled by eosinophils enmeshed in fibrin. In the centre of some of the nodules the alveolar walls are destroyed and the area becomes an 'eosinophil abscess'. In others a central collection of epithelioid cells becomes arranged like a palisade round deeply acidophile hyaline material. Giant cells and fibrosis are a feature of some lesions.

Some authors have described microfilariae in the lung lesions in these cases, and regard the disease as a manifestation of filariasis.[587] In support of this view, the filarial complement fixation test is sometimes positive, with titres of over 1 : 10 and frequently of 1 : 80 or higher, and often there is a dramatic clinical response to the administration of antifilarial drugs such as diethylcarbamazine.

Tropical eosinophilia should be differentiated from eosinophilia due to intestinal worms, trichiniasis, Hodgkin's disease, polyarteritis, asthma, allergic aspergillosis, and skin diseases such as urticaria.

CHRONIC INTERSTITIAL PNEUMONIA AND FIBROSIS OF THE LUNGS

At necropsy, the lungs of most adults show fibrous scars. These are most commonly at the apex of the upper lobe and consist of a narrow band of collapsed, often blackened, fibrotic lung covered by thickened pleura. When such apical scars are accompanied by calcification and pleural adhesions, they are probably tuberculous, but many present neither feature, and their significance remains inadequately explained. A primary tuberculous lesion (Ghon focus) and the corresponding primary lesions of such fungal infections as histoplasmosis are often represented by a subpleural scar, with or without adhesions, in any part of the lungs. Scars also result from infarction, pneumoconiosis and pneumonia. In the last, local failure of resolution leads to carnification and eventual fibrosis.

The persistence of stainable elastic fibres often demonstrates the position of the former alveolar walls in a mass of fibrous tissue.[589] Elastic fibres in healed infarcts may be arranged in whorled and matted tangles rather than in an alveolar pattern. When the scars follow a destructive process, such as tuberculosis or a lung abscess, the elastic tissue within the necrotic area tends to be destroyed. The chronic fibrosis of pneumoconiosis is described on page 380.

In the early days of deep X-ray treatment, overdosage was common, for the dangers were not well appreciated. Fibrosis of the lungs was a frequent sequel. Nowadays, pulmonary fibrosis may be seen in a milder form after irradiation of the breast for carcinoma and, more severely, after irradiation of an intrathoracic neoplasm. Histologically, this form of pulmonary fibrosis is characterized by atypical alveolar lining cells and the formation of hyaline membranes (Fig. 7.56).[590] Patchy oedema, cellular infiltration and necrosis are present in addition. In the later stages the alveolar walls become fibrotic.

Diffuse Fibrosing Alveolitis

The description by Hamman and Rich, in 1935[591] and 1944,[592] of the condition that they referred to as diffuse interstitial fibrosis of the lungs led to

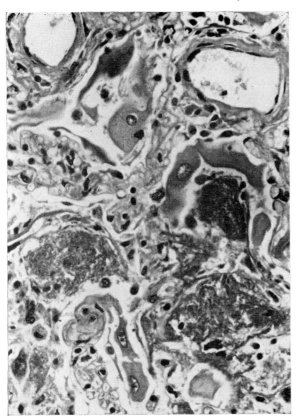

Fig. 7.56.§ Changes in the lung following X-irradiation. The thickened alveolar walls are characteristically covered by atypical alveolar lining cells and there is fibrin in the lumen. *Haematoxylin–eosin.* × 370.

recognition that fibrosis of the lungs, chronic or rapidly progressive, may occur without pneumoconiosis or any systematized 'collagen disorder' or other evident aetiological factor. In British practice, the term diffuse fibrosing alveolitis is widely used for this condition, which is characterized by fibrosis of the alveolar walls, which become much thickened, and by the presence of histiocytes and desquamated epithelial cells within the alveolar lumen.[593, 594] In the United States of America the term 'usual interstitial pneumonia' has been used comparably, although in a broader sense (see page 369).[595]

The patients with this condition complain of progressively worsening breathlessness on exertion, dry cough and loss of weight.[596] The radiological changes comprise coarse mottling of the lungs that spreads upward from the lower zones, with progressive elevation of the diaphragm accompanying the shrinkage of the fibrotic lung tissue. Clubbing of the digits is common, and in the later stages cyanosis and dyspnoea at rest presage death from respiratory or cardiac failure. The mean survival in one series, after the onset of the first symptom, was just under four years, the extremes ranging from less than 12 months to many years in the case of those few patients in whom the progress of the disease was arrested.[597]

The condition is slightly commoner in males. It occurs at any age from childhood to senility and is most frequent in the fourth and fifth decades. It has been observed in twins and quite often in other siblings.[598]

Histopathology.—The histology of the early changes has been studied in biopsy specimens.[599] The alveolar walls are oedematous and thickened by an accumulation of lymphocytes and an increase in the amount of reticulin and collagen (Fig. 7.57). The alveoli contain many histiocytes and detached epithelial cells. Sometimes hyaline membranes form and may become converted into fibrous tissue by organization. There is hyperplasia of lymphoid follicles in the affected parts. In contrast to extrinsic allergic alveolitis (see page 360), there is no granuloma formation.

In the advanced stages the lungs are shrunken and firm. The lower lobes are most severely affected: when the lungs have been pressure-fixed with aqueous formalin the lower lobes particularly have a wrinkled or finely nodular external appearance, somewhat like that of a cirrhotic liver. Even pressure-fixed lungs are shrunken, their volume sometimes being under 1000 ml (the normal left lung, pressure-fixed, has a volume of about 2500 ml): the shrinkage is an important factor in the causation of respiratory failure. The cut surface of the fixed lung shows marked fibrosis and a variable degree of 'honeycombing' (see page 369). Characteristically, the changes are most marked in a subpleural zone, a few centimetres wide, in the posterior basal segment and extending up the back of the lung and forward over its diaphragmatic aspect (Fig. 7.58).

Microscopically, the advanced lesion shows replacement of the normal alveolar structure of the lung by dense collagen enclosing cystically dilated air spaces that are lined by respiratory or flattened epithelium, or, sometimes, by a layer of macrophages, including giant cells (Fig. 7.59). The air spaces contain mucin and numbers of histiocytes and other inflammatory cells; older contents may be marked by cholesterol clefts. The wall of the blood vessels may be thickened. Some inflammatory cells are present also in the fibrous tissue,

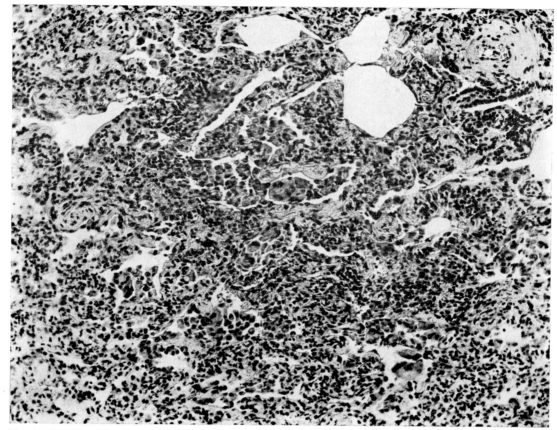

Fig. 7.57.§ Diffuse fibrosing alveolitis. A collapsed piece of lung, taken at operation. The alveolar walls are infiltrated by many lymphocytes and plasma cells. The lumina contain large cells which are histiocytes and type 2 cells. Compare with Fig. 7.59. *Haematoxylin–eosin.* × 160.

but their numbers are seldom as large as in the early stages.

Nature of Diffuse Fibrosing Alveolitis.—It is relevant that some patients with diffuse fibrosing alveolitis have other abnormalities, such as rheumatoid arthritis and polymyositis.[600] As fibrosing alveolitis has been defined here in histological terms, it is important to note that the same histological appearances may be seen in the lungs in some cases of systemic sclerosis and systemic lupus erythematosus. Clinically, the patients may be grouped according to the predominant clinical condition: those in whom the pulmonary changes are not associated with evident disease elsewhere may be said to have diffuse fibrosing alveolitis. It is notable that fibrosing alveolitis has many features in common with the so-called collagen diseases. Hyperglobulinaemia has been reported in some 40 per cent of the patients;[601] non-organ-specific complement-fixing autoantibodies, rheumatoid factor and antinuclear factor are present oftener than in people without fibrosing alveolitis, including patients with extrinsic allergic alveolitis (see page 360) or sarcoidosis.[602, 603]

Immunofluorescent studies sometimes have demonstrated immune complexes in the wall of pulmonary capillaries, suggesting that the damage may be due to autoimmunization in at least some cases.[604] Hepatic fibrosis, with portal infiltration by lymphocytes and plasma cells,[605] and renal tubular acidosis[606] have been present. Some of the patients have developed Hashimoto's thyroiditis or Sjögren's disease.

Diffuse fibrosing alveolitis may be regarded as a complex autoallergic disorder. While attempts should always be made to distinguish between it and the cases of rheumatoid arthritis and the like that are accompanied by diffuse pulmonary fibrosis, the potentially extrapulmonary basis of diffuse fibrosing alveolitis itself must also be appreciated.

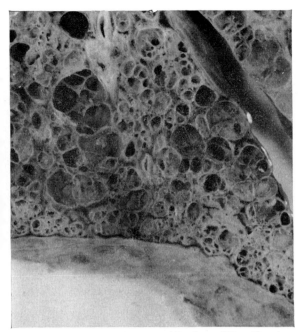

Fig. 7.58.§ 'Honeycomb lung' resulting from diffuse fibrosing alveolitis. Alveoli were absent from this part of the lung, which is composed of dilated small bronchi, non-respiratory bronchioles, and cysts replacing alveoli. Emphysema would affect more distal airways and its lesions do not have the thick fibrous walls seen here. *Pressure fixation; barium sulphate impregnation.* Natural size.

'Honeycomb Lung'[607-609]

It is now recognized that the most frequent cause of the condition that is generally known as 'honeycomb lung' is diffuse fibrosing alveolitis, the advanced stage of which characteristically presents this picture (see above). Only a small proportion of cases is accounted for by other diseases. Among these are pneumonia (including interstitial pneumonia), pulmonary collapse, and the end-results of tuberculosis, especially after treatment with streptomycin. Rarer causes include berylliosis, pulmonary eosinophilia, sarcoidosis, systemic sclerosis and tuberose sclerosis.

Other Forms of Chronic Interstitial Pneumonia

The term interstitial pneumonia has sometimes been used in a general sense to describe any tissue response in the lungs that occurs predominantly in the supporting structures rather than within the alveoli:[610] in such cases any involvement of the lumen of the alveoli is incidental to the interstitial changes.

Acute interstitial pneumonia may be caused by agents that range from fumes to viruses. Most cases of chronic interstitial pneumonia are unexplained: some of them may represent a relatively rare outcome of diffuse damage originating as acute interstitial pneumonia. The term chronic interstitial pneumonia is often used synonymously with chronic fibrosis of the lungs.[611]

Diffuse fibrosing alveolitis (page 366) is, of course, a form of chronic interstitial pneumonia. An American term, *'usual' interstitial pneumonia*, is sometimes applied both to fibrosing alveolitis and to the forms of interstitial pneumonia that are caused by viral infection or that follow pulmonary oedema resulting from exposure to fumes, such as those released during corundum smelting (bauxite lung),[612] or from incorrect use of intermittent positive pressure ventilators (see page 379).[613]

In other cases, chronic interstitial pneumonia is associated with disorders such as rheumatoid arthritis (page 370). Some forms are characterized by the development of granulomas, as in Wegener's disease (page 371). There are also rare types of chronic interstitial pneumonia that remain aetiologically problematical.[610]

Desquamative Interstitial Pneumonia.—This term has been applied to a form of chronic interstitial pneumonia of unknown cause in which there is a relatively inconspicuous thickening of the alveolar walls, with a scanty infiltrate of eosinophils and plasma cells in this situation, while the alveoli are filled with large cells that for the most part are desquamated type 2 pneumonocytes (see page 272).[595] Electron microscopy has shown that histiocytes are present among the type 2 cells:[614] the proportions have varied in different studies, perhaps because the condition has been investigated at different stages in its evolution. In its late stages the disease may progress to 'honeycombing' of the lungs.

It may be noted that some pathologists, we among them, have difficulty in distinguishing the picture described as desquamative interstitial pneumonia from that of diffuse fibrosing alveolitis in its cellular prefibrotic phase (see page 367).[594] Time will tell if this reflects geographical differences in the features of the diseases or results from different interpretations of the histological patterns in a difficult and debatable field of pathology.

Giant Cell Interstitial Pneumonia.[615]—This very rare form of interstitial pneumonia is characterized by a lymphocytic infiltrate in the alveolar

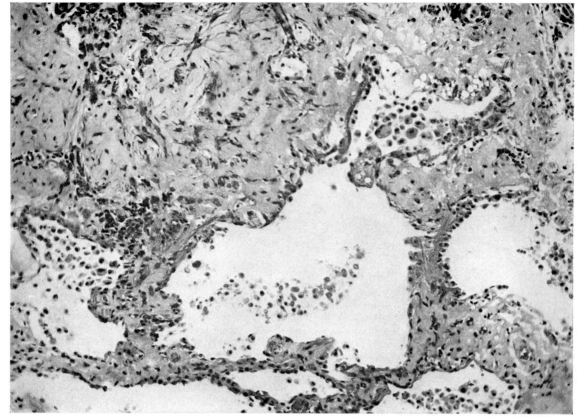

Fig. 7.59.§ Diffuse fibrosing alveolitis. Fibrous stage, showing large air spaces surrounded by dense collagenous tissue. Compare with Fig. 7.57. Note free cells in the air spaces while there are fewer interstitial cells than in the earlier stage illustrated in Fig. 7.57. *Haematoxylin–eosin.* × 160.

septa and numerous, distinctively bizarre giant cells in the alveoli. Its cause is unknown. The presence of the giant cells, recalling the giant cell pneumonia of measles (see page 323), has not been linked with any recognized infective agent.

Lymphocytic Interstitial Pneumonia.[616, 617]—This also is a very rare disease. It is characterized by diffuse infiltration of the interstitial tissue of the lungs by mature lymphocytes. The lymphocytes accumulate in the connective tissue round the bronchioles and also in the alveolar walls; only a few escape into the lumen of the alveoli. Hypergammaglobulinaemia is found in some cases; this is of polyclonal origin, in keeping with the interpretation that the condition is inflammatory rather than neoplastic (the gammaglobulin associated with lymphosarcoma is usually monoclonal).[618] In some cases plasma cells are present as well as lymphocytes: when the two varieties of cell are present in about equal numbers the condition is sometimes described as *lymphoplasmacytic pneumonia.*[619]

The diseases of the lungs that are characterized by accumulation of lymphocytes are, in general, difficult to distinguish from one another. Lymphocytic interstitial pneumonia may be related to the so-called benign lymphoma of the lungs ('pseudolymphoma'—see page 391). The presence of hypergammaglobulinaemia is not specific, since it may occur in cases of Wegener's disease and of rheumatoid lung.[618, 619]

The Lungs in Rheumatoid Arthritis

Various forms of pulmonary lesion may occur in cases of rheumatoid arthritis. Rheumatoid nodules of classic histological appearance may be found (see Chapter 39); if they are near the pleura there may be an accompanying pleural effusion.

Chronic interstitial pneumonia may accompany rheumatoid arthritis.[620] The histological picture is similar to that of diffuse fibrosing alveolitis, although lymphoid nodules may be more numerous than in most cases of the latter. Eventually the lungs become 'honeycombed', especially the subpleural zone of the lower lobes (Fig. 7.60). The condition may be associated with pulmonary arteritis as part of the general arteritis of rheumatoid disease.[621]

A rarer form of rheumatoid lung is characterized by cavitation.[622] This may or may not be associated with pneumoconiosis: when it is, it seems to be unrelated to the condition known as Caplan's syndrome (see below).

Immunofluorescent studies have shown that the lung tissue of patients with rheumatoid lung disease contains rheumatoid factor. This is believed to be significant in the pathogenesis of the lesions.[623]

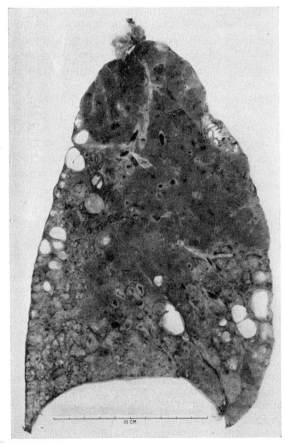

Fig. 7.60.§ Fibrosis of the lung in rheumatoid arthritis. The lung is shrunken and there is a broad zone of 'honeycombing' beneath the pleura of the lower lobe and lingula, with cysts up to 2 cm in diameter. The white material in the cysts is barium sulphate used in preparing the specimen. *Pressure fixation; barium sulphate impregnation.*

Caplan's Syndrome.—When coal-workers' pneumoconiosis and other diseases caused by mineral dusts, such as asbestosis, are associated with rheumatoid arthritis, unusually large and numerous rheumatoid nodules may form in the lungs, giving a striking radiological picture (Caplan's syndrome).[624] The Caplan lesions range from 0·5 to 5 cm across. Macroscopically, they have a distinctive concentric pattern of alternating black and yellowish grey rings.[625] The core of the lesion consists of necrotic debris and may become calcified (Fig. 7.61). It is surrounded by a characteristic layer of 'palisaded' epithelioid cells and fibroblasts; a narrow zone of other inflammatory cells, mostly neutrophils, separates the palisade from the necrotic centre. The successive rings of fibrous tissue and dust that enclose the core indicate a series of phases of activity in the genesis of the lesions. The Caplan lesions must be distinguished from foci of tuberculosis accompanying silicosis: the cellular palisade of the former has the features of the classic rheumatoid granuloma (see Chapter 39) and is further distinguished from tuberculous granulation tissue by the associated zone of neutrophils and the absence of tubercle bacilli. Sometimes, however, the condition is complicated by tuberculosis.

Pulmonary Lesions in Ankylosing Spondylitis.[626, 627] —Changes are found in the lungs in a small proportion of cases of ankylosing spondylitis. The spinal disease appears early in adult life: usually, however, it is not until the fifth decade or so that cough and dyspnoea develop. Radiographs of the chest show mottling in the upper zone on both sides, resembling tuberculosis. Histologically, there is only fibrosis and lymphocytic infiltration: no sign of tuberculosis is found.

Wegener's Granulomatosis[628]

This rare disease of unknown aetiology occurs in previously healthy, young or middle-aged men or women. In about two-thirds it presents with persistent purulent rhinorrhoea and epistaxis, maybe preceded or accompanied by deafness or by ulceration of the gums; in others, it starts with cough and haemoptysis. All the patients have some degree of fever and weakness. Sometimes there is eosinophilia. The lesions progress and ulcers form that involve the nose (see page 213) and the pharynx, larynx, trachea and bronchi. In about half the cases, dense, circular or oval opacities, often showing central cavitation, appear in chest radiographs. Haemorrhagic foci appear in the skin of

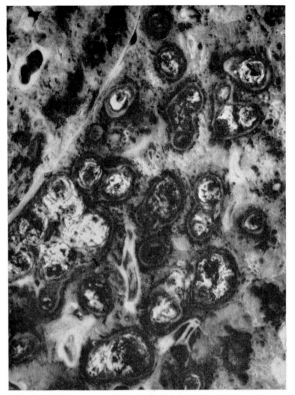

Fig. 7.61.§ The cut surface of the lung in Caplan's syndrome (rheumatoid arthritis in a coal-worker). There are numerous nodules up to 1 cm across, with thick fibrous walls, demarcated inside and out by deposits of coal dust. The specimen is unusual in showing heavy calcification of the centres of the lesions. *Pressure fixation; barium sulphate impregnation.* × 2·5.

the limbs, trunk and face in some cases and may form small ulcers. The patients die from respiratory or renal failure.

At necropsy, the lesions in the lungs are greyish-white areas of consolidation up to 4 cm or so in diameter. As well as these, pale, miliary nodules may be scattered diffusely through all parts of the lungs. Histologically, granulomatous lesions with many giant cells spread from the bronchi and bronchioles into the nearby lung substance. In addition, many of the small arteries and arterioles show fibrinoid necrosis. Later, the lesions become organized and some of the vessels become recanalized.

Vascular changes in Wegener's granulomatosis are not confined to the lungs, for similar lesions occur in the kidneys (see Chapter 24) and may also be found in the heart, spleen, liver and other organs. The condition has affinities with polyarteritis and other 'collagen diseases'. Its main diagnostic feature, however, is ulceration somewhere in the upper or lower reaches of the respiratory tract, with the development of more widespread lesions later. It is this typical clinical course that entitles Wegener's granulomatosis to be regarded as a distinct nosological entity.

Localized Wegener's Granulomatosis.[629]—A limited form of Wegener's disease is sometimes seen, with involvement of one system only, particularly the respiratory system, and sometimes the lungs predominantly or even exclusively. The prognosis is better than in the generalized form. However, other systems, particularly the kidneys and skin, may become affected later. In some such cases there has been an interval of some years between apparently successful treatment of lesions confined to the lungs and the often sudden onset of renal involvement.[630]

The occasional recognition of asymptomatic Wegener's disease as a result of the discovery of a pulmonary lesion presenting as a 'coin' shadow in a chest radiograph, without detectable lesions elsewhere in the body, raises a question whether these are instances of localized disease, in the sense indicated above, or the initial lesion of a condition that, left to itself, tends to become a generalized necrotizing granulomatosis.[630]

In other cases, necrotizing sarcoid, lymphomatoid and bronchocentric granulomatosis have been regarded as variations of the classic histological picture.[631]

Sarcoidosis[632]

The lesions of sarcoidosis (Besnier–Boeck–Schaumann disease) may be confined to a single organ or disseminated widely (see Chapters 9 and 39).[633] The disease usually appears early in adult life in women. The lungs are commonly involved, presenting a multiplicity of small nodules comparable in size with large miliary tubercles. The hilar lymph nodes often form large masses that are readily detectable with X-rays. In many instances, the pulmonary lesions and the lesions in the hilar lymph nodes regress and the patient recovers: sometimes, however, the lungs become progressively infiltrated,[634] and when this happens widespread fibrosis and bronchiectasis may follow.

During their phase of active development sarcoid nodules resemble early tubercles microscopically; they differ from tubercles in that even when large they do not undergo caseation. Multinucleate giant cells, similar to the Langhans cell of tuberculosis, are rarely absent but rarely numerous. They may contain Schaumann bodies and asteroid bodies (see Chapter 9): these are not pathognomonic of sarcoidosis, for they may be found in other forms of granulomatous inflammation.

The aetiology of sarcoidosis is obscure; no single factor is known. Granulomas with the same structure may be found in a variety of conditions, among which some fungal infections and berylliosis are noteworthy. Some authors regard sarcoidosis as an anomalous form of tuberculosis. In the United States, a correlation was observed between the incidence of sarcoidosis and the distribution of pine forests: the suggestion was made that the pulmonary lesions are caused by some inhaled constituent of pine pollen.[635] Further work has not supported this hypothesis.[636]

Many cases of sarcoidosis present anomalous immunological reactions. The intracutaneous tuberculin reaction is generally negative, but the Kveim reaction—the development of a local sarcoid granuloma some weeks after intradermal inoculation of a saline extract of ground-up sarcoid granuloma—is often positive.[637, 638] It may be noted that the Kveim test is often difficult to interpret histologically. This is due in part to the formation of non-specific foreign body granulomas at the site of the inoculation and in part to occasional difficulty in determining the significance of nondescript clusters of epithelioid cells that do not amount to tubercle-like aggregates. There is a considerable subjective element in the interpretation: the results are most reliable when the test is performed in a strictly standardized manner and interpreted by microscopists with special experience and interest in the field.

Other Causes of Pulmonary Granulomas of Sarcoid Type

Granulomatous foci that reproduce the classic structure of the lesion of sarcoidosis are rarely found in the lungs in the absence of that disease. Among the best known causes is berylliosis (see page 386), in which the histological mimicry is particularly close. Similar granulomas in certain infections, including histoplasmosis, leishmaniasis[639] and leprosy,[639] are usually readily distinguishable from sarcoidosis by the demonstrable presence of the causative organisms in the lesions. There remain exceptional cases in which the radiological picture of widespread miliary shadowing in the lung fields, with or without enlargement of the hilar lymph nodes, but in the absence of evidence of disease elsewhere in the body, is shown by biopsy to be due to lesions that are identical with those of sarcoidosis. It is possible, if unlikely, that some such cases are instances of sarcoidosis in which recognizable involvement is confined to the lungs. In other cases it has been suggested that the lesions are a reaction to inhaled matter, perhaps of a particular chemical constitution that causes an epithelioid cell response. Aerosols, such as antiperspirant deodorant solutions and hair-setting sprays,[640] have been blamed (and it may therefore be noted that the frequency of changes in the lungs due to inhalation of hair sprays, particularly the so-called 'hair spray thesaurosis' or histiocytosis has been exaggerated[641]).

LIPID PNEUMONIA

Exogenous Form

Oil may enter the trachea in a variety of circumstances. Most commonly it is liquid paraffin that thus gains access to the lungs, either as a vehicle for drugs administered by a nasal spray or regurgitated after oral administration as a lubricant in constipation.[642] Vegetable oils and animal fats have been concerned in other cases.[643] Regurgitation of ingested oil is especially likely to happen during sleep, or when the oesophagus fails to empty completely into the stomach because of achalasia of the cardia or the presence of a hiatus hernia. Oil may also reach the lungs when given orally to debilitated children with feeding difficulties.[644] While in children the pneumonic condition appears usually to resolve, in adults oils give rise to chronic granulomatous lesions that radiologically may simulate a carcinoma, generally in a lower lobe.

Histologically, there are many large droplets of oil surrounded by a zone of epithelioid and giant cells. The droplets may form a fine sieve-like pattern, but adjoining droplets tend to coalesce, with the result that many alveoli are filled by a single large globule (Fig. 7.62). Since the oil is lost during the preparation of paraffin sections, the presence of the droplets may be unsuspected and the holes mistaken for alveoli on casual inspection. It has to be remembered that liquid paraffin is not shown well by Sudan dyes or osmium tetroxide, as ordinarily used for demonstrating lipids: the fact that it is soluble in chloroform but not in acetone may be useful in its identification.[645]

N

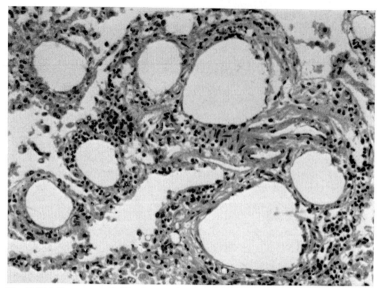

Fig. 7.62.§ Exogenous lipid pneumonia due to the inhalation of liquid paraffin. The oil has been dissolved out in processing the tissue, leaving sharp-edged, rounded holes lined by flattened macrophages and occasional giant cells. Outside these is a thin wall of fibrous tissue lightly infiltrated by lymphocytes. *Haematoxylin–eosin.* × 90.

Pulmonary Fibrosis Complicating Hiatus Hernia.— It has been noted above that a hiatus hernia predisposes to regurgitation of swallowed oil. This may be an appropriate context in which to note that the presence of a hiatus hernia may be associated with fibrosis of the lungs: it seems to be possible that this is the outcome of regurgitation of gastric juice.[646, 647] For this reason, many physicians now consider it worthwhile in all cases of unexplained pulmonary fibrosis to investigate the possibility that the patient has a hiatus hernia, which is generally disclosed by a barium swallow.

Endogenous Form

Exogenous lipid pneumonia, important because largely preventable, has to be distinguished from the endogenous form ('cholesterol pneumonia'). The latter is found oftenest, but not invariably, in the part of a lung peripheral to an obstructing bronchial carcinoma.[648] Chemical analysis of these lesions shows a high concentration of cholesterol and its esters.

Histologically, the endogenous form has a typical appearance (Fig. 7.63). The affected alveoli are stuffed with macrophages with foamy cytoplasm that contains large amounts of fat, much of it sudanophile.[649]

If macrophages obtained in washings from the lung peripheral to a tumour are cultivated *in vitro* for a few hours they yield material that contains a high percentage of dipalmitoyl lecithin, which is a major component of the surfactant produced by type 2 alveolar lining cells (see page 272).[650] This observation may be significant in relation to the pathogenesis of endogenous lipid pneumonia.

PULMONARY ALVEOLAR MICROLITHIASIS

This rare condition is of unknown aetiology.[651] It is characterized by calcification in the lungs that may be so extensive as to produce almost completely opaque fields in radiographs. The condition may be symptomless for many years, and is usually discovered by chance in a routine chest film. No other condition produces a comparable form of miliary shadowing in the lungs. The calcification progresses slowly over many years, until eventually the presence of the concretions leads to severe dyspnoea and death from respiratory and cardiac failure. Functional studies on respiration in these cases show that the diffusion of oxygen and carbon dioxide across the alveolar wall is impaired and that the relative distribution of inspired air and of circulating blood in the lungs is uneven.[652]

At necropsy, the lungs are rock-hard and heavy.[653] In a case that we examined, each lung weighed more than 2 kg; a band saw was needed to cut the

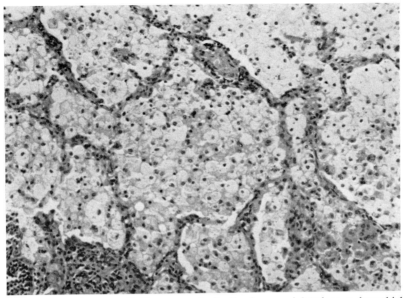

Fig. 7.63.§ Endogenous lipid pneumonia in the lung peripheral to a bronchial carcinoma, showing distension of air spaces by masses of tightly packed, foamy macrophages with small, round or oval nuclei. The lipid has been dissolved out during histological processing of the tissue. *Haematoxylin–eosin.* × 170.

lungs into slices. Histologically, enormous numbers of microliths, each filling most of an alveolus, can be seen as concentrically laminate structures in decalcified sections (Fig. 7.64). The alveolar walls surrounding them show delicate fibrosis. In less advanced areas, only occasional microliths may be scattered among otherwise normal air spaces.

In one reported case, microliths were also present in the bronchial wall, lying in groups between the smooth muscle and surface epithelium and presenting a distinctive nodularity.[654]

Tracheobronchopathia Osteoplastica[655]

This condition is unrelated to alveolar microlithiasis but may be mentioned here. It is a rare disease, affecting men oftener than women and seldom being recognized before the age of 50. Cartilage and bone form in the mucosa of the trachea and, less extensively, of the bronchi, appearing mainly external to the muscularis mucosae but sometimes immediately under the basement membrane of the surface epithelium. Unless the smaller bronchi are affected, with consequent obstruction, the condition is unlikely to endanger the patient. It has been known to interfere with tracheal intubation and the passage of an

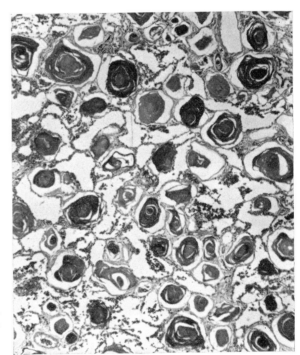

Fig. 7.64.§ Pulmonary alveolar microlithiasis. A severely affected part of the lung showing concentrically laminate microliths in most of the alveoli, and delicate fibrosis of the alveolar walls. *Decalcified tissue; haematoxylin–eosin.* × 40.

endoscope, and in one case fatal mediastinitis followed the resulting injury to the wall of the trachea.[656] The cause of the condition is unknown.

METASTATIC CALCIFICATION OF THE LUNG

Lime salts may be deposited in certain previously normal tissues when the level of serum calcium is intermittently or permanently high.[657, 658] In the lung, this condition must be distinguished from the dystrophic form of calcification that often follows chronic destructive lesions, especially those of tuberculosis and histoplasmosis. Metastatic calcification may occur in chronic renal disease, hyperparathyroidism, hypervitaminosis D, diseases such as Paget's disease of bone and osteopetrosis, primary and secondary tumours in bone, and leukaemia; it may also result from excessive consumption of milk and alkalis[659] and from the administration of large amounts of calcium gluconate.[660] In some cases, no cause is apparent. Deposits of lime salts are usually most conspicuous in the lungs and kidneys, but they may be found histologically in the mucous membrane of the stomach and rectum, and in the dura mater, heart, thyroid, liver, pancreas, tongue, articular tissues and skin. Local tissue alkalosis is thought to explain the localization of calcification in some sites,[661] there being, for example, a loss of carbon dioxide in the lungs and of fixed acids in the gastric mucosa and the kidneys.

Macroscopically, pale firm areas are seen on the cut surface of the lungs. The first impression may be that these are foci of pneumonic consolidation, but inspection through a hand lens reveals empty, fine air spaces with thickened walls. In severe cases, the lungs may be heavy, and feel gritty under the knife. Histologically, the calcium deposit, which stains deep blue with haematoxylin, is seen encrusting the elastic fibres in the alveolar walls, and also the walls of small blood vessels.

AMYLOIDOSIS

In amyloidosis secondary to chronic suppurative and comparable conditions, the lungs may be seen to contain minor deposits of amyloid when examined histologically, but never the large quantities that are found in the liver, spleen and kidneys.

Localized Amyloidosis.—Very rarely, nodules of amyloid form in a bronchus and obstruct the lumen, or are found in the parenchyma, presenting as single or multiple tumour-like shadows in chest radiographs; in neither of these localized forms of amyloidosis is any cause known.[662, 663] These deposits are termed 'amyloid tumours', and are much rarer in the bronchi and lungs than in the larynx (see page 252). Obstructive bronchial deposits may require endoscopic resection, but except when the diagnosis is in doubt there is seldom need to remove the pulmonary masses, for they usually enlarge only slowly. Histologically, the amyloid, which stains by the usual methods, is found mainly in the walls of the bronchi and alveoli. It may extend into the lumen of the alveoli, causing solidification of the parenchyma. Lymphocytes, plasma cells and multinucleate giant cells may be plentiful, and ossification sometimes occurs.[664]

CHEMICAL INJURY TO THE LUNGS

This section is concerned with injury to the lungs by exogenous chemicals other than the dusts that cause pneumoconiosis. The latter are considered in the next section (page 379).

Poisons and Drugs

The lungs can be damaged not only by inhaled fumes and dusts but also by chemical substances that reach them in the blood.[665] These substances may enter the body inadvertently or through therapeutic administration. Some are harmful to all patients who take them; others affect only those who are particularly sensitive, perhaps as a result of previous administration. The changes in the lungs may be part of a widespread reaction, or they may be the only manifestation of the injury. The range of chemicals that may harm the lungs is vast, and more are recognized every year. Some of the most important are described below to illustrate the types of pathological change that may result and that, when no cause has been recognized, may indicate the need to look for a chemical origin of the injury.

Paraquat[666]

This powerful weedkiller has the ecologically and commercially valuable property of being rapidly inactivated on contact with soil. On contact with plants it is reduced by chlorophyll: on reoxidation, it releases forms of oxygen, akin to hydrogen peroxide, that are poisonous to plants. Because it does not poison the soil, new crops can be grown

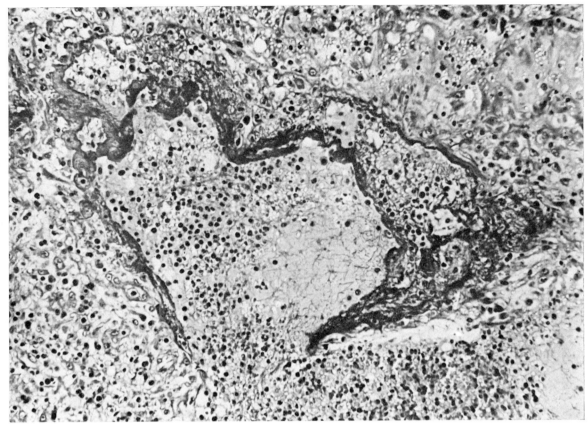

Fig. 7.65.§ Paraquat poisoning. The air space is filled with oedema fluid containing inflammatory cells and fibrin (the fibrin is darkly stained). The wall of the air space (near the edges of the photograph) is thickened by oedema, inflammatory cells and proliferating fibroblasts. *Fibrin stain.* × 200.

on treated sites within a few weeks, saving time and labour. Chemically, paraquat is 1,1′-dimethyl-4,4′-dipyridilium dichloride; it was formerly used as an indicator under the name methyl viologen.

Ingestion of even small quantities of paraquat solution is usually fatal. After initial vomiting, and then a day or more without symptoms, the patient becomes increasingly breathless and dies in extreme respiratory failure after one to three weeks.[667]

At necropsy, the lungs are plum-coloured and firm. The cut surfaces show haemorrhage and fibrosis. Microscopically, there is destruction of the wall of some alveoli and that of others is thickened by an infiltrate of chronic inflammatory cells and proliferating fibroblasts (Fig. 7.65). The lumen of the alveoli is commonly filled with blood, and there is often incipient organization of the clot. There may be fine 'honeycombing' of the lungs. The bronchiolar epithelium is proliferative and may extend into the alveoli.

The changes in the lungs are reproducible in animals.[668] As death is accelerated in experimental studies by keeping the animals in an atmosphere of oxygen, it is thought that the lungs are more susceptible to paraquat than other organs because of the free availability of oxygen, which, as in plants, could be converted into the cytotoxic reactive forms.[669] Electron microscopy of the lesions in animals shows cellular oedema followed by destruction: this is accompanied by a marked increase in the number of macrophages in the lung tissue, and this may lead to the widespread fibroblastic proliferation.[670, 671] Alternatively, paraquat or its products may have an oncogen-like effect on the fibroblasts.

It may be noted that if paraquat were handled sensibly, and stored in appropriately labelled cans instead of lemonade bottles, accidental poisoning might not occur. Fuller's earth, if administered quickly, can neutralize paraquat in the stomach: there is, at present, no antidote once it has been absorbed.

A boy who received a lung transplant in an attempt to save his life after accidental poisoning by paraquat died with similar changes in the transplanted lung, the consequence of paraquat that was still retained in his body.[666]

Iatrogenic Pulmonary Fibrosis ('Iatrogenic Interstitial Pneumonia')

Busulphan.—The alkylating agent busulphan is among the drugs best established in the treatment of chronic myeloid leukaemia. It is also used in treating some other malignant diseases. Its most familiar side effects include thrombocytopenia and bleeding, irreversible depression of haemopoiesis, sterility, and overpigmentation of the skin. A rarer effect is pulmonary fibrosis leading to fatal respiratory failure.[672] The term *busulphan lung* has been applied to this complication.[673]

The changes that characterize busulphan lung are the result of toxic oedema, manifested in a fibrinous, haemorrhagic exudate in the alveoli that becomes organized into fibrous tissue (Fig. 7.66), with obliteration of the lumen. The fibrosis is predominantly intra-alveolar, not interstitial as was

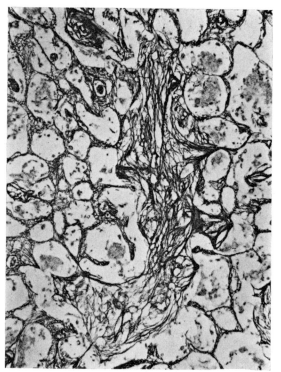

Fig. 7.66.§ Busulphan lung. Across the centre of the field is a broad band of reticular fibrous tissue within an alveolar duct, the result of organization of fibrinous exudate. *Silver impregnation of reticulin.* ×90.

originally reported. Another feature is the presence of large, atypical alveolar lining cells, which are thought to be altered type 2 cells (see page 272). Dysplasia of the bronchial epithelium has been described also.[674]

Busulphan lung is rare. The great therapeutic value of the drug vastly outweighs its dangers.

Hexamethonium.—Hexamethonium bromide was used extensively a few years ago as a ganglion-blocking agent in the treatment of high blood pressure: it has been replaced by drugs that are safer and more effective. It was one of the first drugs to be recognized as a cause of pulmonary fibrosis.[675, 676] Like busulphan, hexamethonium harms the lungs of only a small proportion of the patients who are given it. Fibrinous oedema results and organization leads to intra-alveolar fibrosis. Those patients who survived the acute episode developed scarring of the lungs, bronchiolectasis, and degenerative changes in the pulmonary elastic tissue, with formation of conchoidal bodies resembling the Schaumann bodies of sarcoidosis, and a giant cell reaction in relation to these structures.[676]

Bleomycin.—Bleomycin is an antibiotic with antineoplastic properties.[677] Promising results have been reported following its use in the treatment of squamous carcinomas arising in various parts of the body and also in some types of lymphoma. Death from pulmonary fibrosis was recorded in one per cent of one series of patients who had been treated with the drug;[678] other reports, and experiments on animals, suggest that less severe degrees of fibrosis occur with greater frequency.[679] It has been recommended that, if a patient complains of breathlessness during the course of treatment, the lungs should be examined radiologically every week and the administration of the drug discontinued if infiltrates appear. The histological changes are similar to those of busulphan lung (see above), dense fibrosis resulting in obliteration of the lumen of the alveoli.[680]

Iatrogenic Pulmonary Eosinophilia

Nitrofurantoin.—Nitrofurantoin, used in the treatment of urinary infections, is the therapeutic agent most frequently responsible for pulmonary eosinophilia. Others include aspirin, sodium aminosalicylate, penicillin and sulphonamides (see page 366). The pathological changes differ from those caused by busulphan, hexamethonium and bleo-mycin (see above) in that there are many eosino-phils and histiocytes as well as protein-rich oedema fluid in the air spaces. Sudden fever, dyspnoea and cough are the usual clinical manifestations; patchy shadows are seen in radiographs of the lungs. The illness usually subsides quickly when the drug is withdrawn, but it may persist for weeks and require suppression by corticosteroids.[665]

Oxygen and Ozone

Oxygen Poisoning.—The first demonstration of the toxicity of high concentrations of oxygen at ordinary atmospheric pressure was by Lorrain Smith in Belfast, in 1899.[681] He showed that mice developed severe pulmonary congestion and con-solidation when kept for four days in an atmosphere of 70 to 80 per cent of oxygen.

Patients whose lungs are ventilated with high concentrations of oxygen develop pulmonary oedema, with haemorrhage and the formation of fibrin in the alveoli.[682] There is hyperplasia of the type 2 alveolar lining cells; hyaline membrane formation and organization of the exudate may follow. The changes are similar to those caused by busulphan, hexamethonium and bleomycin (see above).

It is important to recognize that oxygen should not be administered, other than for short emergency periods, at a concentration of more than 40 per cent. Although the harmful effects of oxygen depend on oxygen tension rather than on the pressure *per se*,[683] the therapeutic use of oxygen under increased pressure ('hyperbaric oxygen') may have a toxic side action. Intermittent positive pressure ventila-tion increases the effect (see page 369).[684]

Electron microscopy has shown that the endo-thelial cells of the pulmonary capillaries are damaged more than the alveolar epithelium.[685]

Ozone.—Ozone is an important atmospheric pol-lutant. It is also a potential hazard of supersonic flight, especially at heights over about 12 000 metres (about 40 000 feet). High concentrations of ozone under experimental conditions cause necrosis of bronchiolar epithelium and changes in capillary endothelium, with consequent pulmonary oedema: the effects develop more quickly when animals are exposed to ozone than when they are exposed to hyperbaric oxygen.[686] The damage to the lungs is severest in the centrilobular regions: this has sug-gested that ozone may be a factor in the develop-ment of centrilobular emphysema (see page 291).

OCCUPATIONAL DUST DISEASES OF THE LUNGS

The Pneumoconioses

The injurious effects on the lungs of inhaling certain dusts have been recognized for more than 400 years. Georg Bauer, better known as Georgius Agricola, physician to the mining community of the Sankt Joachimsthal on the Bohemian side of the Ore Mountains, attributed diseases of the lungs in the miners to inhaled dust.[687] The changes that he described are not precisely identifiable from his account, but their association with in-capacity and progressive emaciation is consistent with silicosis, tuberculosis and cancer. Silicosis and accompanying tuberculosis are now known to have been prevalent among the miners in the region of Joachimsthal (Jáchymov, Czechoslovakia), as well as cancer associated with the high level of radio-activity of the ores in some of the silver and gold mines (see page 393).

The occurrence of occupational dust diseases in Britain was recognized soon after the discovery in 1720 that the addition of finely powdered, calcined flint to the 'body', or mixture, from which china is made produced a finer, whiter and tougher ware. The preparation and use of this flint powder was highly dangerous, causing the condition known as potters' rot, one of the first of the many trade names by which silicosis has been known during the two and a half centuries since then.[688]

The name *pneumoconiosis* is now used as a comprehensive term for the group of lung diseases that are caused by the inhalation and retention of industrial dusts. The Industrial Injuries Advisory Council in Britain defined pneumoconiosis in 1973 as 'permanent alteration of lung structure due to the inhalation of mineral dust and the tissue reactions of the lung to its presence', excluding bronchitis and emphysema.[689] Diseases that are caused by organic dusts, such as byssinosis (page 386) and farmers' lung (page 360), are not included among the pneumoconioses: this separate categori-zation is justifiable on the grounds that there are important differences between the effects of these dusts and those of mineral dust.

For lesions in the lung parenchyma to result from the presence of mineral dust the particles must be very small—less than 5 μm in diameter: larger particles are filtered out in the nose or removed by ciliary action from the main respiratory passages.[690] Generally speaking, with dusts of average density, the smaller the particle the likelier it is to be carried into the pulmonary alveoli. Observations on the distribution in the respiratory system of inhaled particles of various sizes have shown that over 80 per cent of those of about 2 μm in diameter reach the alveolar ducts and sacs; in contrast, hardly any of about 20 μm in diameter reach these parts of the lungs, over half being trapped in the trachea and main bronchi.[691] Since the lining cells of the alveolar ducts and sacs possess no cilia, some of those particles that settle in them are likely to be retained (and so ultimately to induce the formation of a chronic local lesion); others will be carried by phagocytes to the regional lymph nodes.[692, 693]

Radiological Grading of Pneumoconiosis

A scheme of grading the radiological appearances in pneumoconiosis has been adopted by the International Labour Organization and is used for all forms of the disease.[694] The smallest opacities (type p) are described as punctiform and measure up to 1·5 mm in diameter; larger lesions up to 3 mm in diameter (type q) are described as micronodular or miliary; and those over 3 mm and up to 1 cm in diameter (type r) are described as nodular. The findings in the films are graded into categories numbered 1 to 3 according to the increasing number and extent of the lesions. Opacities larger than 1 cm in diameter are graded A, B or C according to their extent.

Coal-Workers' Pneumoconiosis

This is the commonest form of pneumoconiosis in Britain. Two types are recognized, simple pneumoconiosis and progressive massive fibrosis ('complicated pneumoconiosis'): the former corresponds to categories 1 to 3 of the International Labour Organization grading (see above) and the latter to categories A to C.

Simple Pneumoconiosis

Simple pneumoconiosis is detected radiologically, usually in miners who are without symptoms unless they have chronic bronchitis or are cigarette smokers. Some degree of black pigmentation (*anthracosis*) of the lungs is common in the general urban population in the United Kingdom, especially in industrial areas.[695] Denser pigmentation is seen in coal miners and other coal-workers: in them the deposits may be dense enough to be recognizable in a chest radiograph. Profuse opacities are related to heavy exposure and a high content of dust in the lungs.[696] At necropsy, the lungs may show

small black lesions, several millimetres in diameter that either are distributed evenly throughout or have a tendency to be more numerous in the upper lobes.[697-699] These foci are called macules, or—if palpable—nodules. Each lesion lies near the centre of a secondary lobule; any respiratory bronchioles that are involved may be dilated ('focal emphysema' —see page 291) (Fig. 7.67).

Large numbers of macrophages laden with coal pigment are present in the alveoli and in the bronchiolar and alveolar walls. There is some associated fibrosis: in macules this takes the form of an increase in the number of reticulin fibres; in nodules the fibrosis is collagenous.[700] The normal clearance mechanism, by which the macrophages that have ingested particles travel toward the centre of the lobule and then escape by the bronchi and the bronchial lymphatics, becomes overloaded as a result of the enormous quantity of dust inhaled; in consequence, the pigment remains in the centre of the secondary lobule (Fig. 7.67). Silica is not concerned in the formation of the lesion of simple pneumoconiosis, and the patient with this condition appears to suffer no disability.

Progressive Massive Fibrosis ('Complicated Pneumoconiosis')

For reasons that are not understood, about 1 per cent of coal miners with simple pneumoconiosis (see above), especially those in categories 2 or 3, develop larger lesions and enter the radiological categories A to C. Disablement slowly—even very slowly—advances, with increasing breathlessness, cough, and, if the lesions cavitate, jet black sputum (melanoptysis); cor pulmonale may develop later. The radiological picture suggests the possibility of tuberculosis or cancer, and steps must usually be taken to exclude these.

At necropsy, besides the small anthracotic macules and nodules of simple pneumoconiosis there are larger, hard, black areas, usually in the upper parts of the lungs posteriorly: these may break down centrally and empty into a bronchus. Microscopically, large amounts of dust are enmeshed in dense, collagenous fibrous tissue that obliterates the air spaces (Fig. 7.68). There may be angitis.

In miners who have been engaged in drilling rock, collagenous nodules containing doubly-refractile crystals of silica are present as well.[701] Their collagen content increases with increasing numbers of visible silica crystals.[702]

Progressive massive fibrosis probably has an

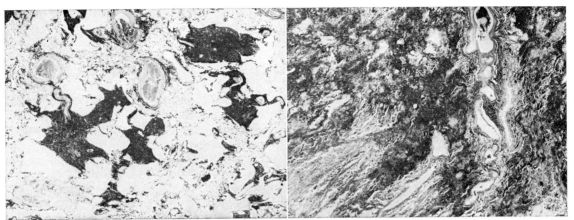

Fig. 7.67.§ Coal-workers' pneumoconiosis. Simple pneumoconiosis, showing heavy deposits of coal dust and surrounding emphysema. *Haematoxylin–eosin.* × 6.

Fig. 7.68.§ Coal-workers' pneumoconiosis. Progressive massive fibrosis, showing obliteration of air spaces by dense collagen and heavy deposits of coal dust. Compare with Fig. 7.67, which is at the same magnification. *Haematoxylin–eosin.* × 6.

immunological basis, but its pathogenesis is not yet understood. It is distinct from the condition that is known as massive conglomerate nodular silicosis (see page 382).

Rheumatoid Disease and Pneumoconiosis.—In some cases of pneumoconiosis in coal-workers the pulmonary disease is complicated by rheumatoid arthritis (see page 371).

Silicosis

This is the commonest and usually the gravest form of pneumoconiosis and is found frequently wherever mining and metal working are widely undertaken. Silica, in one form or another, is used in many trades—in the manufacture of glass and pottery, in the moulds used in iron foundries, as an abrasive in grinding and sandblasting, and as a furnace lining that is refractory to high temperatures. In coal mining in the United Kingdom the heaviest incidence of the disease has been in the anthracite pits in South Wales, where the thinness of the seams requires the removal of a large amount of siliceous rock, known as 'hard heading', to create galleries of a height sufficient for haulage; in recent years, however, the disease has become increasingly recognized in coal fields in other parts of the country as thinner seams come to be worked. The danger to the men in such workings arises from the dust formed during the removal of the siliceous rock. In South Africa, silicosis caused a high mortality among the gold miners on the Witwatersrand, where the metallic ore is embedded in a stratum of quartz.

As a rule, the miner or workman has to be exposed to the silica dust for many years—often some 20 or more—before the symptoms of silicosis first appear: by the time the disease becomes overt clinically, much irreparable damage has been inflicted on the lungs. From then onward, the respiratory disability progresses, until the patient can no longer continue full work and is compelled to seek lighter employment. Ultimately, in advanced cases, there may be distressing dyspnoea with even the slightest exercise.

The pathogenesis of silicosis has been the subject of prolonged study both in man and in experimental animals: it is still far from understood.[703] It seems that the finer particles of silica settle in the alveolar ducts and alveoli of the lungs. They are soon ingested by macrophages and then either expectorated or carried by these cells through lymphatics to the regional lymphoid tissue (the lymphoid nodules in the lungs themselves and, to some extent, the lymph nodes).[704] The silica may remain in these sites for the rest of the patient's life, persistently irritating the nearby tissues, either mechanically or by dissolving gradually to form a toxic substance that stimulates the formation of fibrous tissue.[705] The resulting silicotic nodules enlarge slowly until they form whorled, collagenous foci several millimetres in diameter (Fig. 7.69); in time, some of these may fuse to create the large masses typical of the terminal stages of the disease. The collagen has a hyaline appearance. Most of

N*

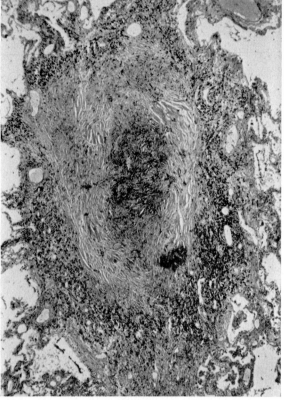

Fig. 7.69.§ Silicotic nodule—an oval area of dense collagen in which there are few nuclei. The dark, granular appearance at the centre and periphery is due to dust, largely carbonaceous, and much of it within macrophages. *Haematoxylin–eosin.* × 40.

the fibroblasts that formed it disappear, leaving only a few cells in the fibrotic tissue. The nodules inevitably impair respiratory function by compression of neighbouring small bronchi and bronchioles: silicotic lungs ultimately become markedly emphysematous—often with the formation of large bullae in their interior and along the free margins. The widespread fibrotic changes in the lungs may lead to obliteration of much of the pulmonary vasculature, perhaps contributing to the pulmonary hypertension that develops and the consequent right ventricular hypertrophy. As a result of the transportation of the coal and silica particles along the pulmonary lymphatics, the regional lymph nodes become enlarged, black and fibrous.

In severe cases, the numerous enlarging nodules may coalesce to form large fibrous masses. This is the condition that is known as *massive conglomerate nodular silicosis*.[706] It is to be distinguished from progressive massive fibrosis (page 380), in which there are no fibrotic nodules.

The first appearance and subsequent enlargement of the silicotic nodules in the lungs can be followed radiologically. Radiographs, especially when compared with standard films exemplifying various grades of silicosis, provide one of the most reliable diagnostic guides, even before there are significant clinical signs of respiratory disability.[707] At this early stage, the patient can change to some less physically arduous employment: but if he continues to be exposed to silica dust, the radiological opacities and his disability grow relentlessly worse. The final physical breakdown may be unexpectedly sudden, sometimes following a minor respiratory infection from which most normal people would recover quickly.

Complications.—One of the commonest and most feared complications of silicosis, which has often given rise to difficulties in the interpretation of the lesions, is chronic respiratory tuberculosis. Once this infection has been added to the silicosis, the prognosis rapidly worsens. It would seem that each condition advances more quickly when associated with the other than when present alone; the bacteria have been thought to destroy the lung substance all the more rapidly because the ingested silica particles interfere with the defensive activity of the macrophages and of the lymphoid tissues. The synergistic action of silica dust has long been held responsible for the inordinately high incidence of respiratory tuberculosis in the mining valleys of South Wales.

Sometimes the development of a distinctive form of pulmonary fibrosis, particularly in miners, is associated with rheumatoid arthritis (see page 371).[708, 709]

Pathogenesis.—The pathogenesis of silicosis is still a subject for speculation.[706] Evidence from electron microscopy suggests that when silica is ingested into a vesicle by a histiocyte, lysosomes inject enzymes into the vesicle, which bursts, liberating the enzymes into the cytoplasm, with consequent death of the cell.[710] Bursting of the vesicles does not happen following ingestion of inert dust particles. The dead histiocytes may be the source of a substance that stimulates fibroblasts to form collagen.[711] An interesting and unexplained phenomenon is that rats that inhale very large amounts of silica dust develop the microscopical changes of alveolar proteinosis (see page 289):[712] this may be due to a reaction involving the type 2 alveolar lining cells.

It is noteworthy that the hyaline fibrous tissue of silicotic foci is rich in globulins. This suggests that there is an abnormal immunological response.[713]

Asbestosis

Because of its fire-resisting properties and the ease with which its long thin fibrils can be spun into yarns and fabrics suitable for thermal and electrical insulation, asbestos has found many applications in industry since it was first widely introduced at the beginning of this century. Instances of pulmonary lesions in work-people were soon reported, sporadically at first and then in growing numbers. As a result of an official investigation, the hazards of work in this industry were recognized and appropriate precautions were recommended.[714]

Four types of asbestos are of commercial importance—chrysotile ('white' asbestos), amosite (brown asbestos), crocidolite (blue or Cape asbestos) and anthophyllite.[715, 716] Of these, chrysotile accounts for more than 90 per cent of the asbestos used in Britain: it has the longest and strongest fibres and can be carded, spun and woven. It is mined in Canada, Cyprus, South Africa and the Soviet Union. Crocidolite, reputedly the most dangerous, is mined in South Africa (Cape Province and the Transvaal); it is said to be no longer imported into Britain. The world production of asbestos has risen rapidly in recent years and is now estimated at over 4 million metric tons annually. It is used in a vast range of trades, particularly for fireproofing, in heat and sound insulation, for strengthening plastics and cement, and in a wide variety of other manufactured forms that make it part of the modern environment. Its near indestructibility accentuates the problems that its ubiquity poses in terms of health. Some of these are touched on again in relation to the aetiology of pleural mesothelioma (see page 408).

In the manufacture of asbestos material, a fine spicular dust is created that may be inhaled by unprotected operatives. As with other dusts, the larger particles are held in the upper respiratory passages and expelled with the sputum; smaller ones, some 20 μm or less in length, are often carried into the bronchioles and alveoli.[717] Once impacted, these sharp fibrils become coated with a film of protein. In time, a distinctive segmentation of the outer layer develops: the structures are then termed *asbestos bodies* (Fig. 7.70). In unstained films of sputum or histological sections asbestos bodies are yellowish. They give the Prussian blue reaction for iron when stained by Perls's method.

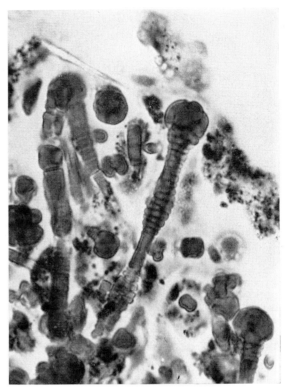

Fig. 7.70.§ A group of asbestos bodies in the lung. Characteristically segmented organic material covers the core of the fibre and forms a knob at its end. An uncovered fibre is present in the upper left quadrant. *Haematoxylin–eosin.* $\times 700$.

In tissue sections they may be found singly or in irregular clumps or stellate clusters.

The clinical signs of respiratory disability in cases of asbestosis develop much as in silicosis. As in that disease, the pulmonary fibrosis may be followed in the course of years by cardiac embarrassment, with enlargement of the right ventricle. Similarly, radiographs of the lungs show an initially fine mottling that in time becomes more coarsely granular.

When the lungs from a patient with advanced asbestosis are seen at necropsy, the pleura is found to be characteristically thickened and almost cartilaginous in toughness (see Fig. 7.71).[718] There is a variable degree of pulmonary fibrosis, especially of the subpleural parts of the lower lobes. Histologically, there is loss of the fine air spaces (Figs 7.72 and 7.73).[719] The few remaining airways, mostly bronchioles, are dilated and lined by tall or flattened epithelial cells or by goblet cells. Sometimes the epithelium is replaced by giant cells and macrophages. Within the lumen are asbestos fibres, asbestos bodies and cell debris. If

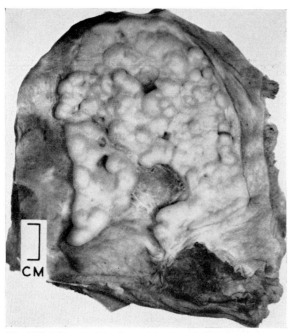

Fig. 7.71.§ Plaque of hyaline thickening of the diaphragmatic pleura in a case of asbestosis.

the bronchioles are very distended, the lung has a honeycomb appearance. Asbestos bodies may also be present in the fibrous tissue.

Complications.—As with silicosis, though less frequently, asbestosis may be complicated by tuberculosis. More important, however, asbestosis predisposes to two varieties of malignant neoplasm: carcinoma of the lung (Fig. 7.74)[720, 721] and mesothelioma of the pleura.[722] In four series reported in England and Germany between 1945 and 1955, carcinoma of the bronchus was found in one in about every six reported cases of asbestosis[723]—an incidence substantially higher than in silicosis. The reason for this difference is obscure; it may be that the small silica particles almost all settle in the alveoli, while the larger asbestos fibres become impacted in the smaller bronchi and bronchioles and damage the lining epithelium. The association of exposure to asbestos and mesothelioma of the pleura is considered on page 408.

Mixed-Dust Pneumoconiosis

This term is used when pneumoconiosis occurs as a result of exposure to a mixture of different types of mineral dust.[724] The mixtures most usually comprise iron and some silica: the occupations concerned include haematite mining, boiler scaling,

foundry work and graphite working. The pathological changes that result from exposure to the mixed dusts are similar to those of coal-workers' pneumoconiosis (see page 380).

Talc Pneumoconiosis ('Talcosis').—This form of pneumoconiosis is included among the mixed-dust pneumoconioses because talc (French chalk), a hydrated magnesium silicate mined in the form of steatite (soapstone), may contain both asbestos (anthophyllite and tremolite) and free silica. Soapstone carvers and polishers in parts of the Americas and of Africa have been known to develop talc pneumoconiosis through long exposure to the dust in unventilated workshops.[725]

Haematite Miners' Lung (Siderosilicosis).—The lungs of haematite miners when seen at necropsy are deeply pigmented with iron oxide and have a rusty colour in consequence; when much silica dust is also present in the workings there may be

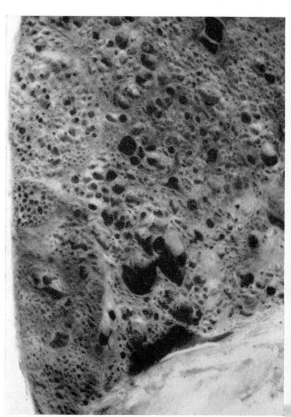

Fig. 7.72.§ Cut surface of the lung in asbestosis. The numerous abnormally large holes in the lung are dilated small bronchi and non-respiratory bronchioles. Dense fibrosis surrounds the dilated structures. *Pressure fixation; barium sulphate impregnation.* × 3.

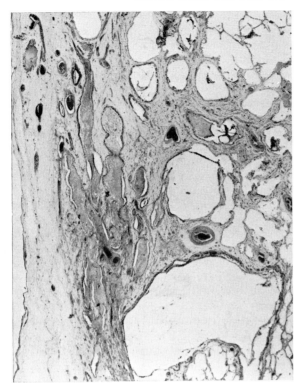

Fig. 7.73.§ Histological appearance of lung in asbestosis, showing dilated bronchioles, dense fibrosis and loss of alveoli. *Haematoxylin–eosin.* × 20.

Industrial Siderosis is both the commonest and the best known of the non-fibrosing forms of pneumo-coniosis.[727, 728] The changes are found in the lungs of workmen in many industries who are exposed for many years to fine iron dust. In arc-welding, iron is volatilized at the high temperatures employed, and the minute particles formed when it condenses may be inhaled as iron oxide by the welders, especially if they are working in a confined space such as the inside of a tank or boiler. Among many other occupations in which excessive amounts of iron dust may be inhaled are metal grinding and turning, and polishing silver with jeweller's rouge.

associated fibrosis.[726] In many cases the pulmonary changes may more correctly be termed 'sidero-silicosis' in view of the mixed nature of the condition. It is noteworthy that an unexpectedly large proportion of haematite miners die with respiratory tuberculosis or bronchial cancer; neither complication is typically a feature of pure siderosis (see below).

Industrial Siderosis

In haematite ore workings the miners are often exposed to atmospheres that are highly polluted with the dust created during extraction and handling (see above).

Much of the iron dust that is inhaled is trapped in the respiratory passages; the sputum is often notably rust-coloured. Some particles may reach the lungs and, after ingestion by alveolar macrophages, be deposited in the lymphoid tissue. Uncomplicated siderosis differs significantly from

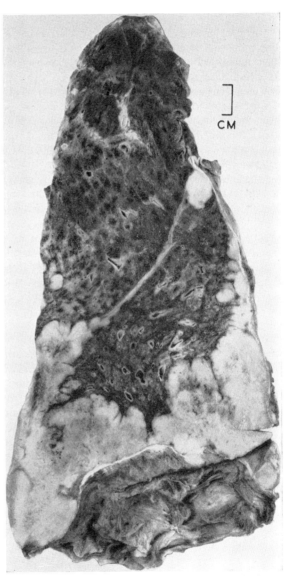

Fig. 7.74.§ Asbestosis and carcinoma of the lung. The lower lobe of this right lung is fibrotic, due to asbestosis, and has been compressed by a tumour growing in the pleural sac. The upper lobe shows centrilobular emphysema.

silicosis in that these focal deposits are not associated with fibrosis and disorganization of lung structure.[729] The reticulation and granular shadows in radiographs in this condition are the result of the natural opacity of iron to X-rays and are not, as in silicosis, due to fibrotic nodules replacing the normally shadowless, air-containing lung substance. It is no matter for surprise, therefore, that patients with uncomplicated siderosis do not present the cardiorespiratory disabilities so typical of silicosis.

Berylliosis

The industrial applications of the metal beryllium have expanded greatly. Its compounds, especially beryllium silicate, were used formerly as phosphors in fluorescent electric lights; mainly because of the danger involved in their manufacture, they have been replaced by other substances. An important use of the metal is in the tubular elements in atomic reactor piles, where its mechanical strength, high melting point, good thermal conductivity and lightness (its specific gravity is 1·86) give it many advantages. Moreover, it is readily penetrated by X-rays, and it is a good source of neutrons on bombardment; with its low atomic number it is an effective moderator for slow-moving neutrons in a reactor pile. Its alloys are becoming widely used, especially those with copper, on which it confers the valuable properties of elasticity and resistance to fatigue. A further use is in the production of refractory materials and crucibles that are to be subjected to particularly high temperatures.

Inhalation of beryllium dust or fumes is now known to be exceedingly dangerous on account of certain toxic properties. Those who worked with beryllium compounds, before precautionary measures were taken to reduce the hazard, suffered a high morbidity and mortality from their effects.[730, 731] Sometimes, the escape of dangerous fumes from the factories was on such a scale that people living in nearby houses, downwind from the places in which these materials were being worked, contracted and occasionally died from berylliosis ('neighbourhood cases'). The ill effects of beryllium compounds usually manifest themselves either as a contact dermatitis and conjunctivitis, or as acute or chronic pulmonary disease. There are good grounds for regarding these lesions as allergic, in part at least, for susceptibility varies widely from person to person, and many of those affected react strongly to skin tests with dilute solutions of beryllium salts. Skin tests in suspected cases must be undertaken with care, for occasionally in a highly sensitized person even so small an exposure may evoke a systemic reaction. Should beryllium enter the subcutaneous tissues through a cut or abrasion, as often happened in the earlier days of fluorescent lamp manufacture, a sarcoid-like granuloma soon appears at the site; in time, the overlying epidermis may break down to form an ulcer (see Chapter 39).

Much the most serious lesions in berylliosis are those produced in the lungs. Pulmonary berylliosis occurs in two forms. One is an acute pneumonia, usually following an attack of nasopharyngitis that appears to be essentially allergic. The other, and commoner, form is a widespread granulomatous pneumonia with a histological picture like that of sarcoidosis. Over a period of several years, with alternating exacerbations and remissions, these sarcoid-like granulomas undergo progressive fibrosis, with consequent grave impairment of pulmonary function.[732] In the later stages, when the disease has become chronic, the dispersal of beryllium from its site of initial absorption may lead to generalization of the disease and to the appearance of similar granulomas elsewhere, particularly in the liver, kidneys, spleen and skin.

Diseases Due to Organic Dusts

Byssinosis

Of the pulmonary diseases that follow exposure to organic dusts in Britain, outstandingly the most serious is byssinosis, which occurs among workers in the Lancashire cotton industry. In the carding of cotton, prior to spinning, a large amount of dust is created, and, although nowadays most of it is removed by ventilation, some is inevitably inhaled by the carders. Winding room workers also face a substantial risk of developing byssinosis.[733] The onset of the disease is gradual; it progresses through a well-defined series of stages, culminating in pronounced disability by middle age.

The dyspnoea of byssinosis is most distressing on resuming work after a short interval of absence —for this reason the disease is known colloquially as 'Monday fever' and 'Monday feeling'. In the younger operatives the feeling of tightness in the chest usually passes off soon after they leave the mill at the end of a shift; in older patients it persists much longer, and after years of exposure the typical symptoms of byssinosis are present almost continuously.

This form of dust disease is not associated with fibrosis of the lungs—the main pathological changes are those of an unspecific chronic bronchitis and emphysema.[734] The nature of the respiratory disturbances has been shown by functional studies: these demonstrate that the dyspnoea is associated with a decline in the maximum breathing capacity (see page 297), attributable to a reduction in the size of the bronchioles and to vesicular emphysema.[735] It was formerly supposed that this arose through allergic sensitization to some constituent of the cotton: more recent studies have suggested that the bronchiolar constriction is brought about by the local action of a histamine liberator present in the dust itself.[736] Either explanation would account for the congestion and oedema of the submucosa and the contraction of the muscle in the bronchial walls.

Bagassosis and Similar Conditions

Many organic dusts cause an extrinsic allergic alveolitis, similar to farmers' lung (see page 360).[737] One of the better known is *bagassosis*, which results from inhalation of the dust of bagasse (sugar cane after extraction of the sugar).[738] Dyspnoea, blood-streaked sputum, fever and mottling of the lungs in chest radiographs are the manifestations. Pulmonary fibrosis, emphysema and bronchiectasis are found at necropsy. Biopsy examination in early cases shows an interstitial pneumonia with giant cells.[739] The cause of the pulmonary changes is uncertain. No fungus or other specific allergen has been identified as consistently present.

Maple Bark Disease.—This affects the men who strip bark from maple logs[740] or others exposed to dust of maplewood and, in Britain,[741] of sycamore. It is essentially a granulomatous allergic reaction to spores of the fungus *Cryptostroma corticale*, which causes 'sooty bark disease', a common epiphytosis disease of trees of the genus *Acer*. Workers in paper mills may develop the disease. The fungus does not grow in animal tissues; it produces its effect through allergic sensitization of the patient.

Paprika Splitters' Lung.—The women who open the fruit of the capsicum in the preparation of Hungarian red pepper are liable to chronic pulmonary fibrosis and bronchiectasis, apparently as an outcome of allergic sensitization to *Mucor stolonifer*, a mould that grows abundantly in the dried fruit without spoiling it.[742] The condition persists now only when paprika is still prepared under cottage industry conditions: it is not a problem in properly ventilated workshops.

Mushroom Growers' Lung.—This condition affects a small proportion of the workers who prepare compost for growing mushrooms.[743] Originally blamed on the formation of nitrogen dioxide during pasteurization of the compost, which might have been expected to affect all, not only some, of those exposed, it is now considered to be due to individual sensitization to some constituent of the compost.

Feather Pickers' Disease ('Duck Fever').—A condition that resembles byssinosis clinically (see opposite) has been observed among French workers who clean and sort the feathers of ducks and geese.[744] While it is evident that dust from the feathers is responsible, the constituent that produces the response has not been identified.

PULMONARY TRANSPLANTATION

A review of 27 cases of human lung transplantation performed by 1971[745] showed that survival generally had been short, fatal respiratory failure supervening early. Infection has been a common complication, predisposed to by the immunosuppressant therapy. In the case of a patient with paraquat poisoning, enough paraquat remained in the body after several days to affect the transplanted lung (see page 378).[746]

Physiological studies after the operation have shown a gross imbalance between the two lungs in the distribution of gas and blood. Most of the gas goes to the patient's own lung and most of the blood to the transplanted one.[747]

TUMOURS OF THE TRACHEA, BRONCHI, LUNGS AND PLEURA

BENIGN TUMOURS AND TUMOUR-LIKE CONDITIONS

It is convenient and appropriate to consider the tumours arising in the trachea and bronchi, lungs and pleura together. When particular tumours have characteristics that are specially related to their origin in one of these different anatomical parts these are noted accordingly.

Benign Epithelial Tumours

Adenoma

An adenoma is rarely found in the bronchial tree. Formerly, the carcinoid tumour (see page 401) was commonly interpreted as adenomatous.

True adenomas of the bronchial mucous glands may closely reproduce the structure of these glands. Others are cystic tumours or benign muco-epidermoid tumours,[748] the latter corresponding to the tumour of salivary glands that goes by that name (see page 401 and Chapter 11).

Papilloma

Papillomas of the bronchial tree are also very rare, which is perhaps surprising in relation to the frequency of carcinomas arising from the same epithelium. Most of the patients with papillomas are young. The growths are commonly multiple.[749] They appear as wart-like projections from the bronchial lining. Microscopically, they are composed of wavy folds of ciliate epithelium or stratified squamous epithelium on a core of connective tissue. They may become malignant.

Paraganglioma (Chemodectoma)

The paraganglioma is a rare tumour.[750] It is usually of microscopical size. It consists of collections of small, round or spindle-shaped cells arranged in relation to a sinusoidal and capillary vasculature resembling that of normal chemoreceptor organs (see page 257 and Chapter 41). Nerve filaments have been demonstrated in the tumours by means of silvering methods.[751]

'Tumourlets'

The so-called tumourlets are microscopical collections of small, tightly packed, proliferating, round or spindle-shaped cells. They are occasional findings in scarred areas of the lungs, especially in relation to bronchiectatic lesions.[752] They are benign and no longer regarded as premalignant. They must be distinguished from carcinoid tumours and chemodectomas, neither of which is associated with evidence of previous damage to the lungs.

Benign Clear Cell Tumour

The origin of the very rare benign tumour composed of closely packed, large, clear cells is uncertain.[753] The cells contain much glycogen.

Endometriosis of the Lungs and Pleura

Although endometriosis is not a neoplastic disease, this is a convenient place to refer to its occurrence in the lungs. Pulmonary endometriosis is very rare and its diagnosis has been considered debatable in some of the published cases.[754] The lesions have been described in the substance of the lungs themselves, in the visceral pleura and in the tracheobronchial tree. If endometrial tissue is found in these situations its genesis is uncertain: it could conceivably result either from embolism of endometrium that has entered the blood stream in the uterus or from metaplasia of pulmonary tissue. In conformity with the metaplastic theory of the development of some cases of pelvic endometriosis (see Chapter 27), it is possible that metaplasia of the pleural mesothelium accounts for pleural endometriosis. Bronchial endometriosis[755] and endometriosis of the parenchyma of the lungs[754] seem unlikely to be explicable on a basis of metaplasia. In one case, recurrent haemoptysis was found to be associated with an endometriotic focus in a main bronchus and extending into the adjoining parenchyma of the lung:[756] the patient had had an abortion by curettage 16 months before the start of the bronchial bleeding, which coincided with menstruation. In another case, biopsy findings that on review were considered to be unquestionably those of endometriosis had originally been interpreted as diagnostic of anaplastic carcinoma, leading to pneumonectomy.[756]

Benign Tumour-like Growths of Mixed Structure

Chondroadenoma

The chondroadenoma,[757, 758] which is a hamartoma, is known also as adenochondroma and mixed tumour. The last of these synonyms is best avoided as it can be confused with the similarly named tumours of bronchial mucosal glands (see page 402). The chondroadenoma is composed mainly of cartilage, but epithelial elements are almost always present. It is commoner in men, and is usually encountered incidentally in radiographs or at necropsy. It usually lies in the substance of the lung, often remote from the major bronchi, and it is commoner in the lower half of the organ. Usually it is from 1 to 3 cm in diameter, but much larger examples have been described. It is somewhat lobulate, and sharply demarcated from the surrounding lung tissue; its cut surface is recognizably cartilaginous in consistency and translucency (Fig. 7 75).

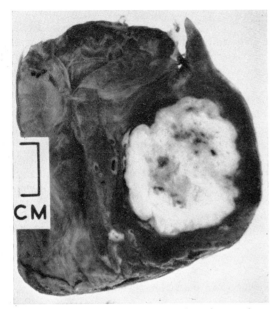

Fig. 7.75.§ Benign chondroadenoma of the lung, a hamartoma of bronchial origin. The tumour was found unexpectedly on X-ray examination of the chest, presenting as a symptomless, peripheral, 'coin' shadow; it was removed surgically.

Histologically, rounded masses of cartilage are enclosed by connective tissue in which there are clefts lined by columnar, ciliate, cubical or flattened epithelium. Less commonly, adipose and lymphoid tissues may be present. Areas of calcification and ossification are sometimes seen. Malignant change occurs exceptionally rarely (see page 407).

Intrabronchial chondroadenomas are much rarer than the extrabronchial tumours just described.[759] They occur in the large bronchi and, more rarely, in the trachea.[760]

Benign Connective Tissue Tumours

Chondroma

The pulmonary chondroma differs from the chondroadenoma (see above) in being composed of cartilage only.[761] It grows from bronchial cartilage and usually protrudes into the lumen, which it may obstruct. Chondrosarcomatous change may occur (see page 407).

Angioma and Arteriovenous Aneurysm

The angiomas of the lungs are hamartomas. They may be solitary or multiple. Often, when very small, they cause no trouble, but if large vessels take part there may be serious shunting of deoxygenated blood from the pulmonary arteries to the pulmonary veins. Lesions of the latter type are essentially arteriovenous aneurysms.[762] The shunt results in cyanosis, polycythaemia and clubbing of the digits. The increased blood volume in cases of pulmonary arteriovenous shunt is due simply to the increased number of circulating red blood cells: the plasma volume is normal and the haematocrit level is raised (in cases of systemic arteriovenous shunt there is an increase in the volume of the plasma as well as in the red cell count, and therefore the haematocrit reading is little if at all altered from normal levels). Cyanosis accompanies a pulmonary arteriovenous aneurysm only if the shunt involves about a fifth of the cardiac output, with a reduced haemoglobin of not less than 5 g/dl of blood.[763]

Pulmonary angiomas are commonly associated with hereditary telangiectasia (Rendu–Osler–Weber syndrome—see page 166): the association is seen in over 35 per cent of those cases in which there is a solitary pulmonary lesion and in almost 60 per cent of those with multiple lesions.[764]

Vascular hamartomas of the tracheal or bronchial mucosa may be the source of uncontrollable bleeding if injured in the course of endoscopy.[765]

'Sclerosing Angioma'

The condition that is generally still referred to as 'sclerosing angioma' is of debatable nature. It was originally believed to be primarily vascular,[766] but the initial change is now believed to be a proliferation of undifferentiated alveolar mesenchymal cells:[767] these cells form buds, protruding into the lumen, with differentiation of a surface layer of cubical cells and a deeper fibroblastic zone into which capillary blood vessels grow. These vessels are the source of bleeding, and the lesion comes to contain much haemosiderin. Many of the patients give a history of haemoptysis, which may have been recurrent over a period of years. The condition is seen most frequently in women; it is particularly rare after the age of 50. It is one of the causes of a 'coin shadow' in radiographs of the lungs. Usually it is situated within the substance of a lung, but sometimes it abuts on the pleura and even protrudes into the pleural cavity: fatal haemorrhage has resulted from injury to a subpleural 'sclerosing angioma' during attempted needle biopsy.[768]

The 'sclerosing angioma' is to be distinguished from the so-called pulmonary histiocytoma (see below). It may also be noted that there is no reason to believe that there is any relation between this lesion of the lungs and the similarly named 'sclerosing haemangioma' or histiocytoma, (dermatofibroma), of the skin (see Chapter 39).

Leiomyoma[769]

Leiomyomas may arise in the trachea or bronchi, causing obstruction,[770] or within the substance of the lung. Microscopically, they closely resemble uterine fibroids. Hyalinization, calcification and ossification may occur. Care has to be taken to exclude the possibility that what appears to be a primary pulmonary leiomyoma is a secondary deposit of a well-differentiated leiomyosarcoma arising in the uterus[771] or elsewhere. It may also be difficult to distinguish histologically between a leiomyoma and a primary leiomyosarcoma of the lungs.

'Granular Cell Myoblastoma'[772]

This is one of the rarest of the tumours that arise in the lungs. Its origin is the wall of the trachea or bronchi. It may cause obstruction. Microscopically, it does not differ from the corresponding tumour elsewhere in the body (see Chapter 39). Most of the patients are adults between 30 and 60. The tumour is not encapsulate but ordinarily it does not extend widely from its site of origin. Direct invasion through the bronchial wall into adjacent lymph nodes has been recorded.[773] Widespread haematogenous metastasis was present in one case.[774]

Fibroma of Lung

This rare tumour may arise in the trachea or bronchi or in the tissue of a lung. Microscopically, its structure is that of any fibroma. When abutting on the pleura it may be difficult to distinguish from a pleural fibroma (see below). Myxomatoid change may occur in part or the whole of the growth.[775]

Fibroma of the Pleura

The pleural fibroma is a distinctive lesion. It may grow into the pleural sac on a pedicle and become very large. In one series of 24 cases, 16 of the patients had changes in joints that simulated rheumatoid arthritis;[776] this arthritis subsides after excision of the pleural tumour and may return if the latter recurs. Histologically, there may be nothing to distinguish a pleural fibroma from any other fibroma. Occasionally, clefts lined by cells resembling mesothelium are found: such

tumours are sometimes referred to as *benign mesotheliomas*—care must be taken to exclude the possibility that the growth is a malignant mesothelioma (see page 407). Some pleural fibromas have a peculiar structure, with palisade or rosette-like arrangements of small, darkly staining, spindle-shaped cells (Fig. 7.76).

Pleural fibromas are generally considered to be true tumours. However, histologically similar masses have been known to follow pneumonia.[777] It has been suggested that encysted or interlobar pleural effusions, such as might accompany a pulmonary infection, may occasionally form a medium in which mesothelial cells can grow, some differentiating to form fibroblasts and others retaining their mesothelial character, lining clefts in the resulting fibromatoid mass.[778]

Neurofibroma and Related Tumours[779]

Neurofibromas and neurolemmomas may arise in the lungs. It can be very difficult to decide whether they are benign or malignant. In some cases the pulmonary tumours are associated with generalized neurofibromatosis (von Recklinghausen's disease of nerves); occasionally there are multiple lesions in

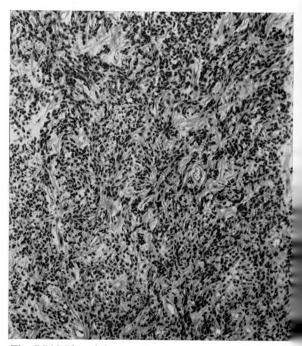

Fig. 7.76.§ Pleural fibroma (benign fibrous mesothelioma). It is composed of closely packed, small, short, spindle-shaped cells, separated by a little collagen. *Haematoxylin-eosin.* × 100.

the lungs and pleura but none elsewhere in the body.[780]

Lipoma

Adipose tissue is sometimes normally present in small amounts under the visceral pleura. More characteristically, it is a normal component of the bronchial wall, between the cartilage rings and the muscularis mucosae.[781] It is also found in some older people within ossified bronchial cartilage. Lipomas may arise in the bronchi[782] and under the pleura.[783] Those in the bronchi tend to protrude in polypoid fashion into the lumen, leading to obstruction and its consequences. Symptoms seldom occur before the fifth decade.

'Histiocytoma' (Plasma Cell Granuloma)[784]

This infrequent benign condition has many synonyms, a consequence of uncertainty about its nature. It has been regarded as an endothelioma,[785] a plasmacytoma[786] and a histiocytoma,[787] but it is probably inflammatory rather than neoplastic. For convenience it may be considered here. It occurs at all ages and in both sexes. The lesion is typically solitary, spherical, encapsulate and situated within the substance of the lung. It is friable or hard and fibrous, and it may be in part calcified. Distinctive yellow areas are usually present on the grey or brownish cut surface.

Microscopically, the structure varies from case to case. There is generally a mixture of fibroblastic tissue, collagen, small blood vessels, foamy and haemosiderin-laden macrophages (histiocytes), and a more or less heavy infiltrate of plasma cells with a variable but smaller proportion of lymphocytes. Russell bodies are sometimes conspicuously numerous: when they are, the possibility of infection by *Klebsiella rhinoscleromatis* (scleroma) may have to be considered (see page 204). When plasma cells are present in very large numbers the diagnosis of plasmacytoma (myeloma) may be suggested, but the conspicuous participation of histiocytes and the collagenous elements distinguish the lesion from the true solitary plasmacytoma (see page 407).

Although some pulmonary 'histiocytomas' have a notable resemblance to the so-called histiocytoma (dermatofibroma) of the skin (see Chapter 39), there is no evidence that these two conditions are of the same nature. There is a history of pneumonia in some cases of pulmonary 'histiocytoma',[788] occasionally with radiographic evidence of the rapid evolution of the spherical lesion during recovery from the acute infection: once it has reached its full size, which rarely exceeds 5 to 6 cm in diameter, it tends to remain unchanged for an indefinite period prior to excision.

Benign 'Lymphoma' (Pseudolymphoma)[789]

The benign pulmonary 'lymphoma' takes the form of a pinkish white consolidation of the parenchyma, with a hazy outline. The hilar lymph nodes are not involved, although they may show simple hyperplastic changes. Microscopically, dense aggregates of mature lymphocytes infiltrate or replace the parenchyma of the affected region; toward the periphery of the lesion the aggregates are less closely packed, and they form interstitial nodules that may have to be distinguished in needle biopsy specimens from foci of predominantly lymphocytic interstitial pneumonia (see page 370). Germinal centres (Flemming centres) are often present. The appearances suggest an inflammatory rather than a neoplastic condition: the name pseudolymphoma was introduced for this reason,[789] and the term solitary lymphocytic granuloma of the lung is also sometimes used.

It may be difficult to distinguish this condition from lymphocytic lymphomas (see page 407). In general, the prognosis after surgical excision is good. However, cases are on record in which there appears to have been a change from 'benign lymphoma' to a malignant condition, such as Hodgkin's disease.[790]

PRIMARY MALIGNANT TUMOURS

A classification of malignant tumours of the lungs was published by the World Health Organization in 1967.[791] It is reproduced in Table 7.10. Its object is to encourage international standardization of nomenclature, so that medical authorities everywhere may compare their results and improve treatment without the serious confusion that is inseparable from the use of different classifications.

Although it is admitted that a generally acceptable, unambiguous classification of tumours is still an unattainable ideal, and that all existing classifications, including the most recent World Health Organization one, are open to argument and debate, the malignant tumours of the lungs will be described in this chapter in the order indicated in the World Health Organization schedule.

Table 7.10. *World Health Organization Classification of the Histological Types of Malignant Tumours Arising in the Lungs**

I. EPIDERMOID CARCINOMAS†

II. SMALL CELL ANAPLASTIC CARCINOMAS
  1. Fusiform cell type
  2. Polygonal cell type
  3. Lymphocyte-like cell ('oat cell') type
  4. Others

III. ADENOCARCINOMAS
  1. Bronchogenic
    a. acinar   } with or without mucin formation
    b. papillary }
  2. Bronchiolo-alveolar

IV. LARGE CELL CARCINOMAS
  1. Solid tumours with mucin-like content
  2. Solid tumours without mucin-like content
  3. Giant cell carcinomas
  4. 'Clear cell' carcinomas

V. COMBINED EPIDERMOID AND ADENOCARCINOMAS

VI. CARCINOID TUMOURS

VII. BRONCHIAL GLAND TUMOURS
  1. Cylindromas
  2. Mucoepidermoid tumours
  3. Others

VIII. PAPILLARY TUMOURS OF THE SURFACE EPITHELIUM
  1. Epidermoid
  2. Epidermoid with goblet cells
  3. Others

IX. 'MIXED' TUMOURS AND CARCINOSARCOMAS
  1. 'Mixed' tumours
  2. Carcinosarcomas of embryonal type ('blastomas')
  3. Other carcinosarcomas

X. SARCOMAS

XI. UNCLASSIFIED

XII. MESOTHELIOMAS
  1. Localized
  2. Diffuse

XIII. MELANOMAS

---

* Kreyberg, L., Liebow, A. A., Uehlinger, E. A., *Histological Typing of Lung Tumours*, pages 19–26. Geneva, 1967.
† In the text of this chapter the tumours that are termed *epidermoid carcinomas* in the World Health Organization classification are referred to as *squamous carcinomas*.

Carcinoma of the Trachea, Bronchi and Lungs

Epidemiology

Bronchial carcinoma has become one of the commonest of pulmonary diseases. The steady, uninterrupted rise in its incidence during the past half-century is one of the most striking features of the mortality statistics in many parts of the world. In 1921, in England and Wales, there were 1240 deaths from lung cancer among men and 481 among women: in 1973 the corresponding figures were 26 032 and 6144.[792] At present, bronchial carcinoma accounts for more deaths among men than any other single form of cancer; it occurs less often among women, but a comparable rise is clearly recognizable (Table 7.11). High as are the

Table 7.11. *Deaths from Cancer of the Bronchus and Lung in England and Wales, 1948 to 1970**

Year	Males	Females
1948	8 403	1 759
1950	10 254	1 987
1952	11 981	2 247
1954	13 995	2 336
1956	15 615	2 571
1958	17 040	2 780
1960	18 882	3 118
1962	20 278	3 501
1964	21 476	3 895
1966	22 538	4 370
1968	23 871	4 911
1970	24 874	5 347
1972	25 728	5 883

* From *The Registrar General's Statistical Reviews of England and Wales for the Years 1948 to 1972;* London, 1949–74.

published returns, it seems likely that they underestimate the real incidence of this generally fatal disease. Indeed, mortality records show that in recent years one in about eight deaths among men aged from 45 to 64 years is attributable to bronchial cancer.[793]

Among the many pitfalls to be avoided in interpreting mortality data, two are always to be borne in mind: first, that changes in terminology have led to the transfer of deaths from one specific disease category to another; and second, that a rise in the recorded incidence may have been spurious, reflecting improvements in diagnostic methods. As regards carcinoma of the bronchus, there is no indication that the increase recorded since the second world war can be ascribed to either source of error.[794] During the period for which figures are shown in Table 7.11, the Registrars General for England and Wales made no change in the method of classifying bronchial cancer. Should any suspicion exist that these records have been affected in this way, the absence of any sharp discontinuities in the rising trends for both sexes—the usual sequel to any important change in methods of classification—should allay it. That any serious errors have arisen from the introduction of improved techniques of diagnosis during this short period seems unlikely, though a minor rise may have followed the greater availability of radiological and bronchoscopic aids to clinical diagnosis. In short, it seems indisputable that a remarkable and very disturbing increase in the incidence of this form of cancer has taken place during the middle period of this century.

Aetiology

While statistical records can, and often do, provide invaluable clues in the search for aetiological factors, it must again be emphasized that this approach is beset with hazards and that anyone who employs it must keep a watchful eye for possible fallacies. Comparisons drawn between the statistics of different countries should be highly suspect; customs and circumstances of life vary so widely that convincing associations of cause and effect can rarely be derived. Even within a single country the differing availability of modern diagnostic techniques always handicaps, and sometimes invalidates, comparisons between the incidence of a disease in urban and rural communities. Evidence of some aetiological connexion becomes most convincing when comparison is made between two population groups selected for their agreement in all respects except for the presence or absence of the factor under suspicion.

Our knowledge of the causation of bronchial cancer gained significantly from studies in occupational medicine. A succession of investigations of the exceptionally high incidence of bronchial cancer among the miners in the Schneeberg and Joachimstal (Jáchymov) provided classic studies of the pathogenesis of the disease. These mines in the Erzgebirge —the Ore Mountains—of Saxony and Bohemia have for centuries been worked for various metals, among them silver, gold, nickel, cobalt, arsenic and, latterly, radium and uranium. Throughout their history they have had a sinister reputation for the high incidence of a distinctive disease among those long employed underground.[795] The neoplastic nature of this pulmonary disease, which develops in early middle life and is always fatal, was first recognized towards the end of the last century; several official commissions confirmed this conclusion.[796] It seems probable that the oncogens are radon gas and radioactive dust that are liberated at rock faces newly exposed by blasting: the shaft with the highest mortality among the drillers and hewers proved to be the one with the highest radioactivity in its galleries. So heavy was the exposure of these men that more than half died, many of them before the age of 40, from cancer of the lung.

The implication that the Schneeberg lung cancer was due to an inhaled oncogenic agent naturally led to the supposition that in other circumstances some comparable, though less potent, factor might be responsible for bronchial cancer. As a result, many of the changing features of modern life have come under review and so a clearer picture of the aetiology of the disease in the general population in western countries has begun to emerge.

In searching for a possible oncogen it was apparent that a factor causing one in every 12 or so deaths of men in Britain cannot be associated with any particular occupation, but must act widely among the adult, male, population. Although it is known that special health hazards are associated with particular industries, such as those in which workers are in close contact with arsenic and asbestos, the total contributions made by such dangerous occupations to national mortality returns for lung cancer are clearly negligible when compared with those that result from some agent that affects people in general. It was because the consumption of tobacco had increased so much during recent decades that suspicion ultimately fell on cigarettes.

Numerous studies have been made in many countries on the possible role of smoking in the causation of bronchial cancer. They have varied widely in quality from an epidemiological standpoint, and the conclusions published have sometimes been affected by other than strictly scientific considerations. Most of them have been retrospective: this means that enquiries have been made into the previous smoking habits of a large number of patients with an established diagnosis of bronchial cancer. Studies of this kind are not free of an intrinsic bias, and wherever possible they should be replaced by prospective investigations. It is noteworthy that retrospective and prospective studies of the relation between smoking and lung cancer have shown good agreement.[797] The principle of a prospective study is that a suspected factor is isolated as far as possible statistically and that its supposed effect on the incidence of the disease in the selected population is examined in the light of mortality returns that are collected subsequently. The main drawback to prospective studies is the length of time, often many years, before sufficient data are obtained to indicate conclusions that fulfil the criteria for statistical significance.

One prospective investigation on smoking and lung cancer—the best of its kind yet undertaken —has been carried out in the United Kingdom.[798] In 1951, 50 000 medical practitioners in this country were sent a questionnaire asking for details of their past and current smoking habits. Forty thousand of them returned usable replies: on the basis of their answers these doctors were classified into a few broad groups. When any of the doctors died, the certified cause of death was obtained from the Registrar General. From the interim report in 1956, which recorded the causes of death of 1714 male doctors aged 35 or over, the results of this survey up to that time may be summed up as follows.[799] Mortality from bronchial cancer is closely correlated with cigarette smoking, less so with smoking pipes and cigars. The annual death rate from this form of cancer ranged from 0·07 per thousand in non-smokers to 2·76 per thousand in heavy cigarette smokers; the likelihood of a medical man in Britain dying from bronchial cancer is thus many times greater in the group of heavy smokers. The death rates for medium and light smokers were correspondingly intermediate between those for heavy smokers and non-smokers. These conclusions have been more than amply confirmed[800] since the interim report appeared.[799] The contrary views are referred to in the more recent appraisal published by the Royal College of Physicians of London[800] and seem clearly to run counter to the vast evidence that has accumulated.

The now widely accepted connexion between tobacco smoking and bronchial cancer[800] has led to many efforts to recover and identify oncogenic products of partial combustion in cigarette smoke. In most instances, the test has been made by painting the skin of mice with preparations of the distilled vegetable tars formed from tobacco at the relatively high temperatures at which cigarettes are designed to burn; in a few studies, animals have been exposed to tobacco smoke in insufflation chambers for long periods. The value of these experiments is questionable, for the susceptibility of different animal species to known oncogenic substances has been found to vary widely: it is doubtful if a substance that is carcinogenic for the mucosal epithelium of the bronchi of man will necessarily be so for the epidermal cells of the mouse. Inferences based on the results of such experiments, whether positive or negative, are manifestly suspect. Further, it should be realized that cigarette smoking may be acting oncogenetically

as a 'promoting' agent rather than as an 'initiating' agent, to use Rous's terms: in either case cigarette smoke remains incriminated as far as bronchial cancer in man is concerned.

The higher incidence of bronchial cancer in urban areas has suggested that some form of atmospheric pollution may play a part in the pathogenesis of the disease. However, the difference in incidence between town and country dwellers is small in comparison with that between smokers and non-smokers. Moreover, this difference may well be exaggerated as a result of the better facilities for diagnosis usually available in urban medical practice. Any difference that remains may be ascribed more to the greater consumption of cigarettes by town people than to air pollution, such as that caused by internal combustion engines. Were the latter important, bronchial cancer might be expected to be commoner among men such as bus drivers and conductors, and garage staff, whose occupation heavily exposes them to the exhaust fumes of petrol and diesel engines: no such raised occupational incidence has been recorded.[801] Finally, in the Channel Islands, where atmospheric pollution is negligible but cigarette consumption high, bronchial cancer is as prevalent as in the United Kingdom; the same is true of Venice and other large cities in Italy.[802]

General Structural Changes in the Lungs in Bronchial Carcinoma

Cancers arise in any part of the lungs, and their progress and prognosis are to some extent related to their site of origin. Their situation is described as hilar when they arise in a named bronchus, intermediate when in a macroscopically visible branch of a named bronchus, and peripheral when arising in one of the smaller bronchi or bronchioles.[803] There is some general correlation between the site of origin and the histological type of a bronchial tumour: squamous carcinomas are commonest in the hilar region and adenocarcinomas in the peripheral zones; 'oat cell' carcinomas occur with roughly equal frequency in the hilar and peripheral zones. 'Oat cell' tumours spread so extensively that it is often difficult to determine their site of origin with certainty. In the intermediate zone, tumours are less common and their histological type varies more widely.

Bronchial carcinoma may spread distally, within the bronchus or along lymphatics in its wall into the related wedge of lung, or centripetally to the regional lymph nodes. In the case of 'oat cell' and squamous carcinomas, such hilar masses are liable to extend into surrounding structures; in particular, the pericardial sac (Fig. 1.4, page 7) and heart are liable to be invaded. Invasion of the pericardium results in a blood-stained effusion; in the heart, the growth may infiltrate and even destroy a large portion of the myocardium, particularly of the atria. Cancers that arise in the main bronchus to the right upper lobe often compress and infiltrate the superior vena cava, which may eventually be closed by the formation of a large thrombus over the affected surface of the intima (Fig. 7.77).

Less often, a carcinoma arises within the lung, producing a discrete mass that is readily visible in radiographs. At necropsy, such growths are seen to infiltrate the surrounding lung substance. They are less apt than hilar tumours to cause bronchial obstruction; they are likelier to spread

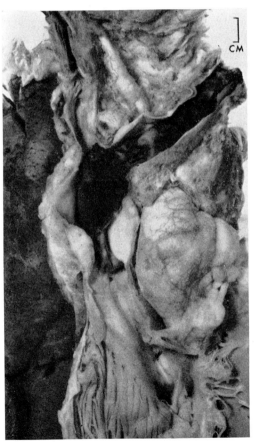

Fig. 7.77.§ Thrombosis of the superior vena cava following encirclement and invasion of the vessel by carcinomatous tissue extending from a primary bronchial growth. The thrombus has extended into both brachiocephalic veins and their tributaries.

toward the periphery of the lung and to involve the chest wall.

A peripheral tumour that arises in the apical part of a lung, sometimes—but not usually—in evident association with the scar of a tuberculous lesion, may extend into the brachial plexus and the cervical portion of the sympathetic nervous chain. This results in the neurological syndrome that has been named after Pancoast, who first described it[804]—pain and muscle wasting in the hand of the affected side, accompanied by the Bernard–Horner syndrome (contracted pupil, ptosis, and ipsilateral facial anhidrosis and vasodilatation).

Squamous Carcinoma

Squamous carcinoma, which is particularly common among the cancers of cigarette smokers, usually arises in the mucosa of a large bronchus. It forms an irregular mass in the wall, and extends partly into the lumen and partly into surrounding structures (Fig. 7.78). The cut surface is almost uniformly white or may enclose black areas that are the remains of pigmented lymph nodes that have become incorporated in the tumour. A distinctive feature is the development of bronchial obstruction at a comparatively early stage: this leads to collapse of the related wedge of lung, often complicated by infection, bronchiectasis, abscess formation and pale yellow areas of lipid pneumonia (see page 374). Infection of the parts of the lobe distal to the obstruction arises partly through inhalation of bacteria in debris detached from the exposed, necrotic surface of the tumour, and partly through interruption of the mucosal pathway along which inhaled organisms and particulate matter are ordinarily removed from the lungs. Because of the tendency to cause early obstruction, squamous carcinoma may become recognizable clinically when still amenable to surgical excision. Squamous cancer accounts for about 60 per cent of all bronchial carcinomas removed at operation, but for only about 20 per cent of those seen at necropsy, when 'oat cell' tumours are commonest.

It has long been known that prolonged irritation of the bronchial mucosa results in *squamous metaplasia* of its ciliate columnar epithelium. This transformation is often seen in bronchi that drain old tuberculous cavities or that have been exposed to the chronic irritation of longstanding suppuration. Detailed studies of the bronchial mucous membrane of smokers and non-smokers have indicated that metaplasia may also arise from prolonged exposure to inhaled tobacco smoke. It

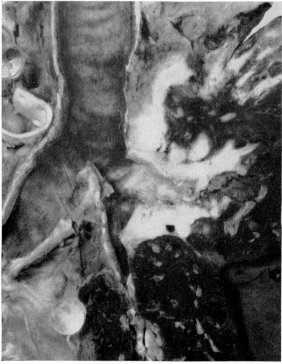

Fig. 7.78.§ Carcinoma of the lung. There is thickening of the wall of the upper part of the right main bronchus by pale tumour tissue that extends into the substance of the upper lobe of the lung. The lumen of the bronchus is narrowed.

appears to take place in a series of stages: at first, the number of cell layers in the surface epithelium increases; then the ciliate columnar superficial cells are replaced by non-ciliate columnar cells; finally, much of the surface comes to consist of a multilayered squamous epithelium, sometimes with keratinization of the superficial cells. This progressive change may be found in the bronchi of elderly non-smokers, but it is commoner in those who have smoked heavily.[805, 806] From the frequency with which the squamous type of bronchial carcinoma is found in heavy smokers, it seems likely that squamous metaplasia is precancerous.[807]

Microscopically, the tumour cells are aggregated into masses typical of squamous carcinoma in general (Fig. 7.79).[808] These masses, in which keratinization and epithelial pearl formation are often present, are commonly traversed by strands of well-developed fibrous stroma. Necrosis is often conspicuous in the larger tumours. The less well differentiated tumours can be identified as squamous by the presence of keratin or of intercellular bridges ('prickles').[809] In fact, the diagnosis of squamous carcinoma should not be made unless at least one

of these features is unequivocally present, for squamoid patterns occur in other tumours.

Poorly differentiated squamous tumours may consist of large spindle-shaped cells and may then resemble sarcomas. It is usually possible to trace transition between squamous and spindle-celled areas in a true squamous carcinoma: in carcino-sarcoma, in contrast, squamous and spindle-celled elements are usually sharply contrasted (see page 402), although the distinction between this tumour and poorly differentiated squamous growths can be difficult.

Electron microscopy of the cells of squamous carcinomas shows the large vesicular nucleus, very large nucleolus, tonofilaments and desmosomes that are characteristic features of stratified squamous epithelium.[810]

Small Cell Anaplastic Carcinomas

The anaplastic tumours are very malignant. The patients often present with symptoms referable to secondary deposits in bone or brain. The 'oat cell' carcinoma—sometimes curiously referred to as the 'lymphocyte-like cell' carcinoma—is the main example of the group (see below): the three variants named in Table 7.10 behave in a similar way. The cells of the fusiform cell tumour have more cytoplasm than those of the 'oat cell' tumour, but the distinction is often difficult to make histologically: in practice, many fusiform cell tumours are classified with the latter. The cells of the polygonal cell carcinomas, although small, are usually distinguished by their fairly abundant cytoplasm and rounded nuclei.

Other small cell anaplastic carcinomas, listed separately in the World Health Organization classification (Table 7.10—'II.4'), differ from the more usual variants in having foci of squamous or glandular structure. Many pathologists include them among the 'oat cell' carcinomas.

'Oat Cell' Carcinoma.—This tumour is composed of small, oval, undifferentiated cells that are intensely haematoxyphile (Fig. 7.80). They have very little cytoplasm. In shape they resemble oat seeds: this gained them the name by which they are generally known to British pathologists. The tumour was for long believed to arise in the hilar lymph nodes, and in consequence was regarded as a mediastinal sarcoma ('oat cell sarcoma'). The change in terminology must be taken into account when long-term statistical studies on the changing

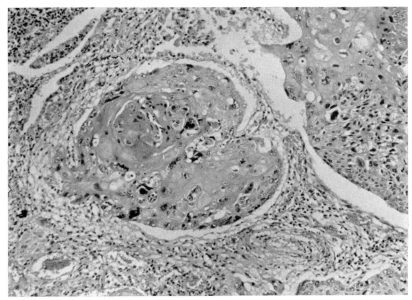

Fig. 7.79.§ Squamous carcinoma of lung. In the centre and on the right are solid masses of fairly well differentiated squamous cells with abundant cytoplasm and some keratin formation. *Haematoxylin–eosin.* × 100.

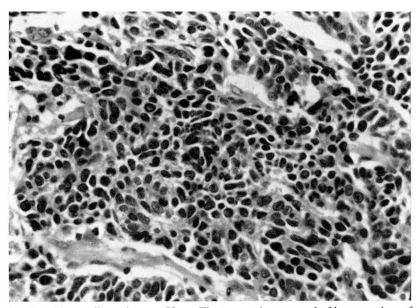

Fig. 7.80.§ 'Oat cell' carcinoma of lung. The tumour is composed of large numbers of tightly packed cells with hyperchromatic, oval nuclei and very little cytoplasm. There is a suggestion of tubule formation in places. Some of the nuclei have been cut transversely and therefore appear round. *Haematoxylin–eosin.* × 370.

incidence of bronchial cancer are considered. It was only when sufficiently exhaustive histological studies were undertaken that the epithelial nature of the malignant cells was recognized.[811, 812] It was then noted that the tumour cells resembled the cells of the germinal layer of the bronchial mucosa (the cells that maintain the physiological regeneration of the more specialized ciliate and mucus-secreting columnar epithelium): this led to the suggestion that these cells were the origin of the tumour.* Electron microscopy has suggested that the 'oat cell' is derived from bronchial cells of the APUD cell series (see below).

The finding of tubules in 'oat cell' tumours should not affect the histological diagnosis. In fact, the presence of streamers, ribbons, rosettes and tubules may be regarded as aids to the identification of the growth: definite tubules may be seen in about 2 per cent of these tumours, and rosettes in about 60 per cent.[813] Mucus may be produced. The wall of blood vessels may stain with haematoxylin, due to deposition of deoxyribonucleic acid.[814]

As might be expected from the poorly differentiated character of the cells, 'oat cell' tumours metastasize early.

Electron microscopy has shown that there are granules of neurosecretory type in the cytoplasm of the cells of 'oat cell' carcinomas. The granules are round, 50 to 240 nm in diameter, and consist of an electron-dense core separated by a clear zone from a thin, ring-like, investing membrane.[815] Similar structures are seen in carcinoid tumours of bronchial origin and in other tumours of the so-called APUD cells (see page 401 and Chapter 16): it is believed that at least some cases of 'oat cell' carcinoma also arise from this series of cells, representatives of which are normally present both in the surface epithelium and in the glands of the normal trachea and bronchi. This view is in keeping with the otherwise unexplained observation of endocrine secretory activity by these tumours (see page 403).

Adenocarcinomas

About a quarter of all bronchial cancers are adenocarcinomas. They account for a larger proportion of cases at necropsy than in surgical series. They are found with almost equal frequency in men and women and are commoner among smokers than non-smokers.

Bronchogenic Adenocarcinoma.—The bronchogenic adenocarcinomas are commonly composed of mucus-secreting columnar cells, grouped in glandular formations (Fig. 7.81). The latter are often

---

* The cells of the basal or germinal layer of the bronchial epithelium are sometimes known as 'reserve cells'. The 'oat cell' carcinoma is consequently sometimes referred to as the 'reserve cell' carcinoma, especially in North America.

distended by retained mucus, sometimes so much so that the secretion breaks through the surrounding epithelium and spreads freely in the neighbouring stroma. However, about a third of bronchial adenocarcinomas cannot be shown to be mucigenic. Squamous metaplasia may be conspicuous in parts of these tumours: its presence does not invalidate the diagnosis if a glandular pattern is present.[816]

It is important to note that secondary deposits of an adenocarcinoma arising elsewhere—for example, in the alimentary tract—may exactly simulate the appearances of a primary bronchogenic adenocarcinoma.

Bronchiolo-Alveolar Adenocarcinoma.[817, 818]—Those adenocarcinomas that arise in the smallest airways extend into the alveoli and may line them with cubical or columnar tumour cells, the alveolar wall remaining intact and forming, in effect, a stroma for the growth. The cells may produce large amounts of mucin, which displaces the air and distends the alveoli, often leading to extensive consolidation. Grossly, the tumour may be confused with lobar pneumonia caused by those type 3 pneumococci that produce abundant mucoid capsular material or by *Klebsiella pneumoniae* (see page 320) and with a rare form of cryptococcosis that is characterized by widespread colonization of the alveoli by highly mucigenic strains of the fungus.

The term bronchiolo-alveolar carcinoma is used to distinguish these very well differentiated tumours from the bronchogenic adenocarcinomas (see above). They are also sometimes known by the terms alveolar cell carcinoma (but see below) and malignant pulmonary adenomatosis.

Before a diagnosis of bronchiolo-alveolar carcinoma can be regarded as certain it is necessary to carry out an exhaustive search for primary adenocarcinomas in other organs, particularly the pancreas, that may metastasize to the lungs and give a similar or identical histological picture.[819, 820] It is not easy to distinguish between bronchioloalveolar and bronchogenic adenocarcinomas, for the latter may also form a columnar cell lining in invaded alveoli.

Non-neoplastic alveolar and bronchiolar epithelium can proliferate to a remarkable degree. The ingrowth of the latter into the alveoli—for example, in collapsed segments of lung—may simulate the picture of bronchiolo-alveolar carcinomas, particularly when the epithelium is mucigenic. Similar non-neoplastic proliferation is seen in the lungs of sheep in the infectious disease

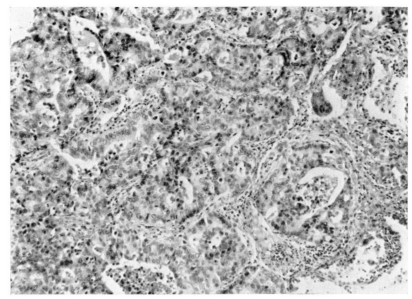

Fig. 7.81.§ Adenocarcinoma of lung. The formation of irregular tubules is seen in most of this field. *Haematoxylin–eosin.* × 100.

that is known by its Afrikaans name, *jaagsiekte.** Electron microscopy in cases of jaagsiekte has shown proliferation of type 2 alveolar epithelial cells in the alveoli and of bronchiolar epithelium in the bronchioles.[821]

It is of interest that small, benign growths in which the pulmonary alveoli are lined by columnar epithelial cells, with or without mucus formation, have been described.[822, 823]

Alveolar Cell Carcinoma. — The bronchiolo-alveolar adenocarcinoma (see above) has some-times been known as an alveolar cell carcinoma: this term is no longer considered to be appropriate for this type of tumour. That there is what may well be a true alveolar cell carcinoma has been disclosed by electron microscopy, which has shown the cytoplasm of the cells of certain tumours to contain laminate inclusions that are characteristic of type 2 alveolar epithelial cells (see page 272).

Large Cell Carcinomas

These tumours are composed of large cells without evidence of epidermoid association (keratinization

* The name *jaagsiekte* means, literally, 'drive disease': it was given to the disease of sheep because this was first observed among flocks being driven to fresh pastures. The affected animals were markedly dyspnoeic and could not keep up with the others, eventually collapsing and dying. Jaagsiekte is believed to be caused by a herpesvirus (Smith, W., MacKay, J. M. K., *J. comp. Path.*, 1969, **79**, 421).

and prickle formation). Their clinical presentation and course are similar to those of the bronchogenic adenocarcinomas.

Solid Large Cell Carcinomas.—The anaplastic large cell carcinoma is probably an undifferentiated adenocarcinoma or squamous carcinoma. The degree of dedifferentiation is such that the cell of origin of the tumour is no longer identifiable: a separate category is therefore required for its classification. It is composed of masses of large cells with a little stroma between them (Fig. 7.82). Mucin can be demonstrated with the help of special stains in some of these tumours but not in all.

Giant Cell Carcinoma.[824]—The only tumours of the lungs that are correctly placed under this heading are very rare growths composed almost wholly of large pleomorphic cells with intensely eosinophile cytoplasm. The cells may be multi-nucleate. They appear to be capable of phagocytosis, for they often contain cell debris in digestion vacuoles and they may be stippled with carbon particles. Such tumours generally arise toward the periphery of the lung. The prognosis is very poor and the clinical course short. Most of the patients have been exceptionally heavy cigarette smokers.

These tumours have to be distinguished from squamous and anaplastic primary carcinomas in which giant cells have appeared as a consequence

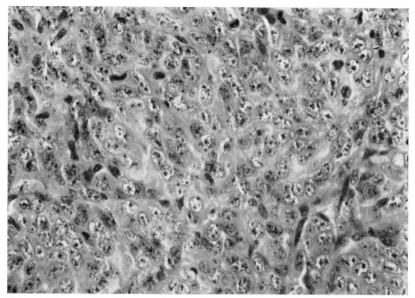

Fig. 7.82.§ Large cell carcinoma of the lung. The tumour cells are poorly differentiated and have large, vesicular, oval nuclei and prominent nucleoli. They are separated in places by a few fibroblasts and capillary endothelial cells. There is no evidence of squamous or glandular differentiation. *Haematoxylin–eosin.* × 370.

of radiotherapy. They must also be distinguished from primary and secondary rhabdomyosarcomas (see page 406) and from secondary deposits of pleomorphic adrenal cortical carcinomas and hepatomas and of anaplastic epidermoid tumours arising in the uterine cervix or elsewhere.

The occurrence of giant cells in localized areas of other types of primary carcinoma of the lungs has been described as *giant cell metaplasia.* Such tumours are not correctly categorized as giant cell carcinomas.

'Clear Cell' Carcinoma.—This is a comparatively rare variety of tumour, accounting for fewer than 5 per cent of lung cancers. The tumour cells are large, with a small, centrally placed nucleus and abundant clear cytoplasm. The cytoplasm appears 'empty' and unstained in haematoxylin–eosin preparations, but when appropriately stained a proportion of the cells in some examples can be shown to contain glycogen.[825] Although the cells appear to be in continuous sheets or clumps in ordinary preparations, staining to show elastic tissue may demonstrate that in their growth they have filled the alveoli and compressed their walls. The presence of occasional tubules in about half the tumours indicates that at least these examples may be regarded as poorly differentiated adenocarcinomas. Areas of necrosis may be present.

Clear cells may be found in some areas of other poorly differentiated adenocarcinomas and in some squamous carcinomas. This does not indicate a special variety of tumour but merely focal clear cell formation in otherwise typical growths.[826] The practical importance of such foci of clear cells is that the tumours in which they occur may be mistaken for metastatic renal tubular adenocarcinomas. In cases of doubt, examination of frozen sections is helpful: abundant sudanophile fat will be seen in the cells of renal adenocarcinomas whereas fat is not found (or is present only in traces) in the clear cells of tumours that arise in the lungs.

Combined Epidermoid Carcinoma and Adenocarcinoma

This rare tumour is characterized by the presence of distinct squamous and tubular areas. The two histological patterns are relatively well differentiated and each contributes significantly to the total extent of the growth. They are intimately combined in the primary tumour and, usually, in secondary deposits. Tumours with this structure have to be distinguished from carcinosarcomas (see page 402) and from squamous carcinomas that include a few tubules.

Carcinoid Tumour

This neoplasm, otherwise known as the carcinoid type of bronchial adenoma, forms about one per cent of all primary tumours of the bronchus. It generally appears at an earlier age than the usual forms of carcinoma; its incidence is the same in both sexes; it grows slowly and metastasizes only rarely; and it sometimes gives rise to the 'carcinoid syndrome' typical of certain tumours of the alimentary tract (see Chapter 16).[827, 828] It causes cough and haemoptysis, and when large enough it may obstruct the airway, with consequent bacterial infection of the bronchial tree distally and collapse of the related parts of the lung.

This tumour almost invariably develops in one of the larger bronchi and can be seen readily by bronchoscopy as a pinkish-red, smooth, mass that protrudes into the lumen and is often moulded to its shape. This appearance, however, is liable to give a misleading impression of the size of the tumour, for it generally extends through the wall of the bronchus to produce an hourglass-shaped mass, most of the tumour lying external to the bronchus. Although the tumour compresses surrounding structures it rarely invades them.

Histologically, most bronchial carcinoids resemble argentaffinomas (carcinoids) of the alimentary tract in being composed of solid columns or masses of small, fairly uniform, polygonal cells in orderly arrangement and with few mitotic figures.[829] Although the similarity between bronchial and intestinal carcinoids has been recognized for years, they were long regarded as different tumours, largely because argentaffin properties had not been demonstrated in the cells of the former. Also, it is only recently that a clear distinction has been made between argentaffin-cell and non-argentaffin endocrine cell tumours of the APUD cell system in various parts of the body (see Chapter 16). It has now been shown that some bronchial carcinoids possess cells with granules that give the argentaffin reaction (reducing silver during the Masson–Fontana procedure).[830] These cells also exhibit yellow autofluorescence in ultraviolet light after formalin fixation—a feature associated with the presence of 5-hydroxytryptamine. These two tests are strongly positive both in normal enterochromaffin (argentaffin) cells and in the cells of argentaffinomas arising in the alimentary tract (see Chapter 16).

Further evidence for the origin of some of these bronchial tumours from argentaffin cells is the demonstration by electron microscopy of the presence of neurosecretory granules in the cytoplasm:[831] the carcinoids of this type are probably related to the 'oat cell' carcinoma in origin (see page 398). Other bronchial carcinoids correspond to the tumours of the non-argentaffin endocrine cells of the APUD cell series (see Chapter 16).

It is rare for a bronchial carcinoid to give rise to fibrosis of the endocardium, as occurs in some cases of metastasizing argentaffinoma of the alimentary tract (see Chapter 16). In the latter cases, it is mainly or exclusively the right side of the heart that is affected: this is ascribed to a direct action of chemical substances liberated into the hepatic venous blood by the cells of secondary deposits in the liver. When the condition accompanies a pulmonary carcinoid it is the endocardium of the chambers of the left side of the heart that is affected, this being the side exposed to the blood coming from the tumour.[832]

Tumours of Bronchial Glands

Adenoid Cystic Carcinoma (Cylindroma).—This tumour was formerly referred to as the cylindroid or cylindromatous type of bronchial adenoma: it is in fact a carcinoma, of low-grade malignancy. It usually arises higher in the tracheobronchial tree than the carcinoid tumour, often involving the region of the carina and sometimes originating in the trachea itself.[833] It is a somewhat translucent, pale, firm growth that has ill-defined outlines and infiltrates diffusely along the tracheobronchial wall, forming polypoid projections that tend to obstruct the lumen. The cartilage of the wall becomes enclosed by tumour tissue, and the adjacent lung may be infiltrated. Metastasis may involve the hilar lymph nodes; it is rare for secondary deposits to develop elsewhere.

Histologically, the tumour resembles the corresponding type of growth arising in salivary glands (see Chapter 11). Small, pleomorphic, deeply staining cells form branching, elongated tubules arranged in a plexiform mass. The tubules are often lined by a double layer of cells (epithelium and myoepithelium). There may be many mitotic figures. Spaces of varying size are often found and are filled with mucus.

Mucoepidermoid Tumours.—Tumours of this type are occasionally seen in the bronchi, arising from mucous glands.[834] They have the same structure as the corresponding tumours of salivary glands (see Chapter 11). They are usually of, at most, a low grade of malignancy.

Papillary Tumours of the Surface Epithelium

Both epidermoid and mucoepidermoid papillary tumours occur in the tracheobronchial tree, usually in the larger bronchi and often near the carina. They may be solitary or multiple.[835] They have stromal stalks of more or less delicate structure. In the epidermoid tumours these stalks support a multilayered growth of squamous cells that vary in differentiation from case to case. Mucigenic goblet cells are present, in addition, in the rarer mucoepidermoid variety.

The prognosis of these tumours varies. Some are notably radiosensitive, which is of particular importance in view of their situation, for they are seldom amenable to excision.

'Mixed' Tumours and Carcinosarcomas

'Mixed' Tumours.—The 'mixed' tumours in the World Health Organization classification (Table 7.10, page 392) are the tumours with a structure resembling that of the familiar pleomorphic tumours of salivary glands (see Chapter 11). Their prognosis is better than that of bronchogenic adenocarcinomas, but they may be difficult to extirpate because of their site, which is usually a main bronchus or the trachea. They tend to recur and they have been known to metastasize.

'Pulmonary Blastoma' (Carcinosarcoma of Embryonal Type).[836]—The so-called pulmonary blastoma is a rare tumour. It arises toward the periphery of the lung, forming a large, rounded, partly necrotic and haemorrhagic mass that generally reaches the pleura. Unlike the carcinomas, its demarcation from the surrounding tissue is sharp. Microscopically, it consists of an embryonic type of connective tissue that contains tubules formed of multilayered, vacuolate, columnar epithelium, resembling fetal bronchioles. Fusiform or strap-like tumour muscle cells, identifiable by cross-striation of their cytoplasm, are present in some areas: they may be sparse, and the striation may be difficult to find. The presence of the muscle cell element indicates that there is no sharp distinction between 'blastoma' and rhabdomyosarcoma (see page 406). The embryonic appearance of the 'blastoma' distinguishes it from the more usual form of carcinosarcoma (see below). The tumour spreads to the hilar lymph nodes and widely in the blood.

Carcinosarcoma.[837]—This type of carcinosarcoma, sometimes referred to as the 'true' carcinosarcoma, is a very rare tumour. It comprises areas that recognizably resemble squamous carcinoma and areas of sarcomatous structure, formed of spindle-shaped cells.[838] Some of these tumours arise in the hilar region and protrude into the bronchial lumen; others are in the peripheral part of the lungs. They are usually slowly growing and the outlook after resection is reasonably good.

The diagnosis of carcinosarcoma is made oftener than is appropriate. It is sometimes applied in cases of squamous carcinoma in which partly differentiated squamous growth and undifferentiated areas formed of spindle-shaped cells are combined. Reticulin impregnation may be helpful in distinguishing this type of squamous carcinoma from carcinosarcoma: reticulin fibres are sparse between cells of the sarcoma-like, undifferentiated parts of the former but outline the individual cells of the sarcomatous parts of the latter.

Dissemination of Bronchial Carcinoma[839]

In the earlier stages of their growth, bronchial carcinomas, like cancers elsewhere, spread by local infiltration. So numerous are the lymphatics and blood vessels in the hilar parts of the lungs, however, and so constantly are the local structures affected by respiratory movements, that local spread of the tumour cells is soon followed by their much more extensive dissemination by these preformed pathways. It is the early and widespread extension of these tumours more than the difficulties inherent in the operative approach to the mass that has rendered the surgical treatment of bronchial carcinomas so unsatisfactory.

Local Spread.—When a bronchial carcinoma is seen at necropsy it has generally become so large, and so merged with the infiltrated hilar lymph nodes, that the separate identity of the primary growth has often been lost. Further, by the time of death the tumour may have extended locally to involve important nearby structures in the mediastinum by direct infiltration.

Lymphatic Spread.—When histological sections are made from the vicinity of the tumour mass, it is often found that many lymphatics are filled with tumour cells; when extensive, this condition is sometimes imprecisely referred to as lymphangitis carcinomatosa (see page 160).[840] Some of the involved lymphatics are in the depths of the bronchial mucosa, but more are generally to be seen in the circumbronchial and circumvascular connective tissues; this infiltration may sometimes be recognizable in radiographs. The neoplastic cells travel along these lymph channels early in the course of the disease, with the result that at the time of lobectomy or pneumonectomy the lymph nodes at the hilum have been invaded in well over half the cases.[841] Once within the nodes, the tumour cells proliferate freely and extend from one node to the next until most of those in the hilar region have been replaced by the growth.

The cancer cells travel in lymphatics not only toward the hilum but also centrifugally, particularly when there is obstruction to the flow of lymph in the other direction. This extension may proceed so far that the cells reach the subpleural lymphatic plexus: there the formation of solid cords of tumour cells within the vessels produces a subserosal network of continuous, fine, white lines. Sometimes, there is more massive infiltration of the pleura, and a bloodstained effusion may collect in the sac, or the visceral and parietal surfaces may adhere to one another by the formation of granulation tissue that becomes infiltrated by tumour cells.

Spread Through the Blood Stream.—Although usually involved less early than the lymphatics, the blood vessels near the tumour are soon invaded. Because their wall is thinner, the pulmonary veins are generally most affected, but pulmonary arteries may also be invaded. In one series of 59 surgical specimens, the veins were seen to be involved in 52 and the arteries in 10.[842] After infiltrating the media and intima, the tumour tissue is in contact with the passing blood: small masses formed of thrombus and tumour cells become detached and are carried away as emboli. It is because the tributaries of the pulmonary veins are so numerous, and their walls so thin and easily penetrated, that distant secondary deposits are particularly numerous in cases of bronchial carcinoma. When an artery is invaded, its consequent obstruction by thrombus sometimes gives rise to infarction in the portion of the lung that it supplies.[843]

The Distribution of Haematogenous Metastasis.—Much attention has been given to the distribution of secondary deposits in cases of bronchial carcinoma, and several studies have been published that record their frequency in the more important organs at necropsy. The findings in two such studies are shown in Table 7.12.

The great frequency of metastasis—which often becomes clinically evident even while the primary tumour itself is still small and unsuspected—provides many difficult clinical problems. Especially

Table 7.12. *Relative Frequency of Secondary Deposits of Bronchial Cancer in Some of the More Important Organs*

	Series A	Series B
Number of cases	866	741
Number with metastasis	620	517
Percentage with metastasis to:		
liver	35	39
adrenals	24	33
brain	17	26
bones	13	15
kidneys	12	15

Series A: Bryson, C. C., Spencer, H., *Quart. J. Med.*, 1951, N.S. **20**, 173.
Series B: Galluzzi, S., Payne, P. M., *Brit. J. Cancer*, 1955, **9**, 511.

noteworthy are the effects of secondary deposits in the brain.[844] Because their situation within the cranial cavity commonly gives rise to early and demanding manifestations, symptoms arising from the primary growth itself may be overlooked.

Syndromes Associated with Carcinoma of the Lung[845]

Besides the effects produced by the presence of the expanding, infiltrating primary growth itself and of secondary deposits in various parts of the body, carcinoma of the lungs occasionally gives rise to endocrine and metabolic effects. These effects, which sometimes are referred to as 'paramalignant' syndromes, are uncommon: for instance, hypercalcaemia, which is among the least infrequent, occurs in only 1 to 5 per cent of cases. However, awareness that such syndromes occur is leading to recognition of many instances that otherwise would be overlooked.

Endocrine Syndromes

The endocrine effects of bronchial and other lung tumours are attributed to synthesis by the tumour cells of polypeptides that have the action of the polypeptide hormones of certain endocrine organs. These substances produced by tumours have been termed 'ectopic hormones' (see Chapters 23 and 29). In many instances the endocrine disturbances regress if the tumour is resected or responds to irradiation or drug therapy: they may, or may not, return when the tumour recurs.

Cushing's Syndrome (Ectopic Corticotrophin Syndrome).—Although basiphil adenoma of the anterior lobe of the pituitary gland (see Chapter 29) and tumours of the adrenal cortex (see Chapter

30) are the best known causes of Cushing's syndrome, it must not be forgotten that tumours arising in other tissues may be accompanied by this condition. The 'oat cell' bronchial carcinoma is the most frequent of these,[846] and lung cancer must be considered as a possible explanation of Cushing's syndrome whenever this develops in adults, particularly men. It is clear that some 'oat cell' tumours produce a substance with corticotrophic activity, adrenal cortical hyperplasia resulting. The consequent secretion of large amounts of cortisol by the adrenals leads to potassium depletion: hypokalaemic alkalosis[847] and muscular weakness are characteristically more marked than in Cushing's syndrome of other causation. Polyuria, intolerance of carbohydrates that may amount to frank diabetes mellitus, and sodium retention with consequent oedema and hypertension are further common features. The corticotrophin-like hormone produced by the tumours is not inhibited by dexamethasone, in contrast to pituitary corticotrophin: the hypercortisolaemia accompanying ectopic secretion of the corticotrophic substance is therefore not reduced by administration of dexamethasone.[848] This may be helpful in distinguishing this condition from other causes of Cushing's syndrome and from hypercortisolaemia occurring as a non-specific 'stress' effect of serious illness, which is a common accompaniment of cancer.[849]

It is possible that the increased output of cortisol may worsen the prognosis of the cancer, since there is some experimental evidence that glucocorticosteroids encourage metastasis.

Syndrome of Inappropriate Secretion of Antidiuretic Hormone.[850]—In this syndrome a bronchial carcinoma, almost always of 'oat cell' type, is accompanied by hyponatraemia due to release of antidiuretic hormone while plasma osmolality is reduced and therefore the availability of the hormone is inappropriate. The antidiuretic substance is elaborated by the tumour cells.[851] There is deficiency in reabsorption of sodium in the proximal part of the renal tubules, with water retention and eventual over-hydration, which leads to cerebral oedema, drowsiness and fits. There may be a more general functional defect of the proximal part of the tubules, manifested in aminoaciduria, glycosuria and phosphaturia, with inability to acidify the urine.[852]

Hypercalcaemia.[853]—Bronchial carcinoma, particularly squamous carcinoma, may secrete para-thyroid hormone or a substance with similar activity. The resulting hypercalcaemia may exceed a level of 20 mg/dl. Muscle weakness, cramps, polyuria, dehydration, renal failure and mental disturbance are among the results. The condition is sometimes termed 'non-metastatic hypercalcaemia', to indicate that it is distinct from hypercalcaemia secondary to extensive destruction of bone by metastatic involvement of the skeleton by the tumour.

Other Hormonal Disturbances.—Other recorded hormonal effects of cancer of the lungs include hyperglycaemia,[849] hypoglycaemia and gynaecomastia. Hypoglycaemia has generally been an accompaniment of large cellular growths, particularly fibrosarcomas:[854] some of these may have been fusiform cell anaplastic bronchial carcinomas, for this type of tumour has been known to be associated with severe hypoglycaemia that disappears on removal of the affected lung, returning with the development of secondary deposits on a widespread scale.[855] The cause of the fall in the blood sugar level in these cases is obscure: it has been attributed to the production of insulin-like substances by tumour cells, or of substances that sensitize the tissues to pancreatic insulin;[856] alternatively, the increased uptake of glucose by very extensive, very cellular tumour tissue may be responsible. Gynaecomastia has usually been associated with production of gonadotrophin-like substances by anaplastic large cell bronchial carcinomas.[857]

It may be noted again that some carcinoid tumours of the bronchi (page 401), like the corresponding tumours of the alimentary tract (Chapter 16), secrete 5-hydroxytryptamine and may be accompanied by the carcinoid syndrome (argentaffinoma syndrome). Other bronchial carcinoids produce substances with corticotrophin-like activity[858] and some 'oat cell' carcinomas produce 5-hydroxytryptamine and may cause the 'carcinoid syndrome':[859] such findings are further evidence of the relation between these two types of bronchial tumour (see page 398).

Neurological Syndromes ('Paramalignant Neuromyopathies')[860]

The neurological and muscular complications of bronchial carcinomas, other than the direct effects of metastatic deposits, include peripheral neuropathy (see Chapter 35), which is the most frequent,[86] encephalopathy and myelopathy (see Chapter 34 and myasthenia (see Chapter 36). It is important to note that neurological and myopathic disturbances often appear even some years before the carcinoma becomes clinically manifest.[862]

The cause of these syndromes is not generally clear. Infection, intoxication, autoimmunity and vitamin deficiency have been suggested. Infection has been incriminated with reasonable evidence only in relation to some cases of progressive multifocal leucoencephalopathy (Chapter 34) in which virions morphologically identical with polyomavirus have been found in the oligodendrocytes.[863] Intoxication by a product of the tumour cells that has an inhibiting effect on the release of acetylcholine at the neuromuscular junctions has been suggested in explanation of the myasthenic syndrome, which ordinarily subsides quickly on excision of the carcinoma.[864] Organ-specific antibodies to the tissues of the central nervous system are present in at least some cases of sensory neuropathy.[865] The suggestion that vitamin deficiencies play a part is not supported by any conclusive evidence.

Other Syndromes Associated with Carcinoma of Lung

Lung cancers are among the tumours that may be accompanied by such general disorders of soft tissues as dermatomyositis[866] and polymyositis (see Chapter 36),[867] systemic lupus erythematosus[868] and systemic sclerosis.[868] Non-infective thrombotic endocardiopathy (see page 56) may occur[869] and may be accompanied by thrombophlebitis migrans;[869] the latter may occur alone. There is also a predisposition to arterial and venous thrombosis, the latter carrying a risk of pulmonary embolism: this predisposition appears to be associated with the presence of an increased amount of antihaemophiliac globulin, possibly resulting from damage to the tissues invaded by the tumour.[870]

Acanthosis nigricans (see Chapter 39)[871] and the rarer but equally distinctive spreading rash described as erythema gyratum repens[872] are more frequently associated with bronchial carcinoma than with tumours arising elsewhere in the body.

Clubbing of the digits, particularly the fingers, may accompany bronchial carcinoma and pleural mesothelioma; it is less commonly associated with metastatic tumours in the lungs. Its explanation is uncertain. The development of direct communication of bronchial veins with pulmonary veins as part of a general increase in the bronchial and pulmonary vascular bed may allow blood containing metabolites of a tumour to bypass the pulmonary capillaries, escaping oxidation and on reaching the digits producing clubbing by a local vasodilator effect.[873] It has been suggested that unreduced ferritin, shunted past the capillary circulation in the lungs and so remaining unoxidized, is responsible for clubbing by its antagonistic effect on the vasoconstrictive action of adrenaline.[874]

Hypertrophic pulmonary osteoarthropathy (see Chapter 37) is likelier to develop in association with peripheral lung tumours than with those arising in the tracheobronchial tree.[875] Although it is often accompanied by clubbing of the digits, this may be relatively minor in degree or even absent. Clubbing, of course, is commonly associated with various benign diseases, both intrathoracic and of other parts: in contrast, hypertrophic osteoarthropathy is almost invariably a manifestation of intrathoracic cancer. The fact that the osteoarthropathy is quickly relieved by vagotomy in certain cases has suggested the possibility of a neural or neurohormonal reflex in its pathogenesis.[876] Gynaecomastia may accompany hypertrophic osteoarthropathy:[877] its explanation is uncertain, and in these cases the tumour is generally not of the large cell type that is associated with this condition when it is not related to the presence of osteoarthropathy (see opposite).

Diagnostic Procedures

Cytological Examination of Sputum.—Malignant cells that are shed from the open surface of tumours involving the trachea, bronchi, bronchioles or alveoli find their way into the sputum and can be recognized microscopically in stained films. Success depends on obtaining specimens of true sputum, not saliva. Thick films are fixed in Schaudinn's fluid and stained with haematoxylin and eosin[878] or by Papanicolaou's method.[879] Alternatively, the wet film can be mixed with a drop of a one per cent solution of methylene blue and examined under a coverslip.[880]

The malignant cells have to be distinguished from others, including squames from the mouth, inflammatory cells, ciliate cells from air passages and histiocytes from the alveoli. Malignant cells of squamous type have large, hyperchromatic, sometimes bizarre, nuclei that vary in size. 'Oat cells' are a little larger than lymphocytes and it is of help in their recognition that there is sometimes flattening at points of contact when the former are close together.[881] Cells of adenocarcinomas may contain mucous vacuoles in the cytoplasm as well as showing nuclear abnormalities.

o

Secondary tumours in the lungs also may shed cells into the sputum.

Cytological examination of sputum is a valuable diagnostic method when the microscopist is experienced in the techniques and in interpreting the findings. When four specimens are competently examined in each case the method gives positive results in about 85 per cent of cases of cancer of the lungs.[882] Unfortunately, it is very time-consuming, and this limits the extent of its use in practice.

Bronchial Biopsy.—A valuable and widely used diagnostic method is biopsy through a broncho-scope.[883] A small piece of tissue is extracted with cup forceps and processed for sectioning in paraffin wax. The method is quick and reliable in those cases in which the tumour is accessible, but the results are often negative—or the procedure is not practicable—when the tumour is toward the periphery of a lung. Cytological examination of sputum is much more helpful in cases of the latter type, giving positive results, in skilled hands, in over 50 per cent of cases of peripheral cancers.

Biopsy specimens from small bronchi, formerly beyond the reach of the ordinary bronchoscope, are now obtainable by means of the fibre-optic bronchoscope.

Mediastinoscopy.—This procedure enables lymph nodes draining the lungs to be removed from the mediastinum by the retrosternal approach. It is much used in some centres and gives valuable information on the extent of spread of carcinoma and lymphoma.[884]

Sarcoma of the Trachea, Bronchi, Lungs and Pleura

The primary sarcomas arising in the tracheo-bronchial tree, lungs and pleura occur with a frequency of one to about every 500 carcinomas of the lungs.

Leiomyosarcoma.[885]—This is the least rare of the sarcomas of the lungs. It may arise in any part of a lung and grow to a large size. It occurs in the same age group as carcinoma and the clinical features in general are also those of carcinoma.[886] Macroscopically, it resembles a primary carcinoma. It may present as a polypoid mass in the lumen of a bronchus or it may arise within the lung. It seldom spreads to the hilar lymph nodes; blood-borne metastasis is less rare. Histologically, it consists of smooth muscle cells that range from well to poorly differentiated. The well-differentiated sarcoma cells differ from the cells of benign leiomyomas (see page 390) in that their nuclei are larger and more pleomorphic. The intrabronchial leiomyosarcoma should be recognizable on biopsy examination, and care must be taken not to mistake it for an un-differentiated squamous carcinoma or fusiform cell anaplastic carcinoma.

Rhabdomyosarcoma.[887]—Primary tumours formed of striated muscle cells are very infrequent in the lungs. Like rhabdomyosarcomas arising elsewhere, they are formed of straplike or bizarrely shaped, sometimes multinucleate, cells with abundant eosinophile cytoplasm that may show cross-striation. The striation may be evident in a large proportion of the cells, or it may not be demonstrated until many sections have been searched. There may be extensive necrosis. In one case the tumour was associated with a primary squamous carcinoma in the other lung:[888] both tumours had metastasized widely, the deposits being composed purely of one or the other type of growth.

Rhabdomyosarcoma is liable to be confused with giant cell carcinoma of lung (see page 399).[889]

Fibrosarcoma.[885]—This is a rare tumour in the lungs. It occurs usually in young people, generally presenting as polypoid projections into the lumen of a large bronchus. The microscopical appearances reproduce the range of structure and differentiation that may be found in fibrosarcomas arising in other parts of the body. In biopsy specimens, carcino-sarcomas (see page 402) may be mistaken for poorly differentiated fibrosarcomas if the carcinomatous element is not represented in the tissue excised. Fusiform cell anaplastic carcinomas and leiomyo-sarcomas may also be confused with fibrosarcoma. The prognosis of pulmonary fibrosarcoma, after excision, is usually good, and depends mainly on the situation of the growth: if it cannot be removed completely the tissue left *in situ* will continue to proliferate. Metastasis occurs late in the course, if at all, and is particularly infrequent when the tumour is well differentiated.

Neurofibrosarcoma.—Neurofibrosarcoma of the lung is usually associated with generalized neuro-fibromatosis (see page 390). Some of the tumours have features of malignant neurolemmoma.[890]

Myxosarcoma.—Sarcomatous change in pulmonary hamartomas, a very rare occurrence, may present microscopical appearances of the type conventionally described as myxosarcomatous.[891] Chondro-sarcomatous change is less rare (see below).

Chondrosarcoma.—In spite of the abundance of cartilage in the tracheobronchial tree, chondro-sarcomas are very rare in the lungs.[892] In fact, most pulmonary chondrosarcomas arise from hamartomas (chondroadenomas—page 388) or chondromas (page 389).

Malignant Lymphomas

Proliferation of lymphocytes characterizes various benign conditions of the lungs and these must be distinguished from malignant lymphomas: the distinction is often difficult. Among the benign diseases that must particularly be kept in mind in this context are lymphocytic interstitial pneumonia (page 370) and benign 'lymphoma' (pseudo-lymphoma—page 391). Malignant lymphomas of the lungs correspond to those occurring elsewhere in the body (see Chapter 9). The lungs are involved at necropsy in about a quarter of all cases of malignant lymphoma arising in other parts.[893] Sometimes the lungs are the primary site of the disease, and some-times they alone are involved.[893, 894]

Lymphocytic Lymphoma.—Primary lymphocytic lymphoma of the lungs is more frequent in women. It forms a grey or yellowish, slightly translucent, moderately firm mass with ill-defined outlines. By the time of diagnosis it often occupies a consider-able part of the lobe in which it has arisen. It is distinguishable from the benign lymphomas by its tendency to involve hilar lymph nodes and extend into adjoining tissues, including the pleura. Some-times it is multifocal in origin. Microscopically, the parenchyma of the lung is densely infiltrated or replaced by small lymphocytes; immunoblasts may be present but are not numerous. In contrast to benign lymphomas, malignant lymphomas in-volve the bronchial cartilages, which may become necrotic.[895]

There are many reports of long survival following excision of a lymphocytic lymphoma of the lung, provided removal has been complete. However, some of these reports evidently relate to benign lymphomas that had been misinterpreted as malig-nant. The distinction between benign and malignant lymphocytic infiltrates in the lungs can be very difficult. The situation is complicated by the fact that some initially benign lesions eventually develop into classic malignant lymphomas.

Other Malignant Lymphomas.[896] — Hodgkin's disease[897] and immunoblastic and histiocytic lym-phomas may arise in the lungs. The prognosis after surgical treatment is less favourable than in cases of primary lymphocytic lymphoma.

Myeloma (plasmacytic lymphoma) may occur in the lungs either as a solitary, localized condition[898] or as a manifestation of myelomatosis. The localized form usually arises apart from the bronchi but may present in the latter situation as an obstructive mass.[899] There may be diagnostic confusion between myeloma and the focal aggregation of plasma cells that occurs in the lungs in some cases of Walden-ström's macroglobulinaemia (see Chapter 9).[900]

Leukaemic Infiltration of the Lungs[901]

It is commonly said that some form of leukaemic lesion is to be found in the lungs in about a quarter of all cases of leukaemia at necropsy although only in some 3 per cent is this accompanied by inter-ference with pulmonary function.[902] In fact, inter-stitial infiltration by leukaemic cells may be found microscopically in almost all cases, particularly round bronchi and the larger blood vessels, but sometimes causing such thickening of the alveolar walls in parts of the lungs as to encroach markedly on the lumen. In some cases the leukaemic cells form macroscopically evident nodules, ranging from 1 mm or so to some 2 cm across.

Unclassified Malignant Tumours

The need for the category of 'unclassified' tumours in the World Health Organization classification (Table 7.10) is self-evident. The proportion of tumours assigned to it by individual pathologists will doubtless vary, reflecting the many factors that influence histological diagnosis. It is in the eventual elucidation of these initially unclassifiable tumours that central registries of lung tumours will have one of their most valuable roles.

Malignant Mesothelioma

The very occurrence of mesothelial tumours was doubted and even denied by experienced patholo-gists, including some specializing in tumour pathology, until 1960, when Wagner and his colleagues published their recognition of primary pleural mesothelioma as an occupational disease of important frequency among the asbestos miners in Cape Province, South Africa.[903] Until that time few such growths had been recorded and there was a tendency to follow the authoritarian view that these could all best be explained as secondary carcinomas. It is now recognized that malignant mesothelioma may arise from the lining of any of the body cavities, pleural mesotheliomas being the most frequent. Whether there is a benign mesothelioma remains debatable (see page 390).

Mesotheliomas are commonly associated with the presence of fibrous plaques in the serosa. Such plaques have long been known to form in the pleura, particularly the parietal pleura, as an accompaniment of asbestosis (see page 383).[904, 905] The fact that comparable plaques are found in at least 4 per cent of all necropsies[906] becomes the more pertinent when it is also considered that asbestos bodies are present in the lungs in over 20 per cent of necropsies in London,[907] their frequency rising in proportion to the increasing age of the patients. The high incidence of asbestos bodies in the community reflects the widespread and continuously growing utilization of asbestos. It is not only the man who works with asbestos— the miner, the labourer involved in its packing and shipping, the worker in the processing and manufacturing plants—who is at risk: his family is exposed to the dust that contaminates his clothing; other people are exposed because they live downwind from asbestos factories[908] and even the home handyman who cuts and drills asbestos sheet or piping is endangering his health and that of others. The association between asbestos and mesothelioma is indisputable. Not surprisingly, it is those with an occupational history of exposure to asbestos who are likeliest to develop the tumour, but mesothelioma may develop also as a result of more casual contamination of the lungs. The tumour arises in the pleura in most cases, but peritoneal mesothelioma is far from rare (27 instances in a series of 83 mesotheliomas in the records of the Institute of Pathology of the London Hospital).[909]

How asbestos causes mesothelioma is uncertain. In cases of pulmonary asbestosis (see page 383) it is unusual to find asbestos fibres in the subserosal connective tissue of the pleura by light microscopy, but very small asbestos fibres can be demonstrated with the electron microscope. Accepting the evidence that asbestos is oncogenic, it still remains to explain why the result is so characteristically a cancer arising in the pleural mesothelium rather than in other tissues of the lungs. The pathogenesis of peritoneal mesotheliomas in association with asbestos is even more problematical. It has been suggested that asbestos fibres migrate through the tissue of the lungs, presumably driven by the natural respiratory movements; the strength and the smooth, fine, filamentous structure of the particles doubtless facilitate such movement. However, although asbestos fibres may be demonstrated, usually in small amounts only, in the fibrotic serosal plaques (see above), they are found only exceptionally rarely in mesotheliomas: the latter observation does not negate a connexion between asbestos and the development of the tumours, which largely grow by displacing the tissues that adjoin them. It has been shown that at least some samples of asbestos, particularly of crocidolite (page 383), contain oncogenic polycyclic hydrocarbons, including 3:4-benzpyrene.[910]

The duration of known occupational exposure to asbestos dust in cases of mesothelioma is of the order of 40 years:[911] this is about 10 years longer than in the cases in which asbestosis is complicated by the development of other lung tumours. The latter are usually bronchial growths, particularly squamous carcinomas; occasionally they are bronchiolo-alveolar adenocarcinomas. In rare instances, asbestos-induced mesothelioma and one or the other of these varieties of carcinoma coexist.

Macroscopical Findings.—The growth usually arises in the parietal pleura near or on the diaphragmatic aspect of the lung. It spreads over the pleural surface and its growth is often accompanied by the formation of a haemorrhagic pleural effusion. At necropsy, the tumour is seen as a thick, white, firm, nodular mass, encasing and compressing the lung and infiltrating its substance. Adjacent structures, such as the pericardial sac, the opposite pleural sac and the chest wall, are invaded. Secondary deposits are commonly found in the regional lymph nodes; less frequently, there is metastasis to other sites, particularly the brain, bones and liver and the other lung.[912] After surgery, the tumour tends to invade the operation site.[913] Surgical intervention seems also to increase the likelihood of haematogenous metastasis.

Microscopical Findings.—Malignant mesotheliomas vary greatly in structure from area to area.[914] One component has an appearance like epithelium and lines clefts or forms sheets, masses, tubules and papillae (see Volume 2, Fig. 20.10). Another component is sarcoma-like, consisting of spindle-shaped cells that may vary widely in the degree of differentiation. There seems to be no particular merit in attempting to define varieties of mesothelioma on a morphological basis, as some authorities have done, recognizing predominantly tubulopapillary, sarcomatous, undifferentiated polygonal cell, and mixed types. When both epithelium-like and sarcoma-like structures are present in a pleural tumour the appearances are accepted by most histopathologists as diagnostic of mesothelioma, but care is needed because a carcinoma of bronchopulmonary or other origin may invade the pleura and lead to the formation of irregular tubules of epithelial cells in a cellular fibromatoid stroma. In some mesotheliomas the epithelium-like element is missing, the picture then being essentially that of a sarcoma.

The presence of abundant mucin that stains strongly with mucicarmine supports a diagnosis of carcinoma. The mucopolysaccharides that are formed by mesotheliomas stain weakly or not at all with mucicarmine. When 'signet ring' cells containing diastase-resistant, periodic-acid/Schiff-positive material are present in a pleural growth they indicate that it is a metastatic adenocarcinoma.[913] The cells of some other types of carcinoma may also give a positive periodic-acid/Schiff reaction: mesothelioma cells do not. In most cases of mesothelioma the lungs contain asbestos bodies (page 383) as evidence of exposure to asbestos dust; pulmonary fibrosis indicative of frank asbestosis in the sense of an established pneumoconiosis is present in only about one-fifth of the cases. It is to be remembered, of course, that the presence of asbestos bodies does not prove that a given tumour is a mesothelioma.

Clinical Background and Prognosis.—The patient with a mesothelioma commonly presents with breathlessness and pain in the chest. The interval between the first exposure to asbestos and the onset of symptoms being so long (see above), the tumour is very rarely recognized in patients who have not reached the fifth decade of life, unless there was exposure to the dust early in childhood. The disease is commoner in men than in women, being mainly a hazard of occupations that are predominantly followed by men, such as asbestos mining and transportation, and work in the ship-building industry.

About half the patients die within a year of the diagnosis being made; about 10 per cent live more than five years. Treatment does not alter these figures greatly.

The incidence of asbestos-induced mesotheliomas is increasing year by year as the use of asbestos increases. Preventive measures appear to have led to disturbingly little abatement of the dangers to workers in the asbestos industry (and industries

making use of its products) and to the community at large.

Malignant Melanoma

Melanomas in the lungs are almost always secondary deposits from a primary growth elsewhere. Only one case of pulmonary melanoma is on record in which thorough post-mortem examination excluded the possibility of origin outside the lungs.[915] The tumour arose in a bronchus, causing obstruction and metastasizing widely.

SECONDARY TUMOURS IN THE LUNGS

The lungs are often the seat of metastasis of malignant tumours, both carcinomas and sarcomas, that arise in organs and tissues that have their venous drainage into the caval vessels.[916] Emboli from the primary tumour, as they break away from sites of vascular infiltration, are carried to the lungs and become impacted in the pulmonary arterioles and capillaries. Few of the cells in these emboli succeed in establishing themselves: the number of recognizable secondary deposits in the lungs represents only a very small fraction of the number of cells that reach them.[917] At the sites where they come to rest the tumour cells are quickly surrounded by fibrin and platelet thrombi. Those that survive attach themselves to the vascular endothelium and may then pass through the vessel wall into surrounding tissues, whence they can make their way into the pulmonary lymphatics. This process of extravasation of the neoplastic cells has been followed experimentally in rabbits injected intravenously with suspensions of carcinoma cells.[918] With the aid of serial photographs taken through transparent chambers previously prepared in their ears, the behaviour of the tumour cells can be watched as they become trapped in the narrowing vessels.

With some tumours, notably carcinoma of the body of the stomach, the obstruction to the pulmonary circulation caused by very large numbers of micro-emboli can be succeeded by pulmonary hypertension and cor pulmonale (see page 283).[919, 920] The subsequent lymphatic permeation from such metastasis may be very extensive, giving rise to the condition of 'lymphangitis carcinomatosa' (see page 160). In this condition, the lymphatics in the connective tissue round the smaller arteries and bronchi are filled with columns of tumour cells. The reaction of the blood vessels to the irritation caused by this nearby cellular infiltrate takes the form of endarteritis obliterans, which adds to the vascular obstruction.

Metastatic deposits in the lungs differ widely in number, size and appearance. They may appear as numerous, small, white nodules, not unlike miliary tubercles; or they may be fewer and larger, forming masses readily detectable by X-rays, such as the 'cannon-ball' deposits of renal adenocarcinoma; others again, such as those from choriocarcinoma and some sarcomas, may form soft, necrotic, and often haemorrhagic, masses. Once they have become established, metastatic tumours in the lungs may in turn invade the pulmonary veins and, by further embolization through the left side of the heart, give rise to tertiary deposits elsewhere.

Surgical resection of an isolated secondary deposit of a carcinoma or sarcoma in a lung is sometimes followed by encouraging results. A proportion as large as one-third of selected patients may survive for more than five years.[921, 922]

THE PLEURA

THE STRUCTURE OF THE PLEURA

The visceral pleura covers the lungs and extends into the fissures. At the hilum it is reflected on to the mediastinal structures; below the hilum this reflexion is extended downward as the pulmonary ligament. The parietal pleura limits the mediastinum and covers the dome of the diaphragm and the inner aspect of the chest wall.

Microscopically, both pleural layers are faced with a single layer of flattened mesothelial cells. Beneath these is a layer of connective tissue that in the visceral pleura is in continuity with the interlobular septa of the lung and in the parietal pleura merges with the extrapleural fat and the epimysium of the intercostal muscles. There is an elastic lamina at the deep aspect of the connective tissue layer of the visceral pleura, abutting on the parenchyma of the lung. Mast cells are numerous in the connective tissue.

The main blood supply of the visceral pleura is from the bronchial arteries, only a small proportion coming from the pulmonary arteries. The parietal pleura is supplied by the intercostal arteries.

Disease affecting the pleural cavities is nearly always secondary to disease in a neighbouring structure. Consequently, most of the conditions that affect the pleura have been considered elsewhere. The following paragraphs merely indicate some of the circumstances in which pleural involvement may acquire notable clinical significance. These pathological states fall broadly into three categories: pleural effusions and pneumothorax; inflammation of the pleural serosa; and pleural tumours.

PLEURAL EFFUSIONS AND PNEUMOTHORAX

Hydrothorax

Normally, the pleural cavities contain a few milli-litres of clear, yellowish fluid that suffices to lubricate the movement of the lungs against the chest wall. The water, though not the protein, of this fluid undergoes constant turnover, its site of entry into the sac being the visceral pleura and its absorption largely taking place through the parietal pleura, whence it returns to the blood through the lymphatics. Even when the sacs contain large amounts of fluid, as in hydrothorax, studies made with heavy water have shown that nearly half of it is exchanged every hour.

Normal pleural fluid contains about 2 g of protein per decilitre. The greater part is plasma albumin. In many effusions the concentration of protein is higher than in the normal fluid.

In most cases of hydrothorax, the collection of fluid is bilateral, but in congestive cardiac failure the right cavity tends to be the more frequently affected. The reason for this is conjectural: it may depend upon a difference in pressure in the right and left pulmonary veins. Although partly accommodated by depression of the diaphragm, the collection of fluid in the thorax necessarily compresses the lungs and impairs pulmonary ventilation. If the volume of fluid much exceeds a litre, the patient may complain of respiratory discomfort, and this increases as the volume rises. It is usually relieved when the amount of fluid is reduced, either by paracentesis or through improvement in the clinical condition of the patient. Some weeks may elapse, however, before the partly collapsed lung again becomes fully aerated.[923] Long continued presence of fluid in the sac may lead to some thickening of the serosa, but unless the condition is complicated by infection no adhesions form between the lung and the chest wall.

Fluid frequently collects in the pleural sac when the serosa has been infiltrated by a malignant neoplasm, which is usually one that arises in lung or breast. In these cases, the effusion is often blood-stained.

The pathogenesis of hydrothorax has much in common with that of oedema generally. In congestive cardiac failure and renal failure, particularly the latter, fluid is retained in the body and collects not only in tissue spaces but also in the serous sacs.[924] The extravasation of fluid in these conditions is probably brought about mainly by an imbalance between the two forces—intravascular blood pressure and plasma colloid osmotic pressure —that are most concerned with maintaining equilibrium of fluid between the blood and the tissues. When the blood pressure is raised or the colloid osmotic pressure lowered, fluid escapes from the plasma into the tissue spaces.

In hydrothorax due to congestive cardiac failure, the fluid probably comes from the smaller pulmonary blood vessels, the pressure in which is raised because of the pulmonary venous hypertension.[925] Any tendency for fluid to collect in the pleural sacs is increased both by a rise in the systemic venous pressure (opposing the normal flow through the mediastinal lymphatics) and by a rise in the colloid osmotic pressure of the effusion through an increase in its protein content.[926] When generalized oedema is due to chronic nephritis or cirrhosis of the liver, the disturbance in fluid equilibrium is increased, if not caused, by the fall in concentration of albumin in the plasma and the consequent decline in the colloid osmotic pressure of the latter. When there is neoplastic infiltration of the pleura, the protein content of the effusion is often substantially raised, with the result that the normal differential between the colloid osmotic pressure of the plasma and that of the fluid is much reduced and re-absorption impaired accordingly.

Occasionally, in cases of ascites, especially the form associated with ovarian fibromas (Meigs' syndrome) or other pelvic tumours, the right pleural sac may fill suddenly, presumably as a result of the development of some communication through the diaphragm (see Chapters 20 and 27).

Haemothorax

Severe haemorrhage into a pleural sac is almost always due to grave trauma to the chest wall or the thoracic viscera. Rarely, it accompanies leakage from an aneurysm of the thoracic aorta. The outcome is grave, and in the latter case the haemothorax is generally terminal. Occasionally, tears in the lungs near adhesions or emphysematous bullae are followed by haemopneumothorax, blood and air escaping simultaneously from the damaged tissue into the sac.

If the volume of blood that escapes is small, it is soon absorbed through lymphatic channels in the pleuropericardial folds.[927] If it is large, the blood coagulates, partly on the surface of the lung and partly in the lower part of the sac. In time, the clot undergoes organization: fibrous adhesions between the lung and chest wall result. In interesting contrast to what is evidently the rule in man, blood that is introduced experimentally into the pleural sac of the rat shrinks to become a very small clot abutting on the mediastinum, where it undergoes organization without the formation of adhesions within the pleural sac.[928]

Chylothorax

Chylothorax is an uncommon condition in which chyle escapes from a major lymph duct into one of the pleural sacs, usually that on the left.[929] In about half the cases the cause is obstruction of the duct by a carcinoma or malignant lymphoma; most of the rest result from surgical or other trauma;[930] some are associated with malformation of the lymphatic system.[931]

Very large amounts of chyle may need to be aspirated at frequent intervals. The possibility of surgical repair of the leaking duct may have to be considered in those cases in which injury is the cause.

Injection of the aspirated chyle intravenously, with the intention of thereby restoring it to the body for utilization, has been undertaken in some cases: this measure is so unsafe that it must never be adopted. It seems that the constituents of chyle undergo changes in concentration and physicochemical properties while in any serosal cavity: inoculation of such chyle into the circulation has caused death from what has seemed in some cases to be an acute anaphylactoid shock and in others a condition that, pathologically, resembles fat embolism very closely.[932]

Pneumothorax

Air may enter the pleural sac either through the chest wall or from the lung itself. In the former case the condition is almost always due to trauma, a fractured clavicle or rib lacerating the parietal pleura and allowing the ingress of air through an associated wound of the skin. Sometimes, the local blood vessels may also be damaged and the condition becomes one of haemopneumothorax. In surgical operations on the thorax the pleural sac is often opened and becomes filled with air. Formerly, chiefly in the treatment of chronic respiratory tuberculosis, air was introduced into the pleural sac to collapse the lung and thus limit its respiratory movements (artificial pneumothorax).

In those forms of pneumothorax that result from the escape of air from the lungs, trauma may again be responsible; more commonly the cause is some pathological change in the lungs. In older patients, spontaneous pneumothorax may complicate chronic bronchitis and emphysema, asthma, tuberculosis and bronchiectasis; less often, it develops in the course of bronchial cancer, silicosis, pulmonary infarction and some rarer disorders. The commonest factor is chronic bronchitis.

In young patients pneumothorax can occur in the absence of such predisposing conditions. In those cases in which thoracotomy has been required in the course of treatment, the usual pathological change has been an area of fibrosis, 2 to 3 cm in its greatest dimension, at the apex of the lung, surmounted by one or more bullae up to 1 cm or so in diameter.[933] A hole may be found in the pleural surface adjoining the bullae, or one of the latter may have a tear in its wall. Microscopical examination shows collapse of the lung parenchyma, with fibrosis and an accumulation of chronic inflammatory cells. The wall of the bulla is fibrotic. It has been suggested that, since most of these patients are tall, thin men, the changes in the apical region of the lungs—demonstrably affected bilaterally in some cases—may be developmental in origin and possibly related to rapid somatic growth. Other possibilities include chronic inflammation, particularly tuberculosis.

Irrespective of its initial pathogenesis, a pneumothorax may be open or closed: in the former, the aperture remains patent, so that air can pass freely into and out of the sac; in the latter, the opening soon becomes sealed, and thus traps the air that has entered. Occasionally—particularly in older people—the tissues near the orifice act as a valve, allowing air to enter but not to escape. In these cases a positive pressure builds up in the sac, displacing the structures of the mediastinum to the opposite side, with consequent grave embarrassment of respiration (*pressure pneumothorax*).

Pneumothorax is usually sudden in onset, and often occurs during physical exertion. It is generally unilateral. Bilateral pneumothorax, which is not uncommon, is more serious since there is interference with the inflation of both lungs. The onset is painful, and quickly followed by shortness of breath, especially in patients with emphysema or other extensive chronic pulmonary disease that already impairs their respiratory capacity. In the cases in which the tissues create a valve at the site of perforation, the pneumothorax may build up slowly without any sudden symptoms; in these instances the displacement of the mediastinum is apt to be greater.

The extent to which the lung collapses in pneumothorax and the degree to which the mediastinal structures become shifted depend largely on the quantity of air that has entered. In some patients, in whom previous chronic adhesions have bound much of the lung to the chest wall, even a large opening in the lung may be associated with only a small entry of air: the presence of the pneumothorax may then add little, if anything, to any pre-existing respiratory distress. Once the air leak has been sealed, the air in the pleural sac is gradually absorbed over the ensuing weeks—oxygen first and nitrogen later.

As with pleural effusions (see page 410), the presence of larger amounts of air in the pleural sacs reduces the vital capacity of the lungs and results in some degree of respiratory disability. This may be lessened in two ways: first, by depression of the dome of the diaphragm, which increases the capacity of the thorax, and second, by a higher rate of respiration, which compensates for the fall in tidal air. These adaptations account for the fact that there is no serious abnormality of the blood gases in such patients while they remain at rest.

INFLAMMATION OF THE PLEURA

Acute Pleurisy

Acute inflammation of the pleural sac can develop in a wide variety of conditions, most of which are infective in origin. In most instances, the serositis is secondary to infection of one of the adjoining intrathoracic or subdiaphragmatic structures, particularly the lungs. Sometimes, as in cases of disseminated lupus erythematosus and other 'collagen diseases', the pathogenetic mechanism is uncertain.

Acute inflammatory reactions in the pleura follow the sequence typical of serositis—hyperaemia of the underlying subserosal tissue, succeeded by the collection of an exudate of fluid and leucocytes in the sac. In its incipient stages, before the exudate has formed, the pleurisy is dry (*fibrinous pleurisy*), and is accompanied by considerable pain on breathing and a rub audible on auscultation. With the development of exudate (*serofibrinous pleurisy*) the visceral and parietal surfaces of the sac become separated and the pain and rub diminish. Should the contents of the sac become infected with bacteria, however, the serofibrinous reaction may be replaced by a suppurative one, in which the cavity becomes filled by pus—the condition known as *empyema thoracis* (see below).

In many cases of serofibrinous pleurisy the inflammation regresses as time or treatment brings about recovery from the underlying disease. In such cases, the exudate is absorbed, and unless the pleura has been extensively denuded of its mesothelium the sac recovers its smooth lining. Where mesothelium has been lost, adhesions may form between the lung and the chest wall: at first the adhesions are fibrinous, but later, through organization, they become fibrous. In this way, part or all of the cavity may be obliterated.

Empyema Thoracis

A bacterial infection of the pleural cavity that converts an initially serofibrinous effusion into a purulent one is a grave complication, although with progress in chemotherapy such progressive suppurative changes are less common than formerly. Of the types of infection that occur nowadays, that due to *Staphylococcus aureus* is the most serious; such infection may complicate staphylococcal pneumonia, especially in children. The greater susceptibility of pneumococci and streptococci to antibiotics has much lessened the frequency with which they cause empyema. When an empyema is due to rupture of a lung abscess into the pleural cavity, the pus may contain a wide variety of bacteria (see page 313).

The pleural sacs may become infected through penetrating injuries to the chest wall, when dirt and pieces of clothing may be introduced into the wound. Sometimes, too, empyema may follow a surgical operation on the lungs, especially lobectomy or pneumonectomy, when infected material may leak from the severed end of a bronchus.

In empyema thoracis the whole or merely a part —usually the lower part—of the sac may be filled with thick, viscous pus. Sometimes the pus is confined to the space between two lobes (*interlobar empyema*—Fig. 7.83). In such instances, organization of parts of the exudate leads to the formation of firm adhesions that restrict the spread of the infection and localize the pus.

Empyema thoracis is a serious condition that, if inadequately treated, has a high mortality. Sometimes the infection is overcome without intervention, and the pus is eventually replaced by granulation tissue and fibrous tissue. Occasionally, the pleural

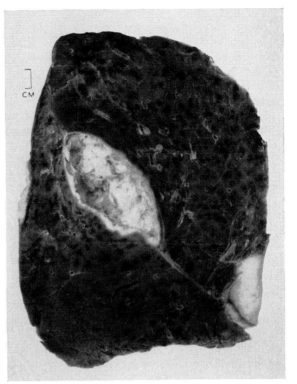

Fig. 7.83.§ Interlobar empyema in the oblique fissure of the left lung, localized by adhesions between the lobes.

infection extends into the chest wall or the lung substance, and the pus is discharged through the opening created. Even in favourable cases the damage to the serosa is severe: when the suppuration subsides, fibrous adhesions develop and eventually obliterate the cavity. The lining of the cavity may undergo calcification during the succeeding years.

Tuberculosis of the Pleura

The visceral pleura may become involved at any stage in the evolution of tuberculosis of the lungs. The pleurisy may become manifest clinically while the pulmonary lesions are quite small; indeed, the appearance of an effusion may be the first indication that the patient has acquired a tuberculous infection. Soon, however, an initially mainly dry, and often painful, pleurisy is succeeded by a large effusion: by this time the pulmonary lesions have, as a rule, made themselves manifest by cough and mild pyrexia.

The effusion may reach a volume of a litre or more. On tapping, a clear, straw-coloured, occasionally blood-tinged, fluid is withdrawn: it contains a little fibrin and numerous lymphocytes. In a proportion of cases, the presence of tubercle bacilli in a centrifuged sample of the fluid can be demonstrated by cultivation on an appropriate medium. Alternatively, the diagnosis can often be made by histological examination of a biopsy specimen of the pleura (see below).

Pleural effusion in children and young adults is nowadays less common than formerly in those countries where the pool of tuberculous infection has been reduced, particularly since the introduction of prophylactic immunization with BCG. Its development has a fairly constant time relation to the primary infection, appearing usually some three to six months after this, and seldom, if ever, after a year has passed.[934]

Histological Changes.—The pleura in cases of effusion accompanying pulmonary tuberculosis is infected with *Mycobacterium tuberculosis*: the condition is not an allergic response to the intrapulmonary tuberculous infection, as formerly was thought. Typical histological changes of tuberculosis can usually be found in pleural biopsy material. If a needle biopsy gives negative results, an open surgical biopsy may be successful.[935]

Course.—In the early stages of a tuberculous pleurisy the appearance of the visceral and parietal serosal surfaces does not differ greatly from that seen in the usual serofibrinous form of pleurisy. Later, however, if the infection does not regress, the pleural surfaces show patches of tuberculous granulation tissue, in which typical tubercles can be seen histologically. Ultimately, the granulation tissue may show areas of caseation; in time, these may undergo calcification and appear as opacities in radiographs.

In the days before effective antituberculosis drugs were available, a simple tuberculous effusion usually disappeared within three to four months, leaving at most a minor degree of obliteration of the costophrenic angle in the radiographs. However, some patients developed dense adhesions and consequent restriction of the pulmonary ventilation: this complication is not seen in cases correctly treated with modern measures.

Tuberculous 'Empyema'

A severer form of tuberculous infection of the pleura may develop in the course of post-primary tuberculosis if a tuberculous cavity erodes into the pleural sac. The result is the condition conventionally described as a tuberculous empyema (Fig. 7.44 —page 343), although the puriform, semifluid matter that collects is caseous and not true pus, except when there is a simultaneous or subsequent infection by pyogenic bacteria. The exudate in the pleural sac becomes encased in a thick, fibrosing layer of tuberculous granulation tissue.

The same condition may result from rupture of a juxtavertebral abscess in cases of tuberculosis of the thoracic part of the spine. Similarly, tuberculosis of a rib may be complicated by pleural effusion or 'empyema'.

Bronchopleural fistula may be present in association with tuberculous 'empyema' and increases the liability to secondary infection. In some cases the latter is caused by fungi. Pleural aspergillosis is the least rare variety of mycosis to develop in these circumstances;[936] candidosis, cryptococcosis and phycomycosis have also been observed.[937]

TUMOURS OF THE PLEURA

Primary Tumours.—Fibroma of the pleura is described on page 390. Malignant mesothelioma is described on page 407.

Secondary Tumours.—The pleural sacs are often the seat of metastatic tumours. The commonest primary growths in such cases are carcinomas, particularly bronchial, mammary and renal carcinomas.[938]

REFERENCES

THE STRUCTURE OF THE NORMAL LUNG
1. *Thorax*, 1950, **5**, 222.
2. Brock, R. C., *The Anatomy of the Bronchial Tree*, 2nd edn. London, 1954.
3. Boyden, E. A., *Segmental Anatomy of the Lungs*. New York, 1955.
4. Boyden, E. A., *Dis. Chest*, 1961, **39**, 1.

5. Hayek, H. von, *The Human Lung*, translated by V. E. Krahl, page 87. New York, 1960.
6. Heard, B. E., *Pathology of Chronic Bronchitis and Emphysema*, page 15. London, 1969.
7. Hayek, H. von, *The Human Lung*, translated by V. E. Krahl, page 202. New York, 1960.

8. Brenner, O., *Arch. intern. Med.*, 1935, **56**, 211, 457, 724, 976, 1189.
9. *Gray's Anatomy*, edited by R. Warwick and P. L. Williams, 35th edn, page 1204. London, 1973.
10. Hayek, H. von, *The Human Lung*, translated by V. E. Krahl, page 127. New York, 1960.
11. Miller, W. S., *The Lung*, 2nd edn, page 31. Springfield, Illinois, 1947.
12. Kohn, H. N., *Münch. med. Wschr.*, 1893, **40**, 42.
13. Van Allen, C. M., Lindskog, G. E., Richter, H. G., *J. clin. Invest.*, 1931, **10**, 559.
14. Cordingley, J. L., *Thorax*, 1972, **27**, 433.
15. Bertalanffy, F. D., *Int. Rev. Cytol.*, 1964, **16**, 233.
16. Bertalanffy, F. D., *Int. Rev. Cytol.*, 1964, **17**, 213.
17. Rhodin, J. A. G., *An Atlas of Ultrastructure*, page 86. Philadelphia, 1963.
18. Rhodin, J., Dalhamn, T., *Z. Zellforsch.*, 1956, **44**, 345.
19. Watson, J. H. L., Brinkman, G. L., *Amer. Rev. resp. Dis.*, 1964, **90**, 851.
20. Clara, M., *Z. mikr.-anat. Forsch.*, 1937, **41**, 321.
21. Low, F. N., Daniels, C. W., *Anat. Rec.*, 1952, **112**, 456.
22. Low, F. N., Daniels, C. W., *Anat. Rec.*, 1952, **113**, 437.
23. Macklin, C. C., *Anat. Rec.*, 1953, **115**, 343.
24. Macklin, C. C., *Anat. Rec.*, 1953, **115**, 431.
25. Klaus, M., Reiss, O. K., Tooley, W. H., Piel, C., Clements, J. A., *Science*, 1962, **137**, 750.
26. Scarpelli, E. M., *The Surfactant System of the Lung*. Philadelphia, 1968.
27. Chase, W. H., *Exp. Cell Res.*, 1959, **18**, 15.
28. Weibel, E. R., Gil, J., *Resp. Physiol.*, 1968, **4**, 42.
29. Gil, J., Weibel, E. R., *Resp. Physiol.*, 1969, **5**, 13.
30. Evans, M. J., Cabral, L. J., Stephans, R. J., *Amer. J. Path.*, 1973, **70**, 175.
31. Hung, K., Hertweck, M. S., Hardy, J. D., Loosli, C. G., *Amer. Rev. resp. Dis.*, 1973, **108**, 328.
32. Lauweryns, J. M., *Amer. Rev. resp. Dis.*, 1970, **102**, 877.
33. Heard, B. E., Salsbury, A., *unpublished studies*.

CONGENITAL MALFORMATIONS
34. Gruenfeld, G. E., Gray, S. H., *Arch. Path. (Chic.)*, 1941, **31**, 392.
35. Wilson, J. G., Roth, C. B., Warkany, J., *Amer. J. Anat.*, 1953, **92**, 189.
36. Arrechon, W., Reid, L., *Brit. med. J.*, 1963, **1**, 230.
37. Neill, C. A., Ferencz, C., Sabiston, D. C., Sheldon, H., *Bull. Johns Hopk. Hosp.*, 1960, **107**, 1.
38. De Jager, H., *J. Path. Bact.*, 1965, **90**, 321.
39. Norris, R. F., Tyson, R. M., *Amer. J. Path.*, 1947, **23**, 1075.
40. Cooke, F. N., Blades, B., *J. thorac. Surg.*, 1952, **23**, 546.
41. Bowden, K. M., *Med. J. Aust.*, 1948, **2**, 311.
42. Laurence, K. M., *J. clin. Path.*, 1959, **12**, 62.
43. Moffat, A. D., *J. Path. Bact.*, 1960, **79**, 361.
44. Fronstin, M. H., Hooper, G. S., Besse, B. E., Ferreri, S., *Amer. J. Dis. Child.*, 1967, **114**, 330.
45. Pryce, D. M., *J. Path. Bact.*, 1946, **58**, 457.
46. Pryce, D. M., Sellors, T. H., Blair, L. G., *Brit. J. Surg.*, 1947–48, **35**, 18.
47. Eade, A. W. T., Stretton, T. B., *Brit. med. J.*, 1961, **1**, 774.
48. Symbas, P. N., Hatcher, C. R., Abbott, O. A., Logan, W. D., *Amer. Rev. resp. Dis.*, 1969, **99**, 406.
49. Iwai, K., Shindo, G., Hajikano, H., Tajima, H., Morimoto, M., Kosuda, T., Yoneuda, R., *Amer. Rev. resp. Dis.*, 1973, **107**, 911.

50. Ch'in, K. Y., Tang, M. Y., *Arch. Path. (Chic.)*, 1949, **48**, 221.
51. Moncrieff, M. W., Cameron, A. H., Astley, R., Roberts, K. D., Abrams, L. D., Mann, J. R., *Thorax*, 1969, **24**, 476.
52. Ellis, F. H., McGoon, D. C., Kincaid, O. W., *Med. Clin. N. Amer.*, 1964, **48**, 1069.
53. Fisher, J. M., Van Epps, E. F., *Amer. Heart J.*, 1959, **58**, 26.
54. Le Roux, B. T., *Quart. J. Med.*, 1959, N.S. **28**, 1.
55. Wagenvoort, C. A., Wagenvoort, N., *Lab. Invest.*, 1967, **16**, 13.
56. Robertson, B., Ivemark, B. I., in *The Anatomy of the Developing Lung*, edited by J. L. Emery, page 170. London, 1969.
57. Hessel, E. A., Boyden, E. A., Stamm, S. J., Sauvage, L. R., *Surgery*, 1970, **67**, 624.
58. Naeye, R. L., *Amer. J. Path.*, 1962, **41**, 287.
59. Naeye, R. L., in *The Lung*, edited by A. A. Liebow and D. E. Smith, page 166. Baltimore, 1968.

VASCULAR DISTURBANCES
60. Parker, B. M., Smith, J. R., *Amer. J. Med.*, 1958, **24**, 402.
61. Hall, C. M., Clark, C. G., *Brit. J. Surg.*, 1971, **58**, 101.
62. Daniel, D. G., Bloom, A. L., Geddings, J. C., Campbell, H., Turnbull, A. C., *Brit. med. J.*, 1968, **1**, 801.
63. Jeffcoate, T. N. A., Miller, J., Roos, F., Tindall, V. R., *Brit. med. J.*, 1968, **4**, 19.
64. Inman, W. H. W., Vessey, M. P., Westerholm, B., Engelund, A., *Brit. med. J.*, 1970, **2**, 203.
65. Wright, H. Payling, Osborn, S. B., Edmonds, D. G., *Lancet*, 1951, **1**, 22.
66. Miller, R., Berry, J. B., *Amer. J. med. Sci.*, 1951, **222**, 197.
67. Cudkowicz, L., Armstrong, J. B., *Thorax*, 1951, **6**, 343.
68. Liebow, A. A., Hales, M. R., Bloomer, W. E., Harrison, W., Lindskog, G. E., *Amer. J. Path.*, 1950, **26**, 177.
69. Roach, H. D., Laufman, H., *Ann. Surg.*, 1955, **142**, 82.
70. Hampton, A. O., Castleman, B., *Amer. J. Roentgenol.*, 1940, **43**, 305.
71. Williams, M. H., Towbin, E. J., *Circulat. Res.*, 1955, **3**, 422.
72. Jackson, C. T., Greendyke, R. M., *Surg. Gynec. Obstet.*, 1965, **120**, 25.
73. Armin, J., Grant, R. T., *Clin. Sci.*, 1951, **10**, 441.
74. Robb-Smith, A. H. T., *Lancet*, 1941, **1**, 135.
75. Gough, J. H., Gough, M. H., Thomas, M. L., *Brit. J. Radiol.*, 1964, **37**, 416.
76. Fraimow, W., Wallace, S., Lewis, P., Greening, R. R., Cathcart, R. T., *Radiology*, 1965, **85**, 231.
77. Jaques, W. E., Mariscal, G. C., *Bull. int. Ass. med. Mus.*, 1951, **32**, 63.
78. Symmers, W. St C., *unpublished studies*, 1938–40.
79. Symmers, W. St C., *Curiosa—A Miscellany of Clinical and Pathological Experiences*, chap. 45. London, 1974.
80. Hopkins, G. B., Taylor, D. G., *Amer. Rev. resp. Dis.*, 1970, **101**, 101.
81. Attwood, H. D., Park, W. W., *J. Obstet. Gynaec. Brit. Cwlth*, 1961, **68**, 611.
82. Savage, M. B., *Amer. J. Obstet. Gynec.*, 1951, **62**, 346.
83. Symmers, W. St C., *unpublished observations*, 1953, 1971.

84. Park, W. W., *J. Path. Bact.*, 1954, **67**, 563.
85. McMillan, J. B., *Amer. J. Path.*, 1956, **32**, 405.
86. Potter, E. L., Young, R. L., *Arch. Path. (Chic.)*, 1942, **34**, 1009.
87. Gruenwald, P., *Amer. J. Path.*, 1941, **17**, 879.
88. Straus, R., *Arch. Path. (Chic.)*, 1942, **33**, 69.
89. Symmers, W. St C., *unpublished case*, 1953.
90. Cole, W. H., McDonald, G. O., Roberts, S. S., Southwick, H. W., *Dissemination of Cancer*, page 166. New York, 1961.
91. Morgan, A. D., *J. Path. Bact.*, 1949, **61**, 75.
92. Hunter, D., *The Diseases of Occupations*, 4th edn, page 839. London, 1969.
93. Attwood, H. D., *J. clin. Path.*, 1956, **9**, 38.
94. Megibow, R. S., Latz, L. N., Steinitz, F. S., *Surgery*, 1942, **11**, 19.
95. Steinberg, B., Mundy, C. S., *Arch. Path. (Chic.)*, 1936, **22**, 529.
96. Holden, W. D., Shaw, B. W., Cameron, D. B., Shea, P. J., Davis, J. H., *Surg. Gynec. Obstet.*, 1949, **88**, 23.
97. Pryce, D. M., Heard, B. E., *J. Path. Bact.*, 1956, **71**, 15.
98. Willis, R. A., *The Spread of Tumours in the Human Body*, 2nd edn, page 173. London, 1952.
99. VonGlahn, W. C., Hall, J. W., *Amer. J. Path.*, 1949, **25**, 575.
100. Heard, B. E., *J. Path. Bact.*, 1952, **64**, 13.
101. Harrison, C. V., *J. Path. Bact.*, 1948, **60**, 289.
102. Daley, R., in *Clinical Disorders of the Pulmonary Circulation*, edited by R. Daley, J. F. Goodwin and R. E. Steiner, page 341. London, 1960.
103. Wood, P., *Diseases of the Heart and Circulation*, 2nd edn, page 828. London, 1956.
104. McGuire, J., Scott, R. C., Helm, R. A., Kaplan, S., Gall, E. A., Biehl, J. P., *A.M.A. Arch. intern. Med.*, 1957, **99**, 917.
105. Yu, P. N., *Ann. intern. Med.*, 1958, **49**, 1138.
106. Harrison, C. V., in *Clinical Disorders of the Pulmonary Circulation*, edited by R. Daley, J. F. Goodwin and R. E. Steiner, page 136. London, 1960.
107. Doyle, A. E., Goodwin, J. F., Harrison, C. V., Steiner, R. E., *Brit. Heart J.*, 1957, **19**, 353.
108. Symmers, W. St C., *J. clin. Path.*, 1952, **5**, 36.
109. Harrison, C. V., *Brit. J. Radiol.*, 1958, **31**, 217, 226.
110. Edwards, J. E., *Circulation*, 1957, **15**, 164.
110a. Liebow, A. A., *Amer. Rev. resp. Dis.*, 1959, **80**, 67.
111. Morgan, A. D., *J. Path. Bact.*, 1949, **61**, 75.
112. Storstein, O., *Circulation*, 1951, **4**, 913.
113. Symmers, W. St. C., *J. Path. Bact.*, 1904, **9**, 237.
114. Shaw, A. F. B., Ghareeb, A. A., *J. Path. Bact.*, 1938, **46**, 401.
115. Marchand, E. J., Marcial-Rojas, R. A., Rodrigues, R., Polanco, G., Diaz-Rivera, R. S., *A.M.A. Arch. intern. Med.*, 1957, **100**, 965.
116. Faria, J. L. de, *J. Path. Bact.*, 1954, **68**, 589.
117. Harrison, C. V., *J. Path. Bact.*, 1951, **63**, 195.
118. Liebow, A. A., in *Pathology of the Heart*, edited by S. E. Gould, 2nd edn, chap. 15. Springfield, Illinois, 1960.
119. Hasleton, P. S., Heath, D., Brewer, D. B., *J. Path. Bact.*, 1968, **95**, 431.
120. Follath, F., Burkart, F., Schweizer, W., *Brit. med. J.*, 1971, **1**, 265.
121. Widgren, S., Kapanci, Y., *Z. Kreisl.-Forsch.*, 1970, **59**, 924.
122. Brunner, H., Stepanek, J., in *Proceedings of the Twelfth Meeting of the European Society for the Study of Drug Toxicity*, edited by S. B. de C. Baker, page 123. Amsterdam, 1971.
123. Heath, D., Scott, O., Lynch, J., *Thorax*, 1971, **26**, 663.
124. Wagenvoort, C. A., Heath, D., Edwards, J. E., *The Pathology of the Pulmonary Vasculature*, pages 94–107. Springfield, Illinois, 1964.
125. Wagenvoort, C. A., Losekoot, G., Mulder, E., *Thorax*, 1971, **26**, 429.
126. *Wld Hlth Org. techn. Rep. Ser.*, No. 213, 1961, 6.
127. Kopelman, H., Lee, G. de J., *Clin. Sci.*, 1951, **10**, 383.
128. Rapaport, E., Kuida, H., Haynes, F. W. Dexter, L., *J. clin. Invest.*, 1956, **35**, 1393.
129. Parker, F., Weiss, S., *Amer. J. Path.*, 1936, **12**, 573.
130. Lendrum, A. C., Scott, L. D. W., Park, S. D. S., *Quart. J. Med.*, 1950, N.S. **19**, 249.
131. Magarey, F. R., *J. Path. Bact.*, 1951, **63**, 729.
132. Wyllie, W. G., Sheldon, W., Bodian, M., Barlow, A., *Quart. J. Med.*, 1948, N.S. **17**, 25.
133. Browning, J. R., Houghton, J. D., *Amer. J. Med.*, 1956, **20**, 374.
134. Wynn-Williams, N., Young, R. D., *Thorax*, 1956, **11**, 101.
135. Parkin, T. W., Rusted, I. E., Burchell, H. B., Edwards, J. E., *Amer. J. Med.*, 1955, **18**, 220.
136. Heptinstall, R. H., Salmon, M. V., *J. clin. Path.*, 1959, **12**, 272.
137. Edwards, J. E., Parkin, T. W., Burchell, H. B., *Proc. Mayo Clin.*, 1954, **29**, 193.
138. Rose, G. A., Spencer, H., *Quart. J. Med.*, 1957, N.S. **26**, 43.
139. Thomas, A. M., *J. clin. Path.*, 1958, **11**, 146.
140. Lilienfield, L. S., Freis, E. D., Partenope, E. A., Morowitz, H. J., *J. clin. Invest.*, 1955, **34**, 1.
141. Lewis, B. M., Houssay, H. E. J., Haynes, F. W., Dexter, L., *Circulat. Res.*, 1953, **1**, 312.
142. Cameron, G. R., Courtice, F. C., *J. Physiol. (Lond.)*, 1946, **105**, 175.
143. Cottrell, T. S., Levine, O. R., Senior, R. M., Wiener, J., Spiro, D., Fishman, A. P., *Circulat. Res.*, 1967, **21**, 783.
144. Cheng, K., *J. Path. Bact.*, 1958, **76**, 241.
145. West, J. B., Dollery, C. T., Heard, B. E., *Circulat. Res.*, 1965, **17**, 191.
146. Hunter, D., *The Diseases of Occupations*, 4th edn, page 667. London, 1969.
147. Grayson, R. R., *Ann. intern. Med.*, 1956, **45**, 393.
148. Lowry, T., Schuman, L. M., *J. Amer. med. Ass.*, 1956, **162**, 153.
149. Doniach, I., Morrison, B., Steiner, R. E., *Brit. Heart J.*, 1954, **16**, 101.
150. Heard, B. E., *J. Path. Bact.*, 1962, **83**, 159.
151. Heard, B. E., Cooke, R. A., *Thorax*, 1968, **23**, 187.
152. Heard, B. E., Steiner, R. E., Herdan, A., Gleason, D., *Brit. J. Radiol.*, 1968, **41**, 161.
153. Hayes, J. A., Shiga, A., *J. Path.*, 1970, **100**, 281.
154. Kerley, P., *Brit. Heart J.*, 1933, **2**, 594.
155. Fleischner, F. G., Reiner, L., *New Engl. J. Med.*, 1954, **250**, 900.
156. Gough, J., *Lancet*, 1955, **1**, 161.
157. Grainger, R. G., *Brit. J. Radiol.*, 1958, **31**, 201.
158. Gleason, D. C., Steiner, R. E., *Amer. J. Roentgenol.* 1966, **98**, 279.

DISORDERS OF RESPIRATORY FUNCTION AT HIGH ALTITUDES

159. Peñazola, D., Sime, F., Banchero, N., Gamboa, R., *Med. thorac.*, 1962, **19**, 449.

160. Hasleton, P. S., Heath, D., Brewer, D. B., *J. Path. Bact.*, 1968, **95**, 431.

161. Hultgren, H. N., Lopez, C. E., Lunberg, E., Miller, H., *Circulation*, 1964, **29**, 393.

162. Saldana, M., in *The Lung*, edited by A. A. Liebow and D. E. Smith, page 259. Baltimore, 1968.

163. Singh, I., Kapila, C. C., Khanna, P. K., Nanda, R. B., Rao, B. D. P., *Lancet*, 1965, **1**, 229.

164. Monge, C., *Arch. intern. Med.*, 1937, **59**, 32.

165. Hurtado, A., *Ann. intern. Med.*, 1960, **53**, 247.

166. Hecht, H. H., Kuida, H., Lange, R. L., Thorne, J. L., Brown, A. M., *Amer. J. Med.*, 1962, **32**, 171.

HYALINE MEMBRANE DISEASE

167. Bound, J. P., Butler, N. R., Spector, W. G., *Brit. med. J.*, 1956, **2**, 1191, 1260.

168. Silverman, W. A., Silverman, R. H., *Lancet*, 1958, **2**, 588.

169. Claireaux, A. E., *Postgrad. med. J.*, 1954, **30**, 338.

170. Tran-Dihn-De, Anderson, G. W., *Obstet. gynec. Surv.*, 1953, **8**, 1.

171. Mahaffey, L. W., Rossdale, P. D., *Lancet*, 1959, **1**, 1223.

172. Feinberg, S. B., Goldberg, M. E., *Radiology*, 1957, **68**, 185.

173. Lauweryns, J. M., *Hum. Path.*, 1970, **1**, 175.

174. Avery, M. E., Mead, J., *A.M.A. J. Dis. Child.*, 1959, **97**, 517.

PULMONARY ALVEOLAR PROTEINOSIS

175. Rosen, S. H., Castleman, B., Liebow, A. A., *New Engl. J. Med.*, 1958, **258**, 1123.

176. Slutzker, B., Knoll, H. C., Ellis, F. E., Silverstone, I. A., *Arch. intern. Med.*, 1961, **107**, 264.

177. Fraimow, W., Cathcart, R. T., Taylor, R. C., *Ann. intern. Med.*, 1960, **52**, 1177.

178. Ray, R. L., Salm, R., *Thorax*, 1962, **17**, 257.

179. Larson, R. K., Gardinier, R., *Ann. intern. Med.*, 1965, **12**, 292.

180. Ramirez, R. J., Harlan, W. R., *Amer. J. Med.*, 1968, **45**, 502.

181. Heppleston, A. G., Wright, N. A., Stewart, J. W., *J. Path.*, 1970, **101**, 293.

182. Gough, J., *Brit. med. J.*, 1967, **1**, 629.

183. Steer, A., *Arch. Path.*, 1969, **87**, 347.

184. Corrin, B., King, E., *Thorax*, 1970, **25**, 230.

185. Andriole, V. T., Ballas, M., Wilson, G. L., *Ann. intern. Med.*, 1964, **60**, 266.

186. Symmers, W. St C., *personal communication*, 1974.

DISTURBANCES OF INFLATION

187. Simmons, D. H., Hemingway, A., *Circulat. Res.*, 1959, **7**, 93.

188. Burton, A. C., Patel, D. J., *J. appl. Physiol.*, 1958, **12**, 239.

189. Patel, D. J., Burton, A. C., *Circulat. Res.*, 1957, **5**, 620.

190. Glaister, D. H., *Brit. J. Hosp. Med.*, 1969, **2**, 635.

191. Tomlin, P. J., *Lancet*, 1968, **1**, 1402.

192. Heard, B. E., *Pathology of Chronic Bronchitis and Emphysema*. London, 1969.

193. Ciba Guest Symposium, *Thorax*, 1959, **14**, 286.

194. American Thoracic Society Statement (Meneely, G. R.,

195. Renzett, A. D., Steele, J. D., Wyatt, J. P., Harris, H. W.), *Amer. Rev. resp. Dis.*, 1962, **85**, 762.

195. Emery, J. L., *Lancet*, 1956, **1**, 405.

196. Liebow, A. A., Stark, J. E., Vogel, J., Schaefer, K. E., *U.S. armed Forces med. J.*, 1959, **10**, 265.

197. Laënnec, R. H. T., *A Treatise on the Diseases of the Chest and Mediate Auscultation*, translated from the 4th edition by J. Forbes, page 141. London, 1834.

198. Heard, B. E., Izukawa, T., *J. Path. Bact.*, 1964, **88**, 423.

199. Gough, J., in *Modern Trends in Pathology*, edited by D. H. Collins, page 286. London, 1959.

200. Leopold, J. G., Gough, J., *Thorax*, 1957, **12**, 219.

201. McLean, K. H., *Aust. Ann. Med.*, 1957, **6**, 124.

202. Heard, B. E., *Thorax*, 1958, **13**, 136.

203. Heard, B. E., *Thorax*, 1959, **14**, 58.

204. Hartroft, W. S., *Amer. J. Path.*, 1945, **21**, 889.

205. Stovin, P. G. I., *Thorax*, 1959, **14**, 254.

206. Wyatt, J. P., *Amer. Rev. resp. Dis.*, 1959, **80**, 94.

207. Waters, A. H. T., *Researches on the Nature, Pathology and Treatment of Emphysema of the Lungs and Its Relation with Other Diseases of the Chest*. London, 1862.

208. Heard, B. E., *Pathology of Chronic Bronchitis and Emphysema*, page 6. London, 1969.

209. Reid, A., Heard, B. E., *Thorax*, 1963, **18**, 201.

210. Gough, J., *Proc. roy. Soc. Med.*, 1952, **45**, 576.

211. Auerbach, O., Stout, A. P., Hammond, E. C., Garfinkel, L., *New Engl. J. Med.*, 1961, **265**, 253.

212. Heard, B. E., *Pathology of Chronic Bronchitis and Emphysema*, page 62. London, 1969.

213. Gross, P., Babyak, M. A., Tolker, E., Kaschak, M., *J. occup. Med.*, 1964, **6**, 481.

214. Hirst, R. N., Perry, H. M., Cruz, M. G., Pierce, J. A., *Amer. Rev. resp. Dis.*, 1973, **108**, 30.

215. Thurlbeck, W. M., Foley, F. D., *Amer. J. Path.*, 1963, **42**, 431.

216. Smith, J. P., Smith, J. C., McCall, A. J., *J. Path. Bact.*, 1960, **80**, 287.

217. Gough, J., *Industr. Med. Surg.*, 1960, **29**, 283.

218. Laurell, C. B., Eriksson, S., *Scand. J. clin. Lab. Invest.*, 1963, **15**, 132.

219. Eriksson, S., *Acta med. scand.*, 1965, suppl. 432, 1.

220. Eriksson, S., *Acta med. scand.*, 1964, **175**, 197.

221. Hutchison, D. C. S., Cook, P. J. L., Barter, C. E., Harris, H., Hugh-Jones, P., *Brit. med. J.*, 1971, **1**, 689.

222. Hutchison, D. C. S., Barter, C. E., Cook, P. J. L., Laws, J. W., Martelli, N. A., Hugh-Jones, P., *Quart. J. Med.*, 1972, N.S. **41**, 301.

223. Schleusener, A., Talamo, R. C., Paré, J. A. P., Thurlbeck, W. M., *Amer. Rev. resp. Dis.*, 1968, **98**, 692.

224. Tarkoff, M. P., Kueppers, F., Miller, W. F., *Amer. J. Med.*, 1968, **45**, 220.

225. Falk, G. A., Siskind, G. W., Smith, J. P., *Amer. Rev. resp. Dis.*, 1971, **103**, 18.

226. Briscoe, W. A., *Clin. Sci.*, 1952, **11**, 45.

227. Briscoe, W. A., Cournand, A., in *Pulmonary Structure and Function*, edited by A. V. S. De Reuck and M. O'Connor, page 304. London, 1962.

228. Donald, K. W., Renzetti, A., Riley, R. L., Cournand, A., *J. appl. Physiol.*, 1952, **4**, 497.

229. Wells, R. E., Walker, J. E. C., Hickler, R. B., *J. clin. Invest.*, 1959, **38**, 1053.

230. Simpson, T., Heard, B. E., Laws, J. W., *Thorax*, 1963, **18**, 361.

231. Hentel, W., Longfield, A. N., Vincent, T. N., Filley,

G. F., Mitchell, R. S., *Amer. Rev. resp. Dis.*, 1963, **87**, 206.

232. Fletcher, C. M., Hugh-Jones, P., McNicol, M. W., Pride, N. B., *Quart. J. Med.*, 1963, N.S. **32**, 33.

233. Laws, J. W., Heard, B. E., *Brit. J. Radiol.*, 1962, **35**, 750.

234. Mounsey, J. P. D., Ritzmann, L. W., Selverstone, M. J., Briscoe, W. A., McLemore, G. A., *Brit. Heart J.*, 1952, **14**, 153.

235. Parkinson, J., Hoyle, C., *Quart. J. Med.*, 1937, N.S. **6**, 59.

236. MacLeod, W. M., *Thorax*, 1954, **9**, 147.

237. Dornhorst, A. C., Heaf, P. J., Semple, S. J. G., *Lancet*, 1957, **2**, 873.

238. Belcher, J. R., Capel, L. H., Pattinson, J. N., Smart, J., *Brit. med. J.*, 1960, **1**, 1654.

239. Reid, L., Simon, G., *Thorax*, 1962, **17**, 230.

BRONCHIAL ASTHMA

240. Unger, L., *Bronchial Asthma*. Springfield, Illinois, 1945.

241. Pepys, J., in *Identification of Asthma*, edited by R. Porter and J. Birch, page 86. Edinburgh and London, 1971.

242. Dunnill, M. S., *J. clin. Path.*, 1960, **13**, 27.

243. Cardell, B. S., Pearson, R. S. B., *Thorax*, 1959, **14**, 341.

244. Gough, J., *Lancet*, 1955, **1**, 161.

245. Naylor, B., *Thorax*, 1962, **17**, 69.

246. Vierordt, O., *Berl. klin. Wschr.*, 1883, **20**, 437.

247. Glynn, A. A., Michaels, L., *Thorax*, 1960, **15**, 142.

248. Williams, D. A., Leopold, J. G., *Acta allerg. (Kbh.)*, 1959, **14**, 83.

249. Heard, B. E., Hossain, S., *J. Path.*, 1973, **110**, 319.

250. Gunther, M., Aschaffenburg, R., Matthews, R. H., Parish, W. E., Coombs, R. R. A., *Immunology*, 1960, **3**, 296.

251. Parish, W. E., Pepys, J., in *Clinical Aspects of Immunology*, edited by P. G. H. Gell and R. R. A. Coombs, page 397. Oxford, 1963.

252. Voorhorst, R., Spieksma-Boezeman, M. I. A., Spieksma, F. Th. M., *Allergie u. Asthma*, 1964, **10**, 329.

253. Voorhorst, R., Spieksma, F. Th. M., Varekamp, H., *House-Dust Atopy and the House-Dust Mite Dermatophagoides Pteronyssinus*, page 86. Leiden, 1969.

254. Hinson, K. F. W., Moon, A. J., Plummer, N. S., *Thorax*, 1952, **7**, 317.

255. Scadding, J. G., *Proc. roy. Soc. Med.*, 1971, **64**, 381.

256. Longbottom, J. L., Pepys, J., *J. Path. Bact.*, 1964, **88**, 441.

257. Perry, K. M. A., in *Chest Diseases*, edited by K. M. A. Perry and T. H. Sellors, vol. 1, page 524. London, 1963.

258. Hunter, D., *The Diseases of Occupations*, 4th edn, pages 1059–1075. London, 1969.

259. Schild, H. O., Hawkins, D. F., Mongar, J. L., Herxheimer, H., *Lancet*, 1951, **2**, 376.

260. De Montreynaud, D. J. M., *Ann. Méd.*, 1950, **51**, 712.

261. Herxheimer, H., West, T., *J. Physiol. (Lond.)*, 1955, **127**, 564.

262. Hall, R., Turner Warwick, M., Doniach, D., *Clin. exp. Immunol.*, 1966, **1**, 285.

263. Turner Warwick, M., Haslam, P., *Clin. exp. Immunol.*, 1970, **7**, 31.

264. Caspary, E. A., Feinmann, E. L., Field, E. J., *Brit. med. J.*, 1973, **1**, 15.

265. Vane, J. R., in *Identification of Asthma*, edited by R. Porter and J. Birch, page 121. Edinburgh and London, 1971.

266. Cardell, B. S., Pearson, R. S. B., *Thorax*, 1959, **14**, 341.

267. *The Registrar General's Statistical Review of England and Wales for the Year 1971*, Part 1. London, 1973.

268. Nelemans, F. A., in *Side Effects of Drugs—A Survey of Unwanted Effects of Drugs Reported in 1968–1971*, edited by L. Meyler and A. Herxheimer, vol. 7, page 227. Amsterdam, 1972.

269. Doll, R., Fraser, P., in *Proceedings of the European Society for the Study of Drug Toxicity*, edited by S. B. de C. Baker, page 133. Amsterdam, 1971.

INFLAMMATION IN THE TRACHEOBRONCHIAL TREE

270. Brumfitt, W., Willoughby, M. L. N., Bromley, L. L., *Lancet*, 1957, **2**, 132.

271. Martin, A. E., Bradley, W. H., *Mth. Bull. Minist. Hlth Lab. Serv.*, 1960, **19**, 56.

272. Stuart-Harris, C. H., *Brit. med. J.*, 1962, **2**, 869.

272a. *The Registrar General's Statistical Review of England and Wales for the Year 1973*, Part 1(A). London, 1975.

273. Feyrter, F., *Frankfurt. Z. Path.*, 1927, **35**, 213.

274. Smith, L. W., *Arch. Path. (Chic.)*, 1927, **4**, 732.

275. Gallavan, M., Goodpasture, E. W., *Amer. J. Path.*, 1937, **13**, 927.

276. Jernelius, H., *Acta paediat. (Uppsala)*, 1964, **53**, 247.

277. McLeod, J. W., Orr, J. W., Woodcock, H. E., *J. Path. Bact.*, 1939, **48**, 99.

278. Smith, W., Andrewes, C. H., Laidlaw, P. P., *Lancet*, 1933, **2**, 66.

279. Leading Article, *Chron. Wld Hlth Org.*, 1957, **11**, 269.

280. Leading Article, *WHO Chron.*, 1959, **13**, 163.

281. Louria, D. B., Blumenfeld, H. L., Ellis, J. T., Kilbourne, E. D., Rogers, D. E., *J. clin. Invest.*, 1959, **38**, 213.

282. Straub, M., *J. Path. Bact.*, 1940, **50**, 31.

283. Hers, J. F. P., *Institute of Preventive Medicine, Leyden*, Monograph No. 26, 1955.

284. Zykov, M. P., *Amer. Rev. resp. Dis.*, 1974, **110**, 537.

285. Greenwood, M., *Epidemics and Crowd Diseases*. London, 1935.

286. Stocks, P., *Lancet*, 1930, **1**, 796.

287. MacLeod, D. R. E., in *Textbook of Virology for Students and Practitioners of Medicine and the Other Health Sciences*, by A. J. Rhodes and C. E. van Rooyen, 5th edn, sect. 4, chap. 7, page 472. Baltimore, 1968.

288. Christensen, P. E., Schmidt, H., Andersen, V., Jordal, B., Jensen, O., Bang, H. O., *Acta med. scand.*, 1953, **144**, 313, 430.

289. Lipsey, A. I., Bolande, R. P., *Amer. J. Dis. Child.*, 1967, **113**, 677.

290. Degen, J. A., *Amer. J. med. Sci.*, 1937, **194**, 104.

291. Roberts, G. B. S., Bain, A. D., *J. Path. Bact.*, 1958, **76**, 111.

292. Wright, J., *Lancet*, 1957, **1**, 669.

293. Baum, H. L., *Ann. Otol. (St Louis)*, 1924, **3**, 782.

294. Peach, A. M., Zaiman, E., *Brit. med. J.*, 1959, **1**, 416.

295. Morris, J. A., Blount, R. E., Jr, Savage, R. E., *Proc. Soc. exp. Biol. (N.Y.)*, 1956, **92**, 544.

296. Beem, M., Wright, F. H., Hamre, D., Egerer, R., Oehme, M., *New Engl. J. Med.*, 1960, **263**, 523.

297. Sandiford, R. R., Spencer, B., *Brit. med. J.*, 1962, **2**, 881.

298. Macmillan, A. S., James, A. E., Stitik, F. P., Grillo, H. C., *Thorax*, 1971, **26**, 696.

299. Fledge, J. B., *Ann. Surg.*, 1967, **166**, 153.

300. Ciba Guest Symposium, *Thorax*, 1959, **14**, 286.

301. Medical Research Council Committee on the Aetiology of Chronic Bronchitis, *Lancet*, 1965, **1**, 775.

302. Stuart-Harris, C. H., *Abstr. Wld Med.*, 1968, **42**, 649, 737.

303. Oswald, N. C., Harold, J. T., Martin, W. J., *Lancet*, 1953, **2**, 639.

304. Turk, D. C., May, J. R., *Haemophilus Influenzae—Its Clinical Importance*, chap. 6. London, 1967.

305. May, J. R., *The Chemotherapy of Chronic Bronchitis and Allied Disorders*, 2nd edn, pages 9–15. London, 1972.

306. Royal College of Physicians of London, *Smoking and Health*, page 27. London, 1962.

307. Doll, R., Hill, A. Bradford, *Brit. med. J.*, 1964, **1**, 1399, 1460.

308. Royal College of Physicians of London, Committee on Smoking and Atmospheric Pollution, *Air Pollution and Health—Summary and Report on Air Pollution and Its Effect on Health*. London, 1970.

309. Crofton, J., Douglas, A., *Respiratory Diseases*, page 300. Oxford and Edinburgh, 1969.

310. Stuart-Harris, C. H., Pownall, M., Scothorne, C. M., Franks, Z., *Quart. J. Med.*, 1953, N.S. **22**, 121.

311. Lawther, P. J., *Proc. roy. Soc. Med.*, 1958, **51**, 262.

312. Martin, A. E., Bradley, W. H., *Mth. Bull. Minist. Hlth Lab. Serv.*, 1960, **19**, 56.

313. Oswald, N. C., in *Recent Trends in Chronic Bronchitis*, edited by N. C. Oswald, page 5. London, 1958.

314. Heard, B. E., *Pathology of Chronic Bronchitis and Emphysema*. London, 1969.

315. Restrepo, G., Heard, B. E., *Amer. Rev. resp. Dis.*, 1964, **90**, 395.

316. Reid, L. M., *Thorax*, 1960, **15**, 132.

317. Restrepo, G., Heard, B. E., *J. Path. Bact.*, 1963, **85**, 305.

318. Restrepo, G., Heard, B. E., *Thorax*, 1963, **18**, 334.

319. McAdams, A. J., *Amer. J. Med.*, 1955, **19**, 314.

320. Simpson, T., *Tubercle (Edinb.)*, 1958, **39**, 307.

321. Laws, J. W., Heard, B. E., *Brit. J. Radiol.*, 1962, **35**, 750.

322. Fletcher, C. M., Hugh-Jones, P., McNichol, M. W., Pride, N. B., *Quart. J. Med.*, 1963, N.S. **32**, 33.

323. Bachman, A. L., Hewitt, W. R., Beekley, H. C., *A.M.A. Arch. intern. Med.*, 1953, **91**, 78.

324. Bodian, M., *Fibrocystic Disease of the Pancreas*. London, 1952.

325. Ruberman, W., Schauffer, I., Biondo, T., *Amer. Rev. Tuberc.*, 1957, **76**, 761.

326. Roberts, J. C., Blair, L. G., *Lancet*, 1950, **1**, 386.

327. Franklin, A. W., Garrod, L. P., *Brit. med. J.*, 1953, **2**, 1067.

328. Ogilvie, A. G., *Arch. intern. Med.*, 1941, **68**, 395.

329. Soulas, A., Mounier-Kuhn, P., *Bronchologie*, 2nd edn, page 502. Paris, 1956.

330. Whitwell, F., *Thorax*, 1952, **7**, 213.

331. Lisa, J. R., Rosenblatt, M. B., *Bronchiectasis: Pathogenesis, Pathology and Treatment*, chap. 6. New York, 1943.

332. Mallory, T. B., *New Engl. J. Med.*, 1947, **237**, 795.

333. Brock, R. C., *The Anatomy of the Bronchial Tree*, 2nd edn, page 13. London, 1954.

334. Pryce, D. M., *J. Path. Bact.*, 1948, **60**, 259.

ACUTE INFECTIONS OF THE LUNGS

335. Stebbins, E. L., Perkins, J. E., Rogers, E. S., Champlin, R. D., Ames, W. R., *Amer. J. publ. Hlth*, 1940, **30**, 349.

336. Smillie, W. G., Jewett, O. F., *Amer. J. publ. Hlth*, 1942, **32**, 987.

337. Wright, G. Payling, Wright, H. Payling, *J. Hyg. (Lond.)*, 1945, **44**, 15.

338. Reimann, H. A., *The Pneumonias*, page 15. St Louis, 1971.

339. Heffron, R., *Pneumonia*, chap. 3. New York, 1939.

340. Stadie, W. C., *J. exp. Med.*, 1919, **30**, 215.

341. Gross, L., *Canad. med. Ass. J.*, 1919, **9**, 632.

342. Porter, W. T., Newburgh, L. H., *Amer. J. Physiol.*, 1916, **42**, 175.

343. Heffron, R., *Pneumonia*, chap. 12. New York, 1939.

344. Heffron, R., *Pneumonia*, page 515. New York, 1939.

345. Reimann, H. A., *The Pneumonias*, page 42. St Louis, 1971.

346. Goslings, W. R. O., Mulder, J., Djajadiningrat, J., Masurel, N., *Lancet*, 1959, **2**, 428.

347. Public Health Laboratory Service, *Brit. med. J.*, 1958, **1**, 915.

348. Briggs, J. N., *Canad. med. Ass. J.*, 1957, **76**, 269.

349. Lowbury, E. J. L., *Brit. med. Bull.*, 1960, **16**, 73.

350. Symmers, W. St C., *personal communication*, 1974.

351. Hirst, L. F., *The Conquest of Plague*, page 222. Oxford, 1958.

352. Pollitzer, R., *Wld Hlth Org. Monogr. Ser.*, No. 22, 1954, 210.

353. Hunter, D., *The Diseases of Occupations*, 4th edn, pages 721–733. London, 1969.

354. Fraenkel, E., *Virchows Arch. path. Anat.*, 1925, **254**, 363.

355. Gleiser, C. A., Berdjis, C. C., Hartman, H. A., Gochenour, W. S., *Brit. J. exp. Path.*, 1963, **44**, 416.

356. Forkner, C. E., Frei, E., Edgcomb, J. H., Utz, J. P., *Amer. J. Med.*, 1958, **25**, 877.

357. Fraenkel, E., *Z. Hyg. Infekt.-Kr.*, 1917, **84**, 369.

358. Williams, R., Williams, E. D., Hyams, D. E., *Lancet*, 1960, **1**, 376.

359. Turner, L. H., *Trans. roy. Soc. trop. Med. Hyg.*, 1967, **61**, 842.

360. Symmers, W. St C., *personal observations*, 1966–72.

361. Reimann, H. A., *The Pneumonias*, page 84. St Louis, 1971.

362. Himmelweit, F., *Lancet*, 1943, **2**, 793.

363. Mulder, J., Verdonk, G. J., *J. Path. Bact.*, 1949, **61**, 55.

364. Hers, J. F. Ph., Masurel, N., Mulder, J., *Lancet*, 1958, **2**, 1141.

365. Smith, W., Andrewes, C. H., Laidlaw, P. P., *Lancet*, 1933, **2**, 66.

366. Winternitz, M. C., Wason, I. M., McNamara, F. P., *The Pathology of Influenza*. New Haven, Connecticut, 1920.

367. Askanazy, M., *Korresp.-Bl. schweiz. Ärz.*, 1919, **49**, 465.

368. Louria, D. B., Blumenfeld, H. L., Ellis, J. T., Kilbourne, E. D., Rogers, D. E., *J. clin. Invest.*, 1959, **38**, 213.

369. Mitus, A., Enders, J. F., Craig, J. M., Holloway, A., *New Engl. J. Med.*, 1959, **261**, 882.

370. Rivers, T. M., *Amer. J. Path.*, 1928, **4**, 91.

371. Sherman, F. E., Ruckle, G., *A.M.A. Arch. Path.*, 1958, **65**, 587.

372. Cohen, S. M., Gordon, I., Rapp, F., Macauley, J. C.,

Bickley, S. M., *Proc. Soc. exp. Biol.* (*N.Y.*), 1955, **90**, 118.

373. Archibald, R. W. R., Weller, R. O., Meadow, S. R., *J. Path.*, 1971, **103**, 27.

374. Akhtar, M., Young, I., *Arch. Path.*, 1973, **96**, 145.

375. Cordy, D. R., *J. Amer. vet. med. Ass.*, 1949, **114**, 21.

376. Hecht, V., *Beitr. path. Anat.*, 1910, **48**, 262.

377. Enders, J. F., McCarthy, K., Mitus, A., Cheatham, W. J., *New Engl. J. Med.*, 1959, **261**, 875.

378. Mitus, A., Enders, J. F., Craig, J. M., Holloway, A., *New Engl. J. Med.*, 1959, **261**, 882.

379. Enders, J. F., *Trans. Stud. Coll. Phycns Philad.*, 1960, **28**, 68.

380. Howat, H. T., Arnott, W. M., *Lancet*, 1944, **2**, 312.

381. Evans, W. H., Foreman, H. M., *Proc. roy. Soc. Med.*, 1963, **56**, 274.

382. Nelson, J. S., Wyatt, J. P., *Medicine* (*Baltimore*), 1959, **38**, 223.

383. Symmers, W. St C., *J. clin. Path.*, 1960, **13**, 1.

384. Heard, B. E., Hassan, A. M., Wilson, S., *J. clin. Path.*, 1962, **15**, 17.

385. Hamperl, H., *Amer. J. Path.*, 1956, **32**, 1.

386. Bedson, S. P., Western, G. T., Simpson, S. L., *Lancet*, 1930, **1**, 235, 345.

387. Page, L. A., *Int. J. system. Bact.*, 1966, **16**, 223.

388. Moulder, J. W., *The Psittacosis Group as Bacteria*. New York, 1964.

389. Meyer, K. F., *Bull. Wld Hlth Org.*, 1959, **20**, 101.

390. Bedson, S. P., *Brit. med. J.*, 1950, **2**, 282.

391. Harding, H. B., Snyder, R. A., *A.M.A. Arch. intern. Med.*, 1960, **105**, 217.

392. Golden, A., *Arch. Path.* (*Chic.*), 1944, **38**, 187.

393. Eaton, M. D., Meiklejohn, G., Herick, W. van, *J. exp. Med.*, 1944, **79**, 649.

394. Evans, A. S., Brobst, M., *New Engl. J. Med.*, 1961, **265**, 401.

395. Goodburn, G. M., Marmion, B. P., Kendall, E. J. C., *Brit. med. J.*, 1963, **1**, 1266.

396. Golden, A., *Arch. Path.* (*Chic.*), 1944, **38**, 187.

397. Derrick, E. H., *Med. J. Aust.*, 1937, **2**, 281.

398. Clinico-Pathological Conference, *Brit. med. J.*, 1963, **1**, 1143.

CHRONIC INFECTIONS OF THE LUNGS

399. Seal, R. M. E., *Brit. J. Hosp. Med.*, 1971, **5**, 783.

400. Runyon, E. H., *Med. Clin. N. Amer.*, 1959, **43**, 273.

401. Runyon, E. H., McDermott, W., *Amer. Rev. resp. Dis.*, 1965, **91**, 289.

402. Marks, J., *Tubercle*, 1969, **50**, suppl., 78.

403. Symmers, W. St C., *unpublished observations*, 1972–73.

404. Crofton, J., *Tubercle*, 1969, **50**, suppl., 65.

405. Steiner, M., Steiner, P., Schmidt, H., *Amer. Rev. resp. Dis.*, 1970, **102**, 75.

406. Pagel, W., Simmonds, F. A. H., Macdonald, N., Nassau, E., *Pulmonary Tuberculosis*, 4th edn. London, 1964.

407. Horne, N. W., *Brit. J. Hosp. Med.*, 1971, **5**, 732.

408. Mahler, H. T., *Bull. int. Un. Tuberc.*, 1970, **43**, 19.

409. Francis, J., *Tuberculosis in Animals and Man*, chap. 5. London, 1958.

410. Hart, P. D'Arcy, Wright, G. Payling, *Tuberculosis and Social Conditions in England with Special Reference to Young Adults* (*A Statistical Study*). London, 1939.

411. *The Registrar General's Statistical Review of England and Wales for the Year 1961*, Part 1. London, 1963.

412. *The Registrar General's Statistical Review of England and Wales for the Year 1973*, Part 1(A). London, 1975.

413. British Thoracic and Tuberculosis Association, *Tubercle*, 1971, **52**, 1.

414. Miller, F. J. W., Seal, R. M. E., Taylor, M. D., *Tuberculosis in Children—Evolution, Control, Treatment*, page 66. London, 1963.

415. Pagel, W., Price, D. S., *Amer. Rev. Tuberc.*, 1943, **47**, 614.

416. Jensen, K. A., Bindaler, G., Holm, J., *Acta tuberc. scand.*, 1935, **9**, 27.

417. Barrie, H. J., *Canad. med. Ass. J.*, 1965, **92**, 1149.

417a. Ghon, A., *Der primäre Lungenherd bei der Tuberkulose der Kinder*. Berlin and Vienna, 1912.

418. Terplan, K., *Amer. Rev. Tuberc.*, 1940, **42**, suppl. 2.

418a. Parrot, J., *C. R. Soc. Biol.* (*Paris*), 1876, sér. 6, **3**, 308.

419. Bentley, F. J., Grzybowski, S., Benjamin, B., *Tuberculosis in Childhood and Adolescence*, chap. 9. London, 1954.

420. Brailey, M., *Bull. Johns Hopk. Hosp.*, 1937, **61**, 258.

421. Sweany, H. C., *Age Morphology of Primary Tubercles*. Springfield, Illinois, 1941.

422. Hirsch, J. G., in *Experimental Tuberculosis*, edited by G. E. W. Wolstenholme, M. P. Cameron and C. M. O'Connor, page 115. London, 1955.

423. Reichle, H. S., Gallavan, M., *Arch. Path.* (*Chic.*), 1937, **24**, 201.

424. Morrison, J. B., *Thorax*, 1970, **25**, 643.

425. Symmers, W. St C., *unpublished observations*, 1966, 1971.

426. Miller, F. J. W., Seal, R. M. E., Taylor, M. D., *Tuberculosis in Children—Evolution, Control, Treatment*, page 53. London, 1963.

427. Eliasberg, H., Newland, W., *Jb. Kinderheilk.*, 1920, **93**, 88.

428. Weigert, C., *Virchows Arch. path. Anat.*, 1882, **88**, 307.

429. Auerbach, O., *Amer. J. Path.*, 1944, **20**, 121.

430. Lurie, M. B., *Amer. J. Med.*, 1950, **9**, 591.

431. Hoyle, C., Vaizey, M., *Chronic Miliary Tuberculosis*. London, 1937.

432. Proudfoot, A. T., Akhtar, A. J., Douglas, A. C., Horn, N. W., *Brit. med. J.*, 1969, **2**, 273.

433. Treip, C., Meyers, D., *Lancet*, 1959, **1**, 164.

434. Brunner, K., Haemmerli, U. P., *Germ. med. Mth.*, 1964, **9**, 372.

435. Naegeli, O., *Virchows Arch. path. Anat.*, 1900, **160**, 426.

436. Uehlinger, E., Blangey, R., *Beitr. Klin. Tuberk.*, 1937, **90**, 339.

437. Hart, P. D'Arcy, *Spec. Rep. Ser. med. Res. Coun.* (*Lond.*), No. 164, 1932.

438. Daniels, M., *Proc. roy. Soc. Med.*, 1952, **45**, 11.

439. Heimbeck, J., *Tubercle* (*Edinb.*), 1936, **18**, 97.

440. Royal College of Physicians, *The Prophit Tuberculosis Survey*, page 138. London, 1948.

441. Long, E. R., *Arch. Path. Lab. Med.*, 1926, **1**, 918.

442. Aronson, J. D., Aronson, C. F., Taylor, H. C., *A.M.A. Arch. intern. Med.*, 1958, **101**, 881.

443. Hyge, T. V., *Acta tuberc. scand.*, 1949, **23**, 153.

444. Chaparas, S. D., Sheagren, J. N., Demeo, A., Hedrick, S., *Amer. Rev. resp. Dis.*, 1970, **101**, 67.

445. Wells, A. Q., *Spec. Rep. Ser. med. Res. Coun.* (*Lond.*), No. 259, 1946.

446. Miller, F. J. W., Seal, R. M. E., Taylor, M. D., *Tuberculosis in Children—Evolution, Control, Treatment*, page 309. London, 1963.

447. Brock, R. C., Hodgkiss, F., Jones, H. O., *Guy's Hosp. Rep.*, 1942, **91**, 131.

448. Davson, J., *J. Path. Bact.*, 1939, **49**, 483.
449. Assmann, H., *Ergebn. ges. Tuberk.- u. Lung.-Forsch.*, 1930, **1**, 115.
450. Rasmussen, V., translated by W. D. Moore, *Edinb. med. J.*, 1868–69, **14**, 385.
451. British Thoracic and Tuberculosis Association, *Tubercle*, 1970, **51**, 227.
452. Siegmund, H., *Beitr. path. Anat.*, 1939, **103**, 431.
453. O'Brien, J. R., *J. clin. Path.*, 1954, **7**, 216.
454. Tchen, P., Hoeven, L. van der, Humphrey, H. I., *Amer. Rev. Tuberc.*, 1957, **76**, 144.
455. Montes, M., Phillips, C., *Amer. Rev. Tuberc.*, 1959, **79**, 362.
456. Skarberg, K. O., Lagerlof, B., Reizenstein, P., *Acta med. scand.*, 1967, **182**, 427.
457. Symmers, W. St C., *personal communication*, 1974.
458. Cook, P. L., Riddell, R. W., Simon, G., *Tubercle*, 1971, **52**, 232.
459. Snijder, J., *J. Path. Bact.*, 1965, **90**, 65.
460. Lloyd, A. C., *Brit. med. J.*, 1968, **3**, 529.
461. Houston, T., Symmers, W. St. C. [Belfast], *unpublished observations, circa* 1908–14.
462. Schonell, M. E., Crofton, J. W., Stuart, A. E., Wallace, A., *Tubercle*, 1968, **49**, 12.
463. Virchow, R., *Virchows Arch. path. Anat.*, 1858, **8**, 103.
464. De Navasquez, S., *J. Path. Bact.*, 1942, **54**, 313.
465. *Human Infection with Fungi, Actinomycetes and Algae*, edited by R. D. Baker. New York, Heidelberg, Berlin, 1971.
466. Georg, L. K., Robertstad, G. W., Brinkman, S. A., Hicklin, M. D., *J. infect. Dis.*, 1965, **115**, 88.
467. Coleman, R. M., Georg, L. K., Rozzell, A. R., *Appl. Microbiol.*, 1969, **18**, 420.
468. Brock, D. W., Georg, L. K., Brown, J. M., Hicklin, M. D., *Amer. J. clin. Path.*, 1973, **59**, 66.
469. Riddell, R. W., in *Chest Diseases*, edited by K. M. A. Perry and T. H. Sellors, vol. 2, page 84. London, 1963.
470. Symmers, W. St C., *Brit. med. J.*, 1973, **4**, 423.
471. Hinson, K. F. W., Moon, A. J., Plummer, N. S., *Thorax*, 1952, **7**, 317.
472. Pepys, J., Riddell, R. W., Citron, K. M., Clayton, Y. M., Short, E. I., *Amer. Rev. resp. Dis.*, 1959, **80**, 167.
473. Pepys, J., Longbottom, J. L., *J. Path. Bact.*, 1964, **88**, 141.
474. Symmers, W. St C., *personal communication*, 1974.
475. Reinhardt, K., *Das Mycetom*. Stuttgart, 1967.
476. Louria, D. B., Lieberman, P. H., Collins, H. S., Blevins, A., *Arch. intern. Med.*, 1966, **117**, 748.
477. McCarthy, D. S., Longbottom, J. L., Riddell, R. W., Batten, J. C., *Amer. Rev. resp. Dis.*, 1969, **100**, 213.
478. Symmers, W. St C., *Curiosa—A Miscellany of Clinical and Pathological Experiences*, page 144. London, 1974.
479. Fors, B., Sääf, J., *Acta chir. scand.*, 1960, **119**, 212.
480. Symmers, W. St C., *unpublished observation*, 1972.
481. Campbell, M. J., Clayton, Y. M., *Amer. Rev. resp. Dis.*, 1964, **89**, 186.
482. Symmers, W. St C., *Proc. roy. Soc. Med.*, 1973, **66**, 1021 [Case 5].
483. Leggat, P. O., De Kretser, D. M. H., *Brit. J. Dis. Chest*, 1968, **62**, 147.
484. Symmers, W. St C., in *Aspergillosis and Farmer's Lung in Man and Animal—Proceedings of the 4th International Symposium, Davos, 1971*, edited by R. de

Haller and F. Suter, page 75. Bern, Stuttgart, Vienna 1974.
485. Symmers, W. St C., *Lab. Invest.*, 1962, **11**, 1073.
486. Owens, A. W., Shacklette, M. H., Baker, R. D., *Sabouraudia*, 1965–66, **4**, 179.
487. Gowing, N. F. C., Hamlin, I. M. E., *J. clin. Path.*, 1960, **13**, 396.
488. Nime, F. A., Hutchins, G. M., *Johns Hopk. med. J.*, 1973, **133**, 183.
489. Winner, H. I., Hurley, R., *Candida Albicans*, chap. 10. London, 1964.
490. Ikeda, K., *Arch. Path. (Chic.)*, 1936, **22**, 62.
491. Shrewsbury, J. F. D., *Quart. J. Med.*, 1936, N.S. **5**, 375.
492. Symmers, W. St C., in *Symposium on Candida Infections*, edited by H. I. Winner and R. Hurley, pages 196–212. Edinburgh and London, 1966.
493. Baker, R. D., in *Human Infection with Fungi, Actinomycetes and Algae*, edited by R. D. Baker, pages 832–918. New York, Heidelberg, Berlin, 1971.
494. Symmers, W. St C., *Ann. Soc. belge Méd. trop.*, 1972, **52**, 365.
495. Symmers, W. St C., *unpublished observation*, 1973.
496. Littman, M. L., Zimmerman, L. E., *Cryptococcosis–Torulosis or European Blastomycosis*. New York, 1956.
497. Campbell, G. D., *Amer. Rev. resp. Dis.*, 1966, **94**, 236.
498. Baker, R. D., Haugen, R. K., *Amer. J. clin. Path.*, 1955, **25**, 14.
499. Symmers, W. St C., *personal communication*, 1974.
500. Schwarz, J., in *Human Infection with Fungi, Actinomycetes and Algae*, edited by R. D. Baker, pages 67–130. New York, Heidelberg, Berlin, 1971.
501. Symmers, W. St C., *Brit. med. J.*, 1956, **2**, 786.
502. Edwards, P. Q., Palmer, C. E., *Publ. Hlth Rep. (Wash.)*, 1963, **78**, 241.
503. Christie, A., *Ann. intern. Med.*, 1958, **49**, 544.
504. Straub, M., Schwarz, J., *Amer. J. clin. Path.*, 1955, **25**, 727.
505. Macleod, W. M., Murray, I. G., Davidson, J., Gibbs, D. D., *Thorax*, 1972, **27**, 6.
506. Symmers, W. St C., *unpublished observation*, 1972.
507. Furcolow, M. L., Brasher, C. A., *Amer. Rev. Tuberc.*, 1956, **73**, 609.
508. Schwarz, J., Baum, G. L., *Arch. Path. (Chic.)*, 1963, **75**, 475.
509. Murray, J. F., Lurie, H. I., Kay, J., Komins, C., Borok, R., Way, M., *S. Afr. med. J.*, 1957, **31**, 245.
510. Reinhard, E. H., McAllister, W. H., Brown, E., Chaplin, H., Garfinkel, L., Harford, C. G., Kobayashi, G., Cate, T., *Amer. J. Med.*, 1967, **43**, 593.
511. Symmers, W. St C., *Ann. Soc. belge Méd. trop.*, 1972, **52**, 435.
512. Cockshott, W. P., Lucas, A. O., *Quart. J. Med.*, 1964, N.S. **33**, 223.
513. Fiese, M. J., *Coccidioidomycosis*. Springfield, Illinois, 1958.
514. *Coccidioidomycosis*, edited by L. Ajello. Tucson, Arizona, 1967.
515. Johnson, J. E., III, Perry, J. E., Fekety, F. R., Kadull, P. J., Cluff, L. E., *Ann. intern. Med.*, 1964, **60**, 941.
516. Symmers, W. St C., in *Coccidioidomycosis*, edited by L. Ajello, page 301 [Case 8]. Tucson, Arizona, 1967.
517. Symmers, W. St C., *Pathology*, 1971, **3**, 1.
518. Huntington, R. W., Jr, in *Human Infection with Fungi,*

Actinomycetes and Algae, edited by R. D. Baker, pages 147–210. New York, Heidelberg, Berlin, 1971.

519. Chick, E. W., in *Human Infection with Fungi, Actinomycetes and Algae*, edited by R. D. Baker, pages 465–506. New York, Heidelberg, Berlin, 1971.

520. Furcolow, M. L., Chick, E. W., Busey, J. F., Menges, R. W., *Amer. Rev. resp. Dis.*, 1970, **102**, 60.

521. Bregant, S., Gigase, P., Bastin, J. P., Vandepitte, J., *Bull. Soc. Path. exot.*, 1973, **66**, 77.

522. Symmers, W. St C., *Amer. J. clin. Path.*, 1966, **46**, 514 [Case 16].

523. Angulo O., A., Pollak, L., in *Human Infection with Fungi, Actinomycetes and Algae*, edited by R. D. Baker, pages 507–576. New York, Heidelberg, Berlin, 1971.

524. Londero, A. T., Ramos, C. D., *Amer. J. Med.*, 1972, **52**, 771.

525. Salfelder, K., Doehnert, G., Doehnert, H.-R., *Virchows Arch. Abt. A*, 1969, **348**, 51.

526. Restrepo, A., Robledo, M., Gutierrez, F., Sanclemente, M., Castaneda, E., Calle, G., *Amer. J. trop. Med. Hyg.*, 1970, **19**, 68.

527. Huang, S.-N., Harris, L. S., *Amer. J. clin. Path.*, 1963, **39**, 167.

528. Morenz, J., in *Human Infection with Fungi, Actinomycetes and Algae*, edited by R. D. Baker, pages 919–952. New York, Heidelberg, Berlin, 1971.

529. Baum, G. L., Donnerberg, R. L., Stewart, D., Mulligan, W. J., Putnam, L. R., *New Engl. J. Med.*, 1969, **280**, 410.

530. Symmers, W. St C., *unpublished cases*, 1967, 1974.

531. Agrawal, S., Sharma, K. D., Shrivastava, J. B., *A.M.A. Arch. Derm.*, 1959, **80**, 22.

532. Koďousek, R., Vortel, V., Fingerland, A., Vojtek, V., Šerý, Z., Hájek, V., Kučera, K., *Amer. J. clin. Path.*, 1971, **56**, 394.

533. Symmers, W. St C., *unpublished case*, 1972.

534. Pepys, J., *J. roy. Coll. Phycns Lond.*, 1967, **2**, 42.

535. Campbell, J. M., *Brit. med. J.*, 1932, **2**, 1143.

536. Thomas, G. C., *Tubercle (Edinb.)*, 1962, **43**, 330.

537. Seal, R. M. E., Hapke, E. J., Thomas, G. O., *Thorax*, 1968, **23**, 469.

538. Hinson, K. F. W., *Hum. Path.*, 1970, **1**, 275.

539. Pepys, J., Riddell, R. W., Citron, K. M., Clayton, Y. M., *Thorax*, 1962, **17**, 366.

540. Williams, J. V., *Thorax*, 1963, **18**, 182.

541. Areán, V. M., in *Pathology of Protozoal and Helminthic Diseases with Clinical Correlation*, edited by R. A. Marcial-Rojas and E. Moreno, chap. 14. Baltimore, 1971.

542. Hamperl, H., *J. Path. Bact.*, 1957, **74**, 353.

543. Chagas, C., *Mem. Inst. Osw. Cruz*, 1909, **1**, 159.

544. Ammich, O., *Virchows Arch. path. Anat.*, 1938, **302**, 539.

545. Vaněk, J., Jírovec, O., *Zbl. Bakt., I. Abt. Orig.*, 1952, **158**, 12.

546. Vaněk, J., Jírovec, O., Lukes, J., *Ann. paediat. (Basel)*, 1953, **180**, 1.

547. Csillag, A., *Acta microbiol. Acad. Sci. hung.*, 1957, **4**, 1.

548. Jírovec, O., *Mschr. Kinderheilk.*, 1960, **108**, 136.

549. Reye, R. D. K., Seldam, R. E. J. ten, *J. Path. Bact.*, 1956, **72**, 451.

550. McKay, E., Richardson, J., *Lancet*, 1959, **2**, 713.

551. Gilbert, C. F., Fordham, C. C., III, Benson, W. R., *Arch. intern. Med.*, 1963, **112**, 158.

552. Symmers, W. St C., *J. clin. Path.*, 1960, **13**, 1.

552a. Henderson, D. W., Humeniuk, V., Meadows, R., Forbes, I. J., *Pathology*, 1974, **6**, 235.

552b. Symmers, W. St C., *Unpublished cases*, 1965, 1974.

553. Takaro, T., Bond, W. M., *Int. Abstr. Surg.*, 1958, **107**, 209.

'OPPORTUNISTIC INFECTIONS'

554. Heard, B. E., in *Recent Advances in Pathology*, 8th edn, edited by C. V. Harrison, pages 369–402. London, 1966.

555. Symmers, W. St C., *Proc. roy. Soc. Med.*, 1965, **58**, 341.

556. Seeliger, H., *Med. Mschr.*, 1954, **8**, 692.

557. Utz, J. P., *Lab. Invest.*, 1962, **11**, 1018.

558. Symmers, W. St C., in *Drug-Induced Diseases—Second Symposium Organized by the Boerhaave Courses for Post-Graduate Medical Education—State University of Leyden, October 1964*, edited by L. Meyler and H. M. Peck, pages 108–151 [Case 6].

METAZOAN INFESTATION

559. El-Gazuyerli, M., in *The Lung*, edited by A. A. Liebow and D. E. Smith, page 245. Baltimore, 1968.

560. Shaw, A. F. B., Ghareeb, A. A., *J. Path. Bact.*, 1938, **46**, 401.

561. Symmers [Egypt], W. St. C., *Lancet*, 1905, **1**, 22.

562. Lopes de Faria, J., *J. Path. Bact.*, 1954, **68**, 589.

563. Azmy, S., *J. Egypt. med. Ass.*, 1932, **15**, 87.

564. Cortes, F. M., Winter, W. L., *Amer. J. Med.*, 1961, **33**, 223.

565. Wagenvoort, C. A., *J. Path. Bact.*, 1959, **78**, 503.

566. El Mallah, S. H., Hashem, M., *Thorax*, 1953, **8**, 148.

567. Symmers, W. St C., *unpublished case*, 1972.

568. Roque, F. T., Ludwick, R. W., Bell, J. C., *Ann. intern. Med.*, 1953, **38**, 1206.

569. Chai Hong Chung, in *Pathology of Protozoal and Helminthic Diseases with Clinical Correlation*, edited by R. A. Marcial-Rojas and E. Moreno, chap. 24. Baltimore, 1971.

570. Dew, H. R., *Hydatid Disease*, chap. 9. Melbourne, 1928.

571. Soulsby, E. J. L., in *Clinical Aspects of Immunology*, edited by P. G. H. Gell and R. R. A. Coombs, page 115. Oxford, 1963.

572. Brown, C. J. Officer, *Postgrad. med. J.*, 1958, **34**, 195.

573. Areán, V. M., Crandall, C. A., in *Pathology of Protozoal and Helminthic Diseases with Clinical Correlation*, edited by R. A. Marcial-Rojas and E. Moreno, chap. 43. Baltimore, 1971.

574. Gelpi, A. P., Mustafa, A., *Amer. J. Med.*, 1967, **44**, 377.

575. Beaver, P. C., Danaraj, T. J., *Amer. J. trop. Med. Hyg.*, 1958, **7**, 100.

576. Symmers, W. St C., *unpublished observations*, 1965–74.

577. Areán, V. M., Crandall, C. A., in *Pathology of Protozoal and Helminthic Diseases with Clinical Correlation*, edited by R. A. Marcial-Rojas and E. Moreno, chap. 44. Baltimore, 1971.

578. Parish, W. E., Pepys, J., in *Clinical Aspects of Immunology*, edited by P. G. H. Gell and R. R. A. Coombs, page 390. Oxford, 1963.

579. Kent, H. N., *Exp. Parasit.*, 1960, **10**, 313.

PULMONARY EOSINOPHILIA

580. Crofton, J. W., Livingstone, J. L., Oswald, N. C., Roberts, A. T. M., *Thorax*, 1952, **7**, 1.

581. Turner-Warwick, M., *Medicine (Lond.)*, 1972–74, Part 14, 889.
582. Löffler, W., *Klin. Wschr.*, 1935, **14**, 297.
583. Reeder, W. H., Goodrich, B. E., *Ann. intern. Med.*, 1952, **26**, 1217.
584. McCarthy, D. S., Pepys, J., *Clin. Allerg.*, 1973, **3**, 339.
585. Viswanathan, R., *Quart. J. Med.*, 1948, N.S. **17**, 257.
586. Vakil, R. J., *Brit. Heart J.*, 1961, **23**, 578.
587. Webb, J. K. G., Job, C. K., Gault, E. W., *Lancet*, 1960, **1**, 835.
588. Danaraj, T. J., *A.M.A. Arch. Path.*, 1959, **67**, 515.

CHRONIC INTERSTITIAL PNEUMONIA AND FIBROSIS OF THE LUNGS
589. Mallory, T. B., *Radiology*, 1948, **51**, 468.
590. Warren, S., *Arch. Path. (Chic.)*, 1942, **34**, 917.
591. Hamman, L., Rich, A. R., *Trans. Amer. clin. climat. Ass.*, 1935, **51**, 154.
592. Hamman, L., Rich, A. R., *Bull. Johns Hopk. Hosp.*, 1944, **74**, 177.
593. Scadding, J. G., *Brit. med. J.*, 1964, **2**, 686, 941.
594. Scadding, J. G., Hinson, K. F. W., *Thorax*, 1967, **22**, 291.
595. Liebow, A. A., Steer, A., Billingsley, J. G., *Amer. J. Med.*, 1965, **39**, 369.
596. Livingstone, J. L., Lewis, J. G., Reid, L., Jefferson, K., *Quart. J. Med.*, 1964, N.S. **33**, 71.
597. Stack, B. H. R., Choo-Kang, Y. F. J., Heard, B. E., *Thorax*, 1972, **27**, 535.
598. Peabody, J. W., Peabody, J. W., Jr, Hayes, E. W., Hayes, E. W., Jr, *Dis. Chest*, 1950, **18**, 330.
599. Hinson, K. F. W., *Hum. Path.*, 1970, **1**, 275.
600. Thompson, P. L., Mackay, I. R., *Thorax*, 1970, **25**, 504.
601. Hobbs, J. R., Turner Warwick, M., *Clin. exp. Immunol.*, 1967, **2**, 465.
602. Turner Warwick, M., Doniach, D., *Brit. med. J.*, 1965, **1**, 886.
603. Turner Warwick, M., Haslam, P., *Clin. Allergy*, 1971, **1**, 83.
604. Turner Warwick, M., Haslam, P., Weeks, J., *Clin. Allergy*, 1971, **1**, 209.
605. Turner Warwick, M., *Quart. J. Med.*, 1968, N.S. **37**, 133.
606. Mason, A. M. S., McIllmurray, M. B., Golding, P. L., Hughes, D. T. D., *Brit. med. J.*, 1970, **4**, 596.
607. Oswald, N., Parkinson, T., *Quart. J. Med.*, 1949, N.S. **18**, 1.
608. Cunningham, G. J., Parkinson, T., *Thorax*, 1950, **5**, 43.
609. Heppleston, A. G., *Thorax*, 1956, **11**, 77.
610. Liebow, A. A., in *The Lung*, edited by A. A. Liebow and D. E. Smith, page 332. Baltimore, 1968.
611. Spencer, H., in *The Lung*, edited by A. A. Liebow and D. E. Smith, page 134. Baltimore, 1968.
612. Wyatt, J. P., Riddell, A. C. R., *Amer. J. Path.*, 1949, **25**, 447.
613. Brewis, R. A., *Thorax*, 1969, **24**, 656.
614. Rhodes, M. L., *Amer. Rev. resp. Dis.*, 1973, **108**, 950.
615. Liebow, A. A., in *The Lung*, edited by A. A. Liebow and D. E. Smith, page 351. Baltimore, 1968.
616. Carrington, C. B., Liebow, A. A., *Amer. J. Path.*, 1966, **48**, 36A.
617. Liebow, A. A., in *The Lung*, edited by A. A. Liebow amd D. E. Smith, page 349. Baltimore, 1968.

618. Greenberg, S. D., Haley, M. D., Jenkins, D. E., Stanton, P. F., *Arch. Path.*, 1973, **96**, 73.
619. Liebow, A. A., Carrington, C. B., *Med. Clin. N: Amer.*, 1973, **57**, 3.
620. Ellman, P., *Proc. roy. Soc. Med.*, 1947, **40**, 332.
621. Cruickshank, B., *Ann. rheum. Dis.*, 1954, **13**, 136.
622. Dumas, L. W., Gregory, R. L., Orzer, F. L., *Brit. med. J.*, 1963, **1**, 383.
623. DeHoratius, R. J., Abruzzo, J. L., Williams, R. C., *Arch. intern. Med.*, 1972, **129**, 441.
624. Caplan, A., *Thorax*, 1953, **8**, 29.
625. Gough, J., Rivers, D., Seal, R. M. E., *Thorax*, 1955, **10**, 9.
626. Hamilton, K. A., *Arch. intern. Med.*, 1949, **31**, 216.
627. Cohen, A. A., Natelson, E. A., Fechner, R. E., *Dis. Chest*, 1971, **59**, 369.
628. Walton, E. W., *Brit. med. J.*, 1958, **2**, 265.
629. Carrington, C. B., Liebow, A. A., *Amer. J. Med.*, 1966, **41**, 497.
630. Symmers, W. St C., *unpublished observations*, 1966–74.
631. Liebow, A. A., *Amer. Rev. resp. Dis.*, 1973, **108**, 1.
632. Scadding, J. G., *Sarcoidosis*. London, 1967.
633. Smellie, H., Hoyle, C., *Quart. J. Med.*, 1960, N.S. **29**, 539.
634. Scadding, J. G., *Brit. med. J.*, 1961, **2**, 1165.
635. Cummings, M. M., Dunner, E., Williams, J. H., *Ann. intern. Med.*, 1959, **50**, 879.
636. Cummings, M. M., *Acta med. scand.*, 1964, suppl. 425, 48.
637. Siltzbach, L. E., *J. Amer. med. Ass.*, 1961, **178**, 476.
638. Mitchell, D. N., in *Recent Advances in Clinical Pathology*, Series 5, edited by S. C. Dyke, chap. 24. London, 1968.
639. Symmers, W. St C., *unpublished observations*, 1973–74.
640. Nevins, M. A., Stechel, G. H., Fishman, S. I., Schwartz, G., Allen, A. C., *J. Amer. med. Ass.*, 1965, **193**, 266.
641. Brunner, M. J., Giovacchini,, R. P., Wyatt, J. P., Dunlap, F. E., Calandra, J. C., *J. Amer. med. Ass.*, 1963, **184**, 851.

LIPID PNEUMONIA
642. Vaidya, M. P., *Postgrad. med. J.*, 1962, **38**, 355.
643. Salva, R., Hughes, E. W., *Thorax*, 1970, **25**, 762.
644. Elston, C. W., *Arch. Dis. Childh.*, 1966, **41**, 428.
645. Wagner, J. C., Adler, D. I., Fuller, D. N., *Thorax*, 1955, **10**, 157.
646. Belcher, J. R., *Thorax*, 1949, **4**, 44.
647. Pearson, J. E. G., Wilson, R. S. E., *Thorax*, 1971, **26**, 300.
648. Sullivan, J. J., Ferraro, L. R., Mangiardi, J. L., Johnson, E. K., *Dis. Chest*, 1961, **39**, 71.
649. Waddell, W. R., Sniffen, R. C., Sweet, R. H., *J. thorac. Surg.*, 1949, **18**, 707.
650. Cohen, A. B., Cline, M. J., *Amer. Rev. resp. Dis.*, 1972, **106**, 69.

PULMONARY ALVEOLAR MICROLITHIASIS
651. Harbitz, F., *Arch. intern. Med.*, 1918, **21**, 139.
652. Thomson, W. B., *Thorax*, 1959, **14**, 76.
653. Sharp, M. E., Danino, E. A., *J. Path. Bact.*, 1953, **65**, 389.
654. Sears, M. R., Chang, A. R., Taylor, A. J., *Thorax*, 1971, **26**, 704.
655. Bowen, D. A. L., *J. clin. Path.*, 1959, **12**, 435.
656. Symmers, W. St C., *unpublished observation*, 1953.

METASTATIC CALCIFICATION

657. Mulligan, R. M., *Arch. Path. (Chic.)*, 1947, **43**, 177.
658. Cheatle, E. L., Sommers, H. M., *Quart. Bull. Northw. Univ. med. Sch.*, 1958, **32**, 55.
659. Wermer, P., Kuschner, M., Riley, E. A., *Amer. J. Med.*, 1953, **14**, 108.
660. Cooke, C. R., Hyland, J. W., *Amer. J. Med.*, 1960, **29**, 363.
661. Hueper, W., *Arch. Path. (Chic.)*, 1927, **3**, 14.

AMYLOIDOSIS

662. Whitwell, F., *Thorax*, 1953, **8**, 309.
663. Cotton, R. E., Jackson, J. W., *Thorax*, 1964, **19**, 97.
664. Zundel, W. E., Prior, A. P., *Thorax*, 1971, **21**, 357.

CHEMICAL INJURY TO THE LUNGS

665. Davies, P. D. B., *Brit. J. Dis. Chest*, 1969, **63**, 57.
666. Matthew, H., Logan, A., Woodruff, M. F. A., Heard, B., *Brit. med. J.*, 1968, **2**, 759.
667. Cooke, N. J., Flenley, D. C., Matthew, H., *Quart. J. Med.*, 1973, N.S. **42**, 683.
668. Clark, D. G., McElligott, T. F., Hurst, E. W., *Brit. J. industr. Med.*, 1966, **23**, 126.
669. Fisher, H. K., Clements, J. A., Wright, R. R., *Amer. Rev. resp. Dis.*, 1973, **107**, 246.
670. Wasan, S. M., McElligott, T. F., *Amer. Rev. resp. Dis.*, 1972, **105**, 276.
671. Modée, J., Ivemark, B. I., Robertson, B., *Acta path. microbiol. scand.*, 1972, **80A**, 54.
672. Oliner, H., Schwartz, R., Rubio, F., Dameshek, W., *Amer. J. Med.*, 1961, **31**, 134.
673. Heard, B. E., Cooke, R. A., *Thorax*, 1968, **23**, 187.
674. Kirschner, R. H., Esterly, J. R., *Cancer (Philad.)*, 1971, **27**, 1074.
675. Doniach, I., Morrison, B., Steiner, R. E., *Brit. Heart J.*, 1954, **16**, 101.
676. Heard, B. E., *J. Path. Bact.*, 1962, **83**, 159.
677. Umezawa, H., Maeda, K., Takeuchi, T., Okami, Y., *J. Antibiot. Ser. A (Tokyo)*, 1966, **19**, 200.
678. Halnan, K. E., Bleehan, N. M., Brewin, T. B., Deeley, T. J., Harrison, D. F. N., Howland, C., Kunkler, P. B., Ritchie, G. L., Wiltshaw, E., Todd, I. D. H., *Brit. med. J.*, 1972, **4**, 635.
679. Fleischman, R. W., Baker, J. R., Thompson, G. R., Schaeppi, U. H., Illievski, V. R., Cooney, D. A., Davis, R. D., *Thorax*, 1971, **26**, 675.
680. Bedrossian, C. W. M., Luna, M. A., Mackay, B., Lichtiger, B., *Cancer (Philad.)*, 1973, **32**, 44.
681. Smith, J. Lorrain, *J. Physiol. (Lond.)*, 1899, **24**, 19.
682. Nash, G., Blennerhassett, J. B., Pontoppidan, H., *New Engl. J. Med.*, 1967, **276**, 368.
683. Heppleston, A. G., Simnett, J. D., *Lancet*, 1964, **1**, 1135.
684. Barter, R. A., Finlay-Jones, L. R., Walters, M. N.-I., *J. Path. Bact.*, 1968, **95**, 481.
685. Kistler, G. S., Caldwell, P. R. B., Weibel, E. R., *J. Cell Biol.*, 1967, **32**, 605.
686. Plopper, C. G., Dungworth, D. L., Tyler, W. S., *Amer. J. Path.*, 1973, **71**, 375, 395.

OCCUPATIONAL DUST DISEASES OF THE LUNGS

687. Agricola, G., [Bauer, G.,] *De Re Metallica*, Book 6. Basel, 1556. [English translation by H. C. Hoover and L. H. Hoover, page 214. London, 1912 (reprinted, New York, 1950).]

688. Hunter, D., *The Diseases of Occupations*, 4th edn, chap. 14. London, 1969.
689. Industrial Injuries Advisory Council, *Pneumoconiosis and Byssinosis*, page 36. London, 1973.
690. Negus, V. E., *Comparative Anatomy and Physiology of the Nose and Paranasal Sinuses*, chap. 13. London, 1958.
691. Davies, C. N., in *Industrial Pulmonary Diseases*, edited by E. J. King and C. M. Fletcher, page 44. London, 1960.
692. McLaughlin, A. I. G., *Lancet*, 1953, **2**, 49, 104.
693. Duguid, J. B., Lambert, M. W., *J. Path. Bact.*, 1964, **88**, 389.
694. International Labour Organization, *International Classification of Radiographs of Pneumoconioses*, revised 1968 (Occupational Safety and Health Series, No. 22). Geneva, 1970.
695. Heard, B. E., Izukawa, T., *J. Path. Bact.*, 1964, **88**, 423.
696. Fletcher, C. M., in *Industrial Pulmonary Diseases*, edited by E. J. King and C. M. Fletcher, page 72. London, 1960.
697. Gough, J., Heppleston, A. G., in *Industrial Pulmonary Diseases*, edited by E. J. King and C. M. Fletcher, page 23. London, 1960.
698. Gough, J., *J. Path. Bact.*, 1940, **51**, 277.
699. Heppleston, A. G., *J. Path. Bact.*, 1947, **59**, 453.
700. Parkes, W. R., *Medicine (Lond.)*, 1973, Part 14, 904.
701. Fletcher, C. M., Gough, J., *Brit. med. Bull.*, 1950, **7**, 42.
702. Naeye, R. L., in *Pulmonary Reactions to Coal Dust— A Review of U.S. Experience*, edited by M. M. Key, L. E. Kerr and M. Bundy, page 93. New York, 1971.
703. Gough, J., in *Recent Advances in Pathology*, 6th edn, edited by G. Hadfield, page 218. London, 1955.
704. Gough, J., Heppleston, A. G., in *Industrial Pulmonary Diseases*, edited by E. J. King and C. M. Fletcher, page 22. London, 1960.
705. Curran, R. C., Ager, J. A. M., *J. Path. Bact.*, 1962, **83**, 1.
706. Steele, R. A., in *Medicine in the Mining Industries*, edited by J. M. Rogan, page 20. London, 1972.
707. Fletcher, C. M., Oldham, P. D., *Brit. J. industr. Med.*, 1951, **8**, 138.
708. Miall, W. E., Caplan, A., Cochrane, A. L., Kilpatrick, G. S., Oldham, P. D., *Brit. med. J.*, 1953, **2**, 1231.
709. Caplan, A., in *Industrial Pulmonary Diseases*, edited by E. J. King and C. M. Fletcher, page 232. London, 1960.
710. Allison, A. C., Harington, J. S., Birbeck, M., Nash, T., in *Inhaled Particles and Vapours—II*, edited by C. N. Davies, page 121. Oxford, 1967.
711. Heppleston, A. G., Styles, J. A., *Nature (Lond.)*, 1967, **214**, 521.
712. Gross, P., de Treville, R. T. P., *Arch. environm. Hlth*, 1968, **17**, 720.
713. Vigliani, E. C., Pernis, B., *Brit. J. industr. Med.*, 1958, **15**, 8.
714. Merewether, E. R. A., Price, C. W., *Report on Effects of Asbestos Dust on the Lungs and Dust Suppression in the Asbestos Industry*. London, 1930.
715. Hunter, D., *The Diseases of Occupations*, 4th edn, page 1009. London, 1969.
716. Industrial Injuries Advisory Council, *Pneumoconiosis and Byssinosis*, pages 22, 25 and 77. London, 1973.
717. King, E. J., Clegg, J. W., Rae, V. M., *Thorax*, 1946, **1**, 188.

718. Lynch, K. M., *A.M.A. Arch. industr. Hlth*, 1955, **11**, 185.

719. Heard, B. E., Williams, R., *Thorax*, 1961, **16**, 264.

720. Doll, R., *Brit. J. industr. Med.*, 1955, **12**, 81.

721. Advisory Committee on Asbestos Cancers, *Brit. J. industr. Med.*, 1973, **30**, 180.

722. Elmes, P. C., McCaughey, W. T. E., Wade, O. L., *Brit. med. J.*, 1965, **1**, 350.

723. McCullough, T. W., *Annual Report of the Chief Inspector of Factories on Industrial Health for the Year 1958.* London, 1959.

724. Industrial Injuries Advisory Council, *Pneumoconiosis and Byssinosis*, page 23. London, 1973.

725. Symmers, W. St C., *personal communication*, 1974.

726. Faulds, J. S., *J. clin. Path.*, 1957, **10**, 187.

727. McLaughlin, A. I. G., *Industrial Lung Diseases of Iron and Steel Foundry Workers.* London, 1950.

728. McLaughlin, A. I. G., in *Industrial Pulmonary Diseases*, edited by E. J. King and C. M. Fletcher, page 146. London, 1960.

729. Harding, H. E., *Brit. J. industr. Med.*, 1945, **2**, 32.

730. Williams, K., *The Natural History of Beryllium Disease.* London, 1959.

731. Symposium on Berylliosis, *A.M.A. Arch. industr. Hlth*, 1959, **19**, 91.

732. Williams, W. J., *Brit. J. industr. Med.*, 1958, **15**, 84.

733. Mekky, S., Roach, S. A., Schilling, R. S. F., *Brit. J. industr. Med.*, 1967, **24**, 123.

734. Schilling, R. S. F., *Lancet*, 1956, **2**, 261, 319.

735. McKerrow, C. B., McDermott, M., Gilson, J. C., Schilling, R. S. F., *Brit. J. industr. Med.*, 1958, **15**, 75.

736. Bouhuys, A., Lindell, S. E., Lundin, G., *Brit. med. J.*, 1960, **1**, 324.

737. Crofton, J., Douglas, A., *Respiratory Diseases*, page 504. Oxford and Edinburgh, 1969.

738. Castleden, L. I. M., Hamilton-Paterson, J. L., *Brit. med. J.*, 1942, **2**, 478.

739. Bradford, J. K., Blalock, J. B., Wascom, C. M., *Amer. Rev. resp. Dis.*, 1961, **84**, 582.

740. Towey, J. W., Sweany, H. C., Huron, W. H., *J. Amer. med. Ass.*, 1932, **99**, 453.

741. Symmers, W. St C., *unpublished observations*, 1972.

742. Kováts, F., Sr, Bugyi, B., *Occupational Mycotic Diseases of the Lung*, page 106. Budapest, 1968.

743. Bringhurst, L. S., Byrne, R. N., Gershon-Cohen, J., *J. Amer. med. Ass.*, 1959, **171**, 15.

744. Plessner, M., *Arch. Mal. prof.*, 1959, **21**, 67.

PULMONARY TRANSPLANTATION

745. Hugh-Jones, P., Macarthur, A. M., Cullum, P. A., Mason, S. A., Crosbie, W. A., Hutchison, D. C. S., Winterton, M. C., Smith, A. P., Mason, B., Smith, L. A., *Brit. med. J.*, 1971, **3**, 391.

746. Matthew, H., Logan, A., Woodruff, M. F. A., Heard, B., *Brit. med. J.*, 1968, **3**, 759.

747. Wildevuur, C. R. H., Benfield, J. R., *Ann. thorac. Surg.*, 1970, **9**, 489.

BENIGN TUMOURS AND TUMOUR-LIKE CONDITIONS

748. Liebow, A. A., *Tumors of the Lower Respiratory Tract* (Atlas of Tumor Pathology, sect. 5, fasc. 17), page 45. Washington, D.C., 1952.

749. Stein, A. A., Volk, B. M., *A.M.A. Arch. Path.*, 1959, **68**, 468.

750. Korn, D., Bensch, K., Liebow, A. A., Castleman, B. *Amer. J. Path.*, 1960, **37**, 641.

751. Barroso-Moguel, R., Costero, I., *Amer. J. Path.*, 1964, **44**, 17a.

752. Whitwell, F., *J. Path. Bact.*, 1955, **70**, 529.

753. Liebow, A. A., Castleman, B., *Amer. J. Path.*, 1963, **43**, 13a.

754. Kovarik, J. L., Toll, G. D., *J. Amer. med. Ass.*, 1966, **196**, 221.

755. Rodman, M. H., Jones, C. W., *New Engl. J. Med.*, 1962, **266**, 805.

756. Symmers, W. St C., *unpublished cases*, 1972.

757. Adams, M. J. T., *Thorax*, 1957, **12**, 268.

758. Perry, D. C., *Brit. med. J.*, 1959, **1**, 1572.

759. Paterson, J. F., *Dis. Chest*, 1956, **30**, 559.

760. Perry, D. C., *Brit. med. J.*, 1959, **1**, 1572.

761. Hochburg, L. A., Schacter, B., *Amer. J. Surg.*, 1955, **89**, 425.

762. Baker, C., Trounce, J. R., *Brit. Heart J.*, 1949, **11**, 109.

763. Sanders, J. A., Martt, J. M., *Circulation*, 1962, **25**, 383.

764. Bosher, L. H., Jr, Blake, D. A., Byrd, B. R., *Surgery*, 1959, **45**, 91.

765. Orr, J. W., *personal communication to W. St C. Symmers*, 1950.

766. Liebow, A. A., Hubbell, D. S., *Cancer (Philad.)*, 1956, **9**, 53.

767. Spencer, H., *Pathology of the Lung (Excluding Pulmonary Tuberculosis)*, 2nd edn, page 935. Oxford, London, Edinburgh, New York, Toronto, Sydney, Paris, Braunschweig, 1968.

768. Symmers, W. St C., *unpublished observation*, 1971.

769. Hirose, F. M., Hennigar, G. R., *J. thorac. Surg.*, 1955, **29**, 502.

770. Turkington, S. I., Scott, G. A., Smiley, T. B., *Thorax*, 1950, **5**, 138.

771. Pierce, W. F., Alznauer, R. L., Rolle, C., *A.M.A. Arch. Path.*, 1954, **58**, 443.

772. Peterson, P. A., Soule, E. H., Bernatz, P. E., *J. thorac. Surg.*, 1957, **34**, 95.

773. Hebert, W. M., Seale, R. H., Samson, P. C., *J. thorac. Surg.*, 1957, **34**, 409.

774. Symmers, W. St C., *unpublished observation*, 1972.

775. Littlefield, J. B., Drash, E. C., *J. thorac. Surg.*, 1959, **37**, 745.

776. Clagett, O. T., McDonald, J. R., Schmidt, H. W., *J. thorac. Surg.*, 1952, **24**, 213.

777. Brown, W. J., Johnson, L. C., *Milit. Surg.*, 1951, **109**, 415.

778. Spencer, H., *Pathology of the Lung (Excluding Pulmonary Tuberculosis)*, 2nd edn, page 926. Oxford, London, Edinburgh, New York, Toronto, Sydney, Paris, Braunschweig, 1968.

779. Neilson, D. B., *J. Path. Bact.*, 1958, **76**, 419.

780. Rubin, E. H., Aronson, W., *Amer. Rev. Tuberc.*, 1940, **41**, 801.

781. Watts, C. F., Clagett, O. T., McDonald, J. R., *J. thorac. Surg.*, 1946, **15**, 132.

782. McCall, R. E., Harrison, W., *J. thorac. Surg.*, 1955, **29**, 317.

783. Shapiro, R., Carter, M. G., *Amer. Rev. Tuberc.*, 1954, **69**, 1042.

784. Spyker, M. A., Kay, S., *J. thorac. Surg.*, 1956, **31**, 211.

785. Edwards, A. T., Taylor, A. B., *Brit. J. Surg.*, 1937–38, **25**, 487.

786. Gordon, J., Walker, G., *Arch. Path. (Chic.)*, 1944, **37**, 222.
787. Bates, T., Hull, O. H., *Amer. J. Dis. Child.*, 1958, **95**, 53.
788. Umiker, W., Iverson, L., *J. thorac. Surg.*, 1954, **28**, 55.
789. Saltzstein, S. L., *Cancer (Philad.)*, 1963, **16**, 928.
790. Greenberg, S. D., Heisler, J. G., Gyorkey, F., Jenkins, D. E., *Sth. med. J. (Bgham, Ala.)*, 1972, **65**, 775.

MALIGNANT TUMOURS
791. Kreyberg, L., Liebow, A. A., Uehlinger, E. A., *Histological Typing of Lung Tumours*. Geneva, 1967.
792. *The Registrar General's Statistical Review of England and Wales for the Year 1973*, Part 1(A). London, 1975.
793. *The Registrar General's Statistical Reviews of England and Wales for the Years 1948–72*, Part 1. London, 1949–74.
794. Case, R. A. M., in *Carcinoma of the Lung*, edited by J. R. Bignall, page 21. London, 1958.
795. Weller, C. V., *Causal Factors in Cancer of the Lung*, chap. 3. Springfield, Illinois, 1956.
796. Hueper, W. C., *Occupational Tumors and Allied Diseases*, page 435. Springfield, Illinois, 1942.
797. Doll, R., in *Carcinoma of the Lung*, edited by J. R. Bignall, page 68. London, 1958.
798. Doll, R., Hill, A. Bradford, *Brit. med. J.*, 1956, **2**, 1071.
799. *Medical Research Council: Report for the Year 1955–56*, page 10. London, 1957.
800. Royal College of Physicians of London, *Smoking and Health Now*, chap. 4. London, 1971.
801. Raffle, P. A. B., *Brit. J. industr. Med.*, 1957, **14**, 73.
802. Wynder, E. L., *Lancet*, 1961, **2**, 1347.
803. Walter, J. B., Pryce, D. M., *Thorax*, 1955, **10**, 117.
804. Pancoast, H. K., *J. Amer. med. Ass.*, 1932, **99**, 1391.
805. Auerbach, O., Gere, J. B., Forman, J. B., Petrick, T. G., Smolin, H. J., Muehsam, G. E., Kassouny, D. Y., Stout, A. P., *New Engl. J. Med.*, 1957, **256**, 97.
806. Hamilton, J. D., Brown, T. C., Sepp, A., Macdonald, F. W., *Canad. med. Ass. J.*, 1957, **77**, 177.
807. Doll, R., Hill, A. Bradford, Kreyberg, L., *Brit. J. Cancer*, 1957, **11**, 43.
808. Glegg, J. W., in *Cancer*, edited by R. W. Raven, vol. 2, page 563. London, 1958.
809. Kreyberg, L., Liebow, A. A., Uehlinger, E. A., *Histological Typing of Lung Tumours*, page 21. Geneva, 1967.
810. Coalson, J. J., Mohr, J. A., Pirtle, J. K., Dee, A. L., Rhoades, E. R., *Amer. Rev. resp. Dis.*, 1970, **101**, 181.
811. Barnard, W. G., *J. Path. Bact.*, 1926, **29**, 241.
812. Brandt, M., *Virchows Arch. path. Anat.*, 1926, **262**, 211.
813. Walter, J. B., Pryce, D. M., *J. Path. Bact.*, 1960, **80**, 121.
814. Azzopardi, J. G., *J. Path. Bact.*, 1959, **78**, 513.
815. Bensch, K. G., Corrin, B., Pariente, R., Spencer, H., *Cancer (Philad.)*, 1968, **22**, 1163.
816. Walter, J. B., Pryce, D. M., *Thorax*, 1955, **10**, 107.
817. Liebow, A. A., *Tumors of the Lower Respiratory Tract* (Atlas of Tumor Pathology, sect. 5, fasc. 17), page 53. Washington, D.C., 1952.
818. Hutchison, H. E., *Cancer (Philad.)*, 1952, **5**, 884.
819. Hewer, T. F., *J. Path. Bact.*, 1961, **81**, 321.
820. Eck, H., *Das sogenannte Alveolarzellkarzinom (Lungenadenomatose)*, page 45. Leipzig, 1957.
821. Nisbet, D. I., MacKay, J. M. K., Smith, W., Gray, E. W., *J. Path.*, 1971, **103**, 157.

822. Spencer, H., Raeburn, C., *J. Path. Bact.*, 1956, **71**, 145.
823. Whitwell, F., *J. Path. Bact.*, 1955, **70**, 529.
824. Nash, A. D., Stout, A. P., *Cancer (Philad.)*, 1958, **11**, 369.
825. Morgan, A. D., Mackenzie, D. H., *J. Path. Bact.*, 1964, **87**, 25.
826. Walter, J. B., Pryce, D. M., *Thorax*, 1955, **10**, 107.
827. Foster-Carter, A. F., *Quart. J. Med.*, 1941, N.S. **10**, 139.
828. Willis, R. A., *Pathology of Tumours*, 4th edn, page 376. London, 1967.
829. Liebow, A. A., *Tumors of the Lower Respiratory Tract* (Atlas of Tumor Pathology, sect. 5, fasc. 17), page 26. Washington, D.C., 1952.
830. Williams, E. D., Azzopardi, J. G., *Thorax*, 1960, **15**, 30.
831. Bensch, K. G., Corrin, B., Pariente, R., Spencer, H., *Cancer (Philad.)*, 1968, **22**, 1163.
832. Roberts, W. C., Sjoerdsma, A., *Amer. J. Med.*, 1964, **36**, 5.
833. Liebow, A. A., *Tumors of the Lower Respiratory Tract* (Atlas of Tumor Pathology, sect. 5, fasc. 17), page 44. Washington, D.C., 1952.
834. Smetana, H. F., cited by A. A. Liebow, *Tumors of the Lower Respiratory Tract* (Atlas of Tumor Pathology, sect. 5, fasc. 17), page 45. Washington, D.C., 1952.
835. Stein, A. A., Volk, B. M., *A.M.A. Arch. Path.*, 1959, **68**, 468.
836. Spencer, H., *J. Path. Bact.*, 1961, **82**, 161.
837. Kakos, G. S., Williams, T. E., Assor, D., Vasko, J. S., *J. thorac. cardiovasc. Surg.*, 1971, **61**, 777.
838. Davis, P. W., Briggs, J. C., Seal, R. M. E., Storring, F. K., *Thorax*, 1972, **27**, 657.
839. Cole, W. H., McDonald, G. O., Roberts, S. S., Southwick, H. W., *Dissemination of Cancer*. New York, 1961.
840. Harold, J. T., *Quart. J. Med.*, 1952, N.S. **21**, 353.
841. Nohl, H. C., *Thorax*, 1956, **11**, 172.
842. Ballantyne, A. J., Clagett, O. T., McDonald, J. R., *Thorax*, 1957, **12**, 294.
843. Hanbury, W. J., Cureton, R. J. R., Simon, G., *Thorax*, 1954, **9**, 304.
844. Galluzzi, S., Payne, P. M., *Brit. J. Cancer*, 1956, **10**, 408.
845. Ross, E. J., *Brit. med. J.*, 1972, **1**, 735.
846. Azzopardi, J. G., Williams, E. D., *Cancer (Philad.)*, 1968, **22**, 274.
847. Bagshawe, K. D., *Lancet*, 1960, **2**, 284.
848. Liddle, G. W., *Amer. J. Path.*, 1966, **48**, 48a.
849. Hatch, H. B., Segaloff, A., Ochsner, A., *Ann. Surg.*, 1965, **161**, 645.
850. Schwartz, W. B., Bennett, W., Curelop, S., Bartter, F. C., *Amer. J. Med.*, 1957, **23**, 529.
851. Amatruda, T. T., Jr, Mulrow, P. J., Gallagher, J. C., Sawyer, W. H., *New Engl. J. Med.*, 1963, **269**, 544.
852. Ross, E. J., *Quart. J. Med.*, 1963, N.S. **32**, 297.
853. Azzopardi, J. G., Whittaker, R. S., *J. clin. Path.*, 1969, **22**, 718.
854. Silverstein, M. N., Wakim, K. G., Bahn, R. C., *Amer. J. Med.*, 1964, **36**, 415.
855. Symmers, W. St C., *unpublished observations*, 1967, 1972.
856. Samols, E., *Postgrad. med. J.*, 1963, **39**, 634.
857. Fusco, F. D., Rosen, S. W., *New Engl. J. Med.*, 1966, **275**, 507.
858. Mason, A. M. S., Ratcliffe, J. G., Buckle, R. M., Mason, A. S., *Clin. Endocr.*, 1972, **1**, 3.

859. Kinloch, J. D., Webb, J. N., Eccleston, D., Zeitlin, J., *Brit. med. J.*, 1965, **1**, 1533.

860. Brain, Adams, R. D., in *The Remote Effects of Cancer on the Nervous System*, edited by Lord Brain and F. Norris, page 216. Baltimore, 1965.

861. Lennox, B., Prichard, S., *Quart. J. Med.*, 1950, N.S. **19**, 97.

862. Morton, D. L., Itabashi, H. H., Grimes, O. F., *J. thorac. cardiovasc. Surg.*, 1966, **51**, 14.

863. Woodhouse, M. A., Dayan, A. D., Burston, J., Caldwell, I., Hume-Adams, J., Melcher, D., Urich, H., *Brain*, 1967, **90**, 863.

864. Lambert, E. H., Rooke, D. E., in *The Remote Effects of Cancer on the Nervous System*, edited by Lord Brain and F. Norris, page 67. Baltimore, 1965.

865. Wilkinson, P. C., Zeromski, J., *Brain*, 1965, **88**, 529.

866. Williams, R. T., *Brit. med. J.*, 1963, **1**, 233.

867. Rose, A. L., Walton, J. N., *Brain*, 1966, **89**, 747.

868. Symmers, W. St C., *personal communication*, 1974.

869. McDonald, R. A., Robbins, S. L., *Ann. intern. Med.*, 1957, **46**, 255.

870. Amundsen, M. A., Spittell, J. A., Thompson, J. H., Owen, C. A., *Ann. intern. Med.*, 1963, **58**, 608.

871. Fox, H., Gunn, A. D. G., *Brit. J. Dis. Chest*, 1965, **59**, 47.

872. Greenberg, E., Divertie, M. B., Woolner, L. B., *Amer. J. Med.*, 1964, **36**, 106.

873. Turner-Warwick, M., *Thorax*, 1963, **18**, 238.

874. Hall, G. H., *Lancet*, 1959, **1**, 750.

875. Yaccoub, M. H., *Thorax*, 1965, **20**, 537.

876. Huckstep, R. L., Bodkin, P. E., *Lancet*, 1958, **2**, 343.

877. Semple, T., McCluskie, R. A., *Brit. med. J.*, 1955, **1**, 754.

878. Bamforth, J., *Cytological Diagnosis in Medical Practice*. London, 1966.

879. Papanicolaou, G. N., *Science*, 1942, **95**, 438.

880. Schuster, N. H., in *Recent Advances in Clinical Pathology*, edited by S. C. Dyke, page 316. London, 1947.

881. Philps, F. R., *A Short Manual of Respiratory Cytology*. London, 1964.

882. Oswald, N. C., Hinson, K. F. W., Canti, G., Miller, A. B., *Thorax*, 1971, **26**, 623.

883. Stradling, P., *Diagnostic Bronchoscopy—An Introduction*. London, 1973.

884. Gibbons, J. R. P., *Brit. J. Dis. Chest*, 1972, **66**, 162.

885. Guccion, J. G., Rosen, S. H., *Cancer (Philad.)*, 1972, **30**, 836.

886. Mason, M. K., Azeem, P. S., *Thorax*, 1965, **20**, 13.

887. Drennan, J. M., McCormack, R. J. M., *J. Path. Bact.*, 1960, **79**, 147.

888. Symmers, W. St C., *unpublished case*, 1972.

889. Conquest, H. F., Thornton, J. L., Massie, J. R., Coxe, J. W., *Ann. Surg.*, 1965, **161**, 688.

890. Crofts, N. F., Forbes, G. B., *Thorax*, 1964, **19**, 334.

891. Stephanopoulos, C., Catsaras, H., *Thorax*, 1963, **18**, 144.

892. Rees, G. M., *Thorax*, 1970, **25**, 366.

893. Robbins, L. L., *Cancer (Philad.)*, 1953, **6**, 80.

894. Sternberg, W. H., Sidransky, H., Ochsner, S., *Cancer (Philad.)*, 1959, **12**, 806.

895. Greenberg, S. D., Heisler, J. G., Gyorkey, F., Jenkins, D. E., *Sth. med. J. (Bgham, Ala.)*, 1972, **65**, 775.

896. Saltzstein, S. L., *Cancer (Philad.)*, 1963, **16**, 928.

897. Monahan, D. T., *J. thorac. cardiovasc. Surg.*, 1965, **49**, 173.

898. Romanoff, H., Milwidsky, H., *Brit. J. Dis. Chest*, 1962, **56**, 139.

899. Kennedy, J. D., Kneafsey, D. V., *Thorax*, 1959, **14**, 353.

900. Furgerson, W. B., Jr, Bachman, L. B., O'Toole, W. F., *Amer. Rev. resp. Dis.*, 1963, **88**, 689.

901. Nathad, D. J., Sanders, M., *New Engl. J. Med.*, 1955, **252**, 797.

902. Resnick, M. E., Berkowitz, R. D., Rodman, T., *Amer. J. Med.*, 1961, **31**, 149.

903. Wagner, J. C., Sleggs, C. A., Marchand, P., *Brit. J. industr. Med.*, 1960, **17**, 260.

904. Gloyne, S. R., *Tubercle (Edinb.)*, 1933, **14**, 445, 493, 550.

905. Heard, B. E., Williams, R., *Thorax*, 1961, **16**, 264.

906. Hourihane, D. O'B., Lessof, L., Richardson, P. C., *Brit. med. J.*, 1966, **1**, 1069.

907. Chang-Hyun Um, *Brit. med. J.*, 1971, **2**, 248.

908. Newhouse, M. L., Thompson, H., *Brit. J. industr. Med.*, 1965, **22**, 261.

909. Hourihane, D. O'B., *Thorax*, 1964, **19**, 268.

910. Harington, J. S., *Nature (Lond.)*, 1962, **193**, 43.

911. Gilson, J. C., *Trans. Soc. occup. Med.*, 1966, **16**, 62.

912. Whitwell, F., Rawcliffe, R. M., *Thorax*, 1971, **26**, 6.

913. Churg, J., Selikoff, I. J., in *The Lung*, edited by A. A. Liebow and D. E. Smith, page 284. Baltimore, 1968.

914. McCaughey, W. T. E., *J. Path. Bact.*, 1958, **76**, 517.

915. Salm, R., *J. Path. Bact.*, 1963, **85**, 121.

916. Willis, R. A., *The Spread of Tumours in the Human Body*, 2nd edn, chap. 15. London, 1952.

917. Roberts, S. S., in *Dissemination of Cancer: Prevention and Therapy*, edited by W. H. Cole, G. O. McDonald, S. S. Roberts and H. W. Southwick, page 190. New York, 1961.

918. Wood, S., *A.M.A. Arch. Path.*, 1958, **66**, 550.

919. Morgan, A. D., *J. Path. Bact.*, 1949, **61**, 75.

920. Trapnell, D. H., *Thorax*, 1964, **19**, 251.

921. Thomford, N. R., Woolner, L. B., Clagett, O. T., *J. thorac. cardiovasc. Surg.*, 1965, **49**, 357.

922. Rees, G. M., Cleland, W. P., *Brit. med. J.*, 1971, **3**, 467.

DISEASES OF THE PLEURA

923. Altschule, M. D., Zamcheck, N., *J. clin. Invest.*, 1944, **23**, 325.

924. Race, G. A., Scheifley, C. H., Edwards, J. E., *Amer. J. Med.*, 1957, **22**, 83.

925. Bedford, D. E., Lovibond, J. L., *Brit. Heart J.*, 1941, **3**, 93.

926. James, A. H., *Clin. Sci.*, 1949, **8**, 291.

927. Ogilvie, A. G., *Thorax*, 1950, **5**, 116.

928. Heard, B. E., *J. Path. Bact.*, 1953, **66**, 359.

929. Macfarlane, J. R., Holman, C. W., *Amer. Rev. resp. Dis.*, 1972, **105**, 287.

930. Judd, E. S., Jr, Nix, J. T., *Surg. Clin. N. Amer.*, 1949, **29**, 1035.

931. Stirlacci, J. R., *J. Pediat.*, 1955, **46**, 581.

932. Symmers, W. St C., *unpublished observations*, 1953, 1968.

933. Lichter, I., Gwynne, J. F., *Thorax*, 1971, **26**, 409.

934. Crofton, J., Douglas, A., *Respiratory Diseases*, page 270. Oxford and Edinburgh, 1966.

935. Mestitz, P., Pollard, A. C., *Brit. J. Dis. Chest*, 1959, **53**, 86.

936. Krakówka, P., Rowińska, E., Halweg, H., *Thorax*, 1970, **25**, 245.

937. Symmers, W. St C., *unpublished observations*, 1965–74.

938. Le Roux, B. T., *Thorax*, 1962, **17**, 111.

ACKNOWLEDGEMENTS FOR ILLUSTRATIONS

Figs 7.2, 13, 14. Reproduced by permission of the editors from: Heard, B. E., Izukawa, T., *J. Path. Bact.*, 1964, **88**, 423. Preparations from the Department of Pathology, Royal Postgraduate Medical School, London; photographs by the Department of Medical Illustration, Royal Postgraduate Medical School.

Figs 7.5, 7, 27, 29, 30, 34, 37, 39, 41–44, 55, 71, 74, 75, 83. Gordon Museum, Guy's Hospital, London; reproduced by permission of the Curator, Mr J. D. Maynard; photographs by Miss P. M. Turnbull, Charing Cross Hospital and Medical School, London.

Figs 7.6, 38, 77, 78. Pathology Museum, Charing Cross Hospital Medical School, London; reproduced by permission of the Curator, Dr B. Fox; photographs by Miss P. M. Turnbull, Charing Cross Hospital and Medical School, London.

Fig. 7.8. Photomicrograph provided by Dr R. E. Rewell, Women's Hospital, Liverpool, Liverpool Maternity Hospital, Royal Liverpool Children's Hospital, and Liverpool Ear, Nose and Throat Infirmary.

Figs 7.9, 10, 12, 15, 19, 21, 23, 26, 28, 31, 40, 53, 54, 56, 58, 60–64, 69, 72, 73, 76, 79–82. Preparations from the Department of Pathology, Royal Postgraduate Medical School, London; photographs by the Department of Medical Illustration, Royal Postgraduate Medical School.

Fig. 7.11. Reproduced by permission of the publishers, Messrs J. & A. Churchill Ltd (Longman Group Ltd), from: Heard, B. E., *Pathology of Chronic Bronchitis and Emphysema*; London, 1969 (Fig. 4.1).

Fig. 7.18. Reproduced by permission of the editor from: Heard, B. E., *Thorax*, 1959, **14**, 286. Preparation from the Department of Pathology, Royal Postgraduate Medical School, London; photograph by the Department of Medical Illustration, Royal Postgraduate Medical School.

Figs 7.16, 17, 20. Reproduced by permission of the editor from: Heard, B. E., *Thorax*, 1959, **14**, 58. Preparations from the Department of Pathology, Royal Postgraduate Medical School, London; photographs by the Department of Medical Illustration, Royal Postgraduate Medical School.

Fig. 7.22. Reproduced by permission of the editor from: Laws, J. W., Heard, B. E., *Brit. J. Radiol.*, 1962, **33**, 750. Preparation from the Department of Pathology, Royal Postgraduate Medical School, London; photograph by the Department of Medical Illustration, Royal Postgraduate Medical School.

Figs 7.24, 32, 33, 35, 47, 48, 51. Photomicrographs provided by W. St C. Symmers.

Fig. 7.25. Reproduced by permission of the editors from: Restrepo, G. L., Heard, B. E., *Amer. Rev. resp. Dis.*, 1964, **90**, 395. Preparation from the Department of Pathology, Royal Postgraduate Medical School, London; photograph by the Department of Medical Illustration, Royal Postgraduate Medical School.

Fig. 7.36. Reproduced by permission of the editor from Heard, B. E., Hassan, A. M., Wilson, S. M., *J. clin. Path.*, 1962, **15**, 17. Preparation from the Department of Pathology, Royal Postgraduate Medical School, London; photograph by the Department of Medical Illustration, Royal Postgraduate Medical School.

Fig. 7.45. Photomicrograph provided by Dr N. S. Plummer and W. St C. Symmers, Charing Cross Hospital and Medical School, London.

Fig. 7.46. Photomicrograph provided by the late Mr K. W. Iles, Charing Cross Hospital Medical School, London.

Fig. 7.49. Reproduced by permission of the editor from: Symmers, W. St C., *Ann. Soc. belge Méd. trop.*, 1964, **44**, 869.

Fig. 7.50. Reproduced by permission of the editor from: Symmers, W. St C., *Nurs. Mirror*, 1963 (Dec. 13), **117**, xi.

Fig. 7.52. Photograph provided by Professor J. Pepys, Cardiothoracic Institute, Brompton Hospital, London.

Figs 7.57, 59. Reproduced by permission of the editor from: Stack, B. H. R., Choo-Kang, Y. F. J., Heard, B. E., *Thorax*, 1972, **27**, 535. Photomicrographs by the Photographic Department, Chester Beatty Research Institute (Institute of Cancer Research: Royal Cancer Hospital), London.

Fig. 7.65. Reproduced by permission of the editor from: Clinicopathological Conference, *Scot. med. J.*, 1971, **16**, 407. Photograph by the Department of Medical Photography, University of Edinburgh.

Fig. 7.66. Reproduced by permission of the editor from Heard, B. E., Cooke, R. A., *Thorax*, 1968, **23**, 187. Photomicrograph by the Department of Medical Illustration, Royal Postgraduate Medical School, London.

Figs 7.67, 68. Preparations provided by Dr K. F. W. Hinson, Brompton Hospital, London. Photomicrographs by the Photographic Department, Chester Beatty Research Institute (Institute of Cancer Research: Royal Cancer Hospital), London.

Fig. 7.70. Reproduced by permission of the editor from Heard, B. E., Williams, R., *Thorax*, 1961, **16**, 264. Preparation from the Department of Pathology, Royal Postgraduate Medical School, London; photograph by the Department of Medical Illustration, Royal Postgraduate Medical School.

Index to Volume 1

compiled by the editor

In some entries there is a cross-reference to other parts of the index where the subject is covered in more detail or under a preferred synonym. To lessen the possible inconvenience, if there is a major account of the topic its page is indicated in parentheses: for example—

When more than one page reference is given in an entry, bold type is used to indicate a main account of the topic, if appropriate.

Reference to an illustration or table is indicated by noting its number in parentheses after the number of the page on which it appears. In general, illustrations and tables are not indexed separately as they are referred to in the pages of the text to which the relevant entry in the index relates.

Terms that American writers generally spell more simply than is traditional in Britain, such as edema (oedema) and etiology (aetiology), should be looked for in the spelling that accords with the latter practice.

Index to Volume 1

H